Nunn's Applied Respiratory Physiology

Nunn's Applied Respiratory Physiology

Fifth edition

Andrew B. Lumb MB BS FRCA
Consultant Anaesthetist St___'s Hospital, Leeds, UK
Senior Clin____ ___ ___aesthesia, University of Leeds, Leeds, UK

Foreword by

JF Nunn MD DSc PhD FRCS FRCA FANZCA(Hon) FFARCSI(Hon)
Formerly Head of the Division of Anaesthesia, Medical Research Council Clinical Research Centre;
Emeritus Consultant Anaesthetist, Northwick Park Hospital, Middlesex; previously Professor of Anaesthesia,
University of Leeds; Dean of the Faculty of Anaesthetists, Royal College of Surgeons of England

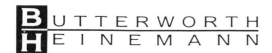

BUTTERWORTH
HEINEMANN

OXFORD AUCKLAND BOSTON JOHANNESBURG MELBOURNE NEW DELHI

Butterworth-Heinemann
Linacre House, Jordan Hill, Oxford OX2 8DP
225 Wildwood Avenue, Woburn, MA 01801–2041
A division of Reed Educational and Professional Publishing Ltd

℞ A member of the Reed Elsevier plc group

First published 1969
Reprinted 1971 (twice), 1972, 1975
Second edition 1977
Reprinted 1978, 1981
Third edition 1987
Reprinted 1989
Fourth edition 1993
Reprinted 1994, 1995, 1997
Fifth edition 2000

British Library Cataloguing in Publication Data
Lumb, Andrew
  Nunn's applied respiratory physiology. – 5th ed.
  1. Respiratory organs
  I. Title
  612.2

Library of Congress Cataloguing in Publication Data
Lumb, Andrew
  Nunn's applied respiratory physiology. – 5th ed./Andrew Lumb:
  foreword by J.F. Nunn.
  p.   cm.
  Rev. ed. of: Nunn's applied respiratory physiology/J.F. Nunn.
  4th ed. 1993.
  Includes bibliographical references and index.
  ISBN 0–7506–3107–4
  1. Respiration.   2. Anesthesia.   3. Respiratory organs –
  Pathophysiology.   I. Nunn, J.F. (John Francis). Nunn's applied
  respiratory physiology.   II. Title.   III. Title: Applied respiratory
  physiology.
  [DNLM: 1. Respiratory Physiology. 2. Respiratory System –
  physiopathology. WF 102 L957n 1999]
  QP121.N75   99–40687
  612.2′024′617–dc21   CIP

ISBN 0 7506 3107 4

Composition by Genesis Typesetting, Laser Quay, Rochester, Kent
Printed and bound in Great Britain by MPG, Bodmin, Cornwall

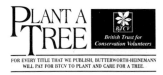

Contents

Foreword to the fifth edition

The first edition of *Applied Respiratory Physiology* was started in 1959 during those exciting years when the post-war advances in human respiratory physiology were seen to have a direct bearing on the well being of patients in many specialties, and not least in anaesthesia. Publication was postponed until 1969, after I became Foundation Professor of Anaesthesia in the University of Leeds.

The first two editions followed the pattern of the present Part I with clinical applications interspersed in various chapters as seemed appropriate. In 1987, the third edition broke new ground with the separation of Applications into Part II, while Part I was confined to Basic Principles. All aspects of the subject increased remorselessly in scope and content, into the fourth edition, in 1993. Non-respiratory functions of the lung were now an important and growing feature of Part I, and the applications considered in Part II expanded to include such topics as the function of the transplanted lung and the effects of zero gravity in space.

The fourth edition was written immediately after my retirement and I determined that it should be my last. However, demand for the book has continued unabated and, happily, Andy Lumb, my last colleague in the old Clinical Research Centre of the Medical Research Council, kindly agreed to take over the book. How fortunate I have been. The time was clearly right for a new and younger look at the whole structure of the book. It has been the greatest pleasure to read every chapter as it was written and watch the pattern unfold.

Many of the changes are very welcome. First of all, division into three parts – Basic Principles, Applied Physiology, and Physiology of Pulmonary Disease – was overdue and provides a much more logical structure. Also it will be seen that the emphasis on pathophysiology is greatly increased, in accord with the specialized knowledge of the new author.

It also required a new author to take the radical step of removing much material that had lingered on since the first edition. This was essential to accommodate the avalanche of new discoveries, without expanding the book beyond reasonable limits. I would have found this a rather painful experience, having lived and worked through the early and exciting discoveries, which are now so well accepted that they no longer merit the space required for the blow-by-blow accounts in the first four editions. The only certainty is that nothing remains the same, and the old must give way to the new.

It is an unusual and very privileged experience to read a book, with which one has lived for thirty years, now rewritten by a colleague. This is especially so when my successor has specialized knowledge which I did not possess, and combines extraordinary organizational ability with a remarkable grasp of the immense literature of pure and applied respiratory physiology. Nevertheless, I confess to a feeling of pleasure that some sections have been retained. I wish Andy Lumb, the publishers and *Nunn's Applied Respiratory Physiology* a long and successful future.

John Nunn

Preface to the fifth edition

Over the past 30 years *Nunn's Applied Respiratory Physiology* has developed into a renowned textbook on respiration, providing both physiologists and clinicians with a unique fusion of underlying principles and their applications. With Dr John Nunn's retirement in 1991 a new author was required, and, as Dr Nunn's final research fellow in the Clinical Research Centre in Harrow, I was honoured to be chosen as his successor. As a practising clinician with a research interest, rather than *vice versa*, the most significant changes to the 5th Edition involve the inclusion of substantially more clinical topics than previously. These changes acknowledge the popularity of the book amongst doctors from many medical specialities and will hopefully provide readers with a scientific background even greater insight into the applications of respiratory physiology.

The evolution of the book has continued with its division into three sections. Part 3, the *Physiology of Pulmonary Disease*, now brings together and expands many existing sections of previous editions. These chapters are not intended to be a comprehensive review of the pulmonary diseases considered, but in each case they provide basic background clinical information alongside a detailed description of the physiological changes which occur. The referencing style has been changed to a numbered system to reduce interruptions to the text flow, and reference lists now appear at the end of each chapter to provide the reader with a snapshot of important literature in each area. The addition of over 800 new references has, by necessity, meant the removal of many older references, though numerous historically important ones are retained.

Advances in respiratory physiology since the last edition are too numerous to mention individually, but mostly involve better understanding of cellular and biochemical mechanisms underlying areas of respiratory physiology which have been described for decades. Notable examples include the neuronal interactions involved in generating breathing in the respiratory centre, the diffusion of gases within the plasma between pulmonary capillary endothelium and erythrocytes, the mechanisms underlying hypoxic cell damage, and the fascinating cellular interactions contributing to lung inflammation in a variety of diseases. The explosion of interest in nitric oxide over recent years has resulted in evidence for its involvement in many disparate areas of respiration, such that 'nitric oxide' now appears in 14 of 33 chapters in this book. Two new chapters have been added. Chapter 18 brings together physiological problems associated with breathing in closed environments, ranging from closed-circuit anaesthesia to long-term space habitation. Chapter 27 considers airway diseases and was conceived in recognition of the increasing prevalence of conditions such as asthma in the world's population, which now approaches 30% in some groups. Many other new topics have been included in the 5th Edition within existing chapters, including physiological aspects of the airway epithelium, automated measurement of lung mechanics, air pollution, flying, regional anaesthesia and several respiratory diseases.

I wish to personally thank the many people who have helped with the preparation of the book, including the numerous colleagues who have encouraged and assisted my acquisition of knowledge in subjects not so close to my own areas of interest. I am also indebted to several colleagues around the world for providing some of the excellent new figures, in particular Dr M Estenne, Prof ER Weibel, Dr I Mortimore, Dr PK Jeffery (whose electron micrograph also appears on the front cover) and to those kind individuals who responded positively to my unsolicited approaches for unpublished information such as Dr M Bagshaw at British Airways. I am especially indebted to Dr Nunn, not only for entrusting me with the responsibility for seeing *Nunn's Applied Respiratory Physiology* into the new millennium, but also for his invaluable comments on each chapter throughout the writing of the 5th edition, and finally for his kind words in the Foreword. Last, but by no means least, I would like to thank my wife Lorraine, and daughters Emma and Jenny, for tolerating a pre-occupied and reclusive husband/father for so long. Jenny, when aged 5, often enquired about my activities in the study, until one evening she nicely summarized my three year's work by reliably informing me that 'if you don't breathe, you die!'. So what were the other 670 pages about?

AL

Preface to the first edition

Clinicians in many branches of medicine find that their work demands an extensive knowledge of respiratory physiology. This applies particularly to anaesthetists working in the operating theatre or in the intensive care unit. It is unfortunately common experience that respiratory physiology learned in the preclinical years proves to be an incomplete preparation for the clinical field. Indeed, the emphasis of the preclinical course seems, in many cases, to be out of tune with the practical problems to be faced after qualification and specialization. Much that is taught does not apply to man in the clinical environment while, on the other hand, a great many physiological problems highly relevant to the survival of patients find no place in the curriculum. It is to be hoped that new approaches to the teaching of medicine may overcome this dichotomy and that, in particular, much will be gained from the integration of physiology with clinical teaching.

This book is designed to bridge the gap between pure respiratory physiology and the treatment of patients. It is neither a primer of respiratory physiology nor a practical manual for use in the wards and operating theatres. It has two aims. First, I have tried to explain those aspects of respiratory physiology that seem most relevant to patient care, particularly in the field of anaesthesia. Secondly, I have brought together in review those studies that seem to me to be most relevant to clinical work. Inevitably there has been a preference for studies of man and particular stress has been laid on those functions in which man appears to differ from laboratory animals. There is an unashamed emphasis on anaesthesia because I am an anaesthetist. However, the work in this specialty spreads freely into the territory of our neighbours.

References have been a problem. It is clearly impracticable to quote every work that deserves mention. In general I have cited the most informative and the most accessible works, but this rule has been broken on numerous occasions when the distinction of prior discovery calls for recognition. Reviews are freely cited because a book of this length can include only a fraction of the relevant material. I must apologize to the writers of multi-author papers. No one likes to be cited as a colleague, but considerations of space have precluded naming more than three authors for any paper.

Chapters are designed to be read separately and this has required some repetition. There are also frequent cross-references between the chapters. The principles of methods of measurement are considered together at the end of each chapter or section.

In spite of optimistic hopes, the book has taken six years to write. Its form, however, has evolved over the last twelve years from a series of lectures and tutorials given at the Royal College of Surgeons, the Royal Postgraduate Medical School, the University of

Leeds and in numerous institutions in Europe and the USA that I have been privileged to visit. Blackboard sketches have gradually taken the form of the figures that appear in this book.

The greater part of this book is distilled from the work of teachers and colleagues. Professor W Melville Arnott and Professor KW Donald introduced me to the study of clinical respiratory physiology and I worked under the late Professor Ronald Woolmer for a further six years. My debt to them is very great. I have also had the good fortune to work in close contact with many gifted colleagues who have not hesitated to share the fruits of their experience. The list of references will indicate how much I have learned from Dr John Severinghaus, Professor Moran Campbell, Dr John Butler and Dr John West. For my own studies, I acknowledge with gratitude the part played by a long series of research fellows and assistants. Some fifteen are cited herein and they come from eleven different countries. Figures 2, 3, 6, 11 and 15 [Figure 5.3 in the fourth edition, and Figures 3.4 and 3.1 in the fifth edition] which are clearly not my blackboard sketches, were drawn by Mr H Grayshon Lumby. I have had unstinted help from librarians, Miss MP Russell, Mr WR LeFanu and Miss EM Reed. Numerous colleagues have given invaluable help in reading and criticizing the manuscript.

Finally, I must thank my wife who has not only borne the inevitable preoccupation of a husband writing a book but has also carried the burden of the paperwork and prepared the manuscript.

JFN

Part 1

Basic Principles

Chapter 1

The atmosphere

Dr JF Nunn

In the solar system, only Earth has an atmosphere that is in chemical disequilibrium (Table 1.1). This is mainly the result of photosynthetic life forms, and oxygen permits the existence of aerobes. Many species have adapted to derive the maximal benefit from the prevailing state of their gaseous environment but, conversely, catastrophic changes in the composition of the atmosphere have probably been responsible for at least some of the mass extinctions that have marked the end of each geological epoch. Major changes in the atmosphere are currently taking place, as a result of human intervention.

Table 1.1 Composition of the atmosphere of Earth and the nearer planets

Planet	Atmosphere			
Mercury	Extremely tenuous			
Venus	Carbon dioxide	96.5%	+ traces: argon, helium, neon,	
	Nitrogen	3.5%	krypton (all <20 ppmv)	
Earth	Nitrogen	78.08%	Water vapour – variable	
	Oxygen	20.95%	Neon	18.2 ppmv
	Argon	0.93%	Helium	5.2 ppmv
	Carbon dioxide	0.036%	Methane	1.7 ppmv
Mars	Carbon dioxide	95.3%	Oxygen	0.13%
	Nitrogen	2.7%	Carbon monoxide	0.27%
	Argon	1.6%	+ traces: neon, krypton, xenon	
Jupiter	Hydrogen	89%	Methane	1750 ppmv
	Helium	11%	+ traces: ammonia, water vapour etc.	
Saturn	Hydrogen	94%	Methane	4500 ppmv
	Helium	6%	+ traces: ethylene, phosphine	

ppmv, parts per million volume.
(Planetary data are from Taylor,[1] reproduced from Nunn[2] by permission of the Geologists' Association.)

3

Evolution of the atmosphere

Much new information has come to light in recent years and, in many places, this section differs radically from the account given in the previous edition of this book. A fuller account with additional references is available in the 1998 review by the author.[2]

Formation of Earth and the pre-biotic atmosphere

Earth is now believed to have been formed by a relatively short-lived, but intense, gravitational accretion of rather large planetesimals, orbiting the newly formed sun some 4600 million years (Ma) ago. The kinetic energy of the impacting bodies was sufficient to raise the temperature to a few thousand degrees Celsius. This would have melted the entire Earth, resulting in loss of the primary atmosphere.

Earth cooled rapidly by radiation when the initial bombardment abated, and the high temperature (Hadean) phase is thought to have lasted no longer than a few hundred Ma. The crust solidified and massive outgassing occurred, resulting in an atmosphere mainly comprising carbon dioxide and steam (Table 1.2), as probably occurred on Venus and Mars. In the case of Earth, the water vapour condensed to surface water, and there is good evidence that oceans existed about 4000 Ma ago and perhaps even earlier.[3] Venus is too hot to retain water, and Mars lacks sufficient gravitational force. Once Earth's crust was cool, and surface water was in existence, it was possible for comets and meteorites to leave a secondary veneer of their contents, including water and a wide range of organic compounds.[4] Carbon dioxide still forms more than 95 per cent of the atmospheres of Venus and Mars (see Table 1.1).

Table 1.2 Average composition of gas evolved from Hawaiian volcanoes

Constituent	Per cent
Water vapour	70.75
Carbon dioxide	14.07
Sulphur dioxide	6.40
Nitrogen	5.45
Sulphur trioxide	1.92
Carbon monoxide	0.40
Hydrogen	0.33
Argon	0.18
Sulphur	0.10
Chlorine	0.05

(Data are from MacDonald and Hubbard,[5] reproduced from Nunn[2] by permission of the Geologists' Association.)

Important physicochemical changes occurred in the primitive atmosphere. Helium and hydrogen tended to be lost from Earth's gravitational field. Ammonia dissociated to nitrogen and hydrogen, the former retained and the latter lost from the atmosphere. Some carbon dioxide might have been reduced by hydrogen to form traces of methane, but very large quantities reacted with surface silicates to became trapped as carbonates while forming silica (weathering). Traces of water vapour underwent photodissociation to hydrogen and oxygen. However, oxygen from this source was present in only minimal quantities. Contrary to earlier views, the early atmosphere is no longer thought to have been strongly reducing.[6]

The initial very high partial pressure of carbon dioxide would have provided a powerful greenhouse effect to offset the initially weak solar radiation before the sun commenced its main sequence of thermonuclear fusion of hydrogen about 3000 Ma ago. Since then solar radiation has been increasing steadily as the sun proceeds remorselessly towards becoming a red giant, which will ultimately envelop the inner planets (Figure 1.1). It is an extraordinary fact that increasing solar radiation has been approximately offset by a diminishing greenhouse effect, owing to decreasing levels of carbon dioxide (see below). As a result, Earth's temperature has permitted the existence of surface water for the last 4000 Ma.

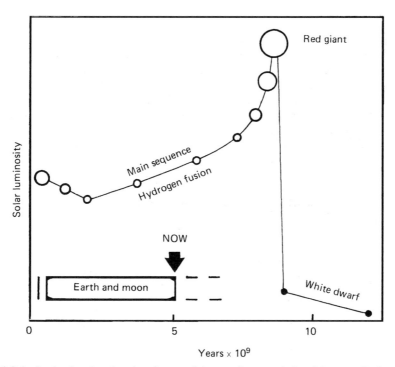

Figure 1.1 Solar luminosity plotted against the age of the sun, the open circles giving a qualitative impression of the diameter of the sun. Superimposed is an indication of the life of Earth and its moon, which is now about half way through the main sequence of the sun deriving its energy from hydrogen fusion to helium. The times can only be very approximate. (After Chapman and Morrison[7].)

Significance of mass of Earth and distance from sun

Small bodies, such as Mercury and most of the planets' satellites, have a gravitational field that is too weak for the retention of any atmosphere at all (Figure 1.2). The large planets (Jupiter, Saturn, Uranus and Neptune) have a gravitational field that is sufficiently strong to retain all gases, including helium and hydrogen, thereby ensuring the retention of a reducing atmosphere. The gravitational field of Earth is intermediate, resulting in a differential retention of the heavier gases (oxygen, carbon dioxide and nitrogen) while permitting the escape of hydrogen and helium. This is essential for the development of an oxidizing atmosphere. Water vapour (molecular weight only 18) would be lost from the atmosphere were it not for the cold trap at the tropopause.

Surface temperature of a planetary body is crucial for the existence of liquid water, which is essential for life and therefore the composition of our atmosphere. To a first approximation, temperature is dependent on the distance of a planet from the sun, and the intensity of solar radiation (Figure 1.2). The major secondary factor is the greenhouse effect of any atmosphere that the planet may possess. Mercury and Venus have surface temperatures far above the boiling point of water. All planets (and their satellites) that are further away from the sun than Earth have a surface temperature too cold for liquid water to exist.

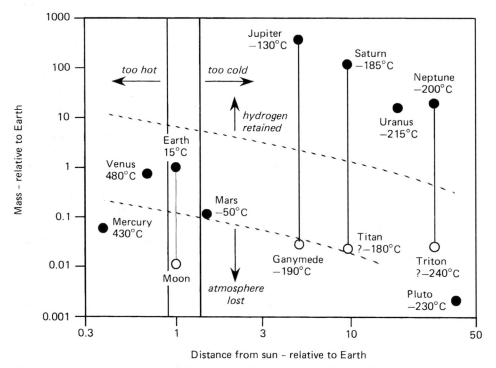

Figure 1.2 The planets and some of their larger satellites, plotted according to distance from sun (abscissa), and mass (ordinate), both scales being logarithmic and relative to Earth. Mean surface temperatures are shown. Potential for life as we know it exists only within the parallelogram surrounding the Earth.

In the solar system, only Earth has a mass that permits retention of an oxidizing atmosphere, and a distance from the sun at which liquid water can exist on the surface. It is difficult to see how there could be life as we know it anywhere in the solar system outside the small parallelogram in Figure 1.2. However, an environment similar to that of Earth's may well exist on a planet of another star in the universe.

Origin of life and its influence on the atmosphere

Until quite recently it was believed that the organic compounds, which were the essential precursors of life, were formed on Earth by abiotic chemical reactions in a strongly reducing atmosphere containing methane and ammonia.[8] However, it now seems unlikely that abiotic synthesis of amino acids could have occurred if Earth's early atmosphere was not strongly reducing, and methane and ammonia were present only in trace concentrations. On the other hand, there is a very wide range of extraterrestrial organic compounds, including amino acids, in many locations, particularly carbonaceous chondrite meteorites and comets. It seems inevitable that, once surface water was present on Earth, the secondary veneer of interstellar dust, meteorites and comets would have provided Earth with a wide range of organic compounds and their precursors.[4]

The next stage in the evolution of life is less easy to explain. An essential feature of life is the synthesis of proteins using a ribonucleic acid (RNA) template, transcribed from the genetic code carried on deoxyribonucleic acid (DNA). There would seem to have been a classic 'chicken and egg' situation. Useful proteins could not be formed without the appropriate sequences in RNA or DNA: RNA and DNA could not be polymerized without appropriate enzymes which are normally proteins. Nevertheless, life did appear, perhaps in the first instance with the genetic code carried on RNA, or even the much simpler peptide nucleic acid (PNA).[9]

The circumstances of the origin of life on Earth remain a mystery, but hydrothermal vents, such as the black smokers along the mid-Ocean ridges, support simple life forms on the basis of chemoautotrophy. They are totally independent of sunlight, and exploit the profound chemical disequilibrium between the emerging hot, reducing and acid water, containing hydrogen sulphide, methane, ammonia, phosphorus and a range of metals, and the surrounding sea water.[10] It is likely that hydrothermal vents have existed on Earth as long as surface water, and chemoautotrophs could have appeared as early as 4000 Ma ago.

It is hard to imagine a more constrained and hazardous environment for life than a hydrothermal vent, with energy supply depending on its continued existence. A much more attractive alternative was to utilize the limitless availability of energy in the form of solar visible light. The most familiar of many photosynthetic reactions is the synthesis of glucose, as follows:

$$6CO_2 + 6H_2O + energy = C_6H_{12}O_6 + 6O_2$$

The biochemical adaptation from thermal detection in hydrothermal vents to photo-synthesis does not seem to have been insuperable,[11] and there is strong palaeontological evidence for the existence of photosynthesizing cyanobacteria (blue–green algae) 3500 Ma ago.[12] These organisms must have released oxygen as a waste product, but this was almost entirely consumed by oxidizing soluble ferrous iron, leached from basalt, and depositing it as ferric iron in the vast banded iron formations.[13] This process prevented the appearance of significant concentrations of oxygen in the oceans or atmosphere until about 2000 Ma ago. Thereafter, banded iron formations seldom appeared, and iron was deposited in red (ferric) beds. Aerobic metabolism then became a possibility. Oxygen accumulated in the oceans and atmosphere, probably reaching a peak 300 Ma ago[14] (Figure 1.3). It then decreased sharply, perhaps contributing to the mass extinction at the end of the Palaeozoic Era, about 250 Ma ago.[2] Thereafter it seems to have risen towards the present atmospheric level. Cyanobacteria probably underwent symbiotic incorporation into the cells of certain eukaryotes to become chloroplasts, which then conferred the biochemical benefits of photosynthesis on their hosts.

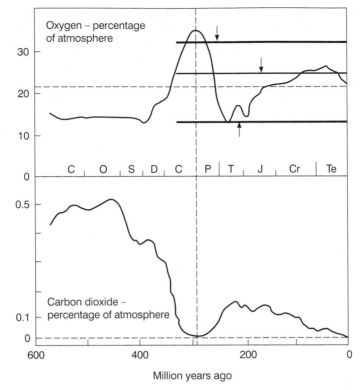

Figure 1.3 Long-term changes in oxygen and carbon dioxide concentrations during the last 600 Ma. Broken horizontal lines show present atmospheric levels. The vertical broken line shows the Carboniferous/Permian boundary. The continuous horizontal lines with arrows show some oxygen limits suggested by the geological record of forest fires.[2,15] Geological periods shown by their capital letters are: Cambrian, Ordovician, Silurian, Devonian, Carboniferous and Permian (Palaeozoic Era), and Triassic, Jurassic, Cretaceous (Mesozoic Era), Tertiary. (From Nunn,[2] after Graham et al.,[14] reproduced by permission of the Geologists' Association.)

Biological consequences of an oxidizing environment

It seems likely that the appearance of molecular oxygen in their environment would have been unwelcome to anaerobic organisms. Chapter 25 describes the toxicity of oxygen and its derived free radicals, against which primitive anaerobes would probably have had no defences. Three lines of response can be identified. Some anaerobes would have sought an anaerobic microenvironment in which to remain and survive. Others developed defences in depth against oxygen and its derived free radicals (page 503). The best response was the development of aerobic metabolism, which gave enormous energetic advantages over organisms relying on anaerobic metabolism (page 282). This required the symbiotic incorporation of mitochondria, but the increased availability of biological energy was essential for the evolution of all forms of life more complex than micro-organisms.

Photosynthesis and aerobic metabolism eventually established a cycle of energy exchange between plants and animals, with its ultimate energy input in the form of solar visible light, which was interrupted only under exceptional circumstances. Such circumstances probably occurred in some of the mass extinctions, which marked the end of certain geological epochs, the best known being the extinction of the dinosaurs at the end of the Mesozoic Era, 65 Ma ago. There is good evidence that this resulted from the impact of an asteroid, probably in the Yucatan, causing a persistent world-wide dust cloud, comparable to the postulated 'nuclear winter', and leaving a one centimetre thick, iridium-rich deposit at the Cretaceous/Tertiary junction throughout the world. The alternative theory is a major volcanic eruption (the flood basalt of the Deccan) but, whatever the cause, it is thought that the dust cloud cut off solar visible life for many consecutive months. This cooled the earth, stopped photosynthesis, interrupted the food chain and resulted in the extinction of an estimated 40 per cent of marine genera.

Changes in carbon dioxide levels

After the major outgassing phase of the newly formed Earth, the concentration of carbon dioxide in the atmosphere probably exceeded 90 per cent at high atmospheric pressure. It declined rapidly, due to weathering and photosynthesis, reaching about 0.5 per cent at the time of the beginning of the overt fossil record (Palaeozoic Era, from 570 Ma ago). A secondary major decline to somewhere near the present atmospheric level occurred during the Carboniferous period, when the coal-forming forests involved photosynthesis and carbon burial on an immense scale. A sharp increase occurred at the end of the Permian Period (the last period of the Palaeozoic Era) about 250 Ma ago, and this 'big belch' of carbon dioxide is considered to be the major factor causing the end-Permian mass extinction.[16] This coincided with the decrease in oxygen concentration mentioned above (Figure 1.3).

Carbon dioxide and the ice ages

Periodic glaciation has been a feature of the last million years of Earth's history. The fundamental causes seem to be largely astronomical, and there are three so-called Milankovitch cycles that appear to influence Earth's temperature. The longest, about 100 thousand years (ka), is the increasing and decreasing ellipticity of Earth's orbit. Next is a cycle of about 41 ka, caused by increasing and decreasing tilt of Earth's axis between 21° 39′ and 24° 36′. The shortest cycle, the 'precession of the equinoxes', has a periodicity cited variously between 21 and 26 ka. The likely effect of these variations on temperature has been calculated and summated to give an estimate of temperature over the last 800 ka. This correlates very well with geological indices of temperature (using the $\delta^{18}O$ index of isotopic ratios of oxygen) obtained from polar ice cores and ocean sediments deposited over the same period.[17]

There is also a remarkably close correlation between temperature and atmospheric concentrations of both carbon dioxide and methane, shown for the last 160 ka in Figure 1.4. It is tempting to think of these gases as the cause of the temperature changes, in view of the current preoccupation with the greenhouse effect of these gases. However, it is difficult to set aside the correlation with the effect of the Milankovitch cycles and, furthermore, the changes in carbon dioxide seem to follow rather than precede the temperature changes. Thus they do not appear to be the prime cause of the transitions between ice ages and interglacials, but rather a consequence. Nevertheless, they would provide positive feedback and amplify the temperature changes.

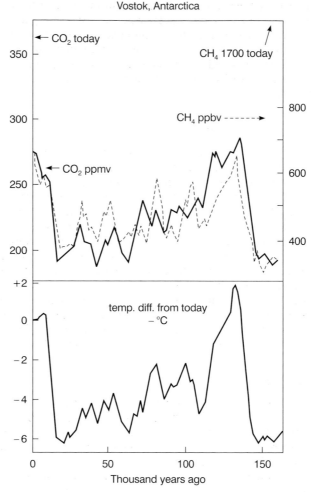

Figure 1.4 Ice core data from Vostok, Antarctica. Gas concentrations were obtained from gas bubbles in the ice, and temperature was derived from the $\delta^{18}O$ index of oxygen isotopes. The actual temperature changes may have been greater than those shown here. (From Nunn,[2] after Raynaud et al.,[18] reproduced by permission of the Geologists' Association.)

Greenhouse effect

The balance of heat gain from solar radiation is the difference between incoming radiation, mainly in the visible wave lengths, and outgoing radiation that is largely infrared. The latter is partially trapped in the troposphere, mainly by water vapour and carbon dioxide. The chilling effect of a clear starlit night is familiar to all, and there is a clear analogy in a greenhouse. The glass transmits incoming visible light, but impedes the loss of infrared radiation from the contents of the greenhouse, which have converted visible light to heat and so emit infrared radiation. It is estimated that the present greenhouse effect raises Earth's mean surface temperature by some 25°C.

The atmospheric concentration of carbon dioxide is a major determinant of the greenhouse effect and must contribute greatly to the very high surface temperature of

Venus (480°C), hotter than Mercury but further from the sun. There is therefore grave concern that excessive burning of fossil fuels will increase atmospheric carbon dioxide concentrations to a level that will result in significant global warming. Not the least serious consequence would be melting of polar ice, which would increase the volume of the oceans by some 2 per cent and cause flooding of low-lying lands. Major changes in sea level have occurred repeatedly in recent geological history, but it is feared the pace of change may now be faster.

Recent changes in carbon dioxide levels

Long-term studies in Hawaii have shown predictable diurnal and annual variations in atmospheric carbon dioxide concentration amounting to some 7 ppm (parts per million). However, against this background it has been possible to demonstrate a linear increase in mean concentration of 1.42 ppm per year between 1973 and 1986.[19] Table 1.3 shows that the mean increase over the last 45 years has been more than 100 times the rate of change at the end of the last ice age (Figure 1.4). The previous section presented evidence for believing that changes in carbon dioxide levels have not been the prime cause of the ice age/interglacial transitions. Nevertheless, this is not to say that present anthropogenic changes will not produce climatic changes quite independent of the Milankovitch cycles. Nevertheless, the current interglacial, which has been the cradle of literate civilization, will not last for ever, and it is conceivable that an enhanced carbon dioxide greenhouse effect could prolong the current interglacial. However, global warming may have disturbing short-term effects on ocean currents, particularly a weakening of the Gulf Stream.[20] It is disconcerting to note that most of the UK lies at the same latitude as Labrador.

Other greenhouse gases

There are no infrared absorption bands for water vapour and carbon dioxide between 7 and 13 μm wavelength, and heat loss in this band is considerable. It follows that any gas or vapour with strong infrared absorption in this range will have a disproportionate greenhouse effect. Such a gas could be considered not so much as thickening the panes in the greenhouse as replacing a missing pane.

Methane is present in the atmosphere at a concentration of only 1.7 ppm. However, it absorbs infrared some 25 times as effectively as carbon dioxide and therefore makes a small but not insignificant contribution to the greenhouse effect. The chlorofluorocarbons

Table 1.3 Recent changes in atmospheric carbon dioxide concentrations

Date	Atmospheric CO_2		Rate of change ppmv per year
	Mass in Gt	ppmv	
18 ka ago	420	200	
10 ka ago	590	280	0.01
1750 AD	590	280	0
1950 AD	650	310	0.15
1995 AD	760	362	1.16

Gt, gigatonne; ka, thousand years; ppmv, parts per million volume.
Data are from various sources.[2] (Reproduced from Nunn[2] by permission of the Geologists' Association.)

have an effect some 10 000 times greater than carbon dioxide. Present atmospheric concentrations are only of the order of 0.003 ppm, so their overall effect is barely one-tenth that of carbon dioxide at present. However, with their long half-life, they cannot be ignored. Nitrous oxide, mainly of biological origin, also makes a small contribution.

Turnover rates of atmospheric gases

Biological and geological turnover rates of carbon dioxide are quantitatively totally different.[2] Living organisms, the atmosphere and surface waters of the oceans contain about 2200 gigatonnes (Gt) of carbon. The annual exchange between photosynthesis and aerobic metabolism is approximately 100 Gt annually, with anthropogenic burning of fossil fuels and deforestation currently releasing about 7 Gt each year (Figure 1.5).

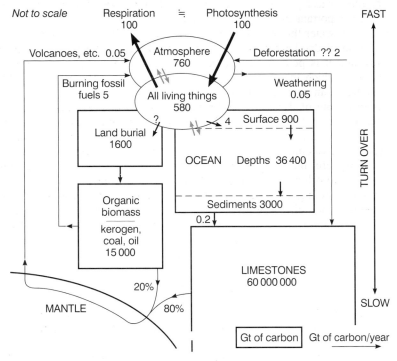

Figure 1.5 Stores and turnover of carbon dioxide. Stores are in gigatonnes (Gt) and turnover in Gt per year. (From Nunn[2] (where sources are cited), reproduced by permission of the Geologists' Association.)

   In stark contrast, geological stores (ocean depths, organic biomass and limestone) have a carbon content in excess of 30 000 000 Gt, but with an annual turnover (volcanoes, weathering, etc.) of less than 0.1 Gt per year. Thus, long-term changes are governed by the geological stores, while very rapid atmospheric changes can occur as a result of imbalance in the biomass or the anthropogenic activities outlined above.
   Atmospheric stores of oxygen are almost 600 times greater than those for carbon dioxide. If oxygen decreased at the same rate as the current increase in carbon dioxide, it would take 40 000 years for sea level P_{O_2} to fall to the level that pertains in Denver today.

Oxygen, ozone and ultraviolet screening

In addition to its toxicity and potential for more efficient metabolism, oxygen had a profound effect on evolution by ultraviolet screening. Oxygen itself absorbs ultraviolet radiation to a certain extent, but ozone (O_3) is far more effective. It is formed in the stratosphere from oxygen that undergoes photodissociation, producing free oxygen atoms. The oxygen atoms then rapidly combine with oxygen molecules to form ozone thus:

$$O_2 \rightleftharpoons 2O$$
$$\downarrow$$
$$O + O_2 \rightleftharpoons O_3$$

The absolute quantity is very small, being the equivalent of a layer of pure ozone only a few millimetres thick. A Dobson unit of ozone is defined as the equivalent of a layer of pure ozone 0.01 mm thick. About 10 per cent of the total atmospheric ozone is in the troposphere, mainly as a pollutant. This also acts as an ultraviolet screen and may become relatively more important in the years to come.

Life evolved in water that provided adequate screening from ultraviolet radiation. The first colonization of dry land by plants and animals was in the late Silurian Period (c. 400 Ma ago), and it is postulated that this coincided with oxygen and ozone reaching concentrations at which the degree of ultraviolet shielding first permitted organisms to leave the shelter of an aqueous environment.

Ozone is in a state of dynamic equilibrium in the stratosphere and its concentration varies markedly from year to year, in addition to displaying a pronounced annual cycle. Ozone can be removed by the action of many free radicals, including chlorine and nitric oxide. Highly reactive chlorine radicals cannot normally pass through the troposphere to reach the stratosphere, but the situation has recently been disturbed by the widespread manufacture of chlorofluorocarbons (e.g. CF_2Cl_2) for use as propellants and refrigerants. These compounds are highly stable in the troposphere with a half-life of the order of 100 years. This permits their diffusion through the troposphere to reach the stratosphere, where they undergo photodissociation to release chlorine radicals, which then react with ozone as follows:

$$Cl + O_3 \rightarrow ClO + O_2$$
$$\uparrow \qquad\qquad \downarrow$$
$$Cl + O_2 \leftarrow ClO + O$$

Chlorine is recycled and it has been estimated that a single chlorine radical will destroy 10 000 molecules of ozone before it combines with hydrogen to form the relatively harmless hydrochloric acid. The Antarctic 'hole' in the ozone layer forms in October of each year, when spring sunlight initiates photochemical reactions. Minimal levels fell from 300 Dobson units in 1960 to 100 in 1994 and are still falling.[21]

Evolution and adaptation

This chapter has outlined the environmental conditions and biological factors under which the atmosphere has evolved to its present composition. In the past nothing has been permanent, and we can expect a continuation of the interaction between organisms and their environment. What is new is that one species now has the power to cause major changes in the environment, and the atmosphere in particular. These will affect a wide range of organisms, and result in the extinction of certain species.

References

1. Taylor SR. *Solar system evolution*. Cambridge: Cambridge University Press, 1992.
2. Nunn JF. Evolution of the atmosphere. *Proc Geol Assoc* 1998; **109**: 1–13.
3. Chang S. The planetary setting of prebiotic evolution. In: Bengston S, ed. *Early life on Earth*. Nobel symposium no. 84. New York: Columbia University Press, 1994; 10–23.
4. Oró J. Early chemical stages in the origin of life. In: Bengston S, ed. *Early life on Earth*. Nobel symposium no. 84. New York: Columbia University Press, 1994; 48–59.
5. MacDonald GA, Hubbard DH. *Volcanoes of the National Parks in Hawaii*, 6th edn. Honolulu: Hawaii Natural History Association, 1972.
6. Kasting JF, Chang S. Formation of the earth and the origin of life. In: Schopf JW, Klein C, eds. *The Proterozoic biosphere*. Cambridge: Cambridge University Press, 1992; 9–12.
7. Chapman CR, Morrison D. *Cosmic catastrophes*. London: Plenum Press, 1989; 97.
8. Miller SL. A production of amino acids under possible primitive earth conditions. *Science* 1953; **117**: 528–529.
9. Böhler C, Nielsen PE, Orgel LE. Template switching between PNA and RNA oligonucleotides. *Nature* 1995; **376**: 578–81.
10. Nisbet EG. Archaean ecology. In: Coward MP, Reis AC, eds. *Early Precambrian processes*. London: Geological Society, 1995; 27–51.
11. Nisbet EG. Origins of photosynthesis. *Nature* 1995; **373**: 479–80.
12. Schopf JW. Paleobiology of the Archaean. In: Schopf JW, Klein C, eds. *The Proterozoic biosphere*. Cambridge: Cambridge University Press, 1992; 25–39.
13. Klein C, Beukes NJ. Time distribution, stratigraphy, and sedimentologic setting, and geochemistry of Precambrian iron formations. In: Schopf JW, Klein C, eds. *The Proterozoic biosphere*. Cambridge: Cambridge University Press, 1992; 139–46.
14. Graham JB, Dudley R, Aguilar NM, Gans C. Implications of the late Palaeozoic oxygen pulse for physiology and evolution. *Nature* 1995; **375**: 117–120.
15. Lovelock JE. *Gaia. A new look at life on earth*. Oxford: Oxford University Press, 1979; 71.
16. Knoll AH, Bambach RK, Canfield DE, Grotzinger JP. Comparative Earth history and late Permian mass extinction. *Science* 1996; **273**: 452–7.
17. Lowe JJ, Walker MJC. *Reconstructing quaternary environments*, 2nd edn. London: Longman, 1997; 8–15.
18. Raynaud D, Jouzel J, Barnola JM, Chappelaz J, Delmas RJ, Lorius C. The ice record of greenhouse gases. *Science* 1993; **259**: 926–41.
19. Thoning KW, Tans PP, Komhyr WD. Atmospheric carbon dioxide at Mauna Loa observatory. *J Geophys Res* 1989; **94**: 8549–65.
20. Broecker WS. Thermohaline circulation, the Achilles heel of our climate system: will man-made CO_2 upset the current balance? *Science* 1997; **278**: 1582–8.
21. Jones AE, Shanklin JD. Continued decline of total ozone over Halley, Antarctica, since 1985. *Nature* 1995; **376**: 409–11.

Chapter 2

Functional anatomy of the respiratory tract

This chapter is not a comprehensive account of respiratory anatomy but concentrates on the aspects that are most relevant to an understanding of function. The respiratory muscles are considered in Chapter 6.

Mouth, nose and pharynx

Breathing is normally possible through either the nose or the mouth, the alternative air passages converging in the oropharynx. Nasal breathing is the norm and has two major advantages over mouth breathing: filtration of particulate matter by the vibrissae hairs and humidification of inspired gas. Humidification by the nose is highly efficient because the nasal septum and turbinates greatly increase the surface area of mucosa available for evaporation and produce turbulent flow, so increasing contact between the mucosa and air. However, the nose may offer more resistance to air flow than the mouth, particularly when obstructed by polyps, adenoids or congestion of the nasal mucosa. Nasal resistance may make oral breathing obligatory, and many children and adults breathe only or partly through their mouths at rest.[1] With increasing levels of exercise in normal adults, the respiratory minute volume increases and at a level of about 35 l.min^{-1} the oral airway is brought into play. Deflection of gas into either the nasal or the oral route is under voluntary control and accomplished with the soft palate, tongue and lips. These functions are best considered in relation to a midline sagittal section (Figure 2.1).

Part (a) of Figure 2.1 shows the normal position for nose breathing, with the mouth closed by occlusion of the lips, and the tongue lying against the hard palate. The soft palate is clear of the posterior pharyngeal wall.

Part (b) shows forced mouth breathing, as for instance when blowing through the mouth, without pinching the nose. The soft palate becomes rigid and is arched upwards and backwards by contraction of tensor and levator palati[2] to lie against a band of the superior constrictor of the pharynx known as Passavant's ridge which, together with the soft palate, forms the palatopharyngeal sphincter. Note also that the orifice of the pharyngotympanic (eustachian) tube lies above the palatopharyngeal sphincter, and the tubes can therefore be inflated by the subject only when the nose is pinched. As the mouth pressure is raised, this tends to force the soft palate against the posterior pharyngeal wall to act as a valve. The combined palatopharyngeal sphincter and valvular action of the soft palate is very strong and can easily withstand mouth pressures in excess of 10 kPa (100 cmH$_2$O).

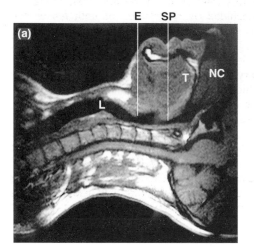
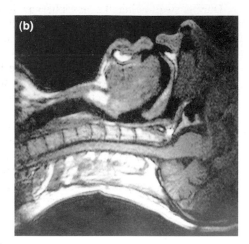
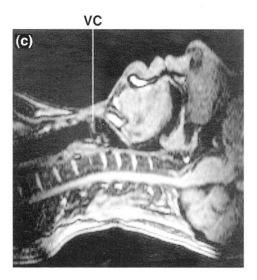

Figure 2.1 Magnetic resonance imaging (MRI) scans showing median sagittal sections of the pharynx in a normal subject. (a) Normal nasal breathing with the oral airway occluded by lips and tongue; (b) Deliberate oral breathing with the nasal airway occluded by elevation and backward movement of the soft palate; (c) A Valsalva manoeuvre in which the subject deliberately tries to exhale against a closed airway. The airway is occluded at many sites. The lips are closed, the tongue is in contact with the hard palate anteriorly, the palatopharyngeal sphincter is tightly closed, the epiglottis is in contact with the posterior pharyngeal wall, and the vocal folds are closed, so becoming visible in this midline section. Data acquisition for scans (a) and (b) took 45 seconds, so anatomical differences between inspiration and expiration will not be visible. Scanning a Valsalva manoeuvre required more rapid data acquisition, so the texture of tissues in scan (c) is different from the previous two. (I am grateful to the staff of the MRI unit at St James's Hospital for performing the scans and to Dr Mark Bellamy for being the subject.) E, epiglottis; L, larynx; NC, nasal cavity; SP, soft palate; T, tongue; VC, vocal folds (cords).

Part (c) shows the occlusion of the respiratory tract during a Valsalva manoeuvre.

During swallowing the nasopharynx is occluded by contraction of both tensor and levator palati. The larynx is elevated 2–3 cm by contraction of the infrahyoid muscles, stylopharyngeus and palatopharyngeus, coming to lie under the epiglottis. In addition, the aryepiglottic folds are approximated, causing total occlusion of the entrance to the larynx.[3] This extremely effective protection of the larynx is capable of withstanding pharyngeal pressures as high as 80 kPa (600 mmHg), which may be generated during swallowing.

Upper airway cross-sectional areas can be estimated from conventional radiographs, magnetic resonance imaging (MRI) as in Figure 2.1 or acoustic reflectometry. In the last-named technique, a single sound pulse of 100 μs duration is generated within the apparatus and passes along the airway of the subject. Recording of the timing and frequency of sound waves reflected back from the airway allows calculation of cross-sectional area, which is then presented as a function of the distance travelled along the airway[4] (Figure 2.2). Acoustic reflectometry has now been developed sufficiently for use in clinical situations with real-time results and good correlation with MRI results.[5]

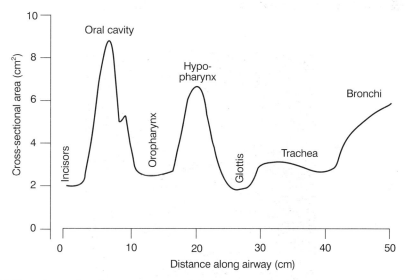

Figure 2.2 Normal acoustic reflectometry pattern of airway cross-sectional area during mouth breathing. Redrawn from references 4 and 5.

Pharyngeal muscles are active during normal breathing, playing an important role in maintaining pharyngeal dimensions during the generation of subatmospheric pressures required for breathing. This aspect of their function is described in Chapter 6.

The larynx

The larynx evolved in the lung fish for the protection of the airway during such activities as feeding and perfusion of the gills with water. Whilst protection of the airway remains important, the larynx now has many other functions, all involving varying degrees of laryngeal occlusion.[3,6]

Speech.[7] Phonation, the laryngeal component of speech, requires a combination of changes in position, tension and mass of the vocal folds (cords). Rotation of the arytenoid cartilages by the posterior cricoarytenoid muscles opens the vocal folds, whilst contraction of the lateral cricoarytenoid and oblique arytenoid muscles opposes this. With the vocal folds almost closed, the respiratory muscles generate a positive pressure of $5-35\,cmH_2O$, which may then be released by slight opening of the vocal folds to produce sound waves. The cricothyroid muscle tilts the cricoid and arytenoid cartilages backwards and also moves them posteriorly in relation to the thyroid cartilage. This produces up to 50 per cent elongation and therefore tensioning of the vocal folds, an action opposed by the thyroarytenoid muscles which draw the arytenoid cartilages forwards toward the thyroid and so shorten and relax the vocal folds. Tensioning of the folds results in both transverse and longitudinal resonance of the vocal fold, allowing the formation of complex sound waves. The deeper fibres of the thyroarytenoids comprise the vocales muscles, which exert fine control over pitch of the voice by slight variations in both the tension and mass of the vocal folds. A more dramatic example of the effect of vocal fold mass on voice production occurs with inflammation of the laryngeal mucosa and the resulting hoarse voice or complete inability to phonate.

Effort closure. Tighter occlusion of the larynx, known as effort closure, is required for making expulsive efforts. It is also needed to lock the thoracic cage and so to secure the origin of the muscles of the upper arm arising from the ribcage, thus increasing the power that can be transmitted to the arm. In addition to simple apposition of the vocal folds described above, the aryepiglottic muscles and their continuation, the oblique and transverse arytenoids, act as a powerful sphincter capable of closing the inlet of the larynx, by bringing the aryepiglottic folds tightly together. The full process enables the larynx to withstand the highest pressures that can be generated in the thorax, usually at least 12 kPa (120 cmH$_2$O) and often more.[6] Sudden release of the obstruction is essential for effective coughing, when the linear velocity of air through the larynx is said to approach the speed of sound.

Swallowing. Effort closure is part of the mechanism involved in the protection of the larynx during swallowing. In addition, the larynx is lifted towards the hyoid bone, elevating the epiglottis which becomes squeezed between the base of the tongue and laryngeal inlet to deflect the food bolus backwards.

  Laryngeal muscles are involved in controlling airways resistance, particularly during expiration, and this aspect of vocal fold function is described in Chapter 6.

The tracheobronchial tree

An accurate and complete model of the branching pattern of the human bronchial tree remains elusive, though several different models have been described.[8] The most useful and widely accepted approach remains that of Weibel,[9,10] who numbered successive generations of air passages from the trachea (generation 0) down to alveolar sacs (generation 23). This 'regular dichotomy' model assumes that each bronchus regularly divides into two approximately equal-size daughter bronchi; it is unlikely to be true in practice where bronchus length is variable, pairs of daughter bronchi are often unequal in size, and trifurcations may be demonstrated. However, as a rough approximation it may be assumed that the number of passages in each generation is double that in the previous generation, and the number of air passages in each generation is approximately indicated

Table 2.1 Structural characteristics of the air passages[9,11]

	Generation (mean)	Number	Mean diameter (mm)	Area supplied	Cartilage	Muscle	Nutrition	Emplacement	Epithelium
Trachea	0	1	18	Both lungs	U-shaped	Links open end of cartilage			
Main bronchi	1	2	12	Individual lungs					
Lobar bronchi	2 → 3	4 → 8	8 → 5	Lobes	Irregular shaped	Helical bands		Within connective tissue sheath alongside arterial vessels	Columnar ciliated epithelium
Segmental bronchi	4	16	4	Segments			From the bronchial circulation		
Small bronchi	5 → 11	32 → 2 000	3 → 1	Secondary lobules					
Bronchioles Terminal bronchioles	12 → 14	4 000 → 16 000	1 → 0.7			Strong helical muscle bands		Embedded directly in the lung parenchyma	Cuboidal
Respiratory bronchioles	15 → 18	32 000 → 260 000	0.4	Pulmonary acinus	Absent	Muscle bands between alveoli	From the pulmonary circulation		Cuboidal to flat between alveoli
Alveolar ducts	19 → 22	520 000 → 4 000 000	0.3			Thin bands in alveolar septa		Form the lung parenchyma	Alveolar epithelium
Alveoli	23	8 000 000	0.2						

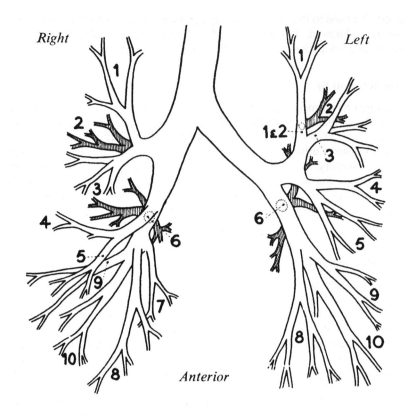

Figure 2.3 Named branches of the tracheobronchial tree, viewed from the front. (Reproduced by permission of the editors of *Thorax*.)

by the number 2 raised to the power of the generation number. This formula indicates one trachea, two main bronchi, four lobar bronchi, 16 segmental bronchi, etc. Table 2.1 traces their essential characteristics progressively down the respiratory tract.

Trachea (generation 0)

The adult trachea has a mean diameter of 1.8 cm and length of 11 cm. It is supported by U-shaped cartilages that are joined posteriorly by smooth muscle bands. The part of the trachea in the neck is not subjected to intrathoracic pressure changes, but it is very vulnerable to pressures arising in the neck due, for example, to tumours or haematoma formation after surgery. An external pressure of the order of 4 kPa (40 cmH$_2$O) is sufficient to occlude the trachea. In the chest, the trachea can be compressed by raised intrathoracic pressure during, for example, a cough, when the decreased diameter increases the linear velocity of gas flow and therefore the efficiency of removal of secretions.

Main, lobar and segmental bronchi (generations 1–4)

The trachea bifurcates asymmetrically, the right bronchus being wider and making a smaller angle with the long axis of the trachea. Foreign bodies therefore tend to enter the right bronchus in preference to the left. Main, lobar and segmental bronchi have firm cartilaginous support in their walls, U-shaped in the main bronchi, but in the form of irregularly shaped and helical plates lower down with bronchial muscle between. Bronchi in this group (down to generation 4) are sufficiently regular to be individually named (Figure 2.3). Total cross-sectional area of the respiratory tract is minimal at the third generation (Figure 2.4).

These bronchi are subjected to the full effect of changes in intrathoracic pressure and will collapse when the intrathoracic pressure exceeds the intraluminar pressure by about 5 kPa (50 cmH$_2$O). This occurs in the larger bronchi during a forced expiration, so limiting peak expiratory flow rate (see Figure 4.7).

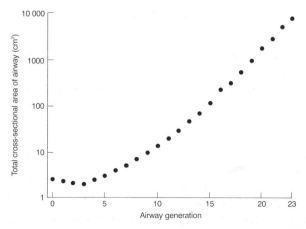

Figure 2.4 The total cross-sectional area of the air passages at different generations of the airways. Note that the minimum cross-sectional area is at generation 3 (lobar to segmental bronchi). The total cross-sectional area becomes very large in the smaller air passages, approaching a square metre in the alveolar ducts. (Redrawn from data in reference 10.)

Small bronchi (generations 5–11)

The small bronchi extend through about seven generations, their diameter progressively falling from 3.5 to 1 mm. Because their number approximately doubles with each generation, the total cross-sectional area increases markedly with each generation to a value (at generation 11) that is about ten times the total cross-sectional area at the level of the lobar bronchi (Figure 2.4). Down to the level of the smallest true bronchi, air passages lie in close proximity to branches of the pulmonary artery in a sheath containing pulmonary lymphatics, which can be distended with oedema fluid that gives rise to the characteristic 'cuffing' that is responsible for the earliest radiographic changes in pulmonary oedema. Because these air passages are not directly attached to the lung parenchyma, they are not subject to direct traction and rely for their patency on cartilage in their walls and on the transmural pressure gradient which is normally positive from lumen to intrathoracic space. In the normal subject, this pressure gradient is seldom reversed and, even during a forced expiration, the intraluminar pressure in the small bronchi rapidly rises to more than 80 per cent of the alveolar pressure, which is more than the extramural (intrathoracic) pressure.

Bronchioles (generations 12–14)

An important change occurs at about the eleventh generation, where the internal diameter is about 1 mm. Cartilage disappears from the wall below this level and ceases to be a factor in maintaining patency. However, beyond this level the air passages are directly embedded in the lung parenchyma, the elastic recoil of which holds the air passages open like the guy ropes of a tent. Therefore, the calibre of the airways below the eleventh generation is influenced mainly by lung volume, because the forces holding their lumina open are stronger at higher lung volumes. The converse of this factor causes airway closure at reduced lung volume (see Chapter 4). In succeeding generations, the number of bronchioles increases far more rapidly than the calibre diminishes (Table 2.1). The total cross-sectional area increases until, in the terminal bronchioles, it is about 100 times the area at the level of the large bronchi (Figure 2.4). Thus the flow resistance of these smaller air passages (less than 2 mm diameter) is negligible under normal conditions.[12] However, the resistance of the bronchioles can increase to very high values when their strong helical muscular bands are contracted by the mechanisms described in Chapters 4 and 30. This can wrinkle the lining epithelium into varying numbers of longitudinal folds and may result in total airway obstruction (see page 72). Down to the terminal bronchiole, the air passages derive their nutrition from the bronchial circulation and are thus influenced by systemic arterial blood gas levels. Beyond this point the smaller air passages rely on the pulmonary circulation for their nutrition.

Respiratory bronchioles (generations 15–18)

Down to the smallest bronchioles, the functions of the air passages are solely conduction and humidification. Beyond this point there is a gradual transition from conduction to gas exchange. In the four generations of respiratory bronchioles there is a gradual increase in the number of alveoli in their walls. Like the bronchioles, the respiratory bronchioles are embedded in lung parenchyma, but they have a well-defined muscle layer with bands that loop over the opening of the alveolar ducts and the mouths of the mural alveoli. There is no significant change in calibre of advancing generations of respiratory bronchioles (about

0.4 mm diameter), and the total cross-sectional area at this level is of the order of hundreds of square centimetres.

Alveolar ducts (generations 19–22)

Alveolar ducts arise from the terminal respiratory bronchiole, from which they differ by having no walls other than the mouths of mural alveoli (about 20 in number). The alveolar septa comprise a series of rings forming the walls of the alveolar ducts and containing smooth muscle. About half the alveoli arise from ducts, and some 35 per cent of the alveolar gas resides in the alveolar ducts and the alveoli that arise directly from them.

Alveolar sacs (generation 23)

The last generation of the air passages differs from alveolar ducts solely in the fact that they are blind. It is estimated that about 17 alveoli arise from each alveolar sac and account for about half of the total number of alveoli.

Pulmonary acinus (*syn.* primary lobule, terminal respiratory unit)

The pulmonary acinus is usually defined as the zone supplied by a first order respiratory bronchiole and includes the respiratory bronchioles, alveolar ducts and alveolar sacs distal to a single terminal bronchiole (Figure 2.5). This represents generations 15–23 above, but in practice the number of generations in a single acinus is quite variable, being between 6 and 12 divisions beyond the terminal bronchiole.[10] A human lung contains about 30 000 acini,[11] each with a diameter of about 3.5 mm and containing about 10 000 alveoli.[13] A single pulmonary acinus is probably the equivalent of the alveolus when it is considered from a functional standpoint, as gas movement in the acinus is by diffusion rather than by tidal ventilation. The path length between the start of the acinus and the most distal alveolus therefore becomes crucial and is between 5 and 12 mm.[11]

Respiratory epithelium[14]

From the nasal cavity to the bronchioles the respiratory tract is lined with a pseudo-stratified columnar ciliated epithelium containing many mucus-secreting (goblet) cells. In the bronchioles the cell height begins to reduce and tends toward cuboidal epithelial cells before gradually flattening further throughout the pulmonary acinus and merging with the alveolar epithelial cells. Goblet cells are present at a density of about $6000.mm^{-2}$ (in the trachea) and are responsible, along with submucosal secretory cells, for producing the thick layer of mucus that lines all but the smallest conducting airways. Mucin, the principal glycoprotein in mucus, is released by rapid (<150 ms) exocytosis from the mucus-secreting cells in response to a range of stimuli, including direct chemical irritation, inflammatory cytokines and neural activity.[15] Both goblet cell numbers and secretions increase in many airway diseases such as asthma,

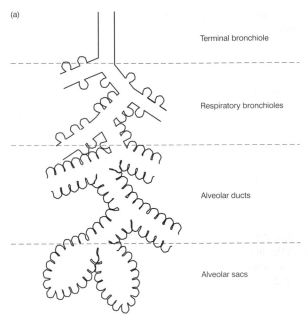

Figure 2.5(a) Schematic diagram of a single pulmonary acinus showing four generations from the terminal bronchiole to the alveolar sacs. The average number of generations in human lung is eight, but may be as many as twelve.[10]

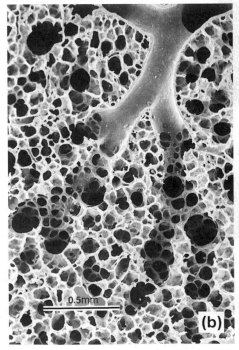

Figure 2.5(b) Thick section of rabbit lung showing respiratory bronchioles leading to alveolar ducts and sacs. Human alveoli would be considerably larger. (Photograph kindly supplied by Professor EM Weibel.)

bronchitis and cystic fibrosis (Chapter 27).[15] The mucous layer is propelled cephalad by the ciliated epithelial cells (Figure 2.6) at a rate of 4 mm.min^{-1}, to be removed by expectoration on reaching the larynx. Each cell is topped by about 250 cilia, which beat at a rate of 12–16 beats per second. Adjacent cells somehow co-ordinate their cilia activity, probably by a physical link between cilia caused by the mucus above. In the mucus there are two layers:[16] a 'sol' layer of low viscosity, containing water and solutes and in which the cilia are embedded; and a 'gel' layer above, containing the viscous mucin in the underside of which the cilia tips intermittently 'grip' the mucous layer.

Other cell types found in the respiratory epithelium are as follows.

Basal cells. These cells lie underneath the columnar cells giving rise to the pseudo-stratified appearance, and are absent in the bronchioles and beyond. They are probably the stem cell responsible for producing new epithelial and goblet cells.

Mast cells. The lungs contain numerous mast cells located below the mucosa of the airways as well as in the alveolar septa. Some also lie free in the lumen of the airways and may be recovered by bronchial lavage. Their important role in bronchoconstriction is described in Chapter 27.

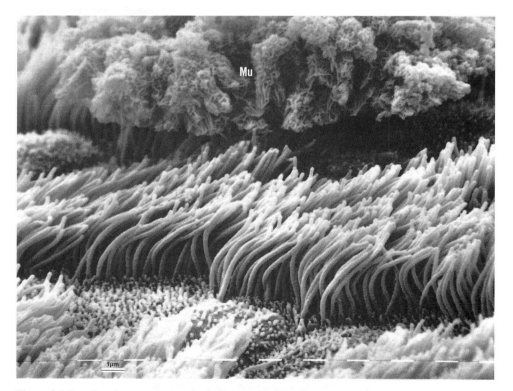

Figure 2.6 Scanning electron micrograph of ciliated epithelial cells beating in the fluid layer beneath the mucus (Mu). (Reproduced by kind permission of Dr PK Jeffery, Imperial College School of Science, Technology and Medicine, London, and the publishers of *Respiratory Medicine*[14].)

Non-ciliated bronchiolar epithelial (Clara) cells. These cells are found in the mucosa of the terminal bronchioles, where they may be the precursor of epithelial cells in the absence of basal cells. They are metabolically active, secreting at least three proteins, including antiproteases and a surfactant apoprotein,[17] and are involved in the metabolism of chemical toxins.

APUD cells. These cells occur in bronchial epithelium and, from morphological considerations, are believed to be part of the APUD series, so named because of their ability to undertake **a**mine and **a**mine-**p**recursor **u**ptake and **d**ecarboxylation. APUD cells elsewhere are known to produce a range of hormones, including ACTH, insulin, calcitonin and gastrin.

Functions of respiratory epithelium

Humidification.[18] The respiratory mucosa acts as a heat and moisture exchanger. During inspiration, relatively cool, dry air causes evaporation of surface water and cooling of the mucosa; then, on expiration, moisture condenses on the surface of the mucosa and warming occurs. Thus only about one-half of the heat and moisture needed to condition (fully warm and saturate) each breath is lost to the atmosphere. With quiet nasal breathing, air is conditioned before reaching the trachea, but, as ventilation increases, smaller airways are recruited until at minute volumes of over $50 \, l.min^{-1}$ airways of 1 mm diameter are involved in humidification.

Chemical barrier and particle clearance. The viscous mucus layer provides a physical barrier to chemical damage of the epithelium, many inhaled irritants simply dissolving in the mucus until exhaled or removed by expectoration. Others are initially metabolized and then conjugated by the underlying cells (particularly Clara cells).[19] Inhaled particles are deposited in the airways either by inertial impaction or by sedimentation depending on their size. Inertial impaction occurs when the airway has a sharp corner (e.g. the pharynx or nose) or when gas flow becomes turbulent (e.g. large bifurcations). Most particles above $8 \, \mu m$ impact on the pharyngeal walls, whilst those between 5 and $8 \, \mu m$ tend to be deposited near large airway divisions. In both cases the particles are either degraded by proteases in the mucosa or removed intact with the mucus. Sedimentation occurs in the respiratory bronchioles and alveoli, where the velocity of gas flow becomes too low for the particle to remain suspended, so depositing particles smaller than $5 \, \mu m$ which are then removed by macrophages.

Defence against infection. Respiratory epithelium is crucial in preventing infection from airborne pathogens. The first line of defence is physical removal of bacterial and viral particles by the mucus. Next, humoral defences in the mucus include immunoglobulins (particularly IgA), complement proteins, protease inhibitors (α_1-antitrypsin), lysozyme, transferrin (which binds iron, an essential cofactor for bacterial proliferation) and endogenous antibiotics (page 536). Thirdly, cellular immunity is in evidence throughout the epithelium with macrophages, neutrophils and lymphocytes all being commonly found during infection in the normal lung.

These functions require quite opposite mucous consistency. For humidification the mucus requires a high water content whilst as a barrier the mucus requires high viscosity and high protein content. The epithelial cells are responsible for balancing these requirements by the secretion and reabsorption of water and solutes as appropriate, and this control must occur quickly to accommodate rapid changes in minute ventilation and air temperature and humidity. It seems likely that the epithelium in small airways secretes fluid into the mucus and that of large airways later absorbs any excess fluid before the mucus is removed from the lung.[16]

The alveoli

The mean total number of alveoli is usually given as 300 million but ranges from about 200 million to 600 million, correlating with the height of the subject.[20] The size of the alveoli is proportional to lung volume but, because of gravity, they are normally larger in the upper part of the lung except at maximal inflation when the vertical gradient in size disappears. At functional residual capacity the mean diameter is 0.2 mm, astonishingly close to the estimate of 1/100 inch (0.25 mm) made by the Reverend Stephen Hales in 1731.[21]

The alveolar septa

The septa are under tension generated partly by elastic fibres but more by surface tension at the air/fluid interface (page 38). They are therefore generally flat, making the alveoli polyhedral rather than spherical. The septa are perforated by small fenestrations, known as the pores of Kohn (Figure 2.7), that provide collateral ventilation between alveoli. Direct communications have also been found between small bronchioles and neighbouring alveoli, adjacent pulmonary acini and, occasionally, intersegmental communications.[22]

On one side of the alveolar wall the capillary endothelium and the alveolar epithelium are closely apposed, with almost no interstitial space, such that the total thickness from gas to blood is about 0.3 µm (Figures 2.8 and 2.9). This may be considered the 'active' side of the capillary, and gas exchange must be more efficient on this side. The other side of the capillary, which may be considered the 'service' side, is usually more than 1–2 µm thick and contains a recognizable interstitial space containing elastin and collagen fibres, nerve endings and occasional migrant polymorphs and macrophages. The distinction between the two sides of the capillary has considerable pathophysiological significance, as the active side tends to be spared in the accumulation of both oedema fluid and fibrous tissue (Chapters 28 and 29).

The fibre scaffold. The alveolar septum contains a network of fibre that forms a continuum between the peripheral fibres and the axial spiral fibres of the bronchioles.[25] The septal fibre is in the form of a network, through which are threaded the pulmonary capillaries, which are themselves a network. Thus the capillaries pass repeatedly from one side of the fibre scaffold to the other (Figure 2.7), the fibre always residing on the thick (or 'service') side of the capillary, allowing the other side to bulge into the lumen of the alveolus. The left side of the capillary in Figure 2.8 is the side with the fibres. At cellular level, the scaffolding for the alveolar septa is provided by the basement membrane.[26] This comprises collagen IV, laminin and heparan sulphate proteoglycan. The first provides a diamond-shaped matrix of great strength relative to its bulk; the other constituents are concerned with cell attachment and regulate the permeability to proteins. These aspects of

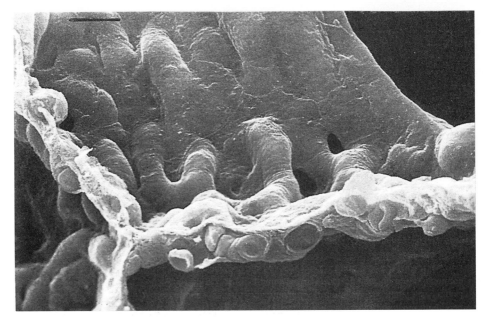

Figure 2.7 Scanning electron micrograph of the junction of three alveolar septa, which are in both surface view and section, showing the polyhedral structure. Two pores of Kohn are seen to the right of centre. Erythrocytes are seen in the cut ends of the capillaries. The scale bar is 10 μm. (Reproduced from reference 23 by permission of the author and the publishers; © Harvard University Press.)

the function of the basement membrane are important. Increases in the capillary transmural pressure gradient above about 3 kPa (30 cmH$_2$O) may cause disruption of endothelium and/or epithelium, while the basement membrane tends to remain intact, sometimes as the only remaining separation between blood and gas.[27]

Alveolar cell types

Capillary endothelial cells.[28] These cells are continuous with the endothelium of the general circulation and, in the pulmonary capillary bed, have a thickness of only 0.1 μm except where expanded to contain nuclei (Figure 2.8). Electron microscopy shows the flat parts of the cytoplasm to be devoid of all organelles except for small vacuoles (caveolae or plasmalemmal vesicles), which may open onto the basement membrane or the lumen of the capillary or be entirely contained within the cytoplasm (Figure 2.9). The lining of the caveolae acts as an extension of the cell membrane beyond its already vast size[29] of about 126 m^2. Surface enzymes are located on the lining of the caveolae as well as on membrane lining the capillaries.[30] The pulmonary capillary endothelium has a metabolic activity approaching that of the liver (Chapter 12). The endothelial cells abut against one another at fairly loose junctions, which are of the order of 5 nm wide.[31] These junctions permit the passage of quite large molecules, and the pulmonary lymph contains albumin at about half the concentration in plasma.[32] Macrophages pass freely through these junctions under normal conditions, and polymorphs can also pass in response to chemotaxis (page 578).

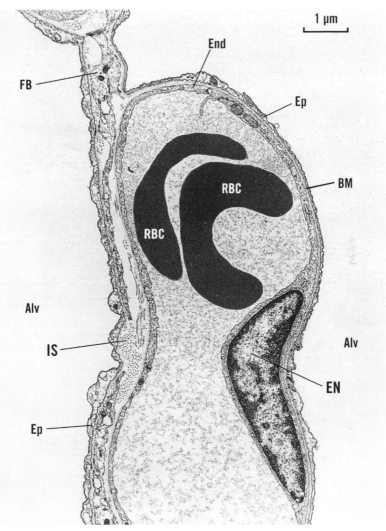

1 µm

End

FB

Ep

RBC

RBC

BM

Alv

IS

Alv

EN

Ep

Figure 2.8. Details of the interstitial space, the capillary endothelium and alveolar epithelium. Thickening of the interstitial space is confined to the left of the capillary (the 'service' side) while the total alveolar/capillary membrane remains thin on the right (the 'active' side) except where it is thickened by the endothelial nucleus. Alv, alveolus; BM, basement membrane; EN, endothelial nucleus; End, endothelium; Ep, epithelium; FB, fibroblast process; IS, interstitial space; RBC, erythrocyte. (Electron micrograph kindly supplied by Professor ER Weibel.)

Alveolar epithelial cells – type I. These cells line the alveoli and also exist as a thin sheet about 0.1 µm in thickness, except where expanded to contain nuclei. Like the endothelium, the flat part of the cytoplasm is devoid of organelles except for small vacuoles. Epithelial cells each cover several capillaries and are joined into a continuous sheet by tight junctions with a gap of only about 1 nm.[31] These junctions may be seen as narrow lines snaking across the septa in Figure 2.7. The tightness of these junctions is crucial for preventing the escape of large molecules, such as albumin, into the alveoli,

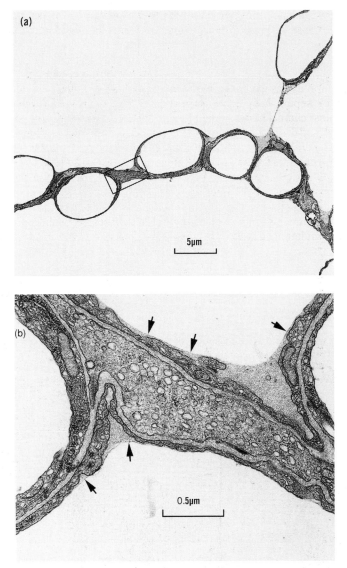

Figure 2.9 (a) Transmission electron micrograph of alveolar septum with lung inflated to 40 per cent of total lung capacity. The section in the box is enlarged in (b) to show alveolar lining fluid, which has pooled in two concavities of the alveolar epithelium and has also spanned the pore of Kohn in (a). There is a thin film of osmiophilic material (arrows), probably surfactant, at the interface between air and the alveolar lining fluid. (Reproduced from reference 24 by permission of the authors and the Editors of *Journal of Applied Physiology*.)

thus preserving the oncotic pressure gradient essential for preventing pulmonary oedema (see page 543). Nevertheless, these junctions permit the free passage of macrophages. Polymorphs may also pass in response to a chemotactic stimulus. Figure 2.9 shows the type I cell covered with a film of alveolar lining fluid, although it has been proposed that the surface is normally dry.[33] Type I cells are end cells and do not divide *in vivo*.

However, they have been cultured *in vitro* with type II cells on a matrix secreted by the latter.[34] They are particularly sensitive to damage from high concentrations of oxygen (Chapter 25).

Alveolar epithelial cells – type II. These are the stem cells from which type I cells arise.[35] They do not function as gas exchange membranes, and are rounded in shape and situated at the junction of septa. They have large nuclei and microvilli (Figure 2.10). The cytoplasm contains characteristic striated osmiophilic organelles that contain stored surfactant (page 41).[36] Type II cells are also involved in pulmonary defence mechanisms in that they may secrete cytokines and contribute to pulmonary inflammation. Type II cells are easily grown in culture and tend to proliferate in lung explant tissue cultures. They are resistant to oxygen toxicity, tending to replace type I cells after prolonged exposure to high concentrations of oxygen (Chapter 25).

Alveolar macrophages. The lung is richly endowed with these phagocytes, which pass freely from the circulation, through the interstitial space and thence through the gaps

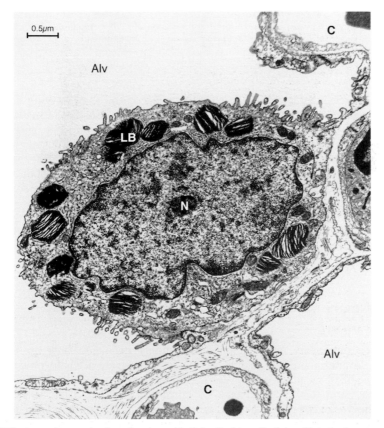

Figure 2.10 Electron micrograph of an alveolar epithelial cell of type II of dog. Note the large nucleus, the microvilli and the osmiophilic lamellar bodies thought to release surfactant. Alv, alveolus; C, capillary; LB, lamellar bodies; N, nucleus. (Reproduced from reference 37 by permission of Professor ER Weibel and the Editors of *Physiological Reviews*.)

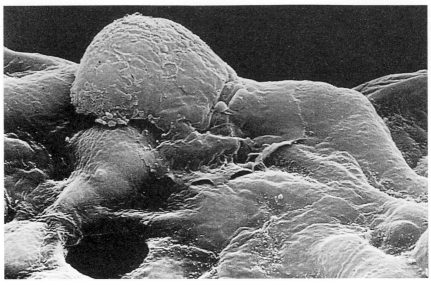

Figure 2.11 Scanning electron micrograph of an alveolar macrophage advancing to the right over epithelial type I cells. The scale bar is 3 μm. (Reproduced from reference 23 by permission of the author and the publishers; © Harvard University Press.)

between alveolar epithelial cells to lie on their surface in the alveolar lining fluid (Figure 2.11). They can re-enter the body but are remarkable for their ability to live and function outside the body. The macrophages are active in combating infection and scavenging foreign bodies such as small dust particles. They contain a variety of destructive enzymes but are also capable of generating oxygen-derived free radicals (Chapter 25). These are highly effective bactericidal agents but the processes used may also rebound to damage the host. Dead macrophages release the enzyme trypsin, which may cause tissue damage in patients who are deficient in the protein α_1-antitrypsin.

Neutrophils. These cells are not normally present in the alveoli but may appear in response to a neutrophil chemotactic factor released from the alveolar macrophages. They are usually present in the alveoli of smokers (Chapter 20).

The pulmonary vasculature

Pulmonary arteries

Although the pulmonary circulation carries roughly the same flow as the systemic circulation, the arterial pressure and the vascular resistance are normally only one-sixth as great. The media of the pulmonary arteries is about half as thick as in systemic arteries of corresponding size. In the larger vessels it consists mainly of elastic tissue but in the smaller vessels it is mainly muscular, the transition being in vessels of about 1 mm diameter. Pulmonary arteries lie close to the corresponding air passages in connective tissue sheaths. Table 2.2 shows a scheme for consideration of the branching of the pulmonary arterial tree.[38] This may be compared with Weibel's scheme for the airways (Table 2.1).

Table 2.2 Dimensions of the branches of the human pulmonary artery

Orders	Numbers	Mean diameter (mm)	Cumulative volume (ml)
17	1	30	64
16	3	15	81
15	8	8.1	85
14	20	5.8	96
13	66	3.7	108
12	203	2.1	116
11	675	1.3	122
10	2 300	0.85	128
9	5 900	0.53	132
8	18 000	0.35	136
7	53 000	0.22	138
6	160 000	0.14	141
5	470 000	0.086	142
4	1 400 000	0.054	144
3	4 200 000	0.034	145
2	13 000 000	0.021	146
1	300 000 000	0.013	151

In contrast to the airways (Table 2.1), the branching is asymmetrical and not dichotomous. Singhal et al.[38] therefore grouped the vessels according to orders and not generation as in Table 2.1.

Pulmonary arterioles

The transition to arterioles occurs at an internal diameter of 100 μm. These vessels differ radically from their counterparts in the systemic circulation, being virtually devoid of muscular tissue. There is a thin media of elastic tissue separated from the blood by endothelium. Structurally there is no real difference between pulmonary arterioles and venules.

Pulmonary capillaries

Pulmonary capillaries tend to arise abruptly from much larger vessels, the pulmonary metarterioles.[39] The capillaries form a dense network over the walls of one or more alveoli, and the spaces between the capillaries are similar in size to the capillaries themselves (Figure 2.7). In the resting state, about 75 per cent of the capillary bed is filled but the percentage is higher in the dependent parts of the lungs. Inflation of the alveoli reduces the cross-sectional area of the capillary bed and increases resistance to blood flow (Chapter 7). One capillary network is not confined to one alveolus but passes from one alveolus to another and blood traverses a number of alveolar septa before reaching a venule. This clearly has a bearing on the efficiency of gas exchange. From the functional standpoint it is often more convenient to consider the pulmonary microcirculation rather than just the capillaries. The microcirculation is defined as the vessels that are devoid of a muscular layer and it commences with arterioles of diameter 75 μm and continues through the capillary bed as far as venules of diameter 200 μm. Special roles of the microcirculation are considered in Chapters 13 and 28.

Pulmonary venules and veins

Pulmonary capillary blood is collected into venules that are structurally almost identical to the arterioles. In fact, Duke[40] obtained satisfactory gas exchange when an isolated cat lung was perfused in reverse. The pulmonary veins do not run alongside the pulmonary arteries but lie some distance away, close to the septa that separate the segments of the lung.

Bronchial circulation[41]

Down to the terminal bronchioles, the air passages and the accompanying blood vessels receive their nutrition from the bronchial vessels that arise from the systemic circulation. The bronchial circulation therefore provides the heat required for warming and humidifying inspired air, and cooling of the respiratory epithelium causes vasodilation and an increase in the flow of bronchial artery blood.[18] Part of the bronchial circulation returns to the systemic venous system but part mingles with the pulmonary venous drainage, thereby constituting a physiological shunt (pages 138 and 182).

Pulmonary lymphatics[42]

There are no lymphatics visible in the interalveolar septa, but small lymph vessels commence at the junction between alveolar and extra-alveolar spaces. There is a well-developed lymphatic system around the bronchi and pulmonary vessels, capable of containing up to 500 ml of lymph, and draining towards the hilum. Down to airway generation 11 the lymphatics lie in a potential space around the air passages and vessels, separating them from the lung parenchyma. This space becomes distended with lymph in pulmonary oedema and accounts for the characteristic butterfly shadow of the chest radiograph. In the hilum of the lung, the lymphatic drainage passes through several groups of tracheobronchial lymph glands, where they receive tributaries from the superficial subpleural plexus. Most of the lymph from the left lung usually enters the thoracic duct whilst the right side drains into the right lymphatic duct. However, the pulmonary lymphatics often cross the midline and pass independently into the junction of the internal jugular and subclavian veins on the corresponding sides of the body. Studies in dogs have indicated that about 15 per cent of the flow in the thoracic duct derives from the lungs.[43] Pulmonary lymphatics are intimately concerned in the pathogenesis of pulmonary oedema (Chapter 28).

References

1. Rodenstein DO, Stanescu DC. The soft palate and breathing. *Am Rev Respir Dis* 1986; **134**: 311–25.
2. Hairston LE, Sauerland EK. Electromyography of the human palate: discharge patterns of the levator and tensor veli palatini. *Electromyogr Clin Neurophysiol* 1981; **21**: 287–97.
3. Fink BR, Demarest RJ. *Laryngeal mechanics*. Cambridge MA: Harvard University Press, 1978.
4. Hoffstein V, Fredberg JJ. The acoustic reflection technique for non-invasive assessment of upper airway area. *Eur Respir J* 1991; **4**: 602–11.
5. Marshall I, Maran NJ, Martin S, Jan MA, Rimmington JE, Best JJK, Drummond GB, Douglas NJ. Acoustic reflectometry for airway measurements in man: implementation and validation. *Physiol Meas* 1993; **14**: 157–69.

6. Bartlett D. Respiratory functions of the larynx. *Physiol Rev* 1989; **69**: 33–57.
7. Bannister LH. Anatomy of Speech. In: Williams PL, ed. *Gray's anatomy*. London: Churchill Livingstone, 1995; 1651–2.
8. Phillips CG, Kaye SR, Schroter RC. A diameter-based reconstruction of the branching pattern of the human bronchial tree. Part I. Description and application. *Respir Physiol* 1994; **98**: 193–217.
9. Weibel ER. *Morphometry of the human lung*. Berlin: Springer, 1963.
10. Weibel ER. Design of airways and blood vessels considered as branching trees. In: Crystal RG, West JB, eds. *The lung: scientific foundations*. New York: Raven, 1991; 711–20.
11. Haefeli-Bleuer B, Weibel ER. Morphometry of the human pulmonary acinus. *Anat Rec* 1988; **220**: 401–14.
12. Macklem PT, Mead J. Resistance of central and peripheral airways measured by a retrograde catheter. *J Appl Physiol* 1967; **22**: 395–401.
13. Weibel ER. Design and morphometry of the pulmonary gas exchanger. In: Crystal RG, West JB, eds. *The lung: scientific foundations*. New York: Raven, 1991; 795–805.
14. Jeffery PK. Microscopic structure of normal lung. In: Brewis RAL, Corrin B, Geddes DM, Gibson GJ, eds. *Respiratory medicine*. London: WB Saunders, 1995; 54–72.
15. Rogers DF. Airway goblet cells: responsive and adaptable frontline defenders. *Eur Respir Journal* 1994; **7**: 1690–1706.
16. Widdicombe JH, Widdicombe JG. Regulation of human airway surface liquid. *Respir Physiol* 1995; **99**: 3–12.
17. Plopper CG, Hyde DM, Buckpitt AR. Clara cells. In: Crystal RG, West JB, eds. *The lung: scientific foundations*. New York: Raven, 1991; 215.
18. McFadden ER Jr. Heat and water exchange in the human airways. *Am Rev Respir Dis* 1992; **146**: S8–10.
19. Dahl AR, Gerde P. Uptake and metabolism of toxicants in the respiratory tract. *Environ Health Perspect* 1994; **102** (Supp 11): 67–70.
20. Angus GE, Thurlbeck WM. Number of alveoli in the human lung. *J Appl Physiol* 1972; **32**: 483–5.
21. Hales S. *Vegetable staticks: analysis of the air*. London, 1731; 240.
22. Topol M. Collateral respiratory pathways of pulmonary acini in man. *Folia Morphologica* 1995; **54**: 61–6.
23. Weibel ER. *The pathway for oxygen*. Cambridge MA: Harvard University Press, 1984.
24. Gil J, Bachofen H, Gehr P, Weibel ER. Alveolar volume–surface area relation in air and saline filled lungs fixed by vascular perfusion. *J Appl Physiol* 1979; **47**: 990–5.
25. Weibel ER, Bachofen H. The fiber scaffold of lung parynchyma. In: Crystal RG, West JB, eds. *The lung: scientific foundations*. New York: Raven, 1991; 787–94.
26. Crouch EC, Martin GR, Brody JS. Basement membranes. In: Crystal RG, West JB, eds. *The lung: scientific foundations*. New York: Raven, 1991; 421
27. Tsukimoto K, Mathieu-Costello O, Prediletto R, Elliott AR, West JB. Ultrastructural appearances of pulmonary capillaries at high transmural pressures. *J Appl Physiol* 1991; **71**: 573–82.
28. Simionescu M. Lung endothelium: structure–function correlates. In: Crystal RG, West JB, eds. *The lung: scientific foundations*. New York: Raven, 1991; 301.
29. Weibel ER. How does lung structure affect gas exchange. *Chest* 1983; **83**: 657–65.
30. Ryan US. Structural basis for metabolic activity. *Am Rev Physiol* 1982; **44**: 223–39.
31. DeFouw DO. Ultrastructural features of alveolar epithelial transport. *Am Rev Respir Dis* 1983; **127**: S9–11.
32. Rippe B, Crone C. Pores and intercellular junctions. In: Crystal RG, West JB, eds. *The lung: scientific foundations*. New York: Raven, 1991; 349.
33. Hills BA. What forces keep the airspace of the lung dry. *Thorax* 1982; **37**: 713–17.
34. Schneeberger EE. Alveolar type I cells. In: Crystal RG, West JB, eds. *The lung: scientific foundations*. New York: Raven, 1991; 229.
35. Uhal BD. Cell cycle kinetics in the alveolar epithelium. *Am J Physiol* 1997; **272**: L1031–45.
36. Mason RJ, Williams MC. Alveolar type II cells. In: Crystal RG, West JB, eds. *The lung: scientific foundations*. New York: Raven, 1991; 235
37. Weibel ER. Morphological basis of alveolar–capillary gas exchange. *Physiol Rev* 1973; **53**: 419.
38. Singhal S, Henderson R, Horsfield K, Harding K, Cumming G. Morphometry of the human pulmonary arterial tree. *Circ Res* 1973; **33**: 190–7.

39. Staub NC. The interdependence of pulmonary structure and function. *Anesthesiology* 1963; **24**: 831–54.
40. Duke HN. The site of action of anoxia on the pulmonary blood vessels of the cat. *J Physiol* 1954; **125**: 373.
41. Widdicombe J. Anatomy and physiology of the airway circulation. *Am Rev Respir Dis* 1992: **146**: S3–7.
42. Staub NC. Pulmonary oedema. *Physiol Rev* 1974; **54**: 678–811.
43. Meyer EC, Ottaviano R. Pulmonary collateral lymph flow: detection using lymph oxygen tensions. *J Appl Physiol* 1972; **32**: 806–11.

Chapter 3

Elastic forces and lung volumes

An isolated lung will tend to contract until eventually all the contained air is expelled. In contrast, when the thoracic cage is opened it tends to expand to a volume about 1 litre greater than functional residual capacity (FRC). Thus in a relaxed subject with an open airway and no air flowing, for example at the end of expiration or inspiration, the inward elastic recoil of the lungs is exactly balanced by the outward recoil of the thoracic cage.

The movements of the lungs are entirely passive and result from forces external to the lungs. In the case of spontaneous breathing the external forces are the respiratory muscles, whilst artificial ventilation is usually in response to a pressure gradient that is developed between the airway and the environment. In each case, the pattern of response by the lung is governed by the physical impedance of the respiratory system. This impedance, or hindrance, has numerous origins, the most important of which are:

1. Elastic resistance of lung tissue and chest wall
2. Resistance from surface forces at the alveolar gas/liquid interface
3. Frictional resistance to gas flow through the airways
4. Frictional resistance from deformation of thoracic tissues (viscoelastic tissue resistance)
5. Inertia associated with movement of gas and tissue.

The last three may be grouped together as non-elastic resistance or respiratory system resistance; they are discussed in Chapter 4. They are measured while gas is flowing in the airways, and work performed in overcoming this 'frictional' resistance is dissipated as heat and lost.

The first two forms of impedance may be grouped together as 'elastic' resistance. These are measured when gas is not flowing within the lung. Work performed in overcoming elastic resistance is stored as potential energy, and elastic deformation during inspiration is the usual source of energy for expiration during both spontaneous and artificial breathing.

This chapter is concerned with the elastic resistance afforded by lungs (including the alveoli) and chest wall – which are considered separately and then together. When the respiratory muscles are totally relaxed, these factors govern the resting end-expiratory lung volume or FRC, and therefore lung volumes are also considered in this chapter.

Elastic recoil of the lungs

Lung compliance is defined as the change in lung volume per unit change in transmural pressure gradient (i.e. between the alveolus and pleural space). Compliance is usually expressed in litres (or millilitres) per kilopascal (or centimetre of water) with a normal value of $1.5 \, l.kPa^{-1}$ ($150 \, ml.cmH_2O^{-1}$). Stiff lungs have a low compliance.

Compliance may be described as static or dynamic, depending on the method of measurement (page 54). Static compliance is measured after a lung has been held at a fixed volume for as long as is practicable, whereas dynamic compliance is usually measured in the course of normal rhythmic breathing. Elastance is the reciprocal of compliance and is expressed in kilopascals per litre. Stiff lungs have a high elastance.

The nature of the forces causing recoil of the lung

For many years it was thought that the recoil of the lung was due entirely to stretching of the yellow elastin fibres present in the lung parenchyma. However, as is so often the case, the workings of the body are far more complex than first impressions suggest. In 1929, von Neergaard[1] showed that a lung completely filled with and immersed in water had an elastance that was much less than the normal value obtained when the lung was filled with air. He correctly concluded that much of the 'elastic recoil' was due to surface tension acting throughout the vast air/water interface lining the alveoli.

Surface tension at an air/water interface produces forces that tend to reduce the area of the interface. Thus the gas pressure in a bubble is always higher than the surrounding gas pressure because the surface of the bubble is in a state of tension. Alveoli resemble bubbles in this respect, although the alveolar gas is connected to the exterior by the air passages. The pressure inside a bubble is higher than the surrounding pressure by an amount depending on the surface tension of the liquid and the radius of curvature of the bubble according to the Laplace equation:

$$P = \frac{2T}{R}$$

where P is the pressure in the bubble ($dyn.cm^{-2}$), T is the surface tension of the liquid ($dyn.cm^{-1}$) and R is the radius of the bubble (cm). In coherent SI units (see Appendix A), the appropriate units would be pressure in pascals (Pa), surface tension in newtons/metre ($N.m^{-1}$) and radius in metres (m).

On the left of Figure 3.1a is shown a typical alveolus of radius 0.1 mm. Assuming that the alveolar lining fluid has a normal surface tension of $20 \, mN.m^{-1}$ ($= 20 \, dyn.cm^{-1}$), the pressure in the alveolus will be 0.4 kPa ($4 \, cmH_2O$), which is rather less than the normal transmural pressure at FRC. If the alveolar lining fluid had the same surface tension as water ($72 \, mN.m^{-1}$), the lungs would be very stiff.

The alveolus on the right of Figure 3.1a has a radius of only 0.05 mm, and the Laplace equation indicates that, if the surface tension of the alveolus is the same, its pressure should be double the pressure in the left-hand alveolus. Thus gas would tend to flow from smaller alveoli into larger alveoli and that lung would be unstable – which, of course, is not the case. Similarly, the retractive forces of the alveolar lining fluid would increase at low lung volumes and decrease at high lung volumes, which is exactly the reverse of what is observed. These paradoxes were clear to von Neergaard in 1929[1] and he concluded that the surface tension of the alveolar lining fluid must be considerably less than would be expected from the properties of simple liquids and, furthermore, that its value must be

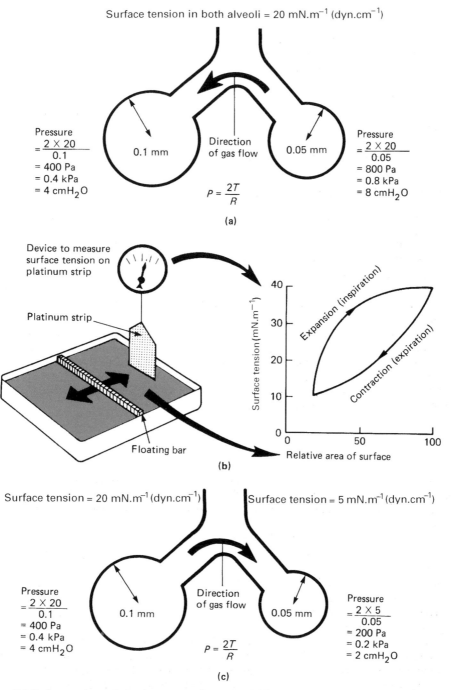

Figure 3.1 Surface tension and alveolar transmural pressure. (a) Pressure relations in two alveoli of different size but with the same surface tension of their lining fluids. (b) The changes in surface tension in relation to the area of the alveolar lining film. (c) Pressure relations of two alveoli of different size when allowance is made for the probable changes in surface tension.

variable. Observations 30 years later confirmed this when alveolar extracts were shown to have a surface tension much lower than water and which varied in proportion to the area of the interface.[2] Figure 3.1b shows an experiment in which a floating bar is moved in a trough containing an alveolar extract. As the bar is moved to the right, the surface film is concentrated and the surface tension changes, as shown in the graph on the right of the figure. During expansion, the surface tension increases to $40 \, mN.m^{-1}$, a value close to that of plasma, but, during contraction, the surface tension falls to $19 \, mN.m^{-1}$, a lower value than any other body fluid. The course of the relationship between pressure and area is different during expansion and contraction, and a loop is described.

The consequences of these changes are very important. In contrast to a bubble of soap solution, the pressure in an alveolus tends to decrease as the radius of curvature is decreased. This is illustrated in Figure 3.1c, where the right-hand alveolus has a smaller diameter and a much lower surface tension than the left-hand alveolus. Gas tends to flow from the larger to the smaller alveolus and stability is maintained.

The alveolar surfactant[3]

The low surface tension of the alveolar lining fluid and its dependence on alveolar radius are due to the presence of a surface-active material. Generally known as the surfactant, it consists mainly of phospholipids, which have the general structure shown in Figure 3.2. The fatty acids are hydrophobic and generally straight, lying parallel to each other and projecting into the gas phase. The other end of the molecule is hydrophilic and lies in the alveolar lining fluid. The molecule is thus confined to the surface where, being detergents, they lower surface tension in proportion to the concentration at the interface. During expiration, as the surface area of the alveolus diminishes, the surfactant molecules are packed more densely and so exert a greater effect on the surface tension, which then decreases as shown in Figure 3.1b.

Composition of surfactant. Some 90 per cent of surfactant consists of lipids, the remainder being proteins and small amounts of carbohydrate.[4] Most of the lipid is phospholipid, of which some 70–80 per cent is dipalmitoyl phosphatidyl choline, the main constituent responsible for the effect on surface tension. The remaining phospholipid is mainly phosphatidyl glycerol, which is not found in such concentrations elsewhere in the body, and traces of phosphatidyl inositol, phosphatidyl ethanolamine and phosphatidyl serine. The role of the other lipids is less certain. The fatty acid chains are mainly saturated and therefore straight. Harlan and Said[5] have advanced the attractive theory that straight fatty acids will pack together in a more satisfactory manner during expiration than would unsaturated fatty acids such as oleic acid which are bent at the double bond.

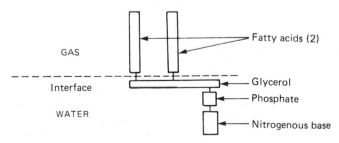

Figure 3.2 General structure of phospholipids.

37

Some 10 per cent of surfactant obtained from bronchoalveolar lavage is protein, most of which are contaminating serum proteins such as albumin and globulin. About 2 per cent of surfactant by weight consists of surfactant proteins (SP), of which there are four types labelled A–D. SP-B and SP-C are small proteins that are vital to the stabilization of the surfactant monolayer, a congenital lack of SP-B resulting in severe and progressive respiratory failure.[6] SP-A and, to a lesser extent, SP-D are involved in the control of surfactant release and possibly in preventing pulmonary infection (see below).[7]

Synthesis of surfactant. Surfactant is both formed in and liberated from the alveolar epithelial type II cell (page 31). The lamellar bodies (see Figure 2.10) contain stored surfactant that is released into the alveolus in response to high volume lung inflation, increased ventilation rate or endocrine stimulation (including adrenaline, thyroid hormones or oestrogens). The alveolar half-life of surfactant is 15–30 hours, most of its components being recycled by type II alveolar cells. Surfactant protein-A is intimately involved in controlling surfactant production. Type II alveolar cells have SP-A surface receptors in which alveolar SP-A exerts a negative feedback on surfactant secretion and increases uptake of surfactant precursors into the cell. Once the surfactant is released into the alveolus, SP-A is again required to establish the functional surfactant layer.

The ability to produce surfactant occurs relatively late in the process of maturation of the fetus. Surfactant levels increase only in the late stages of gestation and are low in babies with the infant respiratory distress syndrome (Chapter 13).

Other effects of surfactant. Pulmonary transudation is also affected by surface forces. Surface tension causes the pressure in the alveolar lining fluid to be less than the alveolar pressure. Because the pulmonary capillary pressure in most of the lung is greater than the alveolar pressure, both factors encourage transudation, a tendency that is checked by the oncotic pressure of the plasma proteins. Thus the surfactant, by reducing surface tension, diminishes one component of the pressure gradient and helps to prevent transudation. A deficiency of surfactant might therefore tip the balance in favour of the development of pulmonary oedema.

There has been a suggestion that the alveolar lining is, in fact, largely dry, the surfactant acting as an anti-wetting agent.[8] This would have implications that run counter to much that has been written above.

Surfactant may also play an important part in the immunology of the lung.[3] The lipid component of surfactant has antioxidant activity, so may attenuate lung damage from a variety of causes, and also suppresses some groups of lymphocytes, so theoretically protecting the lungs from autoimmune damage. Both SP-A and SP-D activate alveolar macrophages, and studies *in vitro* have shown SP-A to bind influenza A virus and increase macrophage recognition of *Mycobacterium tuberculosis*, two very common pulmonary pathogens. However, the contribution of surfactant to pulmonary defences *in vivo* remains unclear.[7]

The transmural pressure gradient and intrathoracic pressure

The transmural pressure gradient is the difference between intrathoracic (or 'intrapleural') and alveolar pressure. The pressure in an alveolus is always greater than the pressure to the surrounding interstitial tissue except when the volume has been reduced to zero. With increasing lung volume, the transmural pressure gradient steadily increases, as shown for the whole lung in Figure 3.3. If an appreciable pneumothorax is present, the pressure gradient from alveolus to pleural cavity provides a measure of the overall transmural pressure gradient. Otherwise, the oesophageal pressure may be used to indicate the pleural pressure, but there are conceptual and technical difficulties. The technical difficulties are considered at the end of this chapter, whilst some of the conceptual difficulties are indicated in Figure 3.4.

The alveoli in the upper part of the lung have a larger volume than those in the dependent parts except at total lung capacity. The greater degree of expansion of the alveoli in the upper parts results in a greater transmural pressure gradient, which decreases steadily down the lung at about 0.1 kPa (or 1 cmH$_2$O) per 3 cm of vertical height; such a difference is indicated in Figure 3.4a. Because the pleural cavity is normally empty, it is not strictly correct to speak of an intrapleural pressure; furthermore, it would not be constant throughout the pleural 'cavity'. One should think rather of the relationship shown in Figure 3.3 as applying to various horizontal strata of the lung, each with its own volume and therefore its own transmural pressure gradient on which its own 'intrapleural' pressure would depend. The transmural pressure gradient has an important influence on many aspects of pulmonary function and so its horizontal stratification confers a regional difference on many features of pulmonary function, including airway closure, ventilation/perfusion ratios and therefore gas exchange. These matters are considered in detail in the appropriate chapters of this book.

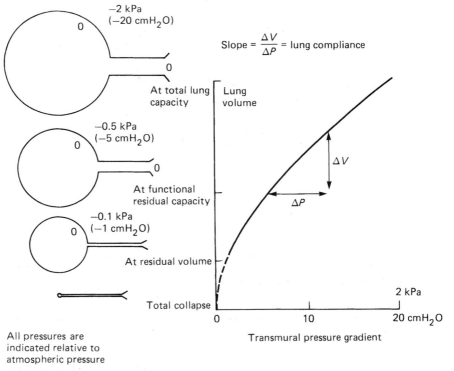

Figure 3.3 Relationship between lung volume and the difference in pressure between the alveoli and the intrathoracic space (transmural pressure gradient). The relationship is almost linear over the normal tidal volume range. The calibre of small air passages decreases in parallel with alveolar volume. Airways begin to close at the closing capacity and there is widespread airway closure at residual volume. Values in the diagram relate to the upright position and to *decreasing* pressure. The opening pressure of a closed alveolus is not shown.

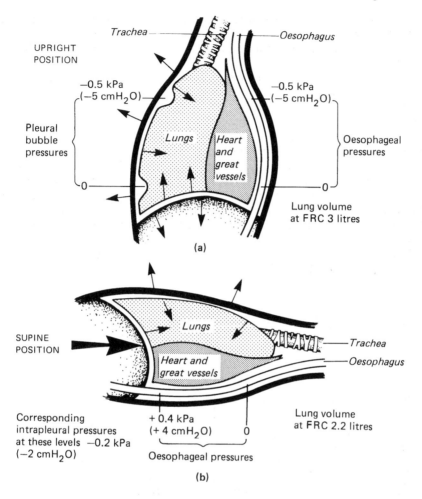

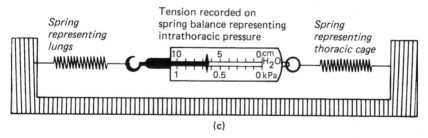

Figure 3.4 Intrathoracic pressures: static relationships in the resting end-expiratory position. The lung volume corresponds to the functional residual capacity (FRC). The figures in (a) and (b) indicate the pressure relative to ambient (atmospheric). The arrows show the direction of elastic forces. The heavy arrow in (b) indicates displacement by the abdominal viscera. In (c) the tension in the two springs is the same and will be indicated on the spring balance. In the supine position: (1) the FRC is reduced; (2) the intrathoracic pressure is raised; (3) the weight of the heart raises the oesophageal pressure above the intrapleural pressure.

At first sight it might be thought that the subatmospheric intrapleural pressure would result in the accumulation of gas evolved from solution in blood and tissues. In fact, the total of the partial pressures of gases dissolved in blood, and therefore tissues, is always less than 1 atmosphere, and this factor keeps the pleural cavity free of gas.

Time dependence of pulmonary elastic behaviour

If an excised lung is rapidly inflated and then held at the new volume, the inflation pressure falls exponentially from its initial value to reach a lower level that is attained after a few seconds. This also occurs in the intact subject. Following inflation to a sustained lung volume, the pulmonary transmural pressure falls from its initial value to a new value some 20–30 per cent less than the original pressure, over the course of about a minute.[9] It is broadly true to say that the volume change divided by the initial change in transmural pressure gradient corresponds to the dynamic compliance whilst the volume change divided by the ultimate change in transmural pressure gradient (i.e. measured after it has become steady) corresponds to the static compliance. Static compliance will thus be greater than the dynamic compliance by an amount determined by the degree of time dependence in the elastic behaviour of a particular lung. The respiratory frequency influences dynamic pulmonary compliance in the normal subject but frequency dependence is much more pronounced in the presence of pulmonary disease.

Hysteresis. If the lungs are slowly inflated and then slowly deflated, the pressure/volume curve for static points during inflation differs from that obtained during deflation. The two curves form a loop that becomes progressively broader as the tidal volume is increased (Figure 3.5). Expressed in words, the loop in Figure 3.5 means that rather more than the expected pressure is required during inflation and rather less than the expected recoil pressure is available during deflation. This resembles the behaviour of perished rubber or polyvinyl chloride, both of which are reluctant to accept deformation under stress but, once deformed, are again reluctant to assume their original shape. This phenomenon is present to a greater or less extent in all elastic bodies and is known as elastic hysteresis.

Causes of time dependence of pulmonary elastic behaviour

There are many possible explanations of the time dependence of pulmonary elastic behaviour, the relative importance of which may vary in different circumstances.

Changes in surfactant activity. It has been explained above that the surface tension of the alveolar lining fluid is greater at larger lung volume and also during inspiration than at the same lung volume during expiration (Figure 3.1b). This is probably the most important cause of the observed hysteresis in the intact lung (Figure 3.5).

Stress relaxation. If a spring is pulled out to a fixed increase in its length, the resultant tension is maximal at first and then declines exponentially to a constant value. This is an inherent property of elastic bodies, known as stress relaxation. Thoracic tissues display stress relaxation and these 'viscoelastic' properties contribute significantly to the difference between static and dynamic compliance[10] as well as forming a component of pulmonary resistance (page 64). The crinkled structure of collagen in the lung is likely to

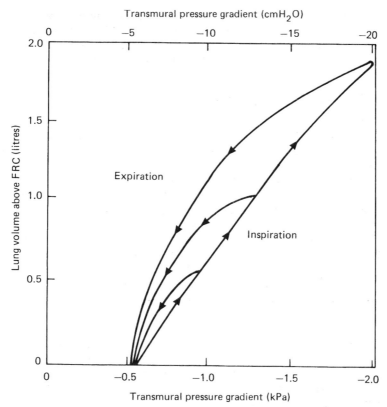

Figure 3.5 Static plot of lung volume against transmural pressure gradient (intra-oesophageal pressure relative to atmospheric at zero air flow). Note that inspiratory and expiratory curves form a loop which gets wider the greater the tidal volume. These loops are typical of elastic hysteresis. For a particular lung volume, the elastic recoil of the lung during expiration is always less than the distending transmural pressure gradient required during inspiration at the same lung volume.

favour stress relaxation, and excised strips of human lung show stress relaxation when stretched.[11] The time course is of the same order as the observed changes in pressure when lungs are held inflated at constant volume, and in 1961 Marshall and Widdicombe[9] concluded that the effect was due to stress relaxation.

Redistribution of gas. In a lung consisting of functional units with identical time constants[†] of inflation, the distribution of gas should be independent of the rate of inflation, and there should be no redistribution when the lungs are held inflated. However, if different parts of the lungs have different time constants, the distribution of inspired gas will depend on the rate of inflation and redistribution ('pendelluft') will occur when inflation is held. This problem is discussed in greater detail on page 165 but for the time being we can distinguish 'fast' and 'slow' alveoli (the term 'alveoli' here referring to functional units rather than the anatomical entity). The 'fast' alveolus has a

[†] Time constants are used to describe the exponential filling and emptying of a lung unit. One time constant is the time taken to achieve 63 per cent of maximal inflation or deflation of the lung unit. See Appendix F for details.

low airway resistance or low compliance (or both) while the 'slow' alveolus has a high airway resistance and/or a high compliance (Figure 3.6b). These properties give the fast alveolus a shorter time constant and are preferentially filled during a short inflation. This preferential filling of alveoli with low compliance gives an overall higher pulmonary transmural pressure gradient. A slow or sustained inflation permits increased distribution of gas to slow alveoli and so tends to distribute gas in accord with the compliance of the different functional units. There should then be a lower overall transmural pressure and no redistribution of gas when inflation is held. The extreme difference between fast and slow alveoli shown in Figure 3.6b applies to diseased lungs and no such differences exist in normal lungs. Gas redistribution is therefore unlikely to be a major factor in healthy subjects, but it can be important in patients with increased airway obstruction, particularly in emphysema, asthma and chronic obstructive pulmonary disease.

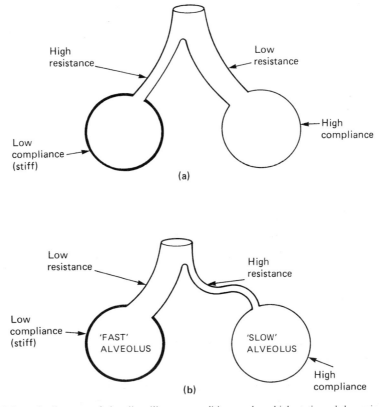

Figure 3.6 Schematic diagrams of alveoli to illustrate conditions under which static and dynamic compliance may differ. (a) represents a theoretically ideal state in which there is a reciprocal relationship between resistance and compliance resulting in gas flow being preferentially delivered to the most compliant regions, regardless of the state of inflation. Static and dynamic compliance are equal. This situation is probably never realized even in the normal subject; (b) illustrates a state that is typical of many patients with respiratory disease. The alveoli can conveniently be divided into 'fast' and 'slow' groups. The direct relationship between compliance and resistance results in inspired gas being preferentially delivered to the stiff alveoli if the rate of inflation is rapid. An end-inspiratory pause then permits redistribution from the fast alveoli to the slow alveoli.

Recruitment of alveoli. Below a certain lung volume, some alveoli tend to close and to reopen only at a considerably greater lung volume, in response to a much higher transmural pressure gradient than that at which they closed. Reopening of collapsed functional units (probably pulmonary acini) may be seen during re-expansion of the lung at thoracotomy. Recruitment of closed alveoli seems at first sight to be a plausible explanation of all the time-dependent phenomena described above, but there are two reasons why this is unlikely. First, the pressure required for reopening a closed unit is very high and is unlikely to be achieved during normal breathing. Secondly, there is no histological evidence for collapsed alveoli in normal lungs at FRC. In the presence of pathological lung collapse, a sustained deep inflation may well cause re-expansion and an increased compliance. This is likely to occur during 'bagging' of patients on prolonged artificial ventilation, but opening and closing of alveoli during a normal respiratory cycle is unlikely in normal lungs although it does occur in injured lungs (page 616).

Displacement of pulmonary blood. A sustained inflation might be expected to displace blood from the lungs and so to increase compliance by reducing the splinting effect of the pulmonary vasculature. The importance of this factor is not known, but experiments with excised lung indicate that all the major time-dependent phenomena are present when the pulmonary vasculature is empty.

Factors affecting lung compliance

Lung volume. It is important to remember that compliance is related to lung volume. This factor may be excluded by relating compliance to FRC to yield the specific compliance (i.e. compliance/FRC), which in humans is almost constant for both sexes and all ages down to neonatal. The relationship between compliance and lung volume is true not only in an individual lung but also between species. Larger animal species have thicker alveolar septae containing increased amounts of collagen and elastin resulting in larger alveolar diameters,[12] so reducing the pressure needed to expand them. An elephant therefore has larger alveoli and so a higher compliance than a mouse.

Posture. Lung volume, and therefore compliance, changes with posture (page 52). There are, however, problems in the measurement of intrapleural pressure in the supine position, and when this is taken into account it seems unlikely that changes of posture have any significant effect on the *specific* compliance.

Pulmonary blood volume. The pulmonary blood vessels probably make an appreciable contribution to the stiffness of the lung. Pulmonary venous congestion from whatever cause is associated with reduced compliance.

Age. One would have expected age to influence the elasticity of the lung as of other tissues in the body. However, no correlation has ever been found between age and compliance, even after allowing for predicted changes in lung volume. This accords with the concept of lung 'elasticity' being largely determined by surface forces.

Restriction of chest expansion. Elastic strapping of the chest reduces both lung volume and compliance. However, when lung volume is returned to normal, either by removal of the restriction or by a more forceful inspiration, the compliance remains reduced. Normal compliance can be restored by taking a single deep breath.[13]

Recent ventilatory history. A period of hypoventilation without periodic deep breaths may lead to a reduction of compliance, particularly in pathological states. Compliance may usually be restored by one or more large breaths corresponding to sighs. This was first observed during artificial ventilation of patients with respiratory paralysis,[14] and these observations led to the introduction of artificial ventilators that periodically administer 'sighs'. There can be no doubt of the importance of periodic expansion of the lungs during prolonged artificial ventilation of diseased lungs, but the case for 'sighs' while ventilating normal lungs (e.g. during anaesthesia) is less convincing.

Bronchial smooth muscle tone. Animal studies[15] have shown that an infusion of methacholine sufficient to result in a doubling of airway resistance decreases *dynamic* compliance by 50 per cent. The airways might contribute to overall compliance or, alternatively, bronchoconstriction could enhance time dependence and so reduce dynamic, but perhaps not static, compliance (Figure 3.6).

Disease. Important changes in lung pressure/volume relationships are found in some lung diseases. Emphysema is unique in that *static* pulmonary compliance is increased, as a result of destruction of pulmonary tissue and loss of both elastin and surface retraction. Although FRC is increased, distribution of inspired gas may be grossly disordered and therefore the *dynamic* compliance is commonly reduced. In asthma the pressure/volume curve is displaced upwards, increasing the FRC, without a change in compliance (Figure 3.7).[16]

Most other types of pulmonary pathology result in decreased lung compliance, both static and dynamic. In particular, all forms of pulmonary fibrosis (e.g. fibrosing alveolitis), consolidation, collapse, vascular engorgement, fibrous pleurisy and especially acute lung injury will reduce compliance and FRC.

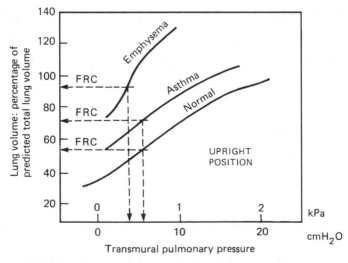

Figure 3.7 Pulmonary transmural pressure/volume plots for normal subjects, patients with asthma in bronchospasm and patients with emphysema. The broken horizontal lines indicate the FRC in each of the three groups and the corresponding point on the abscissa indicates the resting intrathoracic pressure at FRC. (Redrawn from reference 16.)

Elastic recoil of the thoracic cage

The thoracic cage comprises the ribcage and the diaphragm. Each is a muscular structure and can be considered as an elastic structure only when the muscles are relaxed, and that is not easy to achieve except under the conditions of paralysis. Relaxation curves have been prepared relating pressure and volumes in the supposedly relaxed subject, but it is now doubted whether total relaxation was ever achieved. For example, it seems that the diaphragm is not fully relaxed at the end of expiration *in the supine position* but maintains a resting tone to prevent the abdominal contents pushing the diaphragm cephalad.[17]

Compliance of the thoracic cage is defined as change in lung volume per unit change in the pressure gradient between atmosphere and the intrapleural space. The units are the same as for pulmonary compliance. The measurement is seldom made but the value is of the order of $2\,l.kPa^{-1}$ ($200\,ml.cmH_2O^{-1}$).

Factors influencing compliance of the thoracic cage

Anatomical factors include the ribs and the state of ossification of the costal cartilages. Obesity and even pathological skin conditions may have an appreciable effect. In particular, scarring of the skin overlying the front of the chest may result from scalding in children and this may embarrass the breathing.

In terms of compliance, a relaxed diaphragm simply transmits pressure from the abdomen, which may be increased in obesity and abdominal distension. Posture clearly has a major effect and this is considered below in relation to FRC. Compared with the supine posture, thoracic cage compliance is 30 per cent greater in the seated subject, and the total static compliance of the respiratory system is reduced by 60 per cent in the prone position owing to the diminished elasticity of the ribcage and diaphragm in the prone position.

Pressure/volume relationships of the lung plus thoracic cage

Compliance is analogous to electrical capacitance, and in the respiratory system the compliances of lungs and thoracic cage are in series. Therefore the total compliance of the system obeys the same relationship as for capacitances in series, in which reciprocals are added to obtain the reciprocal of the total value, thus:

$$\frac{1}{\text{total compliance}} = \frac{1}{\text{lung compliance}} + \frac{1}{\text{thoracic cage compliance}}$$

typical static values ($l.kPa^{-1}$) for the supine paralysed patient being:

$$\frac{1}{0.85} = \frac{1}{1.5} + \frac{1}{2}$$

Instead of compliance, we may consider its reciprocal, elastance. The relationship is then much simpler:

$$\text{total elastance} = \text{lung elastance} + \text{thoracic cage elastance}$$

corresponding values ($kPa.l^{-1}$) are then:

$$1.17 = 0.67 + 0.5$$

Relationship between alveolar, intrathoracic and ambient pressures

At all times the alveolar/ambient pressure gradient is the sum of the alveolar/intrathoracic (or transmural) and intrathoracic/ambient pressure gradients. This relationship is independent of whether the patient is breathing spontaneously or being ventilated by intermittent positive pressure. Actual values depend on compliances, lung volume and posture; typical values are shown for the upright conscious relaxed subject in Figure 3.8. The values in the illustration are static and relate to conditions when no gas is flowing.

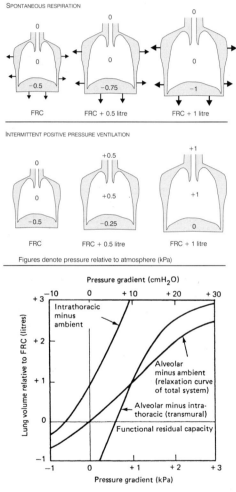

Figure 3.8 Static pressure/volume relations for the intact thorax for the conscious subject in the upright position. The transmural pressure gradient bears the same relationship to lung volume during both intermittent positive pressure ventilation and spontaneous breathing. The intrathoracic-to-ambient pressure difference, however, differs in the two types of ventilation due to muscle action during spontaneous respiration. At all times:

$$\frac{\text{alveolar/ambient}}{\text{pressure difference}} = \frac{\text{alveolar/intrathoracic}}{\text{pressure difference}} + \frac{\text{intrathoracic/ambient}}{\text{pressure difference}}$$

(due attention being paid to the sign of the pressure difference).

Lung volumes

Certain lung volumes, particularly the FRC, are determined by elastic forces. This is therefore a convenient point at which to consider the various lung volumes and their subdivision (Figure 3.9).

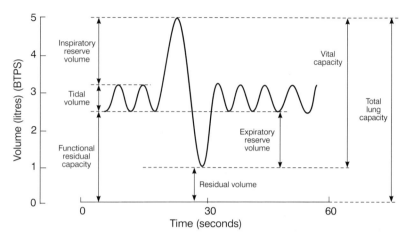

Figure 3.9 Static lung volumes of Dr JF Nunn in 1990. The 'spirometer curve' indicates the lung volumes that can be measured by simple spirometry. These are tidal volume, inspiratory reserve volume, expiratory reserve volume and vital capacity. The residual volume, total lung capacity and functional residual capacity cannot be measured by observation of a spirometer without further elaboration of methods.

Total lung capacity (TLC). This is the volume of gas in the lungs at the end of a maximal inspiration. TLC is achieved when the maximal force generated by the inspiratory muscles is balanced by the forces opposing expansion. It is rather surprising that *expiratory* muscles are also contracting strongly at the end of a maximal inspiration.

Residual volume (RV). This is the volume remaining after a maximal expiration. In the young, RV is governed by the balance between the maximal force generated by expiratory muscles and the elastic forces opposing reduction of lung volume. However, in older subjects closure of small airways may prevent further expiration.

Functional residual capacity. This is the lung volume at the end of a normal expiration. Within the framework of TLC, RV and FRC, other capacities and volumes shown in Figure 3.9 are self-explanatory.

Factors affecting the FRC

So many factors affect the FRC that they require a special section of this chapter. The actual volume of the FRC has particular importance because of its relationship to the closing capacity (page 53).

Body size. FRC is linearly related to height. Estimates range[18,19] from an increase in FRC of 32 ml.cm^{-1} to 51 ml.cm^{-1}. Obesity causes a marked reduction in FRC compared with lean subjects of the same height.

Gender. For the same body height, women have an FRC about 10 per cent less than that in men.[19]

Age. Two studies have shown a slight increase in FRC with age.[18,20] However, Bates and colleagues[19] regard FRC as independent of age in the adult, and pooled preoperative observations of FRC in the supine position derived from many studies (page 430) show no correlation with age.

Diaphragmatic muscle tone. FRC has in the past been considered to be simply the volume at which there is a balance between the elastic forces represented by the inward retraction of the lungs and the outward expansion of the thoracic cage. However, as explained above, it now seems that residual end-expiratory muscle tone is a major factor in the supine position, maintaining the FRC about 400 ml above the volume in the totally relaxed subject, which in practice means paralysed or anaesthetized.

Posture. Figures 3.4 and 3.10 show the reduction in FRC in the supine position, which may be attributed to the increased pressure of the abdominal contents on the diaphragm. Values of FRC in these Figures and Table 3.1 are typical for a subject of 168–170 cm in height, and reported mean differences between supine and upright positions range from 500 to 1000 ml. Teleologically, end-expiratory diaphragmatic tone can be seen as a protection against the weight of the abdominal contents causing an unacceptable reduction of lung volume in the supine position. Values for FRC in other positions are shown in Table 3.1.

Lung disease. The FRC will be reduced by increased elastic recoil of the lungs, chest wall or both. Possible causes include fibrosing alveolitis, organized fibrinous pleurisy, kyphoscoliosis, obesity and scarring of the thorax following burns. Conversely, elastic

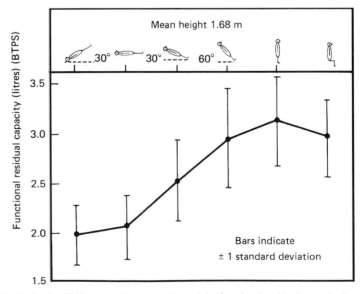

Figure 3.10 Studies by Dr JF Nunn and his co-workers of the functional residual capacity in various body positions.

Table 3.1 Effect of posture on some aspects of respiratory function[21]

Position	FRC (litres) (BTPS)	Ribcage breathing* (%)	Forced expiratory volume in 1 second (litres) (BTPS)
Sitting	2.91†	69.7†	3.79
Supine	2.10	32.3	3.70
Supine (arms up)	2.36†	33.0	3.27
Prone	2.45†	32.6	3.49
Lateral	2.44†	36.5	3.67

Data for 13 healthy males aged 24–64.
* Proportion of breathing accounted for by movement of the ribcage.
† Indicates significant difference relative to the supine position.

recoil of the lungs is diminished in emphysema and asthma and the FRC is usually increased (Figure 3.7). This is beneficial because airway resistance decreases as the lung volume increases.

FRC in relation to closing capacity

In Chapter 4 it is explained how reduction in lung volume below a certain level results in airway closure with relative or total underventilation in the dependent parts of the lung. The lung volume below which this effect becomes apparent is known as the closing capacity (CC). With increasing age, CC rises until it equals FRC at about 66 years in the upright position but only 44 in the supine position (Figure 3.11). This is a major factor in the decrease of arterial P_{O_2} with age (page 276).

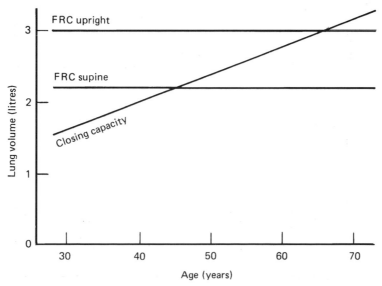

Figure 3.11 Functional residual capacity (FRC) and closing capacity as a function of age. (Redrawn from data in reference 22.)

Principles of measurement of compliance

Compliance is measured as the change in lung volume divided by the corresponding change in the appropriate pressure gradient, there being no gas flow when the two measurements are made. For lung compliance the appropriate pressure gradient is alveolar/intrapleural (or intrathoracic) and for the total compliance alveolar/ambient. Measurement of compliance of the thoracic cage is seldom undertaken but the appropriate pressure gradient would then be intrapleural/ambient. This would be meaningless for measurement of compliance if there were any tone in the respiratory muscles.

Volume may be measured with a spirometer, a body plethysmograph or by integration of a flow rate obtained from a pneumotachogram. Points of zero air flow are best indicated by a pneumotachogram. Static pressures can be measured with a simple water manometer but electrical transducers are now more usual. Intrathoracic pressure is normally measured as oesophageal pressure, which, in the upright subject, is different at different levels. The pressure rises as the balloon descends, the change being roughly in accord with the specific gravity of the lung $(0.3\,\mathrm{g.ml^{-1}})$. It is convention to measure the pressure 32–35 cm beyond the nares, the highest point at which the measurement is free from artefacts due to mouth pressure and tracheal and neck movements. In the supine position the weight of the heart may introduce an artefact (see Figure 3.4) but there is usually a zone some 32–40 cm beyond the nares where the oesophageal pressure is close to atmospheric and probably only about $0.2\,\mathrm{kPa}$ $(2\,\mathrm{cmH_2O})$ above the neighbouring intrathoracic pressure. Alveolar pressure equals mouth pressure when no gas is flowing: it cannot be measured directly.

Static compliance. In the conscious subject, a known volume of air is inhaled from FRC and the subject then relaxes against a closed airway. The various pressure gradients are then measured and compared with the resting values at FRC. It is, in fact, very difficult to ensure that the respiratory muscles are relaxed, but the measurement of lung compliance is valid because the static alveolar/intrathoracic pressure difference is unaffected by any muscle activity.

In the paralysed subject there are no difficulties about muscular relaxation and it is very easy to measure static compliance of the whole respiratory system simply using recordings of airway pressure and respiratory volumes. However, owing to the uncertainties about interpretation of the oesophageal pressure in the supine position (Figure 3.4), there is usually some uncertainty about the pulmonary compliance. For static compliance it is therefore easier to measure *lung* compliance in the upright position, and *total* compliance in the anaesthetized paralysed patient who will usually be in the supine position.

Dynamic compliance. These measurements are made during rhythmic breathing, but compliance is calculated from pressure and volume measurements made when no gas is flowing, usually at end-inspiratory and end-expiratory 'no-flow' points. The usual method involves creation of a pressure–volume loop by displaying simultaneously as X and Y coordinates the required pressure gradient and the respired volume. In the resultant loop, as in Figure 3.12, the 'no-flow' points are where the trace is horizontal and the dynamic compliance is the slope of the line joining these points.

Automated measurement of compliance

In a spontaneously breathing awake patient, lung compliance measurement is difficult because of the requirement to place an oesophageal balloon. However, in anaesthetized patients or in patients receiving intermittent positive pressure ventilation (IPPV) in

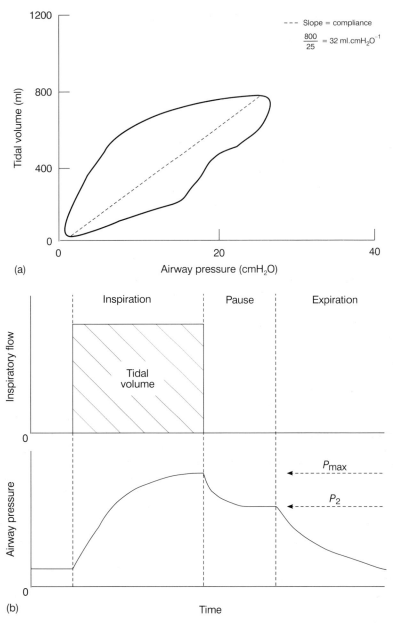

Figure 3.12 Automated measurement of compliance during intermittent positive pressure ventilation. (a) Dynamic compliance. Simultaneous measurement of tidal volume and airway pressure creates a pressure/volume loop. End-expiratory and end-inspiratory 'no-flow' points occur when the trace is horizontal. At this point, airway pressure and alveolar pressure are equal, so the pressure gradient is the difference between alveolar and atmospheric pressure. Total respiratory system compliance is therefore the slope of the line between these points. Note that in this patient compliance is markedly reduced. (b) Static compliance. Following an end-inspiratory pause the plateau pressure is recorded (P_2) and along with tidal volume the static compliance easily derived. This manoeuvre also provides an assessment of respiratory system resistance by recording the pressure drop ($P_{max} - P_2$) and the inspiratory flow immediately before the inspiratory pause (see page 77).

intensive care the measurement of compliance is considerably easier. Many ventilators and anaesthetic monitoring systems now routinely measure airway pressure and tidal volume. This enables a pressure volume loop to be displayed (Figure 3.12a) from which the dynamic compliance of the respiratory system may be calculated on a continuous breath-by-breath basis. When no gas is flowing during IPPV (at the end of inspiration and expiration) the airway pressure equals alveolar pressure. At this point, the airway pressure recorded by the ventilator therefore equals the difference between alveolar and atmospheric pressure, allowing derivation of the total compliance.

Some ventilators will also measure static compliance. The microprocessor will inflate the lung with the patient's usual tidal volume and then pause at end-inspiration for between 0.5 and 2 seconds, until the airway pressure falls to a plateau lasting 300 milliseconds (Figure 3.12b). Static compliance is then calculated from the volume delivered and pressure recorded during the plateau and may be easily compared with dynamic compliance.

Principles of measurement of lung volumes

Vital capacity, tidal volume, inspiratory reserve and expiratory reserve can all be measured with a simple spirometer (see Figure 3.9). Total lung capacity, functional residual capacity and residual volume all contain a fraction (the residual volume) that cannot be measured by simple spirometry. However, if one of these volumes is measured (most commonly the FRC), the others may easily be derived.

Measurement of FRC

Three techniques are available. The first employs nitrogen wash-out by breathing 100 per cent oxygen. The total quantity of nitrogen eliminated is measured as the product of the expired volume collected and the concentration of nitrogen. If, for example, 4 litres of nitrogen are collected and the initial alveolar nitrogen concentration was 80 per cent, the initial lung volume was 5 litres.

The second method uses the wash-in of a tracer gas such as helium, the concentration of which may be measured relatively easily by catharometry.[23] If, for example, 50 ml of helium are introduced into the lungs and the helium concentration is then found to be 1 per cent, the lung volume is 5 litres. Helium is used for this method because of its low solubility in blood. For the technique to be accurate the measurement must be made rapidly or helium dissolving in the tissues and blood will introduce large errors.

The third method uses the body plethysmograph. The subject is totally contained within a gas-tight box and attempts to breathe against an occluded airway. Changes in alveolar pressure are recorded at the mouth and compared with the small changes in lung volume, derived from pressure changes within the plethysmograph. Application of Boyle's law then permits calculation of lung volume.

The last method is the only technique for FRC measurement that includes gas trapped within the lung distal to closed airways.

References

1. von Neergard K. Neue Auffassungen über einen Grundbegriff der Atemmechanik. Die Retraktionskraft der Lunge, abhängig von der Oberflächenspannung in der Alveolen. *Z ges exp Med* 1929; **66**: 373.
2. Brown ES, Johnson RP, Clements JA. Pulmonary surface tension. *J Appl Physiol* 1959; **14**: 717–20.

3. Hamm H, Kroegel C, Hohlfeld J. Surfactant: a review of its functions and relevance in adult respiratory disorders. *Respir Medicine* 1996; **90**: 251–70.

4. van Gold LMG, Batenburg JJ, Robertson B. The pulmonary surfactant system: biochemical aspects and functional significance. *Physiol Rev* 1988; **68**: 374–455.

5. Harlan WR, Said SI. Selected aspects of lung metabolism. In: Bittar EE, Bittar N, eds. *The biological basis of medicine.* New York and London: Academic Press, 1969; Chapter 12.

6. Nogee LM, DeMello DE, Dehner LP, Colten HR. Brief report: deficiency of pulmonary surfactant protein B in congenital alveolar proteinosis. *N Engl J Med* 1993; **328**: 406–10.

7. Mason RJ, Greene K, Voelker DR. Surfactant protein A and surfactant protein D in health and disease. *Am J Physiol* 1998; **275**: L1–13.

8. Hills BA. What forces keep the airspaces of the lung dry ? *Thorax* 1982; **37**: 713–7.

9. Marshall R, Widdicombe JG. Stress relaxation in the human lung. *Clin Sci* 1961; **20**: 19–31.

10. Milic-Emili J, Robatto FM, Bates JHT. Respiratory mechanics in anaesthesia. *Br J Anaesth* 1990; **65**: 4–12.

11. Sugihara T, Hildebrandt J, Martin CJ. Viscoelastic properties of alveolar wall. *J Appl Physiol* 1972; **33**: 93–8.

12. Mercer RE, Russell ML, Crapo JD. Alveolar septal structure in different species. *J Appl Physiol* 1994; **77**: 1060–6.

13. Caro CG, Butler J, DuBois AB. Some effects of restriction of chest cage expansion on pulmonary function in man. *J Clin Invest* 1960; **39**: 573–83.

14. Butler J, Smith BH. Pressure–volume relationships of the chest in the completely relaxed anaesthetised patient. *Clin Sci* 1957; **16**: 125–46.

15. Mitzner W, Blosser S, Yager D, Wagner E. Effect of bronchial smooth muscle contraction on lung compliance. *J Appl Physiol* 1992; **72**: 158–67.

16. Finucane KE, Colebatch HJH. Elastic behaviour of the lung in patients with airway obstruction. *J Appl Physiol* 1969; **26**: 330–8.

17. Muller N, Volgyesi G, Becker L, Bryan MH, Bryan AC. Diaphragmatic muscle tone. *J Appl Physiol* 1979; **47**: 279–84.

18. Cotes JE. *Lung function.* Oxford: Blackwell Scientific, 1975.

19. Bates DV, Macklem PT, Christie RV. *Respiratory function in disease.* Philadelphia and London: WB Saunders, 1971.

20. Needham CD, Rogan MC, McDonald I. Normal standards for lung volumes, intrapulmonary gas mixing and maximum breathing capacity. *Thorax* 1954; **9**: 313–325.

21. Lumb AB, Nunn JF. Respiratory function and ribcage contribution to ventilation in body positions commonly used during anesthesia. *Anesth Analg* 1991; **73**: 422–6.

22. Leblanc P, Ruff F, Milic-Emili J. Effects of age and body position on 'airway closure' in man. *J Appl Physiol* 1970; **28**: 448–53.

23. Hewlett AM, Hulands GH, Nunn JF, Minty KB. Functional residual capacity. I. Methodology. *Br J Anaesth* 1974; **46**: 479–85.

Chapter 4

Respiratory system resistance

Elastic resistance, which occurs when no gas is flowing, results from only two of the numerous causes of impedance to inflation of the lung (considered in the previous chapter). This chapter considers the remaining components, which together are referred to as non-elastic resistance or respiratory system resistance. Most non-elastic resistance is provided by frictional resistance to air flow and thoracic tissue deformation (both lung and chest wall), with small contributions from the inertia of gas and tissue, and compression of intrathoracic gas.[1] Unlike elastic resistance, work performed against non-elastic resistance is not stored as potential energy (and therefore recoverable), but is lost and dissipated as heat.

Physical principles of gas flow and resistance

Gas flows from a region of high pressure to one of lower pressure. The rate at which it does so is a function of the pressure difference and the resistance to gas flow, thus being analogous to the flow of an electrical current (Figure 4.1). The precise relationship between pressure difference and flow rate depends on the nature of the flow, which may be laminar, turbulent or a mixture of the two. It is useful to consider laminar and turbulent flow as two separate entities but mixed patterns of flow usually occur in the respiratory tract. With a number of important caveats, similar basic considerations apply to the flow of liquids through tubes, which is considered in Chapter 7.

Laminar flow

With laminar flow, gas flows along a straight unbranched tube as a series of concentric cylinders that slide over one another, with the peripheral cylinder stationary and the central cylinder moving fastest, the advancing cone forming a parabola (Figure 4.2a).

The advancing cone front means that some fresh gas will reach the end of a tube while the volume entering the tube is still less than the volume of the tube. In the context of the respiratory tract, this is to say that there may be significant alveolar ventilation when the tidal volume is less than the volume of the airways (the anatomical dead space), a fact that was noted by Rohrer in 1915,[2] and is very relevant to high frequency ventilation (page 601). For the same reason, laminar flow is relatively inefficient for purging the contents of a tube.

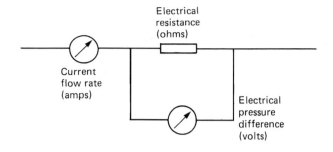

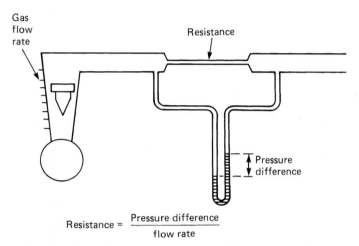

$$Resistance = \frac{Pressure\ difference}{flow\ rate}$$

Figure 4.1 Electrical analogy of gas flow. Resistance is pressure difference per unit flow rate. Resistance to gas flow is analogous to electrical resistance (provided that flow is laminar). Gas flow corresponds to electrical current (amps); gas pressure corresponds to potential (volts); gas flow resistance corresponds to electrical resistance (ohms); Pouseuille's law corresponds to Ohm's law.

In theory, gas adjacent to the tube wall is stationary, so friction between fluid and the tube wall is negligible. The physical characteristics of the airway or vessel wall should therefore not affect resistance to laminar flow. Similarly, the composition of gas sampled from the periphery of a tube during laminar flow may not be representative of the gas advancing down the centre of the tube.

To complicate matters further, laminar flow requires a critical length of tubing before the characteristic advancing cone pattern can be established. This is known as the entrance length and is related to the diameter of the tube and the Reynolds' number of the fluid (see below).

Quantitative relationships. With laminar flow the gas flow rate is directly proportional to the pressure gradient along the tube (Figure 4.2b), the constant being thus defined as resistance to gas flow:

$$\Delta P = \text{flow rate} \times \text{resistance}$$

where ΔP = pressure gradient.

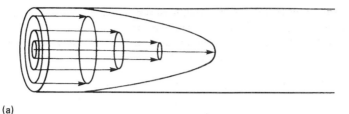

(a)

Pressure gradient (Pa)

40

30

20

10

0

$\dfrac{\text{Pressure}}{\text{gradient}}$ = Resistance × Flow rate

Resistance = 2 Pa litres⁻¹ min = 120 Pa litres⁻¹ s

Resistance = 1 Pa litres⁻¹ min = 60 Pa litres⁻¹ s

Resistance = 0.5 Pa litres⁻¹ min = 30 Pa litres⁻¹ s

0.4

0.3

0.2

0.1

0

Pressure gradient (cmH₂O)

0   10   20   30   40

Gas flow rate (litres.min⁻¹)

(b)

Figure 4.2 Laminar flow. (a) Laminar gas flow down a straight tube as a series of concentric cylinders of gas with the central cylinder moving fastest and the outside cylinder theoretically stationary. This gives rise to a 'cone front' of gas velocity across the tube. (b) The linear relationship between gas flow rate and pressure gradient. The slope of the lines indicates the resistance (1 Pa = 0.01 cmH₂O).

In a straight unbranched tube, the Hagen–Poiseuille equation allows gas flow to be quantified:

$$\text{flow rate} = \frac{\Delta P \times \pi \times (\text{radius})^4}{8 \times \text{length} \times \text{viscosity}}$$

By combining these two equations:

$$\text{resistance} = \frac{8 \times \text{length} \times \text{viscosity}}{\pi \times (\text{radius})^4}$$

In this equation the fourth power of the radius of the tube explains the critical importance of narrowing of air passages. With constant tube dimensions, viscosity is the only property of a gas that is relevant under conditions of laminar flow. Helium has a low density but a viscosity close to that of air. Helium will not therefore improve gas flow if the flow is laminar.

In the Hagen–Poiseuille equation, the units must be coherent. In CGS units, $dyn.cm^{-2}$ (pressure), $ml.s^{-1}$ (flow) and cm (length and radius) are compatible with the unit of poise for viscosity ($dyn.sec.cm^{-2}$). In SI units, with pressure in kilopascals, the unit of viscosity is $newton\ second.metre^{-2}$ (see Appendix A). However, in practice it is still customary to express gas pressure in cmH_2O and flow in $l.s^{-1}$. Resistance usually therefore continues to be expressed as centimetres of water per litre per second ($cmH_2O.l^{-1}.s$).

Turbulent flow

High flow rates, particularly through branched or irregular tubes, result in a breakdown of the orderly flow of gas described above. An irregular movement is superimposed on the general progression along the tube (Figure 4.3a), a square front replacing the cone front of laminar flow. Turbulent flow is almost invariably present when high resistance to gas flow is a problem.

The square front means that no fresh gas can reach the end of a tube until the amount of gas entering the tube is almost equal to the volume of the tube. Turbulent flow is more effective than laminar flow in purging the contents of a tube, and also provides the best conditions for drawing a representative sample of gas from the periphery of a tube. Frictional forces between the tube wall and fluid become more important in turbulent flow.

Quantitative relationships. The relationship between driving pressure and flow rate differs from the relationship described above for laminar flow in three important respects:

1. The driving pressure is proportional to the square of the gas flow rate.
2. The driving pressure is proportional to the density of the gas and is independent of its viscosity.
3. The required driving pressure is, in theory, inversely proportional to the fifth power of the radius of the tube (Fanning equation).

The square law relating driving pressure and flow rate is shown in Figure 4.3b. Resistance, defined as pressure gradient divided by flow rate, is not constant as in laminar flow but increases in proportion to the flow rate. Units such as $cmH_2O.l^{-1}.s$ should therefore be used only when flow is entirely laminar. The following methods for quantifying 'resistance' should be used when flow is totally or partially turbulent.

(a) Two constants. This method considers resistance as comprising two components, one for laminar flow and the other for turbulent flow. The simple relationship for laminar flow given above would then be extended as:

$$\text{pressure difference} = k_1 \text{ (flow)} + k_2 \text{ (flow)}^2$$

k_1 contains the factors of the Hagen–Poiseuille equation and represents the laminar flow component, while k_2 includes factors in the corresponding equation for turbulent flow. Mead and Agostoni[3] summarized studies of normal human subjects in the following equation:

$$\text{pressure gradient (kPa)} = 0.24 \text{ (flow)} + 0.03 \text{ (flow)}^2$$

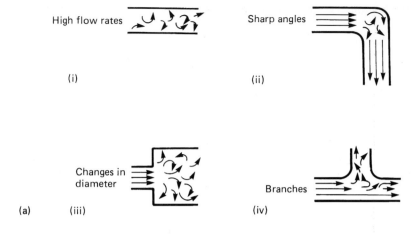

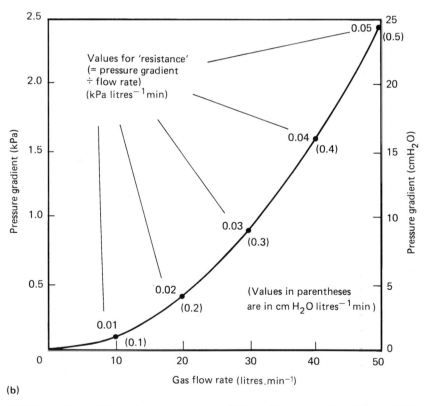

Figure 4.3 Turbulent flow. (a) Four circumstances under which gas flow tends to be turbulent. (b) The square law relationship between gas flow rate and pressure gradient when flow is turbulent. Note that the value for 'resistance', calculated as for laminar flow, is quite meaningless during turbulent flow.

(b) The exponent ^{n}. Over a surprisingly wide range of flow rates, the equation above may be condensed into the following single-term expression with little loss of precision:

$$\text{pressure gradient} = K \, (\text{flow})^n$$

The exponent ^{n} has a value ranging from 1 with purely laminar flow, to 2 with purely turbulent flow, the value of ^{n} being a useful indication of the nature of the flow. The constants for the normal human respiratory tract are:

$$\text{pressure gradient (kPa)} = 0.24 \, (\text{flow})^{1.3}$$

(c) The graphical method. It is often convenient to represent 'resistance' as a graph of pressure difference against gas flow rate, on either linear or logarithmic coordinates. Logarithmic coordinates have the advantage that the plot is usually a straight line whether flow is laminar, turbulent or mixed, and the slope of the line indicates the value of ^{n} in the equation above.

Reynolds' number

In the case of long straight unbranched tubes, the nature of the gas flow may be predicted from the value of Reynolds' number, which is a non-dimensional quantity derived from the expression:

$$\frac{\text{linear velocity of gas} \times \text{tube diameter} \times \text{gas density}}{\text{gas viscosity}}$$

The property of the gas that affects Reynolds' number is the ratio of density to viscosity. When Reynolds' number is less than 2000, flow is predominantly laminar, whereas above a value of 4000, flow is mainly turbulent.[4] Between these values, both types of flow coexist. Reynolds' number also affects the entrance length, that is the distance required for laminar flow to become established, which is derived from:

$$\text{entrance length} = 0.03 \times \text{tube diameter} \times \text{Reynolds' number}$$

Thus for gases with a low Reynolds' number not only will resistance be less during turbulent flow but also laminar flow will become established more quickly after bifurcations, corners and obstructions.

Values for some gas mixtures that a patient may inhale are shown relative to air in Table 4.1. Viscosities of respirable gases do not differ greatly but there may be very large differences in density.

Table 4.1 Physical properties of clinically used gas mixtures relating to gas flow

	Viscosity relative to air	Vapour density relative to air	Vapour density / Viscosity
Oxygen	1.11	1.11	1.00
70% N_2O/30% O_2	0.89	1.41	1.59
80% He/20% O_2	1.08	0.33	0.31

Respiratory system resistance

Airway resistance

This results from frictional resistance in the airways. In the healthy subject, the small airways make only a small contribution to total airway resistance because their aggregate cross-sectional area increases to very large values after about the eighth generation (see Figure 2.4). Overall airway resistance is therefore dominated by the resistance of the larger airways.

Gas flow along pulmonary airways is very complex when compared to the theoretical tubes described above, and consists of a varying mixture of both laminar and turbulent flow. Both the velocity of gas flow and airway diameter (and therefore Reynolds' number) decrease in successive airway generations from a maximum in the trachea to almost zero at the start of the pulmonary acinus (generation 15). In addition, there are frequent divisions with variable lengths of approximately straight airway between. Finally, in large-diameter airways entrance length is normally greater than the length of the individual airway. As a result of these purely physical factors laminar flow cannot become established until approximately the 11th airway generation.[4] Predominantly turbulent flow in the conducting airways has two practical implications. First, the physical characteristics of the airway lining will influence frictional resistance more with turbulent than with laminar flow, so changes in the consistency of mucus that occur in many airway diseases will have a significant effect (Chapter 27). Secondly, gas mixtures containing helium (low Reynolds' number) are beneficial only in overcoming increased resistance in large airways and of no benefit in small airway disease such as asthma.

Tissue resistance

In 1955 Mount identified a component of the work of breathing which he attributed to the resistance caused by tissue deformation.[5] D'Angelo et al.[6] subsequently described how, in anaesthetized and paralysed subjects, the viscoelastic 'tissue' component of respiratory resistance may be measured. They presented a 'spring and dashpot' model that describes this component of respiratory resistance.

Figure 4.4a shows pneumatic and electrical analogues of a simple resistance/capacitance ($\equiv$ compliance) network, which provides an elementary but extremely useful model of the mechanical properties of the respiratory system. Note that in the pneumatic analogue, Boyle's law compression of gases is used to simulate compliance. In each analogue, time constant equals the product of resistance and capacitance ($\equiv$ compliance) (See Appendix F).

Figure 4.4b shows Mount's models, which have secondary capacitances coupled by a second resistance (and with a different time constant). He produced convincing evidence that the additional component was uninfluenced by the viscosity or density of the gas inflating the lung and concluded that it represented tissue deformation that was time dependent. Thus, with a very slow inflation, the additional capacitance ($\equiv$ compliance) becomes available, and this factor contributes to the excess of static over dynamic compliance.

Figure 4.4c shows the 'spring and dashpot model', described by D'Angelo et al.[6] Dashpots here represent resistance, and springs elastance (reciprocal of compliance). Upward movement of the upper bar represents an increase in lung volume, caused by contraction of the inspiratory muscles or the application of inflation pressure as shown in the diagram. There is good evidence that, in humans, the left-hand dashpot represents predominantly airway resistance. The spring in the middle represents the static elastance of the respiratory system. On the right there is a spring and dashpot arranged in series. With a rapid change in lung volume, the spring is extended while the piston is more slowly rising in the dashpot. In due course (approx. 2–3 s) the spring returns to its original length and so ceases to exert any influence on pressure/volume relationships. This spring therefore represents the time-dependent element of elastance. While it is still under tension at end-inspiration, the combined effect of the two springs results in a high elastance of which the reciprocal is the dynamic compliance. If inflation is held for a few seconds and movement of the piston through the right-hand dashpot is completed, the right-hand spring ceases to exert any tension and the total elastance is reduced to that caused by the spring in the middle. The reciprocal of this elastance is the static compliance, which is therefore greater than the dynamic compliance. D'Angelo et al.[6] stress that the system shown in Figure 4.4c is only a simplified scheme to which many further components could be added; nevertheless the model accords well with experimental findings.

(a) Models that ignore time dependence of impedance

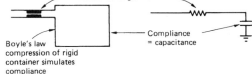

(b) Mount's model incorporating time-dependent tissue resistance

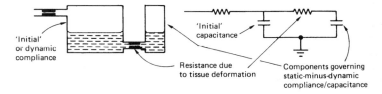

(c) Spring and dashpot model of resistance to breathing

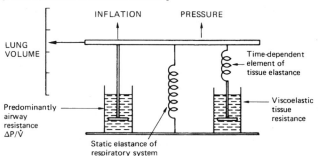

Figure 4.4 (a) Simple pneumatic and electrical models of resistance and compliance (≡ capacitance). Time constant equals the product of compliance and resistance, and is not time dependent. (b) The models now have a second resistance and compliance, which imparts time dependence to the system. Time constant depends on the duration of inflation.[5] (c) The spring and dashpot model of D'Angelo et al.[6] Inflation of the lungs is represented by the bar moving upwards. The springs represent elastance (reciprocal of compliance) and the dashpots resistance. The spring and dashpot in series on the right confers time dependence which is due to viscoelastic tissue resistance.

The time-dependent change in compliance represented by the spring and dashpot in series could be due to many factors. Several workers have now advanced reasons for believing that redistribution of gas makes only a negligible contribution in normal humans and that the major component is due to viscoelastic flow resistance in tissue.[1,6,7]

In anaesthetized patients tissue resistance is of the order of half the respiratory system resistance, depending on lung volume and rate of inflation.[6,7] Tissue resistance originates from both lung and chest wall tissues, some workers suggesting that a significant proportion originates in the chest wall.[8,9] The magnitude and importance of this component has often been underestimated in the past and it is clearly important to distinguish airway resistance from that afforded by the total respiratory system. Separate measurement of tissue resistance is described below.

Inertance as a component of respiratory system resistance

Respired gases, the lungs and the thoracic cage all have appreciable mass and therefore inertia, which must offer an impedance to change in direction of gas flow, analogous to electrical inductance. This component, termed inertance, is extremely difficult to measure, but inductance and inertance offer an impedance that increases with frequency.[10] Therefore, although inertance is generally believed to be negligible at normal respiratory frequencies, it may become appreciable during high frequency ventilation (page 601).

Factors affecting respiratory resistance

In normal lungs respiratory resistance is controlled by changes in airway diameter mainly in small airways and bronchioles. This would be expected to alter only the airways component of respiratory resistance but recent animal work suggests that contraction of bronchial smooth muscle also causes changes in tissue resistance. It is thought that airway constriction distorts the surrounding tissues sufficiently to alter its viscoelastic properties.[11] Airway calibre may be reduced either by physical compression (due to a reversal of the normal transluminal pressure leading to airway collapse) or by contraction of the smooth muscle in the airway wall.

Volume-related airway collapse

Effect of lung volume on resistance to breathing. When the lung volume is reduced, there is a proportional reduction in the volume of all air-containing components, including the air passages. Thus, if other factors (such as bronchomotor tone) remain constant, airway resistance is an inverse function of lung volume (Figure 4.5) and there is a direct relationship between lung volume and the maximum expiratory flow rate that can be attained (see below). Quantifying airway diameter is difficult from these curves. It is therefore more convenient to refer to conductance, which is the reciprocal of resistance and usually expressed as litres per second per centimetre of water. Specific airway conductance (sG_{aw}) is the airway conductance relative to lung volume[12] or the gradient of the line showing conductance as a function of lung volume (Figure 4.5). Because it takes into account the important effect of lung volume on airway resistance, it is a useful index of bronchomotor tone.

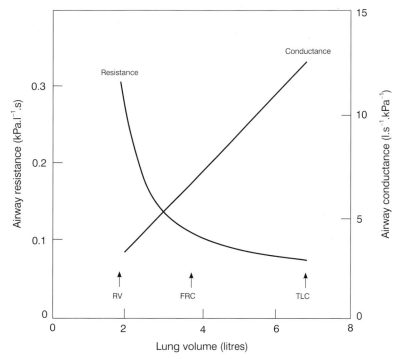

Figure 4.5 Airway resistance and conductance as a function of lung volume (upright). The resistance curve is a hyperbola. Specific conductance (sG_{aw}) is the gradient of the conductance line. RV, residual volume; FRC, functional residual capacity; TLC, total lung capacity.

Gas trapping. At low lung volumes, flow-related airway collapse (see below) occurs more readily because airway calibre and the transmural pressure are less. Expiratory airway collapse gives rise to a 'valve' effect and gas becomes trapped distal to the collapsed airway, leading to an increase in residual volume and FRC. Thus, in general, increasing lung volume reduces airway resistance and helps to prevent trapping. This is most conveniently achieved by the application of continuous positive airway pressure (CPAP) to the spontaneously breathing subject or positive end-expiratory pressure (PEEP) to the paralysed ventilated patient (Chapter 31). Many patients with obstructive airways disease acquire the habit of increasing their expiratory resistance by exhaling through pursed lips. Alternatively, premature termination of expiration keeps the lung volume above FRC (auto-PEEP). Both manoeuvres have the effect of enhancing airway transmural pressure gradient and so reducing airway resistance and preventing trapping.

The closing capacity. In addition to the overall effect on airway resistance shown in Figure 4.5, there are important regional differences. This is because the airways and alveoli in the dependent parts of the lungs are always smaller than those at the top of the lung, except at total lung capacity or at zero gravity when all are the same size. As the lung volume is reduced towards residual volume, there is a point at which dependent airways begin to close, and the lung volume at which this occurs is known as the closing capacity (CC). The alternative term, *closing volume* (CV), equals the closing capacity minus the residual volume (RV) (Figure 4.6). Closing capacity increases with age and is less than the FRC

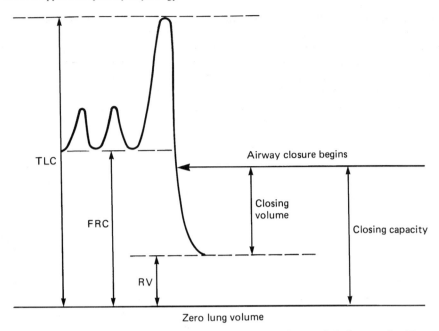

Figure 4.6 Spirogram to illustrate the relationship between closing volume and closing capacity. The example would be in a young adult with closing capacity less than functional residual capacity (FRC). RV, residual volume; TLC, total lung capacity.

in young adults but increases to become equal to FRC at a mean age of 44 years in the supine position and 66 years in the upright position (see Figure 3.11). The closing capacity seems to be independent of body position but the FRC changes markedly with position (see Figure 3.10).

When the FRC is less than the closing capacity, some of the pulmonary blood flow will be distributed to alveoli with closed airways, usually in the dependent parts of the lungs. This will constitute a shunt (page 181), and must increase the alveolar/arterial Po_2 gradient. If the alveolar Po_2 remains the same, the arterial Po_2 must be decreased. This can be seen when volunteers breathe below their FRC, and is particularly marked in older subjects who have a greater closing capacity. Shunting of blood through areas of the lung with closed airways is an important cause of decreasing arterial Po_2 with increasing age (page 276) and changes of position (page 433). Reduction in FRC is closely related to the increased alveolar/arterial Po_2 gradient seen during anaesthesia (page 444).

Flow-related airway collapse

All the airways can be compressed by reversal of the normal transmural pressure gradient to a sufficiently high level. The cartilaginous airways have considerable structural resistance to collapse but even the trachea may be compressed with an external pressure in the range 5–7 kPa (50–70 cmH$_2$O), which may result from neoplasm or haemorrhage. Airways beyond generation 11 have no structural rigidity (see Table 2.1) and rely instead on the traction on their walls from elastic recoil of the lung tissue in which they are embedded. They can be collapsed by a reversed transmural pressure gradient that is considerably less than that which closes the cartilaginous airways.

Reversal of the transmural pressure gradient may be caused by high levels of air flow during expiration. During all phases of normal breathing, the pressure in the lumen of the air passages should always remain well above the subatmospheric pressure in the thorax, so the airways remain patent. During a maximal forced expiration, the intrathoracic pressure rises to well above atmospheric, resulting in high gas flow rates. Pressure drops as gas flows along the airways and there will therefore be a point at which airway pressure equals the intrathoracic pressure. At that point (the equal pressure point) the smaller air passages are held open only by the elastic recoil of the lung parenchyma in which they are embedded or, if it occurs in the larger airways, by their structural rigidity. Downstream of the equal pressure point, the transmural pressure gradient is reversed and at some point may overcome the forces holding the airways open, resulting in airway collapse. This effect is also influenced by lung volume (see above), and the equal pressure point moves progressively down towards the smaller airways as lung volume is decreased.

Flow-related collapse occurs in the larger bronchi during a forced expiration and limits the flow rate. During coughing, the reduction in calibre of the bronchi increases the linear velocity of air flow, thereby improving the scavenging of secretions from the walls of the air passages.[13]

Flow-related collapse is best demonstrated on a flow/volume plot. Figure 4.7 shows the normal relationship between lung volume on the abscissa and instantaneous respiratory flow rate on the ordinate. Time is not directly indicated. In part (a) of the Figure the small loop shows a normal tidal excursion above FRC and with air flow rate either side of zero. Arrows show the direction of the trace. At the end of a maximal expiration the black square indicates residual volume. The lower part of the large curve then shows the course of a maximal inspiration to TLC (black circle). There follow four expiratory curves, each with different expiratory effort and each attaining a different peak expiratory flow rate. Within limits, the greater the effort, the greater is the resultant peak flow rate. However, all the expiratory curves terminate in a final common pathway, which is independent of effort. In this part of the curves, the flow rate is limited by airway collapse and the maximal air flow rate is governed by the lung volume (abscissa). The greater the effort, the greater the degree of airway collapse and the resultant gas flow rate remains the same. Figure 4.7b shows the importance of a maximal inspiration before measurement of peak expiratory flow rate.

Muscular control of airway diameter

Small airways are the site of most of the important causes of obstruction in a range of pathological conditions described in Chapter 27, and as such have been extensively investigated. Only aspects relating to control of airway calibre in normal lung are discussed here.

Four pathways are involved in controlling muscle tone in small bronchi and bronchioles:

1. Neural pathways
2. Humoral (via blood) control
3. Direct physical and chemical effects
4. Local cellular mechanisms.

These may conveniently be considered as discrete mechanisms but in practice there is considerable interaction between them, particularly in disease. Neural control is the most

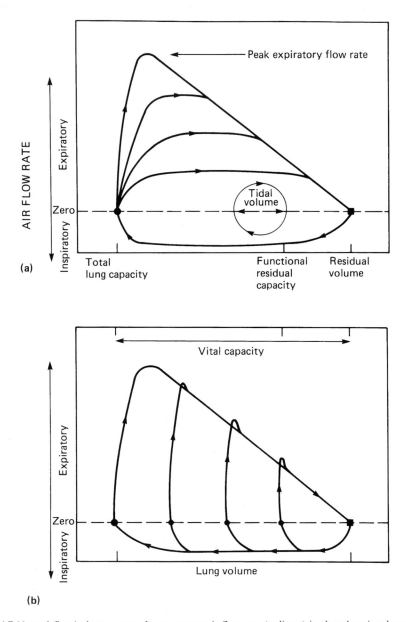

Figure 4.7 Normal flow/volume curves. Instantaneous air flow rate (ordinate) is plotted against lung volume (abscissa). (a) The normal tidal excursion is shown as the small loop. In addition, expiration from total lung capacity at four levels of expiratory effort are shown. Within limits, peak expiratory flow rate is dependent on effort but, during the latter part of expiration, all curves converge on an effort-independent section where flow rate is limited by airway collapse. (b) The effect of forced expirations from different lung volumes. The pips above the effort-independent section probably represent air expelled from collapsed airways.

important in normal lung, with direct stimulation and humoral control contributing under some circumstances. Cellular mechanisms, particularly mast cells, have little influence under normal conditions; they are discussed in detail in Chapter 27.

Neural pathways

Parasympathetic system.[4,14] This system is of major importance in the control of bronchomotor tone. Both afferent and efferent fibres travel to the lung in the vagus nerve with efferent ganglia in the walls of small bronchi. Afferents arise from receptors under the tight junctions of the bronchial epithelium and respond either to noxious stimuli acting directly on the receptors (see below) or from cytokines released by cellular mechanisms such as mast cell degranulation. Efferent nerves release acetylcholine to act at M_3 muscarinic receptors in the bronchial smooth muscle, whilst M_2 pre-junctional muscarinic receptors exert negative feedback.[4] A complex series of second messengers is involved in bringing about smooth muscle contraction in response to acetylcholine. Stimulation of any part of the reflex arc results in bronchoconstriction. Some degree of resting tone is normally present and may therefore permit some degree of bronchodilation when vagal tone is reduced in a similar fashion to vagal control of heart rate.

Sympathetic system. In contrast to the parasympathetic system, the sympathetic system is poorly represented in the lung and not yet proven to be of major importance in humans. Indeed, it seems unlikely that there is any direct sympathetic innervation of the airway smooth muscle, although there may be an inhibitory effect on cholinergic neurotransmission in some species.[14]

Non-adrenergic non-cholinergic (NANC) system.[15] The airways are provided with a third autonomic control that is neither adrenergic nor cholinergic. This is the only potential bronchodilator nervous pathway in humans, though the exact role of the NANC system in humans remains uncertain. The efferent fibres run in the vagus and pass to the smooth muscle of the airway where they cause prolonged relaxation of bronchi. The neurotransmitter is vasoactive intestinal polypeptide (VIP), which produces airway smooth muscle relaxation by promoting the production of nitric oxide (NO). How NO brings about smooth muscle relaxation in the airway is not as fully understood as its effect on vascular smooth muscle. It seems likely that NO has its effect without having to cross the cell membrane by some form of cell surface interaction that produces activation of guanylate cyclase to produce cyclic GMP and muscle relaxation.[16] Resting airway tone does involve bronchodilation by NO, but whether this is from local cellular production of NO or NANC and VIP-mediated release of NO is not clear.

There is also a bronchoconstrictor part of the NANC system. Non-myelinated C-fibres are found in the airway close to, but separate from, the parasympathetic nerves. They are sensory fibres, reacting to direct stimulation by irritants such as cigarette smoke. In addition to their sensory actions, when stimulated the neurones also manufacture and secrete both substance P and neurokinin A, which are potent bronchoconstrictors in normal lung.[16] Although of significance in airways disease, the contribution of this system to normal airway tone is unknown.

Humoral control[4,17]

In spite of the minimal significance of sympathetic innervation, bronchial smooth muscle has plentiful β_2-adrenergic receptors, which are highly sensitive to circulating adrenaline, and once again act via complex second messenger systems.[18] Basal levels of adrenaline probably do not contribute to bronchial muscle tone, but this mechanism is brought into play during exercise or during the sympathetic 'stress response'. There are a few α-adrenergic receptors that are bronchoconstrictor but unlikely to be of much clinical significance.

Adrenergic smooth muscle receptors have been used to therapeutic advantage for many years, and this is probably of greater clinical relevance than their activation by the autonomic nervous system. The β_2-adrenergic receptors are highly sensitive to adrenaline, salbutamol, terbutaline and isoprenaline, which for many years were the mainstay of treatment for bronchospasm.

Physical and chemical effects

Direct stimulation of the respiratory epithelium activates the parasympathetic reflex described above, causing bronchoconstriction. Activation of the bronchoconstrictor path of the NANC system may also play a part. Physical factors known to produce bronchoconstriction include mechanical stimulation of the upper air passages by laryngoscopy and the presence of foreign bodies in the trachea or bronchi. Inhalation of particulate matter, an aerosol of water or just cold air may cause bronchoconstriction, the last being used as a simple provocation test.[19] Many chemical stimuli result in bronchoconstriction, including liquids with low pH such as gastric acid and gases such as sulphur dioxide, ozone and nitrogen dioxide (page 416).

Increased resistance to breathing

Four grades of increased airway resistance may be identified.

Grade 1. Slight resistance is that against which the patient can indefinitely sustain a normal alveolar ventilation.

Grade 2. Moderate resistance is that against which a considerable increase in work of breathing is required to prevent a decrease in alveolar ventilation, with deterioration of arterial gas tensions. Patients vary in their response. Some increase their work of breathing, exhibiting obvious dyspnoea but maintaining normal arterial blood gas tensions. Others do not increase their work of breathing sufficiently to prevent an increase in arterial P_{CO_2} and a decrease in arterial P_{O_2}.

Grade 3. Severe resistance is that against which no patient is able to preserve his alveolar ventilation. Arterial P_{CO_2} is increased up to the level that interferes with the maintenance of consciousness, and there is severe hypoxaemia unless the inspired gas is enriched with oxygen. Because of the very marked effect of changes in the inspired oxygen concentration, the increase in the arterial P_{CO_2} is the best indication of the gravity of the condition (see Chapter 26).

Grade 4. Respiratory obstruction may be defined as an increase in airway resistance that is incompatible with life if it is not relieved as a matter of urgency.

Provided patients remain calm they can withstand surprisingly high resistance. However, once they are alarmed and start to struggle, they may enter a vicious cycle of raised oxygen consumption, increased ventilatory demand and increased work of breathing, leading to a further increase in oxygen consumption that cannot be met.

Causes of increased airway resistance

As in obstruction of other biological systems, it is helpful to think in terms of conducting tubes being blocked by:

1. Material within the lumen.
2. Thickening or contraction of the wall of the passage.
3. Pressure from outside or suction within the air passage.

This classification applies to most of the locations considered below.

External apparatus. Even in ideal circumstances, tracheal tubes and tracheostomies have a greater resistance than the respiratory tract. Normally, this is of little consequence, but severe and potentially lethal increases of resistance can occur when these tubes are blocked, kinked or compressed.

The pharynx and larynx. The lumen may be blocked with foreign material such as gastric contents or blood. Laryngeal obstruction may result from carcinoma, oedema or infections such as diphtheria, croup or epiglottitis. The walls may contract as in laryngeal spasm, or the pharynx may collapse when inspiration is attempted against upstream resistance. The pharynx can withstand an inward transmural pressure gradient of only about $50 \, cmH_2O$ and less in the sleeping or unconscious patient. Anatomical considerations are outlined in Chapter 2 and special consideration is given elsewhere to pharyngeal obstruction during sleep (page 348) and anaesthesia (page 426).

The lower respiratory tract. Intraluminar obstruction may result from mucosal swelling, oedema fluid, secretions, pus, tumour or foreign body. However, much the most important causes of increased resistance in the bronchial tree are airway diseases, which are considered in Chapter 27.

Compensation for increased resistance to breathing

Inspiratory resistance. The normal response to increased inspiratory resistance is increased inspiratory muscle effort with little change in the FRC. Accessory muscles may be brought into play according to the degree of resistance.

There are two principal mechanisms of compensation for increased inspiratory resistance. The first operates immediately and even during the first breath in which resistance is applied. It seems probable that the muscle spindles indicate that the inspiratory muscles have failed to shorten by the intended amount and their afferent discharge then augments the activity in the motor neurone pool of the anterior horn. This is the typical servo operation of the spindle system with which the intercostal muscles are richly endowed. With a severe increase in resistance (added resistance of $8.3 \, kPa.l^{-1}.s$), a second compensatory mechanism develops over about 90 seconds[20] and overacts for a similar period when the resistance is removed.[21] This mechanism is driven by a slight elevation of arterial Pco_2.

Expiratory resistance. Expiration against a pressure of up to 1 kPa ($10 \, cmH_2O$) does not usually result in activation of the expiratory muscles in conscious or anaesthetized subjects. The additional work to overcome this resistance is, in fact, performed by the inspiratory muscles. The subject augments his inspiratory force until he achieves a lung volume (FRC) at which the additional elastic recoil is sufficient to overcome the

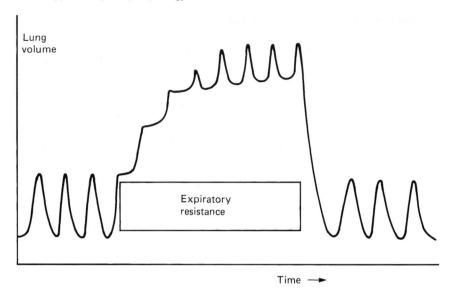

Figure 4.8 Spirogram showing response of an anaesthetized patient to the sudden imposition of an expiratory resistance. Note that there is an immediate augmentation of the force of contraction of the inspiratory muscles. This continues with successive breaths until the elastic recoil is sufficient to overcome the expiratory resistance.[21]

expiratory resistance (Figure 4.8). The mechanism for resetting the FRC at a higher level probably requires accommodation of the intrafusal fibres of the spindles to allow for an altered length of diaphragmatic muscle fibres due to the obstructed expiration. This would reset the developed inspiratory tension in accord with the increased FRC.[21] The conscious subject normally uses his expiratory muscles to overcome expiratory pressures in excess of about 1 kPa (10 cmH$_2$O).

Patients show a remarkable capacity to compensate for acutely increased resistance such that arterial $P\text{CO}_2$ is usually normal. However, the efficiency of these mechanisms in maintaining alveolar ventilation carries severe physiological consequences. In common with other muscles, the respiratory muscles can become fatigued[22] and this is a major factor in the onset of respiratory failure. A raised $P\text{CO}_2$ in a patient with increased respiratory resistance is therefore always serious. Intrathoracic pressure will rise during acutely increased expiratory resistance and so impede venous return and reduce cardiac output (page 611) to the point that syncope may occur.

With long-term increases in airway resistance it is difficult to predict the ventilatory response (Chapter 27). In patients with chronic obstructive airway disease, some allow their arterial $P\text{CO}_2$ to increase (blue bloaters) while others strive to maintain a normal $P\text{CO}_2$ (pink puffers).

Principles of measurement of respiratory resistance and closing capacity

Resistance is determined by the simultaneous measurement of gas flow rate and the driving pressure gradient. In the respiratory tract, the difficulty centres around the measurement of the pressure gradient between mouth and alveolus. Problems also arise

Table 4.2 Components of respiratory system resistance[23]

	Mouth and pharynx	Larynx and large airways	Small airways <3 mm diameter	Alveoli and lung tissue	Chest wall	Total
Contribution (kPa.l⁻¹.s)	0.05	0.05	0.02	0.02	0.12	0.26
Airway resistance		Body plethysmograph Interrupter technique				0.12
Pulmonary resistance		Pressure flow technique				0.14
Respiratory system resistance		Oscillating airflow technique End-inspiratory interruption				0.26

Shaded areas indicate which components contribute to each form of resistance, whilst the text in the shaded boxes states the methodology used to measure each form of resistance.

because of varying nomenclature and different methods for measuring different components of respiratory resistance (Table 4.2).[23,24] In all cases, apparatus resistance must be measured separately and subtracted from the value obtained in the subject.

Normal values for total respiratory resistance are variable because of the large changes with lung volume and methodological differences. Typical values obtained in a normal population at FRC are between 0.14 and 0.4 but values below 0.84 kPa.l⁻¹.s are considered normal.[25]

Pressure–flow technique

In Chapter 3 it was shown how simultaneous measurement of tidal volume and intrathoracic (oesophageal) pressure yielded the dynamic compliance of the lung (see Figure 3.12). For this purpose, pressures were selected at the times of zero air flow when pressures were uninfluenced by air flow resistance. The same apparatus may be employed for the determination of flow resistance by subtracting the pressure component used in overcoming elastic forces (Figure 4.9). The shaded areas in the pressure trace indicate the components of the pressure required to overcome flow resistance, and these may be related to the concurrent gas flow rates.

Alternatively, the intrathoracic-to-mouth pressure gradient and respired volume may be displayed as X and Y coordinates of a loop. Figure 3.12 showed how dynamic compliance could be derived from the no-flow points of such a loop. The area of the loop is a function of the work performed against flow resistance.

The use of an oesophageal balloon makes the method a little invasive, but it does allow continuous measurement of resistance. By measuring intrathoracic pressure, the chest wall component of resistance is excluded, so providing a measure of pulmonary resistance that is airways resistance plus the lung component of tissue resistance.

Oscillating air flow

In this technique, a high frequency oscillating air flow is applied to the airways, with measurement of the resultant pressure and air flow changes. By application of alternating current theory it is possible to derive a continuous measurement of airway resistance.[26,27]

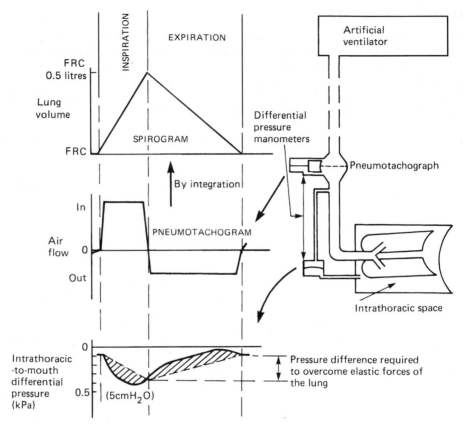

Figure 4.9 The measurement of pulmonary resistance and dynamic compliance by simultaneous measurement of air flow and intrathoracic-to-mouth differential pressure. The spirogram is conveniently obtained by integration of the pneumotachogram. In the pressure trace, the dotted line shows the pressure changes that would be expected in a hypothetical patient with no pulmonary resistance. Compliance is derived as shown in Figure 3.12. Pulmonary resistance is derived as the difference between the measured pressure differential and that which is required for elastic forces (shaded area) compared with the flow rate shown in the pneumotachograph. Note that the pneumotachogram is a much more sensitive indicator of the no-flow points than the spirogram.

The technique measures total respiratory resistance, and may be used throughout a vital capacity manoeuvre and so to display resistance as a function of lung volume and derive specific airway conductance.

The body plethysmograph

During inspiration, alveolar pressure falls below ambient as a function of airway resistance, and the alveolar gas expands in accord with Boyle's law. The increased displacement of the body is then recorded as an increase in pressure in the body plethysmograph. Airway resistance may be derived directly from measurements of air flow and pressure changes. The method requires the subject to perform either a 'panting' respiratory manoeuvre or to deliberately breathe with a small tidal volume, but is generally non-invasive and FRC may be measured at the same time.[23,28]

The interrupter technique

A single manometer may be used to measure both mouth and alveolar pressure if the air passages distal to the manometer are momentarily interrupted with a shutter. The method is based on the assumption that, while the airway is interrupted, the mouth pressure comes to equal the alveolar pressure. Resistance is then determined from the relationship between flow rate (measured before interruption) and the pressure difference between mouth (measured before interruption) and alveoli (measured at the end of the interruption). Interruption duration must be short enough not to disturb the subject's breathing pattern but long enough to allow equilibration of pressure along the airway. In practice, interruption is for 50–100 ms occurring repeatedly throughout the respiratory cycle. The technique is adequate for measuring resistance in normal lungs but it is doubtful if equilibration occurs fully in subjects with diseased airways.[28] The interrupter method measures airway resistance and excludes tissue resistance.

End-inspiratory interruption

This method, first described in 1965 by Don and Robson,[29] has recently become popular as a way to measure the tissue component of respiratory system resistance.[6,8,9,30] The method may be used only in anaesthetized paralysed subjects receiving positive pressure ventilation with accurate control of the respiratory cycle. Following a constant flow inflation of the lung, the airway is occluded for 0.5–3 s before a passive exhalation occurs. To prevent artefacts during the inspiratory pause, numerous successive breaths may be averaged.[8] Figure 4.10 shows the changes in gas flow, transpulmonary pressure (P_L), oesophageal pressure and lung volume averaged over 33 breaths. Immediately before occlusion, P_L reaches a value of P_{max}, which is governed by both elastic and non-elastic resistance. The fall in pressure following occlusion is biphasic. Immediately after airway occlusion, the P_L falls rapidly to P_1 and $P_{max} - P_1$ is referred to as interrupter resistance and believed to reflect airway resistance as in the interrupter method already described.

$$\text{Airway resistance} = \frac{P_{max} - P_1}{\text{flow rate of inflation}}$$

In the second phase, a slower decay in pressure occurs from P_1 to P_2, which represents the loss of the time-dependent element of tissue compliance (due to viscoelastic behaviour) and therefore represents tissue resistance.

$$\text{Tissue resistance} = \frac{P_1 - P_2}{\text{flow rate of inflation}}$$

In practice, the pressure signal may be converted into digital form and computer analysis calculates the three pressures.[8]

Where pressure is recorded determines which component of tissue resistance is measured. In Figure 4.10, transpulmonary pressure (tracheal minus oesophageal pressure) is recorded, so allowing calculation of the tissue resistance of the lung alone. Oesophageal pressure is also recorded, so allowing calculation of the thoracic cage component of tissue resistance. In theory, for oesophageal pressure recordings there should be no contribution from airway resistance and so the pressure decay following interruption should not be biphasic with P_{max} being equal to P_1. For many years this was thought to be the case,[6,9] until averaging of multiple breaths to remove cardiac artefacts revealed a smoother and biphasic oesophageal pressure trace (Figure 4.10). The initial pressure drop is believed to represent 'stress adaptation' of the chest wall.[8]

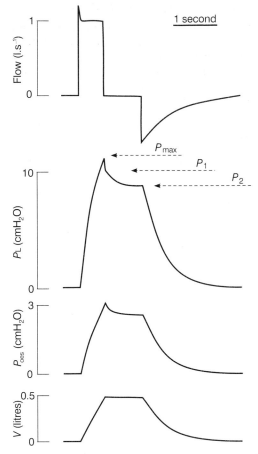

Figure 4.10 End-inspiratory interruption method of measuring resistance. Following a constant flow positive pressure breath, there is an end-inspiratory pause of almost one second before passive exhalation. The peak airway pressure (P_{max}) falls initially very quickly to P_1 and thereafter more slowly to a plateau P_2. Tissue resistance, airway resistance and total resistance can then all be calculated (see text for details). In this example, showing the average of 33 consecutive breaths, both transpulmonary (tracheal minus oesophageal) pressure and oesophageal pressure relative to atmosphere have been measured, allowing lung and chest wall components of tissue resistance to be calculated separately. Flow, airway flow rate; P_L, transpulmonary pressure; P_{oes}, oesophageal pressure; V, change in lung volume. (Redrawn from reference 8)

Finally, measurement of tracheal to atmospheric pressure gradient allows calculation of total respiratory resistance:

$$\text{Respiratory system resistance } = \frac{P_{max} - P_2}{\text{flow rate of inflation}}$$

This technique is used by the current generation of ventilators to calculate respiratory system resistance. The same static respiratory manoeuvre described in the previous chapter for calculating static compliance (Figure 3.12b) also allows measurement of P_{max} and P_2, from which respiratory system resistance is calculated (Figure 4.10).

Tests of ventilatory capacity as a measure of airway resistance

Formal measurement of airway resistance is seldom undertaken in the clinical situation, where the airway resistance is usually inferred from measurement of ventilatory capacity – which is most commonly reduced as a result of increased airway resistance. It must, however, be remembered that there are many other causes of reduction of ventilatory capacity that are nothing to do with airway resistance. Tests of ventilatory capacity and their interpretation are described at the end of Chapter 6.

Measurement of closing capacity[23]

This is perhaps the most convenient place to outline the measurement of closing capacity. It is the maximal lung volume at which airway closure can be detected in the dependent parts of the lungs (page 67). The measurement is made during expiration and is based on having different concentrations of a tracer gas in the upper and lower parts of the lung. This may be achieved by inspiration of a bolus of tracer gas at the commencement of an inspiration from residual volume, at which time airways are closed in the dependent part of the lungs (Figure 4.11). The tracer gas will then be preferentially distributed to the upper parts of the lungs. After a maximal inspiration to total lung capacity, the patient slowly exhales while the concentration of the tracer gas is measured at the mouth. When

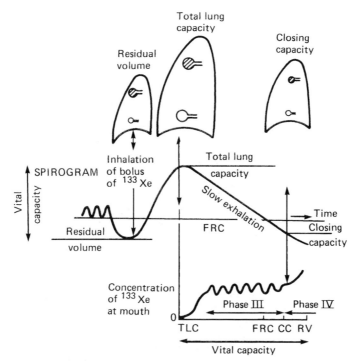

Figure 4.11 Measurement of closing capacity by the use of a tracer gas such as ^{133}Xe. The bolus of tracer gas is inhaled near residual volume and, due to airway closure, is distributed only to the alveoli whose air passages are still open (shown shaded in the diagram). During expiration, the concentration of the tracer gas becomes constant after the dead space is washed out. This plateau (phase III) gives way to a rising concentration of tracer gas (phase IV) when there is closure of airways leading to alveoli that did not receive the tracer gas.

lung volume reaches the closing capacity and airways begin to close in the dependent parts, the concentration of the tracer gas will rise (phase IV) above the alveolar plateau (phase III). Suitable tracers are ^{133}Xe or 100% oxygen (measured as a fall in nitrogen concentration). The technique can be undertaken in the conscious subject who performs the ventilatory manoeuvres spontaneously or in the paralysed subject in whom ventilation is artificially controlled.

References

1. Milic-Emili J, Robatto FM, Bates JHT. Respiratory mechanics in anaesthesia. *Br J Anaesth* 1990; **65**: 4–12.
2. Rohrer F. Der Strömungswiderstand in den menschlichen Atemwegen. *Plügers Arch ges Physiol* 1915; **162**: 225.
3. Mead J, Agostini E. Dynamics of breathing. *Handbook of Physiology, Section 3* 1964; **1**: 1.
4. Burwell DR, Jones JG. The airways and anaesthesia – 1: Anatomy, physiology and fluid mechanics. *Anaesthesia* 1996; **51**; 849–57.
5. Mount LE. The ventilation flow-resistance and compliance of rat lungs. *J Physiol* 1955; **127**: 157–67.
6. D'Angelo E, Calderini E, Torri G, Robatto FM, Bonon D, Milic-Emili J. Respiratory mechanics in anaesthetized paralyzed humans: effects of flow, volume and time. *J Appl Physiol* 1989; **67**: 2556–64.
7. von Neergaard K, Wirz K. Die Messung der Strömungswiderstände in der Atemwege des lebenden Menschen, inbesondere bei Asthma und Emphysem. *Z klin Med* 1927; **105**: 51.
8. D'Angelo E, Prandi E, Tavola M, Calderini E, Milic-Emili J. Chest wall interrupter resistance in anaesthetized paralyzed humans. *J Appl Physiol* 1994; **77**: 883–7.
9. D'Angelo E, Robatto FM, Calderini E, Tavola M, Bono D, Torri G, Milic-Emili J. Pulmonary and chest wall mechanics in anaesthetized paralyzed humans. *J Appl Physiol* 1991; **70**: 2602–10.
10. Dorbin HL, Luchen KR, Jackson AC. Human respiratory input impedance from 4 to 200 Hz: physiologic and modelling considerations. *J Appl Physiol* 1988; **64**; 823–31.
11. Kimmel E, Seri M, Fredberg JJ. Lung tissue resistance and hysteretic modelling of lung parenchyma. *J Appl Physiol* 1995; **79**: 461–6.
12. Lehane JR, Jordan C, Jones JG. Influence of halothane and enflurane on respiratory airflow resistance and specific conductance in man. *Br J Anaesth* 1980; **52**: 773–80.
13. Selsby D, Jones JG. Some physiological and clinical aspects of chest physiotherapy. *Br J Anaesth* 1990; **64**: 621–31.
14. Barnes PJ. Neural control of airway smooth muscle. In: Crystal RG, West JB, eds. *The lung: scientific foundations.* New York: Raven 1991; 903.
15. Widdicombe JG. Autonomic regulation: i-NANC/e-NANC. *Am J Respir Crit Care Med* 1998; **158**: S171–5.
16. Drazen JM, Gaston B, Shore SA. Chemical regulation of pulmonary airway tone. *Annu Rev Physiol* 1995; **57**: 151–70.
17. Thomson NC, Dagg KD, Ramsay SG. Humoral control of airway tone. *Thorax* 1996; **51**: 461–4.
18. Hakonarson H, Grunstein MM. Regulation of second messengers associated with airway smooth muscle contraction and relaxation. *Am J Respir Crit Care Med* 1998; **158**: S115–22.
19. Heaton RW, Henderson AF, Costello JF. Cold air as a bronchial provocation technique. *Chest* 1984; **86**: 810–14.
20. Nishino T, Kochi T. Breathing route and ventilatory responses to inspiratory resistive loading in humans. *Am J Respir Crit Care Med* 1994; **150**: 742–6.
21. Nunn JF, Ezi-Ashi TI. The respiratory effects of resistance to breathing in anaesthetized man. *Anesthesiology* 1961; **22**: 174–85.
22. Moxham J. Respiratory muscle fatigue: mechanisms, evaluation and therapy. *Br J Anaesth* 1990; **65**: 43–53.
23. Cotes JE. *Lung function: assessment and application in medicine.* Oxford: Blackwell Scientific Publications, 1993.
24. Phagoo SB, Watson RA, Silverman M, Pride NB. Comparison of four methods of assessing airflow resistance before and after induced airway narrowing. *J Appl Physiol* 1995; **79**: 518–25.

25. van Altena R, Gimeno F. Respiratory resistance measured by flow-interruption in a normal population. *Respiration* 1994; **61**: 249–54.
26. Hyatt RE, Zimmerman IR, Peters GM, Sullivan WJ. Direct write out of total respiratory resistance. *J Appl Physiol* 1970; **28**: 675–8.
27. Goldman M, Knudson RJ, Mead J, Paterson N, Schwaber JR, Wohl ME. A simplified measurement of respiratory resistance by forced oscillation. *J Appl Physiol* 1970; **28**: 113–16.
28. Freedman S. Mechanics of ventilation. In: Brewis RAL, Corrin B, Gedded DM, Gibson GJ, eds. *Respiratory medicine*. London: WB Saunders, 1995; 116–19.
29. Don HF, Robson JG. The mechanics of the respiratory system during anaesthesia. *Anesthesiology* 1965; **26**: 168–78.
30. Jonson B, Beydon L, Brauer K, Mansson C, Valind S, Grytzell H. Mechanics of the respiratory system in healthy anesthetized humans with an emphasis on viscoelastic properties. *J Appl Physiol* 1993; **75**: 132–40.

Chapter 5

Control of breathing

Early in pregnancy the fetal brainstem develops a 'respiratory centre' that produces uninterrupted rhythmic breathing activity for many years.[1] Throughout life the subject is mostly unaware of this action, which is closely controlled by a combination of chemical and physical reflexes. In addition, when required, breathing may (within limits) be completely overridden by voluntary cortical control or interrupted by swallowing and involuntary non-rhythmic acts such as sneezing, vomiting, hiccuping or coughing. There is progressive realization of the immense complexity of the control system, with its automatic ability to adapt the action of the respiratory muscles to the changing demands of posture, speech, voluntary movement, exercise and innumerable other circumstances that alter the respiratory requirement or influence the performance of the respiratory muscles.

This chapter begins by describing the cellular origin of the underlying respiratory rhythm and the efferent pathways that then bring about respiration. The numerous influences on this underlying pattern of respiration are then described, including CNS connections to the respiratory centre, peripheral inputs from the airways and lung, and finally the chemical control of breathing.

The origin of the respiratory rhythm[2,3]

In 1812, Legallois[4] published reports showing that rhythmic inspiratory movements in animals persisted after removal of the cerebellum and all parts of the brain above the medulla, but ceased when the medulla was removed. During the next 150 years a long series of distinguished investigators carried out more detailed localization of the neurones concerned in the control of respiration and studied their interaction. (For a description of these studies, see previous editions of this book.) These experiments resulted in the description of anatomical regions that when isolated in animals caused a specific respiratory pattern, for example the apneustic and pneumotaxic centres. The complexity of respiratory control in the intact animal is such that this crude anatomical approach to unravelling the various interactions was limited. In addition, human studies of function were mostly impossible.

Recent research has begun to apply modern imaging techniques such as magnetic resonance imaging (MRI)[5] and positron emission tomography (PET)[6] to localizing respiratory regions in normal human subjects, and confirms that much of the historical animal work does apply to humans. The anatomical approach to understanding respiratory patterns has also been succeeded by the biochemical approach. New research methods and the possibility of therapeutic intervention have led to an explosion of interest in the chemical interactions between and within respiratory neurones.

Anatomical location of the 'respiratory centre'

The medulla is accepted as the area of brain where the respiratory pattern is generated and where the various voluntary and involuntary demands on respiratory activity are co-ordinated. There are many neuronal connections both into and out of the medulla, as summarized in Figure 5.1, the functions of which are described below.

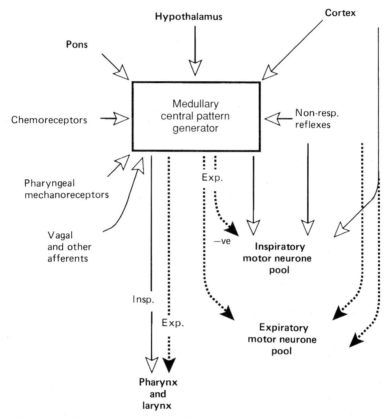

Figure 5.1 Afferent and efferent connections to and from the medullary central pattern generator. The broken lines are expiratory pathways, but the expiratory motor neurone pool normally remains silent during quiet breathing.

Respiratory neurones in the medulla are mainly concentrated in two groups – the ventral and the dorsal respiratory groups – which have numerous interconnections (Figure 5.2).[3]

The dorsal respiratory group lies in close relation to the nucleus tractus solitarius, where visceral afferents from cranial nerves IX and X terminate (Figure 5.2). It is predominantly composed of inspiratory neurones with upper motor neurones passing to the inspiratory anterior horn cells of the opposite side. The dorsal group is primarily concerned with timing of the respiratory cycle.

The ventral respiratory group comprises four nuclei. The most caudal is the nucleus retroambigualis, which is predominantly expiratory with upper motor neurones passing to

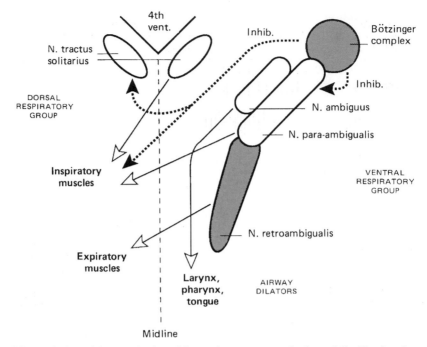

Figure 5.2 Dorsal view of the organization of the respiratory neurones in the medulla. The dorsal respiratory group (nucleus tractus solitarius) is shown on both sides. For clarity, the ventral respiratory group (Bötzinger complex, nucleus ambiguus, nucleus para-ambigualis and nucleus retroambigualis) is shown only on the right side. Areas with predominantly expiratory activity are shaded. Fibres that decussate are shown crossing the midline. The broken lines are expiratory pathways that inhibit inspiratory neurones. See text for details.

the expiratory muscles of the other side. The nucleus ambiguus controls the dilator functions of larynx, pharynx and tongue. The nucleus para-ambigualis (lying parallel to it) is mainly inspiratory and controls the force of contraction of the inspiratory muscles of the opposite side. The Bötzinger complex (within the nucleus retrofacialis) has widespread expiratory functions.

Central pattern generation (CPG)[2,7]

It is no longer sufficient to consider the generation of the respiratory rhythm to be simply oscillating networks of uniform populations of inspiratory and expiratory neurones. The respiratory pattern depends on a complex interaction of at least six groups of neurones with identifiable firing patterns spread throughout the medulla. These include early inspiratory neurones, inspiratory augmenting (ramp) neurones (Iaug), late-inspiratory interneurones (putative 'off-switch' neurones), early expiratory decrementing neurones, expiratory augmenting (ramp) neurones and late expiratory pre-inspiratory neurones. Typical firing patterns and the resulting muscle group activity are shown schematically in Figure 5.3. The resultant respiratory cycle may be divided into three phases, as follows.

Inspiratory phase. A sudden onset is followed by ramp increase in Iaug neurones resulting in motor discharge to the inspiratory muscles, including the pharyngeal dilator muscles.

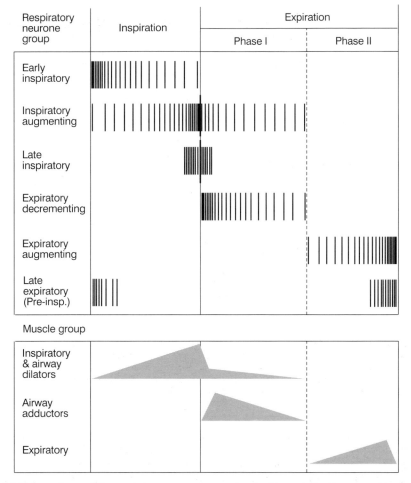

Figure 5.3 Firing patterns of the respiratory neurone groups involved in central pattern generation and the corresponding respiratory muscle group activity. Note that expiration is divided into two phases representing passive (phase I) and active (phase II) expiration. See text for details.

Pharyngeal dilator muscles start to contract shortly before the start of inspiration, possibly by activation of late expiratory (pre-inspiratory) neurones.

Postinspiratory or expiratory phase I. This is characterized by declining discharge of the inspiratory augmenting neurones and therefore motor discharge to the inspiratory muscles. Early expiratory decrementing neurones also produce declining activity in the laryngeal *adductor* muscles. This phase therefore represents passive expiration with a gradual let down of inspiratory muscle tone and an initial braking of the expiratory gas flow rate (page 114) by the larynx.

Expiratory phase II. The inspiratory muscles are now silent and, if required, expiratory augmenting neurones will be activated to produce a gradual increase in expiratory muscle activity.

Alterations in the rate at which spontaneous neuronal activity increases or decreases and the point at which the next group of neurones are activated allows an infinite variation of respiratory patterns. For example, during quiet breathing in the supine position, early expiratory neurones will reduce activity slowly and expiratory augmenting neurones will be active only briefly, resulting in almost totally passive exhalation. The converse situation will arise following exercise or at a minute volume in excess of about 40 l.min^{-1} when expiration will be immediately and almost totally active.

In practice, many such rhythm-generating networks are represented in parallel, so it is difficult to destroy the respiratory rhythm by isolated electrical or cold lesions.[8] The system is thus very robust.

Cellular mechanisms of central pattern generation.[2] Respiratory neurones that exhibit spontaneous activity achieve this by a combination of intrinsic membrane properties and excitatory and inhibitory feedback mechanisms requiring neurotransmitters. In practice, neurotransmitters (both inhibitory and excitatory) have a dual effect: they recruit other cells by direct activation and modulate the spontaneous activity of a single cell by effects on its own membrane ion channels.

In a fashion similar to rhythm generation in cardiac tissue, a combination of potassium and calcium ion channels are involved. For instance, in a single Iaug neurone slow membrane depolarization occurs, so producing a spontaneous discharge. These cells then 'recruit' other Iaug cells by excitatory postsynaptic potentials (EPSPs) and a crescendo of Iaug activity develops. Calcium-dependent potassium channels then begin to be activated and repolarize the cells, so 'switching off' the Iaug respiratory group. Activation of other cell groups, for instance expiratory augmenting neurones, will result in activation of inhibitory postsynaptic potentials (IPSPs) on the Iaug neurones to hyperpolarize the neurone and inhibit the next wave of inspiratory activity. Similar membrane effects occur in all the respiratory neurone groups shown in Figure 5.3.

Neurotransmitters involved in CPG and respiratory control[2,9]

These are summarized in Figure 5.4.

Central pattern generation (CPG) requires a combination of excitatory and inhibitory neurotransmitters. Excitatory amino acids (usually glutamate) activate several different receptors. These are divided into two groups: *N*-methyl-D-aspartate (NMDA) receptors, which are fast-acting ion channels; and non-NMDA receptors, which are slower reacting receptors involving G-protein-mediated effects. Inhibitory neurotransmitters include glycine and GABA (γ-aminobutyric acid) acting via specific glycine receptors and GABA$_A$ receptors respectively to hyperpolarize the neurone and thereby inhibit its activity. These two inhibitory transmitters act quite independently during different phases of CPG.

Neuromodulators are substances that can influence the CPG output, but are not themselves involved in rhythm generation. There are numerous neuromodulators of respiration, many of which have several subtypes of receptors. Their exact role in normal human respiration remains unclear, but they are of undoubted relevance in both normal and abnormal breathing. For example, exogenous opioids are known to have an enormous effect in depressing respiratory activity in humans, indicating the presence of opioid receptors in the respiratory centre (which inhibit glutamate activity).[9] However, administration of the opioid antagonist naloxone has no effect on respiration in resting normal subjects but does increase the ventilatory response to chemical stimuli (hypoxia or hypercapnia), indicating that endogenous opioids have a damping effect on some reflex stimuli of respiration.

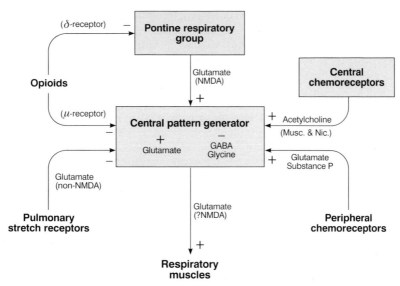

Figure 5.4 Neurotransmitters and neuromodulators in the respiratory centre. Boxes indicate functional neuronal groups and bold type represents other influences on the respiratory centre. Substances involved in neurotransmission are shown with the most likely receptor subtype, in parentheses, if known. + indicates excitatory effect increasing respiratory activity; – indicates inhibitory activity decreasing respiration. Many of the connections shown may not be active during normal resting conditions (see text for details). (After references 2 and 8.)

Other neuromodulators include acetylcholine, which acts via both muscarinic and nicotinic receptors to mediate the effect of central chemoreceptors on respiration. Serotonin (5-hydroxytryptamine) has many conflicting effects on respiration as a result of the numerous receptor subtypes present. Glutamate acts as a neuromodulator via both NMDA and non-NMDA receptors to mediate the pontine influence on CPG, and is also involved in the influence of pulmonary stretch receptors and peripheral chemoreceptors on the respiratory pattern. Substance P also has an excitatory influence, resulting in an increase in tidal volume in response to peripheral chemoreceptor activity.

Efferent pathways from the respiratory centre

Respiratory motor neurones in the brainstem are pooled into two separate areas, corresponding to inspiratory and expiratory muscle activity (see Figure 5.1). The complex integration of respiratory control seen in the CPG neurones continues to take place at the junction of the upper motor neurone with the anterior horn cell of the lower motor neurone.[10] Three groups of upper motor neurones converge on the anterior horn cells supplying the respiratory muscles. The first group of upper motor neurones is from the dorsal and ventral respiratory groups of the medulla and are concerned with both inspiratory and expiratory output from the CPG. The second group is concerned with voluntary control of breathing (speech, respiratory gymnastics, etc.) and the third group with involuntary non-rhythmic respiratory control (swallowing, cough, hiccup, etc.). Each group of upper motor neurones occupies a specific anatomical location in the spinal cord. Experimental selective cordotomies can interfere with rhythmic but not voluntary respiration, particularly during sleep; Newsom Davis in 1974 described a patient with partial transverse cervical myelitis who had normal rhythmic breathing but could not voluntarily alter his ventilation.[11]

Neuronal control of the respiratory muscles is described in Chapter 6.

Central nervous system connections to the respiratory centre

The pons[2]

There is no doubt of the existence of pontine neurones firing in synchrony with different phases of respiration, now referred to as the pontine respiratory group (PRG). Previously known as the pneumotaxic centre, three groups of neurones were identified (inspiratory, expiratory and phase-spanning) which were believed to be involved in controlling the timing of the respiratory cycle. The PRG is no longer considered to be essential for the generation of the respiratory rhythm, but does nevertheless influence the medullary respiratory neurones via a multisynaptic pathway contributing to fine control of the respiratory rhythm as, for example, in setting the lung volume at which inspiration is terminated. There are many central afferent pathways into the PRG, including connections to the hypothalamus, the cortex and the nucleus tractus solitarius. These connections suggest that the pons regulates the respiratory effects of numerous CNS activities, including cortical control, peripheral sensory information (odour, temperature) and visceral/cardiovascular inputs. ∮ medulla

Cerebral cortex[12]

Breathing can be voluntarily interrupted and the pattern of respiratory movements altered within limits determined mainly by changes in arterial blood gas tensions. This is essential for such acts as speaking, singing, sniffing, coughing, expulsive efforts and the performance of tests of ventilatory function. There is now some evidence that the neurones involved in this cortical 'override' of respiration may completely bypass the respiratory centre and act directly on the respiratory muscle lower motor neurones.[13]

Volitional changes in respiration are common, and in some circumstances overcome the usual chemical control of respiration. Douglas and Haldane in 1909 observed periods of apnoea following voluntary hyperventilation[14] by subjects aware of the classic paper of Haldane and Priestley four years earlier[15] describing the major role of carbon dioxide in the regulation of breathing. The apnoea was ascribed to reduction of $P\text{co}_2$ below the apnoeic threshold (see below). However, in 1961 Fink[16] found that 13 conscious subjects who were unaware of the role of $P\text{co}_2$ all continued to breathe rhythmically during recovery from reduction of end-expiratory $P\text{co}_2$ to 3.3 kPa (25 mmHg) or less. Conscious drive may well maintain breathing in subjects following hyperventilation, as apnoea may be consistently produced by moderate hypocapnia in anaesthetized patients.[17]

There are usually minor changes in the respiratory pattern when subjects focus their attention on their breathing, as when physiological mouthpieces or breathing masks are used.[18]

In addition to volitional changes in the pattern of breathing, there are numerous other suprapontine reflex interferences with respiration such as sneezing, swallowing and coughing. Reflex control of respiration during speech is a complex process.[19] During prolonged conversation, respiratory rate and tidal volume must be maintained approximately normal to prevent biochemical disturbance. In addition, for speech to be easily understood, pauses to allow inspiration must occur at appropriate boundaries in the text –

for example, between sentences. There is now evidence that the brain performs complex assessments of the forthcoming speech to select appropriate size breaths to prevent cumbersome interruptions. This is easier to achieve during reading aloud when 88 per cent of breaths are taken at appropriate boundaries in the text,[20] compared with a figure of only 63 per cent during spontaneous speech.[19]

Ondine's curse (primary alveolar hypoventilation syndrome)

In 1962 Severinghaus and Mitchell[21] described three patients who exhibited long periods of apnoea, even when awake, but who breathed on command. They termed the condition 'Ondine's curse' from its first description in German legend. The water nymph, Ondine, having been jilted by her mortal husband, took from him all automatic functions, requiring him to remember to breathe. When he finally fell asleep, he died. The condition is seen in adults with primary alveolar hypoventilation occurring as a feature of many different diseases, including chronic poliomyelitis and cerebrovascular accidents.[22] Characteristics include a raised P_{CO_2} in the absence of pulmonary pathology, a flat CO_2/ventilation response curve and periods of apnoea which may be central or obstructive. A similar condition is also produced by overdosage with opiates.

Ondine's curse is also used to describe the rare condition of congenital central hypoventilation syndrome in which babies are born with a permanent defect in automatic respiratory control, leading to apnoea and hypoventilation during sleep.[23,24] In addition, these children have abnormal respiratory responses to exercise[25] and, in keeping with the German legend, also have abnormalities of cardiac control.[26] In spite of such severe abnormalities, non-invasive methods of nocturnal ventilation and diaphragmatic pacing have allowed almost normal lives in many of these children.[24]

Peripheral input to the respiratory centre and non-chemical reflexes
Pulmonary stretch reflexes

There are a large number of different types of receptors in the lungs[27,28] sensitive to inflation, deflation, mechanical and chemical stimulation, afferents from which are mostly conducted by the vagus although some fibres may be carried in the sympathetic nerves. The stretch receptors are predominantly in the airways rather than in the alveoli, with slowly adapting receptors in the tracheobronchial smooth muscle and rapidly adapting receptors[29] in the superficial mucosal layer. These receptors have attracted much attention since the associated inflation and deflation reflexes were described by Hering[30] and Breuer[31] in 1868. Breuer was a clinical assistant to Professor Hering but apparently the work was at his own instigation. However, Hering, who was a corresponding member of the Vienna Academy of Science, published Breuer's work under his own name, in accord with the custom of the time.[30] Breuer's role was clearly stated in Hering's paper but he was not a co-author. Later the same year, Breuer published a much fuller account of his work under his own name.[31] The extent of the individual contributions of Hering and Breuer has been discussed by Ullmann,[32] who also appended an English translation of the original papers.

The inflation reflex consists of inhibition of inspiration in response to an increased pulmonary transmural pressure gradient (as in sustained inflation of the lung). An exactly similar effect may be obtained by obstructing expiration so that an inspiration is retained in the lungs.

The significance of the Hering–Breuer reflex in humans remains controversial.[33] There seems to be a most important species difference between humans and the laboratory animals in which the reflex is so easy to demonstrate. In 1961, Widdicombe[34] compared the strength of the inflation reflex in eight species and found the reflex weakest in humans, concluding that '. . . caution must be exercised before ascribing any important role to the Hering–Breuer reflexes in modifying the pattern of breathing in healthy man'. This is borne out in studies showing no effect of bilateral vagal block on breathing patterns in volunteers,[35] and it is also clear that patients have essentially normal ventilatory patterns after bilateral lung transplant when both lungs must be totally denervated (Chapter 33). It has also been noted (page 73) that end-expiratory obstruction *augments* the force of the inspiratory muscles. Although the Hering–Breuer inflation reflex therefore appears to have minimal functional significance in humans, its existence has been demonstrated in adults,[34,36] and it is widely accepted as being present in neonates and infants.[37]

The deflation reflex consists of an augmentation of inspiration in response to deflation of the lung and can be demonstrated in humans.[38] These results were consistent with the hypothesis that lung deflation has a reflex excitatory effect on breathing, but that the threshold is higher in humans than for other mammalian species.

The inflation and deflation reflexes were the basis of the *Selbsteuerung* (self-steering) hypothesis of Hering and Breuer. This concept has played a major role in theories of the control of breathing and, even though its role in humans may be questionable, it remains a classic example of a physiological autoregulating mechanism.

Head's paradoxical reflex. Head, working in Professor Hering's laboratory, described a reversal of the inflation reflex.[39] This could be elicited during partial block of the vagus nerves in the rabbit when inflation of the lung caused strong maintained contractions of an isolated diaphragmatic slip. Many authors have reported that, with normal vagal conduction, sudden inflation of the lungs of many species may cause a transient inspiratory effort before the onset of apnoea due to the inflation reflex.[34] A similar response may also be elicited in newborn infants,[40] but it has not been established whether this 'gasp reflex' is analogous to Head's paradoxical reflex. All anaesthetists are aware that, after administration of respiratory depressants, transient increases in airway pressure often cause an immediate deep gasping type of inspiration. There is a possible relationship between the reflex and the mechanism of sighing, which may be considered a normal feature of breathing.[41]

Other pulmonary afferents

C-fibre endings. These endings lie in close relationship to the capillaries: one group is in relation to the bronchial circulation and the other to the pulmonary microcirculation. The latter correspond to Paintal's juxtapulmonary capillary receptors (J receptors, for short).[29,42,43,44]

These receptors are relatively silent during normal breathing but are stimulated under various pathological conditions. They seem to be nociceptive and activated by tissue damage, accumulation of interstitial fluid and release of various mediators.[28] In the laboratory they can be activated by intravascular injection of capsaicin to produce the so-called pulmonary chemoreflex which comprises bradycardia, hypotension, apnoea or shallow breathing,[29] bronchoconstriction and increased secretion of mucus. They may well be concerned in the dyspnoea of pulmonary vascular congestion and the ventilatory

response to exercise and pulmonary embolization. C-fibre endings have been characterized in physiological studies but have never been identified histologically, although
non-myelinated nerve fibres are seen in the alveolar walls.

Phrenic nerve afferents[45]

Approximately one-third of neurones in the phrenic nerve are afferent, with the majority
arising from muscle spindles and tendon organs forming the spinal reflex arc described on
page 122. However, some afferent neurones continue through the ipsilateral spinal cord to
the brainstem and somatosensory cortex. Experimental stimulation of phrenic afferent
fibres generally results in a reduction of respiratory efferent activity known as phrenic-to-
phrenic inhibition, but stimulation of some smaller afferent fibres has the opposite effect.
Thus the physiological role of phrenic afferents remains obscure, but it is unlikely that
they have any influence on normal breathing. The sensory information provided by
phrenic afferents is believed to be important in the perception of, and compensation for,
increased inspiratory loads and these afferents are important in the 'breaking point'
following a breath hold (page 105).

Reflexes arising from the upper respiratory tract[27,29,46]

The nose. Water and stimulants such as ammonia or cigarette smoke may cause apnoea as
part of the diving reflex (page 402). Irritants can initiate sneezing which, unlike coughing,
cannot be undertaken voluntarily. There are also cold receptors that initiate bronchoconstriction in sensitive subjects.

The pharynx. Mechanoreceptors that respond to pressures play a major role in activation
of the pharyngeal dilator muscles (page 113). There is ample evidence that local
anaesthesia of the pharynx impairs their action. Irritants may cause bronchodilatation,
hypertension, tachycardia and secretion of mucus in the lower airway.

The larynx. The larynx has a dense sensory innervation with fibres from the subglottal
region in the recurrent laryngeal nerve and those from the supraglottic region in the
internal branch of the superior laryngeal nerve. Most reflexes arise from the supraglottic
area, as section of the latter nerve abolishes almost all reflex activity. There are three
groups of receptors. Mechanoreceptors respond to changes in transmural pressure or
laryngeal motion and result in increased pharyngeal dilator muscle activity, particularly
during airway obstruction. Cold receptors are found superficially on the vocal folds and
activation generally results in depression of ventilation. The importance of this reflex in
adult humans is uncertain, but these receptors may produce bronchoconstriction in
susceptible individuals (see Chapter 27). Irritant receptors respond to many substances
such as distilled water, cigarette smoke and halothane, and, in a fashion similar to
direct mechanical stimulation of the larynx, cause cough, laryngeal closure and
bronchoconstriction.

The cough reflex may be elicited by chemical or mechanical stimuli arising in the larynx,
trachea, carina or main bronchi. Which of these sites is responsible for the initiation of a
cough is difficult to determine. For chemical stimuli the larynx may be of less importance,
as superior laryngeal nerve block has little effect on cough stimulated by inhalation of
citric acid,[47] and in patients following heart–lung transplant the inhalation of the normally

potent stimulant distilled water results in little or no cough.[48] Coughing can be undertaken voluntarily but the reflex is complex and comprises three main stages:

1. An inspiration, which takes into the lungs a volume of air sufficient for the expiratory activity.
2. Build-up of pressure in the lungs by contraction of expiratory muscles against a closed glottis.
3. Forceful expiration occurs through narrowed airways, resulting in high linear velocity of gas flow, which sweeps irritant material up towards the pharynx.

Transient changes of pressure up to 40 kPa (300 mmHg) may occur in the thorax, arterial blood and the cerebrospinal fluid (CSF) during the act of coughing.

Baroreceptor reflexes

The most important groups of arterial baroreceptors are in the carotid sinus and around the aortic arch. These receptors are primarily concerned with regulation of the circulation, but a large decrease in arterial pressure produces hyperventilation, whereas in animals a substantial rise in arterial pressure causes respiratory depression and, ultimately, apnoea.

Afferents from the musculoskeletal system

A variety of mechanical stimuli applied to the gastrocnemius muscle of the dog can produce a reflex increase in ventilation.[49] This occurred when afferents from the pressure–pain receptors were blocked by antidromic stimulation. Afferents from the musculoskeletal system probably do not contribute to normal resting ventilation but have an important role in the hyperventilation of exercise (Chapter 14).

The influence of carbon dioxide on respiratory control[50,51]

Pflüger, in his classic paper of 1868, gave the first convincing evidence that breathing could be stimulated either by a reduction of oxygen content or by an increase of carbon dioxide content of the arterial blood.[52] However, the importance of the role of carbon dioxide was not fully established until the work of Haldane and Priestley[15] in 1905. In one paper they presented their technique for sampling alveolar gas, showed the constancy of the alveolar P_{CO_2} under a wide range of circumstances, and also demonstrated the great sensitivity of ventilation to small changes in alveolar P_{CO_2}.

Until recently it was generally believed that the respiratory centre itself was sensitive to carbon dioxide. However, it is now known that the central chemoreceptors, as they have come to be called, are actually separate from the respiratory neurones of the medulla although located only a short distance away. About 85 per cent of the total respiratory response to inhaled carbon dioxide originates in these medullary chemoreceptors.[53]

More recently, attention has been turned to the role of the CSF in the control of breathing. This followed the important studies of Leusen (in the 1950s) who showed that the ventilation of anaesthetized dogs was stimulated by perfusion of the ventriculocisternal system with mock CSF of elevated P_{CO_2} and reduced pH.[54,55]

Localization of the central chemoreceptors

Leusen's work touched off a long series of studies aimed at localizing central chemoreceptors. They were thought to lie superficially and in contact with one or other of the reservoirs of CSF, because it seemed unlikely that changes in the composition of the CSF could influence the respiratory neurones within the substance of the medulla in the few minutes required for full development of the ventilatory response to inhaled carbon dioxide.

It has now been shown that the central chemosensitive areas are on the anterolateral surfaces of the medulla, close to the origins of the glossopharyngeal and vagus nerves, and crossed by the anterior inferior cerebellar arteries.[56] In the cat, there are bilateral rostral (Mitchell) and caudal (Loeschcke) areas that are sensitive to pH (Figure 5.5). It seems likely that their connections pass through a third intermediate area, as all chemosensitivity is lost if the intermediate areas are destroyed.[57]

More recently, c-fos immunochemistry has been used in animals to identify the medullary neurones that responded to stimulation by carbon dioxide.[59] Evidence of stimulation was found in the rostral and caudal areas of the anterior medulla, and the most stimulated cells lay within 0.2 mm of the surface. In addition, MRI and PET scanning techniques during CO_2-stimulated breathing in humans have confirmed that the surface of the anterior medulla is the primary site of chemosensitive neurone activity.[5,6] Other areas of the CNS that display increased neural activity with CO_2 stimulation include other regions of the medulla, the midline pons, small areas in the cerebellum, and the limbic system,[5,6] though the contribution of these areas to respiratory control is unclear at present.

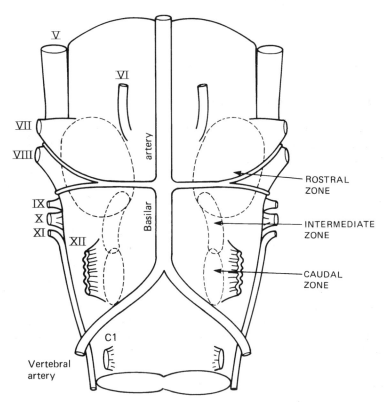

Figure 5.5 Location of the chemoreceptor zones on the anterolateral surface of the medulla of the cat. (After reference 58 by permission of the Editors of the *Bulletin de Physio-Pathologie Respiratoire*.)

Mechanism of action

An elevation of arterial P_{CO_2} causes an approximately equal rise of CSF, cerebral tissue and jugular venous P_{CO_2}, which are all about 1.3 kPa (10 mmHg) more than the arterial P_{CO_2}. In the short term, and without change in CSF bicarbonate, a rise in CSF P_{CO_2} causes a fall in CSF pH, and it was postulated by Mitchell in 1963[56] that the reduction in pH stimulated the respiratory neurones indirectly through receptors in the chemosensitive area. The theory was especially attractive because the time course of change in CSF pH accorded with the well-known delay in the ventilatory response to a change in arterial P_{CO_2}. The blood/brain barrier (operative between blood and CSF) is permeable to carbon dioxide but not hydrogen ions, and in this respect resembles the membrane of a P_{CO_2}-sensitive electrode (page 242). In both cases, carbon dioxide crosses the barrier and hydrates to carbonic acid, which then ionizes to give a pH inversely proportional to the log of the P_{CO_2}. A hydrogen ion sensor is thus made to respond to P_{CO_2}. This accords with the old observation that the ventilatory response to respiratory acidosis is greater than that to a metabolic acidosis with the same change in *blood* pH. Ventilation is, in fact, a single function of CSF pH in both conditions.[60]

The precise mechanism by which a change in pH causes stimulation of neurones is not firmly established, but it could clearly influence the action of an enzyme. Decreased pH inhibits the metabolism of acetylcholine by choline esterase, and it has been observed that atropine blocks the CO_2 sensitivity of the central chemoreceptors, which effect has been shown to occur at M_2 muscarinic receptors.[61]

Compensatory bicarbonate shift in the CSF. If the P_{CO_2} of CSF is maintained at an abnormal level, the CSF pH gradually returns towards normal over the course of many hours as a result of changes in the CSF bicarbonate level. This is analogous to and proceeds in parallel with the partial restoration of blood pH in patients with chronic hyper- or hypocapnia. The mechanism of the shift in bicarbonate was originally thought to be due to active transport of bicarbonate ion.[62] However, it was later found that compensatory changes were similar in both CSF and blood,[63,64] suggesting that bicarbonate shift could result from passive ion distribution, although the possibility of active ion transfer cannot be completely excluded.[65,66,67,68]

A shift in CSF bicarbonate occurs during prolonged periods of hypocapnic artificial ventilation and contributes to the early partial reversal of the hypocapnia that occurs in response to hypoxia at altitude (page 362). As would be expected from a passive ion transfer system, the speed at which bicarbonate shift compensates the CSF pH depends on the magnitude of the change in P_{CO_2}. After commencing passive hyperventilation the CSF bicarbonate would in theory be significantly reduced after only 1 hour,[69] and CSF pH has been reported to have returned to normal after 30 hours of hyperventilation in humans following cerebrovascular accidents.[70] A substantial resetting of the CSF pH occurs within 4.5 hours of a step increase in the ventilation of an anaesthetized paralysed dog.[68] This offers one reason why patients receiving artificial hyperventilation often continue to hyperventilate after resumption of spontaneous breathing.

Compensatory changes in CSF bicarbonate and the restoration of its pH are not confined to respiratory alkalosis, but are also found in chronic respiratory acidosis and metabolic acidosis and alkalosis.[71] In this study of patients with a variety of pathological acid–base disturbances, values of CSF pH did not differ by more than 0.011 units from the normal value (7.326) in spite of mean arterial pH values ranging from 7.334 to 7.523.

If the bicarbonate concentration in CSF is itself altered by pathological factors, the pH is changed and ventilatory disturbances follow. For example, after intracranial haemorrhage patients may spontaneously hyperventilate,[72] and in these cases the CSF pH and bicarbonate have been shown to be below the normal values. It was postulated that this was due to the metabolic breakdown products of blood which contaminated the CSF, and the correction of hyperventilation by intrathecal administration of 3–5 mmol of bicarbonate has been reported.[73]

The P_{CO_2}/ventilation response curve

Following a rise in arterial P_{CO_2}, respiratory depth and rate increase until a steady state of hyperventilation is achieved after a few minutes. The response is linear over the range that is usually studied and may therefore be defined in terms of two parameters: slope and intercept (see Appendix F):

$$\text{ventilation} = S(P_{CO_2} - B)$$

where S is the slope ($l.min^{-1}.kPa^{-1}$ or $l.min^{-1}.mmHg^{-1}$), and B is the intercept at zero ventilation (kPa or mmHg). The heavy continuous line in Figure 5.6 is a typical normal curve with an intercept (B) of about 4.8 kPa (36 mmHg) and a slope (S) of about 15 $l.min^{-1}.kPa^{-1}$ (2 $l.min^{-1}.mmHg^{-1}$). There is in fact a very wide individual variation in P_{CO_2}/ventilation response curves, and the response may be decreased by normal hormonal changes, disease or drugs. The broken curve in Figure 5.6 shows the effect of changing ventilation on arterial P_{CO_2} when the inspired carbon dioxide concentration is negligible,

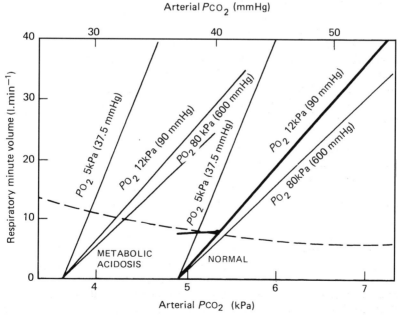

Figure 5.6 Two fans of P_{CO_2}/ventilation response curves at different values of P_{O_2}. The right-hand fan is at normal metabolic acid–base state (zero base excess). The left-hand fan represents metabolic acidosis. The broken line represents the P_{CO_2} produced by the indicated ventilation for zero inspired P_{CO_2}, at basal metabolic rate. The intersection of the broken curve and any response curve indicates the resting P_{CO_2} and ventilation for the relevant metabolic acid–base state and P_{O_2}. The heavy curve is the normal response. See text for details.

and is a section of a rectangular hyperbola. The normal resting Pco_2 and ventilation are indicated by the intersection of this curve with the normal Pco_2/ventilation response curve, which is usually obtained by varying the carbon dioxide concentration in the inspired gas.

Figure 5.6 shows two possible extensions to the response curves below the dotted curve, which defines the effect of ventilation on Pco_2. These extensions are of two types. The first is an extrapolation of the curve to intersect the X axis (zero ventilation) at a Pco_2 known as the apnoeic threshold. If Pco_2 is depressed below this point, apnoea may result, and this represents Haldane's post-hyperventilation apnoea. The second type of extension is shown on the middle line of the right-hand fan. It is horizontal and to the left, like a hockey stick, representing the response of a subject who continues to breathe regardless of the fact that his Pco_2 has been reduced (see above). The resting arterial point at resting ventilation is in fact 0.3 kPa to the left of the extrapolated response curve.[74]

As Pco_2 is raised, a point of maximal ventilatory stimulation is reached, probably in the range 13.3–26.7 kPa (100–200 mmHg), beyond which respiratory fatigue and CO_2 narcosis intervene (Chapter 22). The ventilatory stimulation is reduced until, at very high Pco_2, the ventilation is actually depressed below the control value and finally apnoea results, at least in the dog and almost certainly in humans as well.

The Pco_2/ventilation response curve is the response of the entire respiratory system to the challenge of a raised Pco_2. Apart from reduced sensitivity of the central chemoreceptors, the overall response may be blunted by partial neuromuscular blockade or by obstructive or restrictive lung disease. These factors must be taken into account in drawing conclusions from a reduced response, and diffuse airway obstruction is a most important consideration. Nevertheless, the slope of the Pco_2/ventilation response curve remains one of the most valuable parameters in the assessment of the responsiveness of the respiratory system to carbon dioxide and its depression by drugs.

Time course of Pco_2/ventilation response.[75] As described above, the initial ventilatory response to elevated Pco_2 is extremely rapid, taking place in just a few minutes, at which time about 75 per cent of the final ventilatory response has occurred. With sustained hypercapnia, the minute ventilation continues to increase for a further hour before reaching a plateau, which is sustained for at least 8 hours in healthy subjects.

The influence of oxygen on respiratory control[76]

Until 1926 it was thought that changes in the chemical composition of the blood influenced ventilation solely by direct action on the respiratory centre, which was presumed to be sensitive to these influences although direct experimental proof was lacking. However, between 1926 and 1930 there occurred a major revision following the histological studies of de Castro,[77] which led him to suggest a chemoreceptor function for the carotid bodies. These receptors were found to be sensitive to hypoxia, and the role of the carotid bodies in the control of breathing was clearly established by Heymans,[78] who received a Nobel prize in 1938 for his work.

Peripheral chemoreceptors

The peripheral chemoreceptors[79] are fast-responding monitors of the arterial blood, responding to a fall in Pa_{O_2}, a rise in Pa_{CO_2} or H^+ concentration, or a fall in their perfusion rate. An increase in ventilation is the result of stimulation. The bilaterally paired carotid bodies, rather than the aortic bodies, are almost exclusively responsible for the respiratory response. Each is only about 6 mm^3 in volume and they are located close to the bifurcation of the common carotid artery. The carotid bodies undergo hypertrophy and hyperplasia under conditions of chronic hypoxia and are usually lost in the operation of carotid endarterectomy (see below).

Histology. The carotid bodies contain large sinusoids with a very high rate of perfusion – about ten times the level that would be proportional to their metabolic rate, which is itself very high.[80] Therefore the arterial/venous Po_2 difference is small. This accords with their role as a sensor of arterial blood gas tensions, and their rapid response which is within the range 1–3 seconds.[81]

At cellular level, the main feature is the glomus or type I cell, which is in synaptic contact with nerve endings derived from an axon with its cell body in the petrosal ganglion of the glossopharyngeal nerve (Figure 5.7). These endings are mainly postsynaptic to the glomus cell. Type I cells are partly encircled by type II or sheath cells whose function is still obscure. Efferent nerves, which are known to modulate receptor afferent discharge, include preganglionic sympathetic fibres from the superior cervical ganglion, amounting to 5 per cent of the nerve endings on the glomus cell.

Discharge rate in the afferent nerves from the carotid body increases in response to the following forms of stimulation.

Decrease of arterial Po_2. Stimulation is by decreased Po_2 and not by reduced oxygen content (at least down to about half the normal value). Thus there is little stimulation in anaemia, carboxyhaemoglobinaemia or methaemoglobinaemia. Quantitative aspects of the hypoxic ventilatory response are discussed in detail below.

Decrease of arterial pH. Acidaemia of perfusing blood causes stimulation, the magnitude of which is the same whether it is due to respiratory or metabolic acidosis. Quantitatively, the change produced by elevated Pco_2 on the peripheral chemoreceptors is only about one-sixth of that caused by the action on the central chemosensitive areas (see below). This response does, however, occur very rapidly,[75] and develops only when a 'threshold' value of arterial Pco_2 is exceeded.[82]

Respiratory oscillations of Pco_2. A series of square waves of raised Pco_2 in the carotid artery of the dog results in a higher level of ventilation than is obtained when the Pco_2 is maintained steady at the same mean value.[83] Central chemoreceptors are too slow to respond to these changes, but the output of the peripheral chemoreceptor in the sinus nerve has been found to vary during the respiratory cycle. The timing of the nerve discharge suggests that the response is to the rate of rise of Pco_2 as well as to its magnitude. In contrast to animal experiments, there is no evidence that the overall ventilation in humans is higher than it would be with the same mean Pco_2 held at a steady level, and this applies even to hypoxic conditions. However, if the Pco_2 is made to rise sharply during inspiration, an augmentation of ventilation occurs.[84] This mechanism may have relevance to hyperventilation of exercise when the increased mixed venous/arterial Pco_2 difference causes a more abrupt rise in arterial Pco_2 during expiration.

Hypoperfusion of peripheral chemoreceptors causes stimulation, possibly by causing a 'stagnant hypoxia' of the chemoreceptor cells. Hypoperfusion may result from severe hypotension (systolic blood pressure less than 60 mmHg).

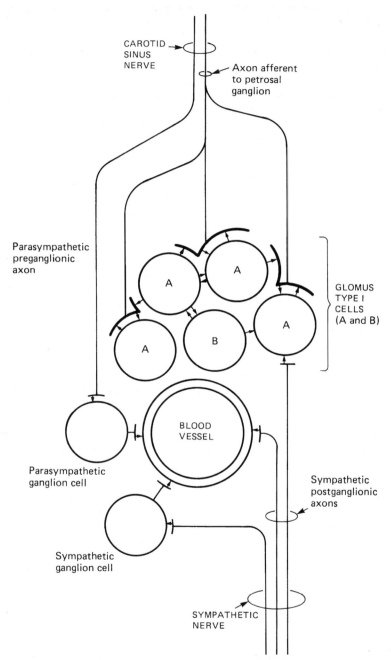

Figure 5.7 Schematic representation of the histology of the carotid bodies. Glomus type I cells are grouped around a blood vessel in the carotid body. Numerous nerve cells are also shown. This grouping would be surrounded by a sheath cell (not shown), and is sometimes termed a glomoid.

Blood temperature elevation causes stimulation of breathing via the peripheral chemoreceptors. In addition, the ventilatory responses to both hypoxia and carbon dioxide are enhanced by a modest (1.4°C) rise in body temperature.[85]

Chemical stimulation by a wide range of substances is known to cause increased ventilation through the medium of the peripheral chemoreceptors. These substances fall into two groups. The first comprises agents such as nicotine and acetylcholine, which stimulate sympathetic ganglia. The second group of chemical stimulants comprises substances such as cyanide and carbon monoxide, which block the cytochrome system and so prevent oxidative metabolism. Respiration is also stimulated through the carotid bodies by the drugs doxapram and almitrine.

Mechanism of action of peripheral chemoreceptors

In 1926, de Castro[77] postulated that glomus cells excited the carotid sinus nerve endings by products of their own metabolism in response to hypoxia (the so-called 'metabolic hypothesis'). His view has stood the test of time. In type I cells arterial hypoxaemia causes a reduction in the intracellular level of adenosine triphosphate (ATP) at levels of P_{O_2}, which have little effect elsewhere in the body. In addition, in response to hypoxia there is a graded increase in intracellular calcium concentration following its release from mitochondria, indicating that the mitochondrial membrane is the ultimate site of oxygen responsiveness.[86] Oxygen-sensitive potassium channels have been described, as have haem-based intracellular proteins that respond to changes in local P_{O_2}.[87] Stimulation of the chemoreceptors by an increased P_{CO_2} depends on carbonic anhydrase (present in the type I cell) and there is therefore the possibility of both raised P_{CO_2} and decreased arterial pH acting through an increase in intracellular hydrogen ion concentration. However, for hypoxia, raised P_{CO_2} and decreased pH, the full trans-ductive cascade of events between the stimulus and activation of the carotid sinus nerve afferents is not yet clear.

Various neurotransmitters have been identified in the carotid body, including dopamine, noradrenaline, acetylcholine, substance P and enkephalins, but the role of each is also unclear.[80] For example, dopamine is abundant in type I cells, and both carotid sinus nerve endings and type I cells have dopamine D_2 receptors. Exogenous low-dose dopamine inhibits carotid sinus nerve activity and reduces the acute hypoxic ventilatory response,[88] and selective D_2 dopamine antagonists augment the response to hypoxia[89] – indicating that dopamine has an inhibitory or 'regulatory' role in the carotid bodies. Similarly, the α_2-adrenoceptor agonist clonidine reduces the ventilatory response to acute hypoxia, indicating that noradrenaline also has an inhibitory effect.[90] It is therefore impossible at this stage to define any one critical neurotransmitter between the type I cell and the carotid sinus nerve endings. No single receptor blocker prevents the hypoxic ventilatory response.

The gain of the carotid bodies is under nervous control. There is an efferent pathway in the sinus nerve that, on excitation, decreases chemoreceptor activity. Excitation of the sympathetic nerve supply to the carotid body causes an increase in activity.[91]

Other effects of stimulation. Apart from the well-known increase in depth and rate of breathing, peripheral chemoreceptor stimulation causes a number of other effects, including bradycardia, hypertension, increase in bronchiolar tone and adrenal secretion. Stimulation of the carotid bodies has predominantly respiratory effects, whilst the aortic bodies have a greater influence on circulation.

Time course of the ventilatory response to constant isocapnic hypoxia[92]

By controlling the concentration of inhaled oxygen, arterial oxygen saturation can be reduced and then maintained at a constant level of hypoxia, usually with a Sao_2 of about 80 per cent. In order to separate the effects on ventilation of hypoxia and Pco_2, most studies use isocapnic conditions, where the subject's alveolar Pco_2 is maintained at their control (resting ventilation) level by addition of CO_2 to the inspired gas. The interaction of Pco_2 and hypoxia in ventilatory control is discussed below. With a moderate degree of sustained hypoxia the ventilatory response is triphasic as shown in Figure 5.8. The three phases are described separately.

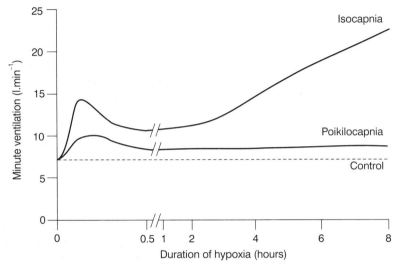

Figure 5.8 Time course of the ventilatory response to hypoxia ($Sao_2 \approx 80\%$). Practical problems prevent the continuous and rapid measurement of minute volume and respiratory gases for 8 hours, so the curves are produced from combining the data from three studies. When arterial Pco_2 is maintained at normal levels, or isocapnia, the response is triphasic. When arterial Pco_2 is not controlled, or poikilocapnia, the magnitude of the response is damped because the hypoxia-induced hyperventilation reduces Pco_2 and therefore respiratory drive. See Figure 16.3 for respiratory effects of prolonged hypoxia. (After references 93, 94 and 95.)

Acute hypoxic response is the first immediate and rapid increase in ventilation. Sudden imposition of hypoxia results in stimulation of ventilation within the lung-to-carotid body circulation time (about 6 s), but in most studies the response seems slower because of the delay between reducing inspired oxygen and the reduction in alveolar and arterial Po_2. Ventilation continues to increase for between 5 and 10 minutes, rapidly reaching high levels.

Many factors affect the acute ventilatory response. There are wide variations between individuals, within an individual on different days,[96] between male and female subjects, and with the hormonal changes of the menstrual cycle.[97] A small number of otherwise normal subjects lack a measurable ventilatory response to hypoxia when studied at normal Pco_2. This is of little importance in normal circumstances, because the Pco_2 drive from the central chemoreceptors will normally ensure a safe level of Po_2. However, in certain therapeutic and abnormal environmental circumstances, it could be dangerous. Such people would certainly do badly at high altitude.

Hypoxic ventilatory decline (HVD). Shortly after the acute hypoxic response reaches a peak, minute ventilation begins to decline, reaching a plateau level – still above the resting ventilation – after 20–30 minutes (Figure 5.8). This effect was first described in neonates, and only relatively recently described in adults.[94] The degree of HVD in a single subject correlates with the acute hypoxic response: the greater the initial increase in ventilation, the greater the subsequent decline.[94] Though not yet completely elucidated, the mechanism of HVD seems to have a significant centrally mediated component.[98] In neonates, HVD is reversed by naloxone, but this effect is not seen in adults.[99] In animals, central glutamate release is involved in the acute hypoxic response, whilst GABA is implicated in producing HVD.[100] Whether the trigger for release of these transmitters is from the peripheral chemoreceptors or a direct central effect of hypoxia remains unclear.

Ventilatory response to sustained hypoxia. Once HVD is complete, continued isocapnic hypoxia results in a second, slower, rise in ventilation over several hours (Figure 5.8).[95] Ventilation continues to increase for at least 8 hours,[95] and reaches a plateau by 24 hours.[101] Species differences in this response again make elucidation of the mechanism in humans difficult, but the most likely explanation is a direct effect of hypoxia on the carotid bodies.[95]

Hypoxia for more than 2–3 days occurs only after ascent to altitude (the effects of this are discussed in Chapter 16). Finally, over many years there is a loss of hypoxic drive, which is grossly attenuated in residents at very high altitude.[102]

Ventilatory response to progressive hypoxia

Instead of maintaining a constant degree of hypoxia, ventilation may be measured during a progressive reduction in Po_2. Once again, by controlling inspired gas concentrations, alveolar Po_2 may be reduced from 16 to 5 kPa (120 to 40 mmHg) over 15 minutes,[103] and ventilation increases progressively throughout this period. The response in these circumstances probably equates to the acute hypoxic response. If alveolar Po_2 is plotted against minute ventilation, a Po_2/ventilation response curve is produced (Figure 5.9). A Po_2/ventilation response curve approximates to a rectangular hyperbola (see Appendix F), asymptotic to the ventilation at high Pa_{O_2} (zero hypoxic drive) and to the Pa_{O_2} at which ventilation theoretically becomes infinite (known as 'C', and about 4.3 kPa). Figure 5.9 shows a typical example but there are very wide individual variations. Note that there is a small but measurable difference in ventilation between normal and very high Po_2.

The initial ventilatory response to Po_2 may be expressed as:

$$\frac{W}{Pa_{O_2} - C}$$

where W is a multiplier (i.e. the gain of the system) and partly dependent upon the Pco_2. The ventilatory response here is the difference between the actual ventilation and the ventilation at high Po_2, Pco_2 being unchanged.

The inconvenience of the non-linear relationship between ventilation and Po_2 may be overcome by plotting ventilation against oxygen saturation. The relationship is then linear with a negative slope, at least down to a saturation of 70 per cent.[106] This approach is the basis of a simple non-invasive method of measurement of the hypoxic ventilatory response (see below).

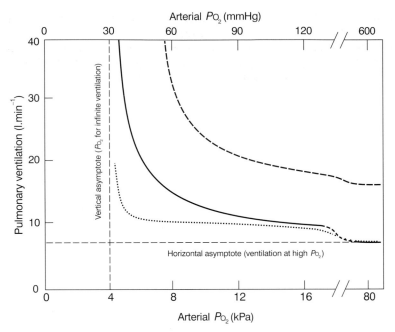

Figure 5.9 Ventilatory response to progressive hypoxia. The heavy curve represents the normal P_{O_2}/ventilation response under isocapnic conditions, that is with P_{CO_2} maintained at the resting value. It has the form of a rectangular hyperbola asymptotic to the ventilation at high P_{O_2} and the P_{O_2} at which ventilation becomes infinite. The curve is displaced upwards by both hypercapnia and exercise at normal P_{CO_2} (dashed line). Hypocapnia displaces the curve downwards (dotted line) regardless of whether the hypocapnia results from not controlling P_{CO_2} (poikilocapnia) or by deliberately reducing P_{CO_2}. (Drawn from data in references 103, 104 and 105)

Iatrogenic loss of peripheral chemoreceptor sensitivity

Nerves from the carotid bodies are usually divided during bilateral carotid endarterectomy,[107] which provides evidence that the carotid bodies are not essential for the maintenance of reasonably normal breathing under conditions of rest and mild exercise. Indeed, there is some evidence that the common finding of atheromatous disease at the carotid bifurcation may itself reduce chemoreceptor function and that a careful 'nerve sparing' carotid endarterectomy can increase the ventilatory response to hypoxia.[108] Deliberate abolition of the hypoxic ventilatory response by carotid endarterectomy has been advocated as a treatment for incapacitating dyspnoea in severe respiratory disease.[109]

Anaesthetics have a depressant effect on the initial ventilatory response to hypoxia (Chapter 21), and all patients without peripheral chemoreceptor sensitivity are dangerously at risk if exposed to low partial pressures of oxygen or if they also lose their central chemosensitivity.

Central hypoxic depression of breathing

In addition to its effects on peripheral chemoreceptors, hypoxia also has a direct effect on the respiratory centre. Central respiratory neurones are depressed by hypoxia, and apnoea follows severe medullary hypoxia whether due to ischaemia or to hypoxaemia. With denervated peripheral chemoreceptors, phrenic motor activity becomes silent when the medullary P_{O_2} falls to about 1.7 kPa (13 mmHg).[110] More intense hypoxia causes a resumption of breathing with an abnormal pattern, possibly driven by a 'gasping' centre. This pattern of central hypoxic depression seems to be particularly marked in neonates and may be the relic of a mechanism to prevent the fetus from attempting to breathe *in utero*.

Mechanisms of hypoxic depression of ventilation. Medullary P_{CO_2}, and therefore ventilation, may be reduced by increased cerebral blood flow induced by hypoxia, and severe hypoxia causes depletion of high energy phosphates. However, it has also been shown that neonatal hypoxia results in decreased levels of excitatory neurotransmitters (glutamate and aspartate) and increased levels of inhibitory substances, particularly GABA and endogenous opioids, both powerful respiratory depressants.

Other cerebral regions that contribute to respiratory control, for example the hypothalamus, are also sensitive to changes in P_{O_2} but the functional significance of this observation is not yet known.[12]

Integration of the chemical control of breathing

The two main systems contributing to chemical control of breathing have been described quite separately, but in the intact subject this is not possible. For example, the peripheral chemoreceptors respond (slightly) to changes in P_{CO_2}, and hypoxia affects the respiratory centre directly as well as via the carotid body receptors. An overall view of the chemical control of breathing is shown schematically in Figure 5.10.

It was originally thought that the various factors interacted according to the algebraic sum of the individual effects caused by changes of P_{CO_2}, P_{O_2}, pH, etc. Hypoxia and hypercapnia were, for example, thought to be simply additive in their effects, but it is now realized that this was a very simplistic view of a complex system.

Effects of P_{CO_2} and pH on the hypoxic ventilatory response[103]

The acute hypoxic response is enhanced at elevated P_{CO_2} as shown by the upper dashed curve in Figure 5.9, the mechanism being indicated by broken line B in Figure 5.10. This interaction contributes to the ventilatory response in asphyxia being greater than the sum of the response to be expected from the rise in P_{CO_2} and the fall in P_{O_2} if considered separately.

Responses to both acute and prolonged hypoxia are depressed by hypocapnia, as shown in the lower dotted curve in Figure 5.9. This results from opposing effects on the CPG of increased chemoreceptor input and decreased central chemoreceptor drive. On prolonged exposure to hypoxia at altitude, this effect continues until acclimatization takes place (page 360).

Poikilocapnic conditions occur when no attempt is made to control P_{CO_2} during hypoxic ventilation, and the hypoxia-induced hyperventilation immediately gives rise to hypocapnia. Though rarely studied, this situation is important, because poikilocapnia will occur in clinical situations. Early studies of the effects of P_{CO_2} on hypoxic ventilation showed that without control of P_{CO_2} the hypoxia-driven increase in ventilation is almost exactly counteracted by the P_{CO_2}-driven depression of ventilation, resulting in no change in minute volume until breathing less than 10% oxygen.[104,105] Many earlier studies were,

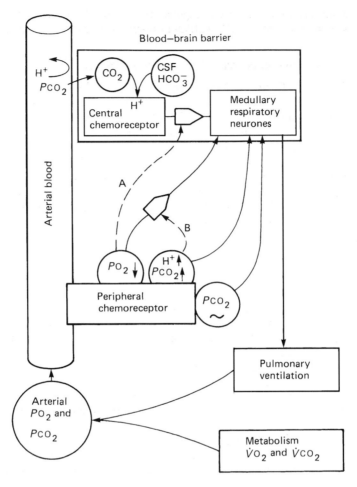

Figure 5.10 Scheme of connections between individual aspects of chemical control of breathing. See text for details.

however, performed before technology allowed elucidation of the time course of hypoxic ventilation, and may have been measuring the plateau of ventilation after hypoxic ventilatory decline rather than the acute hypoxic response. More recent studies have shown that poikilocapnic conditions attenuate, but do not abolish, the first two phases of the ventilatory response to constant hypoxia (see Figures 5.8 and 5.9).[93,94] Increasing ventilation with sustained (over 1 hour) hypoxia is abolished during poikilocapnia but the minute volume remains above resting levels (Figure 5.8).[95]

Exercise enhances the response to hypoxia even if the P_{CO_2} is not raised,[111] possibly due to lactic acidosis, oscillations of Pa_{CO_2}, afferents from muscle, or perhaps to catecholamine secretion. The upper broken curve in Figure 5.9 would also correspond to the response during exercise at an oxygen consumption of about 800 ml.min^{-1}. It is important to note that the slope of the curve at normal P_{O_2} is considerably increased in both these circumstances, so there will then be an appreciable 'hypoxic' drive to ventilation at normal Po_2. Enhanced response to Po_2 during exercise seems to be an important component in the overall ventilatory response to exercise (Chapter 14).

Effects of Pa_{O_2} and pH on central chemoreceptor response[82]

The broken line (A) in Figure 5.10 shows the influence of the peripheral chemoreceptor drive on the gain of the central ventilatory response to Pco_2. Typical quantitative relationships are shown in Figure 5.6, with hypoxia at the left of the fan and hyperoxia on the right. The curve marked Po_2 80 kPa represents total abolition of chemoreceptor drive obtained by the inhalation of 100% oxygen.

Metabolic acidosis displaces the whole fan of curves to the left, as shown in Figure 5.6. The intercept (B) is reduced but the slope of the curves at each value of Po_2 is virtually unaltered. Display of the fan of Pco_2/ventilation response curves at different Po_2 is a particularly complete method for representing the state of respiratory control in a patient, but it is unfortunately laborious to determine.

Breath holding

Influence of Pco_2 and Po_2

When the breath is held after air breathing, the arterial and alveolar Pco_2 are remarkably constant at the breaking point and values are normally close to 6.7 kPa (50 mmHg). This does not mean that Pco_2 is the sole or dominant factor, and concomitant hypoxia is probably more important. Preliminary oxygen breathing delays the onset of hypoxia, and breath-holding times may be greatly prolonged with consequent elevation of Pco_2 at the breaking point. The relationship between Pco_2 and Po_2 at breaking point, after starting from different levels of oxygenation, is shown in Figure 5.11. The breaking point curve is displaced upwards and to the left by carotid body resection.[112] Breath holding is prolonged after the vagus and glossopharyngeal nerves are blocked, but the workers who performed this study advanced cogent reasons for believing that this was not due primarily to block of the chemoreceptor[113] (see below). Oxygen breathing would also reduce the chemoreceptor drive but this did not prolong breath holding to the same extent as the nerve block.

On the basis of changing blood gas tensions and the great variability of individuals' responses, it might be predicted that subjects with 'flat' ventilatory responses to oxygen and carbon dioxide would be able to hold their breath longer. Elite breath-hold divers have been shown to have a blunted response to carbon dioxide but not to hypoxia (page 381).[114]

Effect of lung volume

Breath-holding time is directly proportional to the lung volume at the onset of breath holding, partly because this has a major influence on oxygen stores. There are, however, other effects of lung volume and its change, which are mediated by afferents arising from the chest wall, the diaphragm and the lung itself. Prolongation of breath-holding times are seen after bilateral vagal and glossopharyngeal nerve block.[113] As a sequel to these studies, Campbell et al. in 1967–9 reported prolongation of breath-holding time following curarization of conscious subjects.[115,116] Their explanation was that much of the distress leading to the termination of breath holding is caused by frustration of the involuntary contractions of the respiratory muscles, which increase progressively during breath

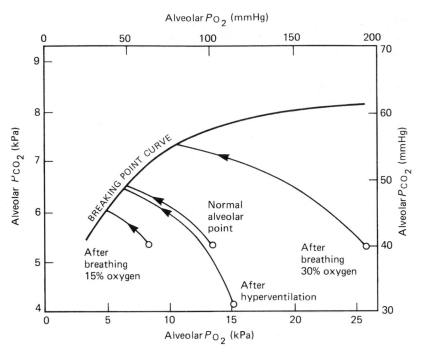

Figure 5.11 The 'breaking point' curve defines the coexisting values of alveolar P_{O_2} and P_{CO_2}, at the breaking point of breath holding, starting from various states. The normal alveolar point is shown and the curved arrow shows the changes in alveolar gas tensions that occur during breath holding. Starting points are displaced to the right by preliminary breathing of oxygen-enriched gases, and to the left by breathing mixtures containing less than 21% oxygen. Hyperventilation displaces the point representing alveolar gas to the right and downwards. The length of arrows from starting point to the breaking point curve gives an approximate indication of the duration of breath hold. This can clearly be prolonged by oxygen breathing or by hyperventilation, maximal duration occurring after hyperventilation with 100% oxygen.

holding. It seems that the inappropriateness arises in the diaphragm rather than in the intercostals.[117]

Fowler's experiment in 1954 demonstrated the importance of frustration of involuntary respiratory movements.[118] After normal air breathing, the breath is held until breaking point. If the expirate is then taken in a bag and immediately reinhaled, there is a marked sense of relief although it may be shown that the rise of P_{CO_2} and fall of P_{O_2} are uninfluenced.

Extreme durations of breath holding may be attained after hyperventilation and preoxygenation. Times of 14 minutes have been reached, and the limiting factor is then reduction of lung volume to residual volume, as oxygen is removed from the alveolar gas.

Outline of methods for assessment of factors in control of breathing

In assessing the control of breathing under ideal conditions, arterial blood gas tensions would be measured continuously. In practice, this is invasive and rapid measurements are impossible, so in almost all cases end-tidal gas concentrations are measured and converted to partial pressure. In normal healthy subjects with reasonably slow respiratory rates, these measurements will equate well to alveolar and therefore arterial tension, but this may not be the case in patients.

Sensitivity to carbon dioxide

A lack of ventilatory response to carbon dioxide may result from impaired function of the respiratory system anywhere between the medullary neurones and the mechanical properties of the lung (see Figure 26.2). Thus it cannot be assumed that a decreased ventilation/P_{CO_2} response is necessarily due to failure of the central chemoreceptor mechanism.

The steady state method requires the simultaneous measurement of minute volume and P_{CO_2} after P_{CO_2} has been raised by increasing the concentration of carbon dioxide in the inspired gas. The ventilation is usually reasonably stable after 5 minutes of inhaling a fixed concentration of carbon dioxide. Severinghaus's pseudo steady state method[119] measures ventilation after 4 minutes and is a useful compromise giving highly repeatable results.[74] Several points are needed to define the P_{CO_2}/ventilation response curve and it is a time-consuming process, which may be distressing to some patients.

The rebreathing method introduced by Read in 1967 has greatly simplified determination of the slope of the P_{CO_2}/ventilation response curve.[120] The subject rebreathes for up to 4 minutes from a 6-litre bag originally containing 7% carbon dioxide and about 50% oxygen, the remainder being nitrogen. The carbon dioxide concentration rises steadily during rebreathing while the oxygen concentration should remain above 30 per cent. Thus there should be no appreciable hypoxic drive and ventilation is driven solely by the rising arterial P_{CO_2}, which should be very close to the P_{CO_2} of the gas in the bag. Ventilation is measured by any convenient means and plotted against the P_{CO_2} of the gas in the bag. An automated technique may be used by which the P_{CO_2}/ventilation response curve is automatically determined and presented on an X–Y plotter.[121]

The P_{CO_2}/ventilation response curve measured by the rebreathing technique is displaced to the right by about 0.7 kPa (5 mmHg) compared with the steady state method, but the slope agrees closely with the steady state method.[74,120]

The $P_{CO_2}/P_{0.1}$ response. It has been suggested that a better indication of the output of the respiratory centre may be obtained by measuring the effect of P_{CO_2} on the subatmospheric pressure developed in the airways when obstructed for 0.1 second at the beginning of inspiration ($P_{0.1}$).[122] This eliminates any effect due to increased airway resistance or reduced compliance. Nevertheless, it is still influenced by impaired performance in the lower motor neurones or respiratory muscles.

Sensitivity to hypoxia

There is often some reluctance to test sensitivity to hypoxia because the patient is exposed to a reduction in P_{O_2}. Various approaches to the problem have been described,[123] of which three are used (albeit rarely) in practice.

The steady state method is the classic technique and is best undertaken by preparing P_{CO_2}/ventilation response curves at different levels of P_{O_2}, which are presented as a fan (see Figure 5.6). The spread of the fan is an indication of peripheral chemoreceptor sensitivity but it is also possible to present the data in the form of the rectangular hyperbola (see Figure 5.9) by plotting the ventilatory response for different values of Po_2 at the same Pco_2 (intercepts of components of the fan with a vertical line drawn through a particular value of Pco_2). The parameters of the hyperbola may then be derived as outlined above.

A minimum of 5 minutes is required to reach a steady state for Pco_2, although it is possible to speed up the process by varying Po_2 while keeping Pco_2 constant. Alternatively, the ventilation may be kept approximately constant while both Pco_2 and Po_2 are raised by appropriate amounts so that the Pco_2 stimulus increases by the same amount as the hypoxic drive diminishes. Nevertheless, it is a laborious undertaking to determine the oxygen response by these methods and patients may be distressed, particularly by the run at low Po_2 and high Pco_2.

The rebreathing method has been adapted to measure the response to hypoxia.[106] The oxygen concentration of the rebreathed gas is reduced by the oxygen consumption of the subject, but active steps have to be taken to maintain the Pco_2 at a constant level. Calculation of the response is greatly simplified by measuring the oxygen saturation (usually non-invasively by means of an ear oximeter) and plotting the response as ventilation against saturation. This normally approximates to a straight line and the slope is a function of the chemoreceptor sensitivity. However, even if Pco_2 is held constant, the response is directly influenced by the patient's sensitivity to Pco_2.

Intermittent inhalation of high oxygen concentration. This method avoids exposing subjects to hypoxia. Temporary withdrawal of peripheral chemoreceptor drive by inhalation of oxygen should reduce ventilation by about 15 per cent. This may be used as an indication of the existence of carotid body activity but clearly it is much less sensitive than the steady state method.

References

1. Blanco CE. Maturation of fetal breathing activity. *Biol Neonate* 1994; **65**: 182–8.
2. Bianchi AL, Denavit-Saubie M, Champagnat J. Central control of breathing in mammals: neuronal circuitry, membrane properties, and neurotransmitters. *Physiol Rev* 1995; **75**: 1–31.
3. von Euler C. Neural organization and rhythm generation. In: Crystal RG, West JB, eds. *The lung: scientific foundations*. New York: Raven, 1991; 1307.
4. Leggallois C. *Experiences sur le Principe de la Vie*. Paris: d'Hautel, 1912.
5. Gozal D, Hathout GM, Konrad AT, Tang H, Woo MS, Zhang J et al. Localization of putative neural respiratory regions in the human by functional magnetic resonance imaging. *J Appl Physiol* 1994; **76**: 2076–83.
6. Corfield DR, Fink GR, Ramsay SC, Murphy K, Harty HR, Watson JDG et al. Evidence for limbic system activation during CO_2-stimulated breathing in man. *J Physiol (Lond)* 1995; **488**: 77–84.
7. Richter DW, Ballanyi K, Schwarzacher S. Mechanisms of respiratory rhythm generation. *Curr Opin Neurobiol* 1992 **2**: 788–93.
8. Speck DF, Beck ER. Respiratory rhythmicity after extensive lesions of the dorsal and ventral respiratory groups in the decerebrate cat. *Brain Res* 1989; **482**: 387–92.
9. Bonham AC. Neurotransmitters in the CNS control of breathing. *Respir Physiol* 1995; **101**: 219–30.
10. Mitchell RA, Berger AJ. Neural regulation of respiration. In: Hornbein TF, ed. *Regulation of breathing*, Part I. New York: Marcel Dekker, 1981.
11. Newsom-Davis J. Control of the muscles in breathing. In: *Respiratory physiology*. London: Butterworths, 1974; 221.
12. Horn EM, Waldrop TG. Suprapontine control of respiration. *Respir Physiol* 1998; **114**: 201–11.

13. Corfield DR, Murphy K, Guz A. Does the motor cortical control of the diaphragm 'bypass' the brain stem respiratory centres in man? *Respir Physiol* 1998; **114**: 109–17.

14. Douglas CG, Haldane JS. The causes of periodic or Cheyne–Stokes breathing. *J Physiol (Lond)* 1909; **38**: 401–19.

15. Haldane JS, Priestley JG. The regulation of the lung ventilation. *J Physiol (Lond)* 1905; **32**: 225–66.

16. Fink BR. Influence of cerebral activity in wakefulness on regulation of breathing. *J Appl Physiol* 1961; **16**: 15–20.

17. Hanks EC, Ngai SH, Fink BR. The respiratory threshold for carbon dioxide in anesthetized man. *Anesthesiology* 1961; **22**: 393–7.

18. Western PJ, Patrick JM. Effects of focussing attention on breathing with and without apparatus on the face. *Respir Physiol* 1988; **72**: 123–30.

19. Winkworth AL, Davis PJ, Adams RD, Ellis E. Breathing patterns during spontaneous speech. *J Speech Hear Res* 1995; **38**: 124–44.

20. Winkworth AL, Davis PJ, Ellis E, Adams RD. Variability and consistency in speech breathing during reading: lung volumes, speech intensity and linguistic factors. *J Speech Hear Res* 1994; **37**: 535–6.

21. Severinghaus JW, Mitchell RA. Ondine's curse: failure of respiratory centre automaticity while asleep. *Clin Res* 1962; **10**: 122.

22. Vingerhoets F, Bogousslavsky J. Respiratory dysfunction in stroke. *Clin Chest Med* 1994; **15**: 729–37.

23. Commare MC, Francois B, Estournet B, Barois A. Ondine's curse: a discussion of five cases. *Neuropediatrics* 1993; **24**: 313–18.

24. Weese-Mayer DE, Silvestri JM, Menzies LJ, Morrow-Kenny AS, Hunt CE, Hauptman SA. Congenital central hypoventilation syndrome: diagnosis, management, and long-term outcome in thirty-two children. *J Pediatr* 1992; **120**: 381–7.

25. Silvestri JM, Weese-Mayer DE, Flanagan EA. Congenital central hypoventilation syndrome: cardio-respiratory responses to moderate exercise, simulating daily activity. *Pediatr Pulmonol* 1995; **20**: 89–93.

26. Woo MS, Woo MA, Gozal D, Jansen MT, Keens TG, Harper RM. Heart rate variability in congenital central hypoventilation syndrome. *Pediatr Res* 1992; **31**: 291–6.

27. Sant'Ambrogio G, Sant'Ambrogio FB. Reflexes from the airway, lung, chest wall and limbs. In: Crystal RG, West JB, eds. *The lung: scientific foundations.* New York: Raven, 1991; 1383.

28. Widdicombe JG. Nervous receptors in the respiratory tract. In: Hornbein TF, ed. *Regulation of breathing,* Part I. New York: Marcel Dekker, 1981.

29. Widdicombe JG. Afferent receptors in the airways and cough. *Respir Physiol* 1998; **114**: 5–15.

30. Hering E. Die Selbsteuerung der Athmung durch den Nervus vagus. *Sber Akad Wiss Wien* 1868; **57**: 672.

31. Breuer J. Die Selbsteuerung der Athmung durch den Nervus vagus. *Sber Akad Wiss Wien* 1868; **58**: 909.

32. Ullman E. About Hering and Breuer. In: Porter R, ed. *Breathing: Hering–Breuer Centenary Symposium.* Edinburgh and London: Churchill Livingstone, 1970; 3.

33. Gaudy JH. The Hering–Breuer reflex in man? *Br J Anaesth* 1991; **66**: 627–8.

34. Widdicombe JG. Respiratory reflexes in man and other mammalian species. *Clin Sci* 1961; **21**: 163–70.

35. Guz A, Noble MIM, Trenchard D, Cochrane HL, Makey AR. Studies on the vagus nerves in man: their role in respiratory and circulatory control. *Clin Sci* 1964; **27**: 293–304.

36. Gautier H, Bonora M, Gaudy JH. Breuer–Hering inflation reflex and breathing pattern in anaesthetized humans and cats. *J Appl Physiol* 1981; **51**: 1162–8.

37. Rabbette PS, Fletcher ME, Dezateux CA, Soriano-Brucher H, Stocks J. Hering–Breuer reflex and respiratory system compliance in the first year of life: a longitudinal study. *J Appl Physiol* 1994; **76**: 650–6.

38. Guz A, Noble MIM, Eisle JH, Trenchard D. The effect of lung deflation on breathing in man. *Clin Sci* 1971; **40**: 451–61.

39. Head H. On the regulation of respiration. *J Physiol (Lond)* 1889; **10**: 1–70.

40. Cross KW, Klaus M, Tooley WH, Weisser K. The response of the new-born baby to inflation of the lungs. *J Physiol (Lond)* 1960; **151**: 551–65.

41. Bendixen HH, Smith GM, Mead J. Pattern of ventilation in young adults. *J Appl Physiol* 1964; **19**: 195–8.

42. Paintal AS. Lung and airway receptors. In: Pallot DJ, ed. *Control of Respiration.* London: Croom Helm, 1983.

43. Coleridge JCG, Coleridge HM. Afferent vagal C fibre innervation of the lungs and airways and its functional significance. *Rev Physiol Biochem Pharmacol* 1984; **99**: 1–98.
44. Paintal AS. Some recent advances in studies on J receptors. *Adv Exp Med Biol* 1995; **381**: 15–25.
45. Frazier DT, Revelette WR. Role of phrenic nerve afferents in the control of breathing. *J Appl Physiol* 1991; **70**: 491–6.
46. Sant'Ambrogio G, Tsubone H, Sant'Ambrogio FB. Sensory information from the upper airway: role in the control of breathing. *Respir Physiol* 1995; **102**: 1–16.
47. Stockwell M, Lang S, Yip R, Zintel T, White C, Gallagher CG. Lack of importance of the superior laryngeal nerves in citric acid cough in humans. *J Appl Physiol* 1993; **75**: 613–7.
48. Higginbottam T, Jackson M, Woolman P, Lowry R, Wallwork J. The cough response to ultrasonically nebulised distilled water in heart–lung transplantion patients. *Am Rev Respir Dis* 1989; **140**: 58–61.
49. Kalia M, Senapati JM, Parida B, Panda A. Reflex increase in ventilation by muscle receptors with nonmedullated fibers (C-fibers). *J Appl Physiol* 1972; **32**: 189–93.
50. Bledsoe SW, Hornbein TF. Central chemosensors and the regulation of their chemical environment. In: Hornbein TF, ed. *Regulation of breathing*, Part I. New York: Marcel Dekker, 1981.
51. Loeschcke HH. Central chemoreceptors. In: Pallot DJ, ed. *Control of respiration*. London: Croom Helm, 1983.
52. Pflüger E. Ueber die Urasche der Athembewegungen, sowie der Dyspnoë und Apnoë. *Arch Ges Physiol* 1868; **1**: 61.
53. Cunningham DJC. The control system regulating breathing in man. *Q Rev Biophys* 1974; **6**: 433–83.
54. Leusen IR. Chemosensitivity of the respiratory centre. Influence of CO_2 in the cerebral ventricles on respiration. *Am J Physiol* 1954; **176**: 39–44.
55. Leusen IR. Influence du pH du liquide cephalo-rachidien sur la respiration. *Experientia* 1950; **6**: 272.
56. Mitchell RA, Loeschcke HH, Massion WH, Severinghaus JW. Respiratory responses mediated through superficial chemosensitive areas on the medulla. *J Appl Physiol* 1963; **18**: 523–33.
57. Berger AJ, Hornbein TF. Control of respiration. In: Patton HD, Fuchs AF, Hille B, Scher AM, eds. *Physiology and biophysics*, vol 2, 21st edn. Philadelphia: WB Saunders, 1986.
58. Schläfke ME, Pokorski M, See WR, Prill RK, Loeschcke HH. Chemosensitive neurons on the ventral medullary surface. *Bull Physio-Pathol Respir* 1975; **11**: 277.
59. Sato M, Severinghaus JW, Basbaum AI. Medullary CO_2 chemoreceptor neuron identification by c-fos immunochemistry. *FASEB J* 1991; **5**: A1120.
60. Fencl V, Miller TB, Pappenheimer JR. Studies on the respiratory response to disturbances of acid–base balance, with deductions concerning the ionic composition of cerebral interstitial fluid. *Am J Physiol* 1966; **210**: 459–72.
61. Dev NB, Loeschcke HH. Topography of the respiratory and circulatory responses to acetylcholine and nicotine of the ventral surface of the medulla oblongata. *Pflüger's Archiv* 1979; **379**: 19–27.
62. Severinghaus JW, Mitchell RA, Richardson BW, Singer MM. Respiratory control at high altitude suggesting active transport regulation of CSF pH. *J Appl Physiol* 1963; **18**: 1155–66.
63. Dempsey JA, Forster HV, doPico GA. Ventilatory acclimatization to moderate hypoxaemia in man. *J Clin Invest* 1974; **53**: 1091–100.
64. Forster HV, Dempsey JA, Chosy LW. Incomplete compensation of CSF [H^+] in man during acclimatization to high altitude. *J Appl Physiol* 1975; **38**: 1067–72.
65. Pavlin EG, Hornbein TF. Distribution of H^+ and HCO_3^- between CSF and blood during respiratory acidosis in dogs. *Am J Physiol* 1975; **228**: 1145–8.
66. Pavlin EG, Hornbein TF. Distribution of H^+ and HCO_3^- between CSF and blood during metabolic acidosis in dogs. *Am J Physiol* 1975; **228**: 1134–40.
67. Pavlin EG, Hornbein TF. Distribution of H^+ and HCO_3^- between CSF and blood during metabolic alkalosis in dogs. *Am J Physiol* 1975; **228**: 1141–4.
68. Hornbein TF, Pavlin EG. Distribution of H^+ and HCO_3^- between CSF and blood during respiratory alkalosis in dogs. *Am J Physiol* 1975; **228**: 1149–54.
69. Semple SLG. Respiration and the cerebrospinal fluid. *Br J Anaesth* 1965; **37**: 262–7.
70. Christensen MS. Acid–base changes in cerebrospinal fluid and blood, and blood volume changes, following prolonged hyperventilation in man. *Br J Anaesth* 1974; **46**: 348–57.
71. Mitchell RA, Carman CT, Severinghaus JW, Richardson BW, Singer MM, Snider S. Stability of cerebrospinal fluid pH in chronic acid–base disturbances in blood. *J Appl Physiol* 1965; **20**: 443–52.

72. Froman C, Crampton-Smith A. Hyperventilation associated with low pH of cerebrospinal fluid after intracranial haemorrhage. *Lancet* 1966; **1**: 780–2.
73. Froman C. Correction of cerebrospinal fluid metabolic acidosis by intrathecal injection of bicarbonate. *Br J Anaesth* 1966; **39**: 90.
74. Lumb AB, Nunn JF. Ribcage contributions to CO_2 response during rebreathing and steady state methods. *Respir Physiol* 1991; **85**: 97–110.
75. Tansley JG, Pedersen MEF, Clar C, Robbins PA. Human ventilatory response to 8 h of euoxic hypercapnia. *J Appl Physiol* 1998; **84**: 431–4.
76. Lahiri S. Physiological responses: peripheral chemoreceptors. In: Crystal RG, West JB, eds. *The lung: scientific foundations*. New York: Raven, 1991; 1333.
77. de Castro F. Sur la structure et l'innervation de la glande intercarotidienne. *Trab Lab Invest Biol Univ Madrid* 1926; **26**: 365.
78. Heymans C, Bouckaert JJ, Dautrebande L. Sinus carotidien et réflexes respiratoire. *Arch Int Pharmacodyn Ther* 1930; **39**: 400.
79. McDonald DM. Peripheral chemoreceptors. In: Hornbein TF, ed. *Regulation of breathing*, Part I. New York: Marcel Dekker, 1981.
80. Fidone SJ, Gonzalez C, Dinger B, Gomez-Nino A, Obeso A, Yoshizaki K. Cellular aspects of peripheral chemoreceptor function. In: Crystal RG, West JB, eds. *The lung: scientific foundations*. New York: Raven, 1991; 1319.
81. Ponte J, Purves MJ. Frequency response of carotid body chemoreceptors in the cat to changes of Pa_{O_2}, Pa_{CO_2}, and pH_a. *J Appl Physiol* 1974; **37**: 635–47.
82. Mohan R, Duffin J. The effect of hypoxia on the ventilatory response to carbon dioxide in man. *Respir Physiol* 1997; **108**: 101–15.
83. Dutton RE, Fitzgerald RS, Gross N. Ventilatory response to square wave forcing of carbon dioxide at the carotid bodies. *Respir Physiol* 1968; **4**: 101–8.
84. Cunningham DJC, Howson MG, Pearson SB. The respiratory effects in man of altering the time profile of alveolar CO_2 and O_2 within each respiratory cycle. *J Physiol (Lond)* 1973; **234**: 1–28.
85. Petersen ES, Vejby-Christenson H. Effects of body temperature on ventilatory response to hypoxia and breathing pattern in man. *J Appl Physiol* 1977; **42**: 492–500.
86. Biscoe TJ, Duchen MR. Cellular basis of transduction in carotid chemoreceptors. *Am J Physiol* 1990; **258**: L271–8.
87. Acker H. Cellular oxygen sensors. *Ann N Y Acad Sci* 1994; **718**: 3–10.
88. Ward DS, Bellville JW. Reduction of hypoxic ventilatory drive by dopamine. *Anesth Analg* 1982; **61**: 333–7.
89. Delpierre S, Fornaris M, Guillot C, Grimaud C. Increased ventilatory chemosensitivity induced by domperidone, a dopamine antagonist, in healthy humans. *Bull Eur Physiopath Respir* 1987; **23**: 31–5.
90. Foo IT, Warren PM, Drummond GB. Influence of oral clonidine on the ventilatory response to acute and sustained isocapnic hypoxia in human males. *Br J Anaesth* 1996; **76**: 214–20.
91. Biscoe TJ, Willshaw P. Stimulus-response relationships of the peripheral arterial chemoreceptors. In: Hornbein TF, ed. *Regulation of breathing*, Part I. New York: Marcel Dekker, 1981.
92. Powell FL, Milsom WK, Mitchell GS. Time domains of the hypoxic ventilatory response. *Respir Physiol* 1998; **112**: 123–34.
93. Huang SY, Alexander JK, Grover RF, Maher JT, McCullough RE, McCullough RG et al. Hypocapnia and sustained hypoxia blunt ventilation on arrival at high altitude. *J Appl Physiol* 1984; **56**: 602–6.
94. Easton PA, Slykerman LJ, Anthonisen NR. Ventilatory response to sustained hypoxia in normal adults. *J Appl Physiol* 1986; **61**: 906–11.
95. Howard LSGE, Robbins PA. Ventilatory response to 8 h of isocapnic and poikilocapnic hypoxia in humans. *J Appl Physiol* 1995; **78**: 1092–7.
96. Sahn SA, Zwillich CW, Dick N, McCullough RE, Lakshminarayan S, Weil JV. Variability of ventilatory responses to hypoxia and hypercapnia. *J Appl Physiol* 1977; **43**: 1019–25.
97. White DP, Douglas NJ, Picket CK, Weil JV, Zwillich CW. Sexual influence on the control of breathing. *J Appl Physiol* 1983; **54**: 874–9.
98. Robbins PA. Hypoxic ventilatory decline: site of action. *J Appl Physiol* 1995; **78**: 373–4.
99. Kagawa S, Stafford MJ, Waggener TB, Severinghaus JW. No effect of naloxone on hypoxia-induced ventilatory depression in adults. *J Appl Physiol* 1982; **52**: 1030–4.

100. Soto-Arape I, Burton MD, Kazemi H. Central amino acid neurotransmitters and the hypoxic ventilatory response. *Am J Respir Crit Care Med* 1995; **151**: 1113–20.

101. Cruz JC, Reeves JT, Grover RF, Maher JT, McCullough RE, Cymerman A, Denniston JC. Ventilatory acclimatization to high altitude is prevented by CO_2 breathing. *Respiration* 1980; **39**: 121–30.

102. Weil JVW, Byrne-Quinn E, Sodal IE, Filley GF, Grover RF. Acquired attenuation of chemoreceptor function in chronically hypoxic man at high altitude. *J Clin Invest* 1971; **50**: 186–95.

103. Weil JV, Byrne-Quinn E, Sodal IE, Friesen WO, Underhill B, Filley GF, Grover RF. Hypoxic ventilatory drive in normal man. *J Clin Invest* 1970; **49**: 1061–72.

104. Dripps RD, Comroe JH. The effect of the inhalation of high and low oxygen concentrations on respiration, pulse rate, ballistocardiogram and arterial oxygen saturation (oximeter) of normal individuals. *Am J Physiol* 1947; **149**: 277–91.

105. Cormack RS, Cunningham DJC, Gee JBL. The effect of carbon dioxide on the respiratory response to want of oxygen in man. *Q J Exp Physiol* 1957; **42**: 303–16.

106. Rebuck AS, Campbell EJM. A clinical method for assessing the ventilatory response to hypoxia. *Am Rev Respir Dis* 1974; **109**: 345–50.

107. Wade JG, Larson CP, Hickey RF, Ehrenfeld WK, Severinghaus JW. Effect of carotid endarterectomy on carotid chemoreceptor and baroreceptor function in man. *New Engl J Med* 1970; **282**: 823–9.

108. Vanmaele RG, De Backer WA, Willeman MJ, Van Schil PE, De Maeseneer G, Van Look RF, Bosmans EJ. Hypoxic ventilatory response to carotid endarterectomy. *Eur J Vasc Surg* 1992; **6**: 241–4.

109. Vanmaele RG, De Leersnijder, Bal J, Van Kerkhoven W, Bongaerts P, Vaerenberg C. One year follow-up after bilateral carotid body resection for COPD. *Eur J Respir Dis* 1983; **64** (Supp 126): 470.

110. Edelman NH, Neubauer JA. Hypoxic depression of breathing. In: Crystal RG, West JB, eds. *The lung: scientific foundations*. New York: Raven, 1991; 1341.

111. Weil JVW, Byrne-Quinn E, Sodal IE, Kline JS, McCullough RE, Filley GF. Augmentation of chemosensitivity during mild exercise in normal man. *J Appl Physiol* 1972; **33**: 813–19.

112. Davidson JT, Whipp BJ, Wasserman K, Koyal SN, Lugliani R. Role of carotid bodies in breath holding. *N Engl J Med* 1974; **290**: 819–22.

113. Guz A, Noble MIM, Widdicombe JG, Trenchard D, Mushin WW, Makey AR. The role of the vagal and glossopharyngeal afferent nerves in respiratory sensation, control of breathing and arterial pressure regulation in conscious man. *Clin Sci* 1966; **30**: 161–70.

114. Grassi B, Ferretti G, Costa M, Ferrigno M, Panzacchi A, Lundgren CE et al. Ventilatory responses to hypercapnia and hypoxia in elite breath-hold divers. *Respir Physiol* 1994; **97**: 323–32.

115. Campbell EJM, Freedman S, Clark TJH, Robson JG, Norman J. The effect of muscular paralysis induced by tubocurarine on the duration and sensation of breath holding. *Clin Sci* 1967; **32**: 425–32.

116. Campbell EJM, Godfrey S, Clark TJH, Freedman S, Norman J. The effect of muscular paralysis induced by tubocurarine on the duration and sensation of breath holding during hypercapnia. *Clin Sci* 1969; **36**: 323–8.

117. Noble MIM, Eisle JH, Frankel HL, Else W, Guz A. The role of the diaphragm in the sensation of holding the breath. *Clin Sci* 1971; **41**: 275–83.

118. Fowler WS. Breaking point of breath-holding. *J Appl Physiol* 1954; **6**: 539–45.

119. Severinghaus JW. Proposed standard determination of ventilatory responses to hypoxia and hypercapnia in man. *Chest* 1976; **70**: 129s.

120. Read DJC. A clinical method for assessing the ventilatory response to carbon dioxide. *Australas Ann Med* 1967; **16**: 20–32.

121. Milledge JS, Minty KB, Duncalf D. On-line assessment of ventilatory response to carbon dioxide. *J Appl Physiol* 1974; **37**: 596–9.

122. Whitelaw WA, Derenne J-P, Milic-Emili J. Occlusion pressure as a measure of respiratory center output in conscious man. *Respir Physiol* 1975; **23**: 181–99.

123. Rebuck AS, Slutsky AS. Measurement of ventilatory responses to hypercapnia and hypoxia. In: Hornbein TF, ed. *Regulation of breathing*, Part I. New York: Marcel Dekker, 1981.

Chapter 6

Pulmonary ventilation: mechanisms and the work of breathing

Breathing consists of rhythmic changes in lung volume brought about by the medullary respiratory neurones described in Chapter 5. Several muscle groups are involved in effecting the change in lung volume. First, muscles of the pharynx and larynx control upper airway resistance; secondly, the diaphragm, ribcage, spine and neck muscles bring about inspiration; and finally, muscles of the abdominal wall, ribcage and spine are used when active expiration is required. Many of these muscle groups have common origins and attachments such that their activity is complex and dependent both on each other and on many non-respiratory factors such as posture, locomotion and voluntary activity.

Upper airway muscles

During inspiration through the nose, the pressure in the pharynx must fall below atmospheric by an amount equal to the product of inspiratory gas flow rate and the flow resistance afforded by the nose (see Figure 4.1). This development of only a few kilopascals of subatmospheric pressure in the pharynx tends to pull the tongue backwards and cause the pharynx to collapse.

Pharyngeal obstruction in response to these pressure changes during inspiration is opposed by reflex contraction of pharyngeal dilator muscles during inspiration. The best known, largest and easiest to study is genioglossus, but many other pharyngeal dilator muscles show tonic contraction and/or phasic inspiratory activity. The afferent side of the reflex arises from mechanoreceptors in the pharynx and larynx, which respond in a graded manner to subatmospheric pressure.[1] The reflex is extremely rapid, both genioglossus[1] and tensor palati[2] electromyographic (EMG) activity increasing less than 50 ms after a negative pressure is applied to the pharynx. This compares with a reaction time for voluntary tongue movements of 190 ms.[1] Airway diameters are well maintained down to pressures of 1.5 kPa (15 cmH$_2$O) below atmospheric, during active but not passive breathing manoeuvres.[3] Pulmonary stretch receptors may also contribute to the reflex as pharyngeal cross-sectional area correlates directly with lung volume.[4]

There is no significant narrowing of the airway when changing from the erect to the supine posture in the normal subject.[5] Genioglossus EMG activity is increased by 34 per cent in the supine position, presumably to counteract the effect of gravity on the tongue.[6,7] Anatomical considerations suggest that patency of the nasopharynx in the supine position is maintained by tensor palati, palatoglossus and palatopharyngeus, and tonic but not phasic respiratory activity has been detected in levator palati.[8] The soft palate tends to fall back against the posterior pharyngeal wall in the supine position without contraction of these muscles.

Failure of the various mechanisms to preserve the pharyngeal airway may occur in sleep, hypoxia or anaesthesia; their occurrence and prevention are discussed in Chapters 15 and 21.

Laryngeal control of airway resistance. During quiet breathing, movement of the vocal folds is used as a choke for fine control of airway resistance.[9] On inspiration, phasic activity of the posterior cricoarytenoid muscles, acting by rotating the arytenoid cartilages, abducts the vocal folds to minimize resistance.[10] A greater effect occurs during expiration, when phasic electrical activity in thyroarytenoid muscles indicates adduction of the vocal folds,[11] and therefore an increase in resistance. This may help to prevent collapse of the lower airways (page 68).

Respiratory muscles of the trunk

Nomenclature in this area can be confusing, different authors using different terms. The trunk (referred to as chest wall in some studies) may be divided into the ribcage and abdomen. These two compartments are separated by the diaphragm and both are therefore greatly influenced by its activity.

The diaphragm

The diaphragm is a membranous muscle separating the abdominal cavity and chest, and in adults has a total surface area[12] of approximately $900\,cm^2$. It is the most important inspiratory muscle, with motor innervation solely from the phrenic nerves (C3,4,5). In comparison with other skeletal muscles, the diaphragm is extremely active. Muscle fibres in the diaphragm can reduce their length by up to 40 per cent between residual volume and total lung capacity,[12] and spend 45 per cent of each day contracting, compared with only 14 per cent for the soleus muscle.[13] The diaphragm has considerable reserve of function, and unilateral phrenic block causes little decrement of overall ventilatory capacity. Despite the importance of the diaphragm to respiration, bilateral phrenic interruption is still compatible with good ventilatory function.[14]

Mechanics of diaphragmatic function. The origins of the crural part of the diaphragm are the lumbar vertebrae and the arcuate ligaments, whilst the costal parts arise from the lower ribs and xiphisternum. Both parts are inserted into the central tendon. In normal circumstances, a zone of apposition exists around the outside of the diaphragm where it is in direct contact with the internal aspect of the ribcage, with no lung in between but the parietal pleura still allowing free movement of the diaphragm. At upright FRC in humans, about 55 per cent of the diaphragm surface area is in the zone of apposition.[12,15] During inspiration, the origins and insertion are approximated, resulting in shape changes, descent of the diaphragm, and elevation and rotation of the lower ribs (increasing the cross-sectional area of the lower ribcage). The upper ribs, in contrast, are drawn inwards when the diaphragm contracts in isolation.[16]

Recent studies of human subjects using MRI scans, illustrated in Figure 6.1, have enabled the *in vivo* actions of the diaphragm to be defined.[12,15,17,18] There are many ways in which diaphragm contraction may bring about an increase in lung volume,[19] and these

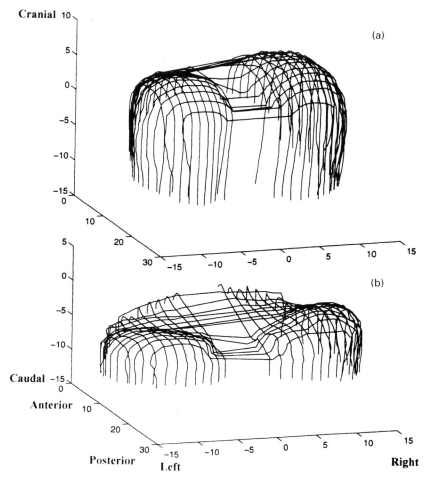

Figure 6.1 Three-dimensional reconstructions of the human diaphragm at FRC using fast CT scanning (dimensions in cm). (a) Normal subject showing extensive zone of apposition and normal curvature of the diaphragm domes. (b) Patient with hyperinflated chest as a result of chronic obstructive pulmonary disease (page 533). Note the reduced zone of apposition and the flattened diaphragm domes. (After reference 18 by permission of the authors and the publishers of *American Journal of Respiratory and Critical Care Medicine*.)

are illustrated schematically in Figure 6.2. They may be considered using a 'piston in a cylinder' analogy, the trunk representing the cylinder and the diaphragm the piston (Figure 6.2a). Figure 6.2b illustrates the first possible mechanism, involving downward movement of the diaphragm simply by shortening the zone of apposition around the whole cylinder and leaving the dome shape unchanged. This is a pure 'piston-like' action and has the advantage of very efficient conversion of diaphragm muscle fibre shortening into changes in lung volume. Figure 6.2c illustrates 'non-piston-like' behaviour in which the zone of apposition remains unchanged but an increase in the tension of the diaphragm domes reduces the curvature, so expanding the lung. In this situation, the diaphragm behaves like a bubble and Laplace's law dictates the change in trans-diaphragmatic pressure (or lung volume) with changes in diaphragmatic tension. This is likely to be less efficient than

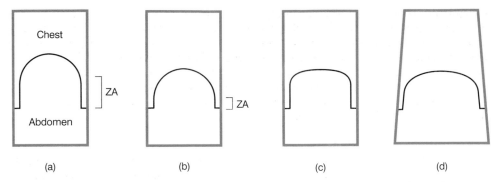

Figure 6.2 'Piston in a cylinder' analogy of the mechanisms of diaphragm actions on the lung volume. (a) Resting position. (b) Inspiration with pure piston-like behaviour. (c) Inspiration with pure non-piston-like behaviour. (d) Combination of non-piston-like behaviour and piston-like behaviour in an expanding cylinder. See text for details. ZA, zone of apposition.

piston-like behaviour, as much of the muscle tension developed simply opposes the opposite side of the diaphragm rather than moving the diaphragm downwards, such that, in theory, when the diaphragm becomes flat, further contraction will have no effect on lung volume. Finally, Figure 6.2d incorporates both types of behaviour already described and expansion of the lower ribcage that occurs with diaphragmatic contraction (known as 'piston in an expanding cylinder'), and represents a simple description of the situation *in vivo*.

In the supine position, diaphragm action is a combination of all the above mechanisms as well as a change in shape involving a tilting and flattening of the diaphragm in the anteroposterior direction.[12]

Ribcage muscles[20]

As already described, the ribcage may be regarded as a cylinder with length governed primarily by the diaphragm and secondarily by flexion and extension of the spine. The cross-sectional area of the cylinder is governed by movement of the ribs. This movement involves mainly rotation of the neck of the rib about the axis of the costovertebral joints, and their shape is such that elevation of the ribs in this way increases both the lateral and the anteroposterior diameter of the ribcage.[16] Elevation of the ribs by the intercostal muscles tends to result in a 'bucket-handle' action, whilst elevation of the anterior ribcage by, for example, the sternomastoid muscle elevating the sternum results in a 'pump-handle' type of movement. These two actions tend to occur together, and depend also on other requirements such as posture and upper limb movements. Upper ribs are inserted into the sternum and do not necessarily behave in quite the same way as the lower 'floating' ribs, which are inserted into the more flexible costal cartilage.

The intercostal muscles. These muscles are divided into the external group (deficient anteriorly), the less powerful internal group (deficient posteriorly) and the feeble strands of intercostalis intima. Internal intercostal muscles of the upper ribcage become thicker anteriorly, where they are known as the parasternal intercostal muscles. In 1749, mechanical considerations led Hamberger to suggest that the external intercostals were primarily inspiratory, and the internal intercostals primarily expiratory.[21] Though an oversimplification,[16] this has generally been confirmed by electromyography. The parasternal portion of the internal intercostals are inspiratory in both humans and animals,[22] and the inspiratory activity of external intercostals, though minimal during quiet breathing,[20] becomes increasingly important during stimulated breathing. Posture plays an important role in intercostal activity in humans. For example, during the rather extreme postural challenge of rotating the trunk, which changes the mechanical properties of the ribs, the respiratory activity of internal and external intercostals is reversed, the internal intercostals becoming expiratory and *vice versa.*[23]

Scalenes are not accessory respiratory muscles as was originally thought, but are active in inspiration during quiet breathing in humans,[22] particularly when upright. Their role is to elevate the ribcage and this counteracts the tendency of the diaphragm to cause inward displacement of the upper ribs (see above). Innervation is from C1 to C5.

Accessory muscles are silent in normal breathing in humans but, as ventilation increases, the inspiratory muscles contract more vigorously and accessory muscles are recruited. Considerable hyperventilation (about $50\ 1.min^{-1}$) or severe increases in respiratory loading are usually present before the accessory muscles become active. Accessory muscles include the sternocleidomastoids, extensors of the vertebral column, pectoralis minor, trapezius and the serrati muscles. Many of these muscles, for example the pectorals, reverse their usual origin/insertion and help to expand the chest, provided the arms and shoulder girdle are fixed by grasping a suitable support.

The abdominal muscles

With the exception of gas within the bowel lumen, the abdomen is an incompressible volume held between the diaphragm and the abdominal muscles. Contraction of either will cause a corresponding passive displacement of the other. Thus abdominal muscles are generally expiratory.

Rectus abdominis, external oblique, internal oblique and tranversalis muscles are the most important expiratory muscles, whilst the muscles of the pelvic floor have a supportive role. Contraction of this muscle group results in an increase in abdominal pressure, displacing the diaphragm in a cephalad direction. In addition, their insertion into the costal margin results in a caudad movement of the ribcage, so assisting expiration by opposing the ribcage muscles. External oblique is usually monitored as an indication of expiratory muscle activity but gastric pressure is also a valuable index of their activity because they cannot contract without causing an increase in intra-abdominal pressure.

In the supine position, the abdominal muscles are normally silent during quiet breathing and become active only when the minute volume exceeds about $40\ 1.min^{-1}$, in the face of substantial expiratory resistance, during phonation or when making expulsive efforts. When upright, their use in breathing is complicated by their role in the maintenance of posture.

Integration of respiratory muscle activity[16,24]

Breathing

Figure 6.3 shows the radiographic appearance of the ribcage at residual volume, at the normal expiratory level and at maximal inspiration, and illustrates the enormous range of movement within the semi-rigid ribcage. Expiration normally proceeds passively to the

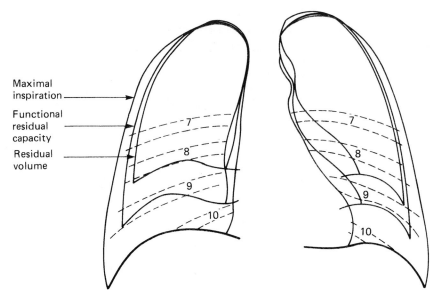

Figure 6.3 Outlines of chest radiographs of a normal subject at various levels of lung inflation. The numbers refer to ribs as seen in the position of maximal inspiration. (With thanks to Dr RL Marks, who was the subject.)

functional residual capacity (FRC), which may be considered as the equilibrium position governed by the balance of elastic forces, unless modified by residual end-expiratory tone in certain muscle groups. Inspiration is the active phase, entering the inspiratory capacity but normally leaving a substantial volume unused (the inspiratory reserve volume). Similarly, there is a substantial volume (the expiratory reserve volume) between FRC and the residual volume (see Figure 3.9). By voluntary effort it is possible to effect a satisfactory tidal exchange anywhere in the vital capacity, but the work of breathing is minimal at FRC.

Although we tend to think of the respiratory muscles individually, it is important to remember that they act together in an extraordinarily complex interaction that is influenced by factors including posture, minute volume, respiratory load, disease and anaesthesia. Figure 6.4 illustrates some features of the interaction; it has been developed from the model proposed by Hillman and Finucane[25] and further developed by Drummond.[26]

Inspiration. In Figure 6.4 it can be seen that the ribcage inspiratory muscles and diaphragm act in parallel to inflate the lungs, with posture affecting which muscle group is dominant (see below). In either position, diaphragm activity alone results in a widening of the lower ribcage and an indrawing of the upper ribcage (often seen with spontaneous respiration during general anaesthesia), which must be countered by the intercostal and neck muscles contracting simultaneously. Inspiratory muscle activity does not terminate abruptly at the end of inspiration. There is a gradual let-down of muscle tone during early expiration (see Figure 5.3), which does not therefore assume the pattern of exponential decay as seen in the paralysed patient.

The inspiratory muscles are not easy to access for electromyographic or other methods of study, and this has greatly hampered elucidation of their pattern of contraction.

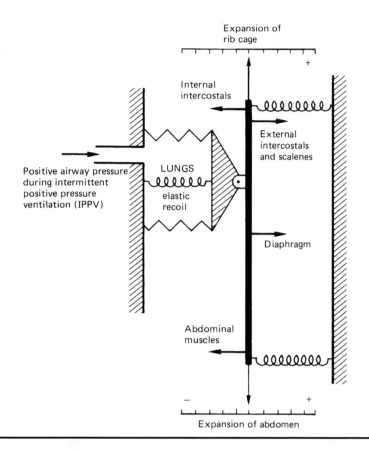

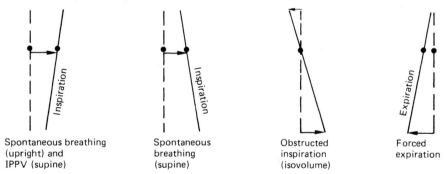

THE BROKEN LINE REPRESENTS FUNCTIONAL RESIDUAL CAPACITY

Figure 6.4 A model of the balance of static and dynamic forces acting on the respiratory system. The central bar, attached to the lungs, is floating freely, held in equilibrium by the elastic forces at the end-expiratory position as shown. It may be displaced by the actions of the various muscles shown, with movement to the right generally indicating inspiration and *vice versa*. Action of the various inspiratory or expiratory muscles causes changes, not only in the lung volume but also in the inclination of the bar, which represents relative changes in the cross-sectional area of the ribcage and abdomen. See text for details. (Derived from references 25 and 26.)

Measurement of pressure difference between the thorax and abdomen is particularly useful to distinguish between active and passive movements of the diaphragm. Radiographic and a wide range of other imaging and stethographic methods will indicate the change in shape of the confines of thorax, abdomen and lungs, but do not necessarily indicate the muscle groups responsible for the observed changes (Figure 6.4).

Expiration requires no muscular activity during quiet breathing in the supine position, because the elastic recoil of the lungs provides the energy required, aided by the weight of the abdominal contents pushing the diaphragm in a cephalad direction. In the upright posture and during stimulated ventilation the internal intercostal muscles and the abdominal wall muscles are active in returning the ribcage and diaphragm to the resting position. In extreme hyperventilation, for example following exercise, the expiratory muscles become progressively more important until ventilation assumes a quasi sine wave push–pull pattern.

Separation of volume contribution of ribcage and abdomen

In 1967 Konno and Mead proposed that the separate contributions to tidal volume of changes in ribcage (RC) and abdomen (AB) could be measured.[27] Essentially similar results may be obtained by measuring anteroposterior distance (magnetometers), circumference (strain gauge) or cross-sectional area (respiratory inductance plethysmography – RIP[28]). The sum of RC and AB correlates well with tidal volume and provides an excellent non-invasive measure of ventilation. RC/(RC + AB) indicates the proportion of total ventilation that can be attributed to expansion of the ribcage (usually expressed as %RC). However, such is the complexity of the muscular system described above that changes in %RC cannot be attributed to changes in the force of contraction of any particular muscle. Figure 6.5 shows RIP traces during normal breathing in different positions; also shown is a spontaneous sigh occurring in the prone position and resulting entirely from ribcage expansion.

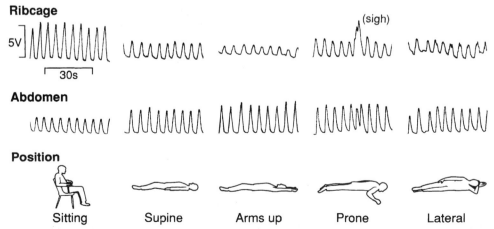

Figure 6.5 Normal respiratory inductance plethysmography (RIP) traces. The amplitude (in volts) of the RIP signal reflects the cross-sectional area of the ribcage (RC) and abdomen (AB). The sum of the RC and AB signals correlates closely with tidal volume. The Figure shows normal breathing in five different positions, demonstrating the predominantly RC contribution when upright and AB contribution in all horizontal positions. (After reference 29 by permission of the publishers of *Anesthesia and Analgesia*.)

Effect of posture on respiratory muscles

Upright posture, whether standing or sitting, is associated with greater expansion of the ribcage,[29] such that %RC is around 67 per cent (Figure 6.5). To account for this, increased EMG activity has been demonstrated in the scalene muscles[30] and the parasternal intercostals,[31] and probably therefore also occurs in the external intercostals.

Supine position. When upright, the weight of the abdominal contents pulls the diaphragm downwards, so that in the supine position the diaphragm tends to lie some 4 cm higher –which accords with the reduction in FRC when supine (see Figure 3.10). Whether or not the diaphragm displays resting (expiratory) tone to resist pressure from the abdominal contents is disputed, two studies of diaphragmatic EMG giving opposite results.[31,32] With the diaphragm higher in the chest, its fibre length is greater and it can therefore contract more effectively, counteracting the tendency to airway closure at the reduced FRC. The dimensions of the ribcage are probably little altered, and the increased diaphragm activity therefore results in a reduced %RC of about 33 per cent in the supine position.[29] In the prone and lateral position, RC contribution does not differ significantly from that in the supine position (Figure 6.5).[29]

Lateral position. In this position (Figure 6.6), only the lower dome of the diaphragm is pushed higher into the chest by the weight of the abdominal contents while the upper

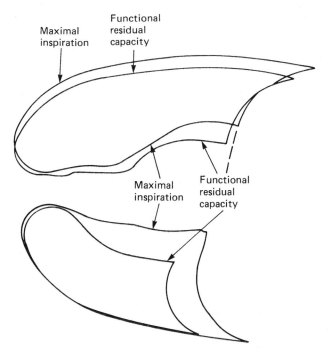

Figure 6.6 Radiographic outlines of the lungs at two levels of lung volume in a conscious subject during spontaneous breathing in the lateral position (right side down). This is the same subject as in Figure 6.3: comparison will show that, in the lateral position at FRC, the lower lung is close to residual volume while the upper lung is close to inspiratory capacity. The diaphragm therefore lies much more cephalad in the lower half of the chest. Both these factors contribute to the greater volume changes that occur in the lower lung during inspiration. The mediastinum seems to rest on a pneumatic cushion at FRC and rises during inspiration.

dome is flattened. It follows that the lower dome can contract more effectively than the upper, and the ventilation of the lower lung is about twice that of the upper. This is fortunate because gravity causes a preferential perfusion of the lower lung (page 169). As in other horizontal positions, abdominal expansion is predominant in the lateral position (Figure 6.5).

Chemoreceptor activation

In animals, clear differences have been demonstrated in the respiratory muscle response to hyperventilation induced either by hypoxia or hypercapnia.[33] For an equivalent minute volume, hypoxia stimulates mostly inspiratory muscles whilst hypercapnia stimulates both inspiratory and expiratory groups. Similar responses occur in humans, diaphragm EMG activity increasing in response to both hypercapnia and hypoxia but more rapidly in the latter, and expiratory muscle activity increasing almost exclusively during hypercapnic hyperventilation.[30,34] Hyperventilation in response to hypercapnia in the supine position results in a small increase in RC contribution (0.13% per kPa P_{CO_2} or 1% per mmHg P_{CO_2}).[35]

Neuronal control of respiratory muscles

The respiratory muscles, in common with other skeletal muscles, have their tension controlled by a servo mechanism mediated by muscle spindles. They seem to play a more important role in the intercostal muscles than in the diaphragm, and there was some doubt about the existence of spindles in the human diaphragm until a small number were demonstrated in humans.[32] Their function is largely inferred from knowledge of their well-established role in other skeletal muscles not concerned with respiration.

Two types of cell can be distinguished in the motor neurone pool of the anterior horn cell. The alpha motor neurone has a thick efferent fibre (12–20 μm diameter) and passes in the ventral root directly to the neuromuscular junction of the muscle fibre (Figure 6.7a). The gamma motor neurone has a thin efferent fibre (2–8 μm), which also passes in the ventral root but terminates in the intrafusal fibres of the muscle spindle. Contraction of the intrafusal fibres alone (without overall shortening of the muscle) increases the tension in the central part of the spindle (the nuclear bag), causing stimulation of the annulospiral endings. Impulses so generated are then transmitted via fibres that lie in the dorsal root to reach the anterior horn, where they have an excitatory effect on the alpha motor neurones. It will be seen that an efferent impulse transmitted by the gamma system may cause reflex contraction of the main muscle mass by means of an arc through the annulospiral afferent and the alpha motor neurone. Thus contraction of the whole muscle may be controlled entirely by efferents travelling in the gamma fibres, and this has been suggested in relation to breathing.[36]

Alternatively, muscle contraction may in the first instance result from discharge of both the alpha and the gamma motor neurones. If the shortening of the muscle is unopposed, main (extrafusal) and intrafusal fibres will contract together and the tension in the nuclear bag of the spindle will be unchanged. If, however, the shortening of the muscle is opposed, the intrafusal fibres will shorten more than the extrafusal fibres, causing the nuclear bag to be stretched (Figure 6.7b). The consequent stimulation of the annulospiral endings results in afferent activity that raises the excitatory state of the motor neurones, causing the main muscle fibres to increase their tension until the resistance is overcome, allowing the muscle to shorten and the tension in the nuclear bag of the spindle to be reduced (Figure 6.7c).

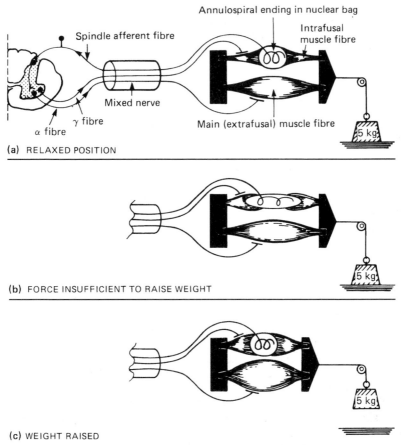

Figure 6.7 Diagrammatic representation of the servo mechanism mediated by the muscle spindles. (a) The resting state with muscle and intrafusal fibres of spindle relaxed. (b) The muscle is attempting to lift the weight following discharge of both alpha and gamma systems. The force developed by the muscle is insufficient: the weight is not lifted and the muscle cannot shorten. However, the intrafusal fibres are able to shorten and stretch the annulospiral endings in the nuclear bag of the spindle. Afferent discharge causes increased excitation of the motor neurone pool in the anterior horn. (c) Alpha discharge is augmented and the weight is finally lifted by the more powerful contraction of the muscle. When the weight is lifted, the tension on the nuclear bag is relieved and the afferent discharge from the spindle ceases. This series of diagrams relates to the lifting of a weight but it is thought that similar action of spindles is brought into play when inspiratory muscles contract against increased airways resistance.

By this mechanism, fine control of muscle contraction is possible. The message from the upper motor neurone is in the form: 'muscles should contract with whatever force may be found necessary to effect such and such a shortening', and not simply: 'muscles should contract with such and such a force'. The former message is typical of input into a servo system and far more satisfactory when the load is not known in advance.

Campbell and Howell in 1962 presented evidence for believing that a spindle servo system governs the action of the respiratory muscles.[37] According to this belief, the message conveyed by the efferent tract from the inspiratory neurones of the medulla would be in the form: 'inspiratory muscles should contract with whatever force may be necessary to effect such and such a change in length (corresponding to a certain tidal volume)' and not simply: 'inspiratory muscles should contract with such and such a force'.

The spindle servo mechanism also provides an excellent mechanism for rapid response to sudden changes in airway resistance. The nature and magnitude of the response of the inspiratory muscles to added resistance to breathing is described in Chapter 4, and the immediate response is easily explicable in terms of muscle spindles.

Neuronal firing patterns[38]

Respiratory muscles are also similar to other skeletal muscle with respect to the action potential (AP) patterns in their motor neurones. The tension generated in a muscle is directly related to the frequency of APs in the motor nerve. Even in supine resting subjects, nerves supplying the parasternal intercostals display a continuous 'train' of APs at a frequency of 8 Hz during expiration, increasing to 12 Hz during inspiration. Occasionally superimposed on this pattern are 'doublets' of APs, which are pairs of APs only 8 ms apart. In non-respiratory muscle, doublets are believed to cause a sudden step increase in muscle tension, but their role in respiration is unclear and they may be related only to voluntary chest movements.

Muscle fibre subtypes

Respiratory muscles, like all skeletal muscle, contain two different types of muscle fibre. Slow twitch (type I) fibres contain large numbers of mitochondria and, as their name suggests, they contract slowly, can maintain tension for long periods using aerobic metabolic pathways and are fatigue resistant. In contrast, fast twitch fibres (type II) rely mainly on glycolytic metabolic pathways for energy supply, contraction is quicker and stronger in bursts of activity, and they fatigue. The proportions of type I and type II fibres in a muscle therefore reveal the sort of work normally undertaken by the muscle; for example, in muscles mainly involved in maintaining posture, type I fibres predominate, whilst in those requiring intermittent activity such as hand muscles, type II fibres predominate. In human respiratory muscle it is unclear which type of fibres are responsible for different respiratory muscle activities. In animal respiratory muscles, which tend to have fewer type II fibres than humans, both eupnoeic and stimulated breathing can be achieved solely by using type I fibres, and type II fibres are required only for expulsive efforts such as gagging, sneezing and coughing.[13] In the human diaphragm there are 50 per cent type I fibres,[39] and intercostal muscles, whether inspiratory or expiratory, have over 60 per cent type I fibres.[39] This high proportion of type I fibres indicates that they are probably responsible for both posture and respiration in humans, and that type II fibres are required only for expulsive efforts and active movements, for instance during running, jumping, etc.

The work of breathing[40]

When expiration is passive during quiet breathing, the work of breathing is performed entirely by the inspiratory muscles. About half of this work is dissipated during inspiration as heat in overcoming the frictional forces opposing inspiration. The other half is stored as potential energy in the deformed elastic tissues of lung and chest wall. This potential energy is thus available as the source of energy for expiration and is then dissipated as heat in

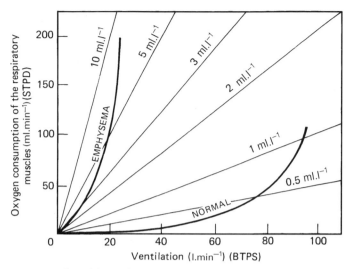

Figure 6.8 Oxygen consumption of the respiratory muscles plotted against minute volume of respiration. The isopleths indicate the oxygen cost of breathing in millilitres of oxygen consumed per litre of minute volume. The curve obtained from the normal subject shows the low oxygen cost of breathing up to a minute volume of $70\,l.min^{-1}$. Thereafter the oxygen cost rises steeply. In the emphysematous patient, the oxygen cost of breathing is not only much higher at the resting minute volume but also rises steeply as ventilation increases. At a minute volume of $20\,l.min^{-1}$, the respiratory muscles are consuming 200 ml of oxygen per minute, and a further increase of ventilation would consume more oxygen than it would make available to the rest of the body. (After reference 41 by permission of the *Journal of Applied Physiology.*)

overcoming the frictional forces resisting expiration. Energy stored in deformed elastic tissue thus permits the work of *expiration* to be transferred to the *inspiratory* muscles. This remains true with moderate increases of either inspiratory or expiratory resistance, lung volume and therefore elastic recoil being increased in the latter condition (page 74).

The actual work performed by the respiratory muscles is very small in the healthy resting subject. In these circumstances the consumption of oxygen by the respiratory muscles is only about $3\,ml.min^{-1}$, or less than 2 per cent of the metabolic rate. Furthermore, the efficiency of the respiratory muscles is only about 10 per cent. The efficiency is further reduced in many forms of respiratory disease, certain deformities, pregnancy and when the minute volume is increased (Figure 6.8). When maximal ventilation is approached, the efficiency falls to such a low level that additional oxygen made available by further increases in ventilation will be entirely consumed by the respiratory muscles.

Units of measurement of work

Work is performed when a force moves its point of application, and the work is equal to the product of force and distance moved. Similarly, work is performed when force is applied to the plunger of a syringe raising the pressure of gas contained therein. In this case the work is equal to the product of the mean pressure and the change in volume, or alternatively the product of the mean volume and the change in pressure. The units of work are identical whether the product is *force × distance* or *pressure × volume*. A multiplicity of units have been used for measuring work; they are listed in Appendix A.

Power is a measure of the rate at which work is being (or can be) performed. The term 'work of breathing', as it is normally used and when expressed in watts, is thus a misnomer because we are referring to the rate at which work is being performed and *power* is the correct term. 'Work of breathing' would be appropriate for a single event such as one breath, and joules would then be the appropriate units.

Dissipation of the work of breathing

The work of breathing overcomes two main sources of impedance. The first is the elastic recoil of the lungs and chest wall (Chapter 3) and the second is the non-elastic (mainly frictional) resistance to gas flow (Chapter 4).

Work against elastic recoil. When an elastic body is deformed, no work is dissipated as heat and all work is stored as potential energy. Figure 6.9a shows a section of the alveolar

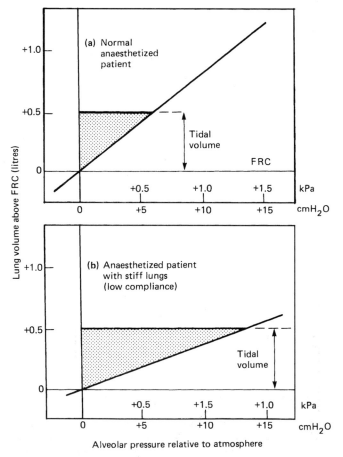

Figure 6.9 Work of breathing against elastic resistance during passive inflation. The lines show pressure/volume plots of the lungs of anaesthetized patients (conscious subjects are shown in Figure 3.8). The length of the pressure/volume curve covered during inspiration forms the hypotenuse of a right-angled triangle whose area equals the work performed against elastic resistance. Note that the area is greater when the pressure/volume curve is flatter (indicating stiffer or less compliant lungs).

pressure/volume plot for the total respiratory system (see Figure 3.8). As the lungs are inflated, the plot forms the hypotenuse of a triangle, whose area represents the work done against elastic resistance. The area of the triangle (half the base times the height) will thus equal either half the tidal volume times the pressure change or the mean pressure times the volume change. Either product has the units of work or energy (joules) and represents the potential energy available for expiration. In Figure 6.9b, the pressure/volume curve is flatter, indicating stiffer or less compliant lungs. For the same tidal volume, the area of the triangle is increased. This indicates the greater amount of work performed against elastic resistance and the greater potential energy available for expiration.

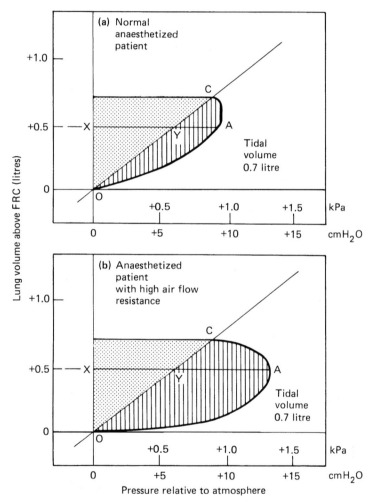

Figure 6.10 Work of breathing against air flow resistance during passive inflation. The sloping line OYC is the alveolar pressure/volume curve. The curve OAC is the mouth pressure/volume curve during inflation of the lungs. The area shaded with vertical stripes indicates the work of inspiration performed against air flow resistance. This work is increased in the patient with high resistance (b). At the point when 500 ml gas has entered the patient, XY represents the pressure distending the lungs, while YA represents the pressure overcoming air flow resistance. XA is the inflation pressure at that moment. The stippled areas represent the work done against elastic resistance (see Figure 6.9).

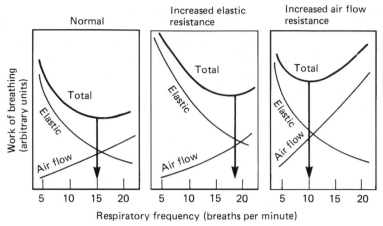

Figure 6.11 Minimal work of breathing. The diagrams show the work done against elastic and air flow resistance separately and summated to indicate the total work of breathing at different respiratory frequencies. The total work of breathing has a minimum value at about 15 breaths per minute under normal circumstances. For the same minute volume, minimum work is performed at higher frequencies with stiff (less compliant) lungs and at lower frequencies when the air flow resistance is increased.

Work against resistance to gas flow. Frictional resistance was ignored in Figure 6.9. Additional pressure is required to overcome frictional resistance to gas flow that is reflected in the mouth pressure, which, during inspiration, is above the alveolar pressure by the driving pressure required to overcome frictional resistance. When mouth pressure is plotted as in Figure 6.10, the inspiratory curve is bowed to the right, and the area shaded with vertical lines to the right of the pressure volume curve indicates the additional work performed in overcoming inspiratory frictional resistance. Figure 6.10b represents a patient with increased airway resistance. The expiratory curve, not shown in Figure 6.10, would be bowed to the left as the mouth-to-alveolar pressure gradient is reversed during expiration.

The minimal work of breathing

For a constant minute volume, the work performed against elastic resistance is increased when breathing is slow and deep. Conversely, the work performed against air flow resistance is increased when breathing is rapid and shallow. If the two components are summated and the total work is plotted against respiratory frequency, it will be found that there is an optimal frequency at which the total work of breathing is minimal (Figure 6.11). If there is increased elastic resistance (as in patients with pulmonary fibrosis), the optimal frequency is increased, whilst in the presence of increased air flow resistance the optimal frequency is decreased. Humans and animals tend to select a respiratory frequency close to that which minimizes respiratory work. This applies to different species, different age groups and also to pathological conditions.

Respiratory muscle fatigue and disuse[42]

The diaphragm, like other striated muscles, is subject to fatigue – defined as an inability to sustain tension with repeated activity.[42] For non-respiratory skeletal muscle, fatigue may be 'central' – that is, the subject is not trying hard enough (either consciously or subconsciously) – but this is unlikely to be significant in respiration where subjects with respiratory failure usually have a high central respiratory drive. Peripheral fatigue occurs when the frequency of motor nerve APs becomes chronically increased in an attempt to increase muscle tension. Eventually, when working against an unsustainable load, striated muscle shows a progressive loss of the high frequency component of the electromyogram (EMG) relative to lower frequencies. A reduction in the high/low frequency ratio of the EMG is an indication of impending fatigue. Finally, relaxation of the muscle fibre, the energy-requiring part of contraction, becomes prolonged and the muscle is unable to respond to the next AP in order to generate the required tension. In the diaphragm, resistive loads less than 40 per cent of maximum may be sustained indefinitely, but loads greater than 40 per cent of maximum can be sustained for only a short time.[43]

It seems probable that respiratory muscle fatigue may be an important factor in ventilatory failure and failure to wean from artificial ventilation. Although the clinical significance of respiratory muscle fatigue is still unclear, steps can be taken to minimize the oxygen demand of patients, to minimize respiratory impedance, to optimize the efficiency of the ventilatory pump and to rest the respiratory muscles by the use of assisted ventilation.

Blood supply to respiratory muscles may be important in fatigue.[44,45] Animal studies have shown that increased cardiac output and diaphragmatic blood flow (stimulated with noradrenaline) augment the contractility of fatigued diaphragm. In addition, patients with severe congestive cardiac failure, and therefore low cardiac output, have weakened respiratory muscles compared with matched controls, despite having similar muscle strength in the arms.[46] The high rate of activity of respiratory muscles seems to render them more susceptible to weakness in the face of reduced oxygen supply when compared with other muscles, a situation that often causes problems in intensive care when trying to wean patients from artificial ventilation before their cardiovascular function is adequate (page 604).

Effect of disuse[13]

The diaphragm may be rested by artificial ventilation with or without neuromuscular blockade, and the effect on diaphragmatic performance is clearly important. In adult hamsters, two weeks of unilateral phrenic nerve block resulted in ipsilateral hypertrophy of type I fibres whereas type II fibres were atrophied.[47] The functional result of these changes is a decrease in maximal contractile strength but increased resistance to fatigue. If, as in animals, breathing is accomplished using only type I fibres (page 124), then following disuse the hypertrophied respiratory muscles should be relatively efficient, although type II fibre atrophy may make coughing less effective.

The minute volume of pulmonary ventilation

The primary function of the respiratory system is to ensure the normality of oxygen and carbon dioxide partial pressures in the arterial blood. The adequacy of minute volume depends on the corresponding alveolar ventilation, which equals the product of respiratory frequency and (tidal volume less dead space). Dead space is considered in detail on pages 175 et seq. As alveolar ventilation increases, the composition of the alveolar gas tends to approach that of the inspired gas. The difference between inspired and alveolar gas concentrations is equal to the ratio of the output (or uptake) of the gas to the alveolar ventilation according to the universal alveolar air equation:

$$\begin{array}{c} \text{alveolar} \\ \text{concentration} \\ \text{of gas X} \end{array} = \begin{array}{c} \text{inspired} \\ \text{concentration} \\ \text{of gas X} \end{array} + (\text{or} -) \ \frac{\text{output (or uptake) of gas X}}{\text{alveolar ventilation}}$$

Note:

1. The equation is only approximate and does not correct for any difference between inspired and expired minute volumes. Corrections for this factor are considered on page 193.
2. The sign on the right-hand side is + for output of a gas (e.g. carbon dioxide) and – for uptake (e.g. oxygen).
3. The tension or partial pressure of gas X may be obtained by multiplying the fractional concentration by the dry barometric pressure (page 250).

Alveolar P_{CO_2} and P_{O_2} (the latter for different values of inspired oxygen concentration) are plotted against alveolar ventilation in Figure 6.12, and receive individual consideration for carbon dioxide on page 234 and for oxygen on page 251. The curves are rectangular hyperbolas (explained in Appendix F) and have great practical and clinical relevance, making clear many aspects of the effect of changes in ventilation.

Rectangular hyperbolas relating alveolar gas concentrations to alveolar ventilation all obey the following general rules:

1. The vertical asymptote is zero alveolar ventilation.
2. The horizontal asymptote is the inspired concentration of the gas under consideration (i.e. effectively zero for carbon dioxide and approximately 21 kPa (or 21 per cent) for oxygen while breathing air).
3. The curve is concave upwards for gases being eliminated from the body and concave downwards for gas being taken up into the body.
4. The curves move away from the intersection of the asymptotes as the volume of the gas being exchanged increases.

Failure of ventilation is considered in Chapter 26.

Measurement of ventilation

Volume may be measured either directly or by the continuous integration of instantaneous gas flow rate (Figure 6.13).

Direct measurement of respired volumes

Inspiratory and expiratory tidal volumes (and therefore minute volume) may be markedly different, and the difference is important in calculations of gas exchange. The normal respiratory exchange ratio of about 0.8 means that inspiratory minute volume is about 50 ml larger than the expiratory minute volume in the resting subject. Much larger differences can arise during exercise and during uptake or wash-out of an inert gas such as nitrogen or, to a greater extent, nitrous oxide.

Water-sealed spirometers provide the reference method for the measurement of ventilation (Figure 6.13), and may be precisely calibrated by water displacement. They provide

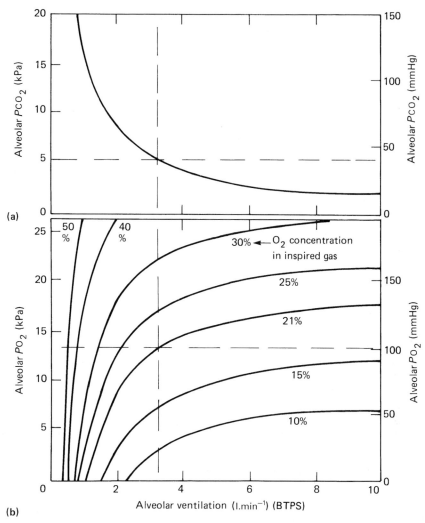

Figure 6.12 Alveolar gas tensions produced by different levels of alveolar ventilation. (a) The hyperbolic relationship between alveolar P_{CO_2} and alveolar ventilation. (b) The relationship between P_{O_2} and alveolar ventilation for different levels of oxygen concentration in the inspired gas. The broken vertical line indicates an alveolar ventilation of 3.2 l.min^{-1}. Dry barometric pressure, 95 kPa = 713 mmHg; carbon dioxide output, 150 ml.min^{-1} (STPD) = 180 ml.min^{-1} (BTPS); oxygen uptake, 190 ml.min^{-1} (STPD) = 225 ml.min^{-1} (BTPS). No allowance has been made for the difference between inspired and expired minute volumes.

negligible resistance to breathing and, by suitable design, may have a satisfactory frequency response up to very high respiratory frequencies.

Dry spirometers are hinged bellows, usually with electrical read-out of both volume and instantaneous flow rate. Their accuracy approaches that of a water-filled spirometer and they are far more convenient in use.

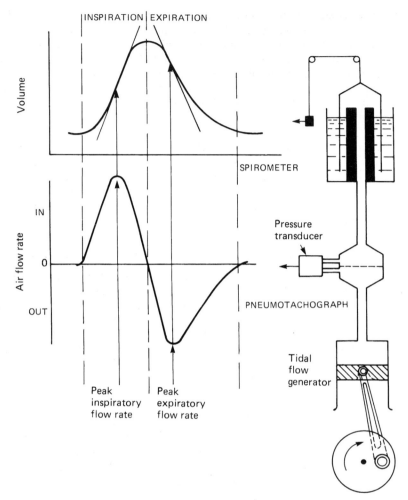

Figure 6.13 Relationship between volume and flow rate. The upper graph shows volume plotted against time; this type of tracing is obtained from a spirometer. The lower graph shows instantaneous air flow rate plotted against time; this type of tracing is obtained from a pneumotachograph. At any instant, the flow-rate trace indicates the slope of the volume trace, while the volume trace indicates the cumulative area under the flow-rate trace. *Flow* is the differential of volume; *volume* is the integral of flow rate. Differentiation of the spirometer trace gives a 'pneumotachogram'; integration of the pneumotachogram gives a 'spirometer' trace.

The wet gas meter consists of a type of paddle wheel that is sealed with water. These instruments are rather cumbersome but are highly accurate for the measurement of a volume that is passed steadily through the meter. It is particularly suitable for the measurement of the expired volume collected in a Douglas bag.

Dry gas meters are based on two bellows that alternately drive a spindle by means of cranks. The principle is similar to the long-established design of meters used for measuring domestic gas consumption. They are not accurate for small volumes such as a single tidal volume but are very reliable for the measurement of larger volumes such as the volume exhaled over a few minutes.

Impellers and turbines. The best known of these instruments is the respirometer developed by Wright in 1955.[48] Alternating gas flow is mechanically rectified and the dead space (22 ml) is sufficiently small for the patient to breathe to and fro through it. The essential mechanism is entirely mechanical with indication of volume on a dial, but the output may be converted to an electrical signal to indicate either tidal volume or minute volume. In general, the respirometer is accurate and tends to read low at low minute volumes and high at high minute volumes.[49] Departure from normality is thus exaggerated and the instrument is essentially safe.

Respiratory inductance plethysmography. Reference has been made above (page 120) to this method of measurement of cross-sectional area of ribcage (RC) and abdomen (AB).[28] The sum of RC and AB signals correlates well with lung volume and, following calibration against a spirometer, changes in the summated signals provide a very useful non-invasive method of measurement or monitoring of ventilation, uninfluenced by the presence of a mouthpiece or mask, and feasible during sleep (Figure 6.5b).

Measurement of ventilatory volumes by integration of instantaneous gas flow rate

Technical advances in electronic circuitry have increased the attractions of measuring ventilatory volumes by integration of instantaneous flow rate. There are many methods of measurement of rapidly changing gas flow rates, of which the original was pneumo-tachography. This employs measurement of the pressure gradient across a laminar resistance, which ensures that the pressure drop is directly proportional to flow rate. This is illustrated in Figure 6.13 where the resistance is a wire mesh screen. It is necessary to take precautions to prevent errors due to different gas composition and temperature, and to prevent condensation of moisture on the screen. The pressure drop need not exceed a few millimetres of water and the volume can be very small. The pneumotachograph should not therefore interfere with respiration.

Alternative flow detectors include Venturi tubes (which give a pressure signal proportional to the square of flow), Pitot tubes and the hot wire anemometer. The last device depends on the cooling of a very thin platinum wire heated to about 400°C. The hot wire anemometer is capable of considerable accuracy when run at high temperature and is little influenced by the temperature of the gas.

Most ventilators and anaesthetic machines currently in use can measure respiratory volumes. A pneumotachograph or electronic turbine system is used, normally on the expired limb of the breathing system, and designed to be of very low resistance to allow measurements during spontaneous respiration. In this way, each expired tidal volume may be measured from which respiratory rate and minute volume can be derived, and a useful method of detecting apnoea or disconnection is therefore provided.

Measurement of ventilatory capacity

Measurement of ventilatory capacity is the most commonly performed test of respiratory function. The ratio of ventilatory capacity to actual ventilation is a measure of ventilatory reserve and of the comfort of breathing.

Maximal breathing capacity (MBC)

Also referred to as maximal voluntary ventilation, MBC is defined as the maximal minute volume of ventilation that the subject can maintain for 15 seconds. In the normal subject,

MBC is about 15–20 times the resting minute volume. The subject simply breathes in and out of a spirometer without the need for removal of carbon dioxide; although simple, the test is exhausting to perform and is now seldom used. Dyspnoea ensues when ventilation reaches about a third of MBC. The average fit young male adult should have an MBC of about 170 $l.min^{-1}$ but normal values depend on body size, age and gender, the range being 47–253 $l.min^{-1}$ for men and 55–139 $l.min^{-1}$ for women.[50]

Forced expiration

A more practical test of ventilatory capacity is the forced expiratory volume in 1 second (FEV_1), which is the maximal volume exhaled in the first second starting from a maximal inspiration. A simple spirometer is all that is required. It is far more convenient to perform than the MBC and less exhausting for the patient. It correlates well with the MBC, which is normally about 35 times the FEV_1.

Peak expiratory flow rate

Most convenient of all the indirect tests of ventilatory capacity is the peak expiratory flow rate. This can be measured with simple and inexpensive hand-held devices. It is most commonly done with the Wright peak flow meter, described in its original form by Wright and McKerrow in 1959.[51] Alternatively, the peak flow may be derived from a pneumotachogram but this is sensitive to very short transients and may give a spuriously high value. The Wright peak flow meter tends to give values about 5.7 times the MBC. Interpretation of measurements of maximal expirations may be misleading. It should be remembered that these tests measure active expiration, which plays no part in normal breathing. They are most commonly performed as a measure of airway obstruction, and are used extensively in asthma and chronic obstructive airway disease. However, the results also depend on many other factors, including chest restriction, motivation and muscular power. The measurements may also be inhibited by pain. A more specific indication of airway resistance is the ratio of FEV_1 to vital capacity. This should exceed 75 per cent in the normal subject.

Assessment of the respiratory muscles[52,53]

Severe abnormalities of muscle function may be assessed by simple observation of spontaneous breathing. During inspiration, paradoxical movements of the trunk may occur, such as inward displacement of the abdominal wall (diaphragm failure) or inward movement of the upper chest (intercostal failure). Fluoroscopy or ultrasound imaging of the diaphragm provides a more subtle form of observation, and is helpful in detecting phrenic nerve damage – particularly if unilateral, when the body surface changes will be less obvious.

Vital capacity (VC) (see Figure 3.9) is now accepted as the best 'bedside' monitor of respiratory muscle function, particularly when performed supine.[52] Performance of a VC manoeuvre requires patient cooperation and coordination, and a single low reading is non-specific. However, repeated measurement allows the observation of a trend in VC to be followed, and a 25 per cent reduction is unequivocally abnormal. In spite of the many causes of a reduced VC, this method of assessing respiratory muscle function is very useful for monitoring the development of progressive muscle weakness in conditions such as myasthenia gravis and Guillain-Barré syndrome (page 516).

Pressure measurements, when breathing against an imposed resistance, are used to assess both inspiratory and expiratory muscle strength. All require some patient compliance and involve a degree of respiratory discomfort, so these tests, though more specific than VC for respiratory muscle function, are not widely used. Mouth pressure may be measured while a slow inspiration or expiration is performed against a moderate respiratory resistance, or mouth pressure may be measured during a rapid 'sniff' procedure in which the nasal airway acts as the resistance. Finally, using either of the above imposed resistances, the more invasive oesophageal and intragastric pressures may be measured to obtain transdiaphragmatic pressure, which is the best assessment of diaphragm force generation.

References

1. Horner RL, Innes JA, Guz A. Reflex pharyngeal dilator muscle activation by stimuli of negative airway pressure in awake man. *Sleep* 1993; **16** (Supp 8): S85–6.
2. Wheatley JR, Tangel DJ, Mezzanotte WS, White DP. Influence of sleep on response to negative airway pressure of tensor palatini muscle and retropalatal airway. *J Appl Physiol* 1993; **75**: 2117–24.
3. Wheatley JR, Kelley WT, Tully A, Engel LA. Pressure–diameter relationships in the upper airway in awake supine subjects. *J Appl Physiol* 1991; **70**: 2242–51.
4. Burger CD, Stanson AW, Daniels BK, Sheedy PF, Shepard JW. Fast CT evaluation of the effect of lung volume on upper airway size and function in normal men. *Am Rev Respir Dis* 1992; **146**: 335–9.
5. Yildirim N, Fitzpatrick MF, Whyte KF, Jalleh R, Wightman AJA, Douglas NJ. The effect of posture on upper airway dimensions in normal subjects and in patients with the sleep apnea/hypopnea syndrome. *Am Rev Respir Dis* 1991; **144**: 845–7.
6. Douglas NJ, Jan MA, Yildirim N, Warren PM, Drummond GB. Effect of posture and breathing route on genioglossal EMG activity in normal subjects and in patients with the sleep apnea/hypopnea syndrome. *Am Rev Respir Dis* 1993; **148**: 1341–5.
7. Pae EK, Lowe AA, Sasaki K, Price C, Tsuchiya M, Fleetham JA. A cephalometric and electromyographic study of upper airway structures in the upright and supine positions. *Am J Orthod Dent Facial Orthop* 1991; **106**: 52–9.
8. Tangel DJ, Mezzanotte WS, White DP. Influence of sleep on tensor palatini EMG and upper airway resistance in normal men. *J Appl Physiol* 1991; **70**: 2574–81.
9. Gal TJ. Is glottic function the key to improved gas exchange? *Chest* 1990; **98**: 9–10.
10. Brancatisano TP, Dodd DS, Engel LA. Respiratory activity of posterior cricoarytenoid muscle and vocal cords in humans. *J Appl Physiol* 1984; **57**: 1143–9.
11. Kuna ST, Insalaco G, Woodson GE. Thyroarytenoid muscle activity during wakefulness and sleep in normal adults. *J Appl Physiol* 1988; **65**: 1332–9.
12. Gauthier AP, Verbanck S, Estenne M, Segebarth C, Macklem PT, Paiva M. Three-dimensional reconstruction of the in vivo human diaphragm shape at different lung volumes. *J Appl Physiol* 1994; **76**: 495–506.
13. Sieck GC. Physiological effects of diaphragm muscle denervation and disuse. *Clin Chest Med* 1994; **15**: 641–59.
14. Eisele JH, Noble MIM, Katz J, Fung DL, Hickey RF. Bilateral phrenic nerve block in man. *Anesthesiology* 1972; **37**: 64–9.
15. Paiva M, Verbanck S, Estenne M, Poncelet B, Segebarth C, Macklem PT. Mechanical implications of in vivo human diaphragm shape. *J Appl Physiol* 1992; **72**: 1407–12.
16. De Troyer A. Respiratory muscle function. In: Brewis RAL, Corrin B, Gedded DM, Gibson GJ, eds. *Respiratory medicine*. London: WB Saunders, 1995; 125–33.
17. Loring SH. Invited editorial on 'Three-dimensional reconstruction of the in vivo human diaphragm shape at different lung volumes'. *J Appl Physiol* 1994; **79**: 493–4.
18. Cassart M, Pettiaux N, Gevenois PA, Paiva M, Estenne M. Effect of chronic hyperinflation on diaphragm length and surface area. *Am J Respir Crit Care Med* 1997; **156**: 504–8.

19. Petroll WM, Knight H, Rochester DF. A model approach to assess diaphragmatic volume displacement. *J Appl Physiol* 1990; **69**: 2175–82.

20. Han JN, Gayan-Ramirez G, Dekhuijzen R, Decramer M. Respiratory function of the rib cage muscles. *Eur Respir J* 1993; **6**: 722–8.

21. Hamberger GE. *De Respirirationis Mechanismo et usu genuino.* Jena, 1749.

22. De Troyer A, Estenne M. Coordination between rib cage muscles and diaphragm during quiet breathing in humans. *J Appl Physiol* 1984; **57**: 899–906.

23. Rimmer KP, Ford GT, Whitelaw WA. Interaction between postural and respiratory control of human intercostal muscles. *J Appl Physiol* 1995; **79**: 1556–61.

24. De Troyer A. Respiratory muscles. In: Crystal RG, West JB, eds. *The lung: scientific foundations.* New York: Raven, 1991; 869.

25. Hillman DR, Finucane KE. A model of the respiratory pump. *J Appl Physiol* 1987; **63**: 951–61.

26. Drummond GB. Chest wall movements in anaesthesia. *Eur J Anaesthesiol* 1989; **6**: 161–96.

27. Konno K, Mead J. Measurement of the separate volume changes of rib cage and abdomen during breathing. *J Appl Physiol* 1967; **22**: 407–22.

28. Milledge JS, Stott FD. Inductive plethysmography – a new respiratory transducer. *J Physiol (Lond)* 1977; **267**: 4–5P.

29. Lumb AB, Nunn JF. Respiratory function and ribcage contribution to ventilation in body positions commonly used during anaesthesia. *Anesth Analg* 1991; **73**: 422–6.

30. Xie S, Takasaki Y, Popkin J, Orr D, Bradley TD. Chemical and postural influence on scalene and diaphragmatic activation in humans. *J Appl Physiol* 1991; **70**: 658–64.

31. Druz WS, Sharp JT. Activity of respiratory muscles in upright and recumbent humans. *J Appl Physiol* 1981; **51**: 1552–61.

32. Muller N, Volgyesi G, Becker L, Bryan MH, Bryan AC. Diaphragmatic muscle tone. *J Appl Physiol* 1979; **47**: 279–84.

33. Cooke IRC, Soust M, Berger PJ. Differential recruitment of inspiratory muscles in response to chemoreceptor drive. *Respir Physiol* 1993; **92**: 167–81.

34. Takasaki Y, Orr D, Popkin J, Xie A, Bradley TD. Effect of hypercapnia and hypoxia on respiratory muscle activation in humans. *J Appl Physiol* 1989; **67**: 1776–84.

35. Lumb AB, Nunn JF. Ribcage contribution to CO_2 response during rebreathing and steady state methods. *Respir Physiol* 1991; **85**: 97–110.

36. Robson JG. The respiratory centres and their responses. In: Evans FT, Gray TC, eds. *Modern Trends in Anaesthesia – 3.* London: Butterworths, 1967.

37. Campbell EJM, Howell JBL. Proprioceptive control of breathing. In: de Rueck AVS, O'Connor M, eds. *Ciba Foundation symposium on pulmonary structure and function.* Edinburgh and London: Churchill Livingstone, 1962.

38. Whitelaw WA, Watson TWJ. Spike trains from single motor units in human parasternal intercostal muscles. *Respir Physiol* 1992; **88**: 289–98.

39. Mizuno M. Human respiratory muscles: fibre morphology and capillary supply. *Eur Respir J* 1991; **4**: 587–601.

40. Milic-Emili J. Work of breathing. In: Crystal RG, West JB, eds. *The lung: scientific foundations.* New York: Raven, 1991; 1065–75.

41. Campbell EJM, Westlake EK, Cherniak RM. Simple methods of estimating oxygen consumption and the efficiency of the muscles of breathing. *J Appl Physiol* 1957; **11**: 303–8.

42. Moxham J. Respiratory muscle fatigue: mechanisms, evaluation and therapy. *Br J Anaesth* 1990; **65**: 43–53.

43. Roussos C, Macklem PT. Diaphragmatic fatigue in man. *J Appl Physiol* 1977; **43**: 189–97.

44. Fujii Y, Toyooka H, Amaha K. Diaphragmatic fatigue and its recovery are influenced by cardiac output. *J Anesth* 1991; **5**: 17–23.

45. Supinski GS, DiMarco AF, Gonzalez J, Altose MD. Effect of norepinephrine on diaphragm contractility and blood flow. *J Appl Physiol* 1990; **69**: 2019–28.

46. Hammond MD, Bauer KA, Sharp JT, Rocha RD. Respiratory muscle strength in congestive cardiac failure. *Chest* 1990; **98**: 1091–4.

47. Zhan W, Sieck GC. Adaptations of diaphragm and medial gastrocnemius muscles to inactivity. *J Appl Physiol* 1992; **72**: 1445–53.

48. Wright BM. A respiratory anemometer. *J Physiol* 1955; **127**: 25P.
49. Nunn JF, Ezi-Ashi TI. The accuracy of the respirometer and ventigrator. *Br J Anaesth* 1962; **34**: 422–32.
50. Cotes JE. *Lung function: assessment and application in medicine.* Oxford: Blackwell Scientific Publications, 1993; 122.
51. Wright BM, McKerrow CB. Maximum forced expiratory flow rate as a measure of ventilatory capacity. *BMJ* 1959; **2**: 1041–7.
52. Polkey MI, Green M, Moxham J. Measurement of respiratory muscle strength. *Thorax* 1995; **50**: 1131–5.
53. Clanton TL, Diaz PT. Clinical assessment of the respiratory muscles. *Phys Ther* 1995; **75**: 983–95.

Chapter 7

The pulmonary circulation

Evolution first led to the development of a separate pulmonary circulation in amphibians, though in this case both systemic and pulmonary circulations are supplied by a single ventricle and there is therefore a great deal of mixing of blood between the two. The occurrence of warm-blooded animals led to a tenfold increase in oxygen requirements, which may be achieved only by having a pulmonary circulation almost completely separate from the systemic circulation.[1] As early as 1553, in a theological writing, Michael Servetus was the first to suggest that venous blood did not pass through the middle wall of the heart, as was generally believed, but followed a long course through the lungs, starting from the right side of the heart.[2]

The entire blood volume passes through the lungs during each circulation. This is an ideal arrangement for gas exchange but is equally suitable for the filtering and metabolic functions of the lungs, which are considered in Chapter 12.

Pulmonary blood flow

The flow of blood through the pulmonary circulation is approximately equal to the flow through the whole of the systemic circulation. It therefore varies from about $6 \, \text{l.min}^{-1}$ under resting conditions, to as much as $25 \, \text{l.min}^{-1}$ in severe exercise. It is remarkable that such an increase can normally be achieved with minimal increase in pressure. Pulmonary vascular pressures and vascular resistance are much less than those of the systemic circulation. Consequently the pulmonary circulation has only limited ability to control the distribution of blood flow in the lung fields and is markedly affected by gravity, which results in overperfusion of the dependent parts of the lung fields. Maldistribution of the pulmonary blood flow has important consequences for gaseous exchange, and these are considered in Chapter 8.

In fact, the relationship between the inflow and outflow of the pulmonary circulation is much more complicated (Figure 7.1). The lungs receive a significant quantity of blood from the bronchial arteries, which usually arise from the arch of the aorta. Blood from the bronchial circulation returns to the heart in two ways. From a plexus around the hilum, blood from the pleurohilar part of the bronchial circulation returns to the superior vena cava via the azygos veins, and this fraction may thus be regarded as normal systemic flow, neither arising from nor returning to the pulmonary circulation.

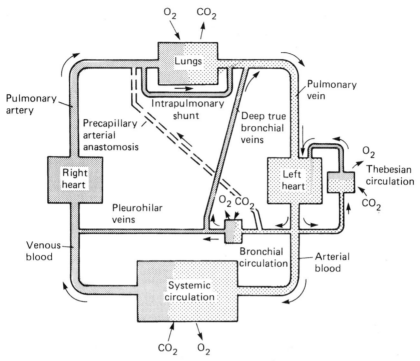

Figure 7.1 Schema of bronchopulmonary anastomoses and other forms of venous admixture in the normal subject. Part of the bronchial circulation returns venous blood to the systemic venous system while another part returns venous blood to the pulmonary veins and so constitutes venous admixture. Other forms of venous admixture are the thebesian circulation of the left heart and flow through atelectatic parts of the lungs. It will be clear from this diagram why the output of the left heart must be slightly greater than that of the right heart.

However, another fraction of the bronchial circulation, distributed more peripherally in the lung, passes through postcapillary anastomoses to join the pulmonary veins, constituting an admixture of venous blood with the arterialized blood from the alveolar capillary networks.[3]

The situation may be further complicated by blood flow through precapillary anastomoses from the bronchial arteries to the pulmonary arteries. The communications (so-called 'sperr arteries') have muscular walls and are thought to act as sluice gates, opening when increased pulmonary blood flow is required.[4] Their functional significance in normal subjects is unknown, but they may be vital in situations involving pulmonary oligaemia, of which congenital pulmonary atresia is the most important natural cause. It should be noted that a Blalock–Taussig shunt operation achieves the same purpose for palliation of patients with cyanotic congenital heart disease.

There are many possible abnormal communications between the pulmonary and systemic circulations. It is not unusual for aberrant pulmonary veins to drain into the right atrium. Furthermore, flow may be reversed through normally occurring channels. Thus, in pulmonary venous hypertension due to mitral stenosis, pulmonary venous blood may traverse the bronchial venous system to gain access to the azygos system.

Pulmonary blood volume

As a first approximation the right heart pumps blood into the pulmonary circulation, while the left heart pumps away the blood that returns from the lungs. Therefore, provided that the output of the two sides is the same, the pulmonary blood volume will remain constant. However, very small differences in the output of the two sides must result in large changes in pulmonary blood volume if they are maintained for more than a few beats.

Factors influencing pulmonary blood volume

Posture. Pulmonary blood volume is directly influenced by posture.[5] Change from the supine to the erect position decreases the pulmonary blood volume by 27 per cent, which is about the same as the corresponding change in cardiac output. Both changes are probably due to pooling of blood in dependent parts of the systemic circulation.

Drugs. Because the systemic circulation has much greater vasomotor activity than the pulmonary circulation, an overall increase in vascular tone will tend to squeeze blood from the systemic into the pulmonary circulation. This may result from the administration of vasoconstrictor drugs, from release of endogenous catecholamines or from passive compression of the body in a G-suit. The magnitude of the resulting volume shift will depend on many factors such as position, overall blood volume and activity of the numerous humoral and nervous mechanisms controlling pulmonary vascular tone at the time (see below). Conversely, it seems likely that pulmonary blood volume would be diminished when systemic tone is diminished, as for example by sympathetic ganglion blockade or, in particular, following regional anaesthesia when systemic vascular resistance is decreased with no effect on the autonomic supply to the pulmonary vasculature.

Left heart failure. Pulmonary venous hypertension (due, for example, to mitral stenosis) would be expected to result in an increased pulmonary blood volume. There has, however, been difficulty in the experimental demonstration of any significant change.

Pulmonary vascular pressures

Pulmonary arterial pressure is only about one-sixth of systemic arterial pressure, although the capillary and venous pressures are not greatly different for the two circulations (Figure 7.2). There is thus only a small pressure drop along the pulmonary arterioles and therefore a reduced potential for active regulation of the distribution of the pulmonary blood flow. This also explains why there is little damping of the arterial pressure wave, and the pulmonary capillary blood flow is markedly pulsatile.

Consideration of pulmonary vascular pressures carries a special difficulty in the selection of the reference pressure. Systemic pressures are customarily measured with reference to ambient atmospheric pressure, but this is not always appropriate when considering the pulmonary arterial pressure, which is relatively small compared with the intrathoracic and pulmonary venous pressures. This may be important in two circumstances. First, the extravascular (intrathoracic) pressure may have a major influence on the intravascular pressure and should be taken into account. Secondly, the driving pressure through the pulmonary circulation may be markedly influenced by the pulmonary venous pressure, which must be taken into account when measuring pulmonary vascular resistance. We must therefore distinguish between pressures within the pulmonary circulation expressed in the three different forms listed below. Measurement techniques may be adapted to indicate these pressures directly (Figure 7.3).

SYSTEMIC CIRCULATION		PULMONARY CIRCULATION
12 (90)	Arteries	2.2 (17)
	Arterioles	
4 (30)		1.7 (13)
	Capillaries	
1.3 (10)		1.2 (9)
	Veins	
0.3 (2)		0.8 (6)
	Atria	

Figure 7.2 Comparison of typical mean pressure gradients along the systemic and pulmonary circulations. (Mean pressures relative to atmosphere in kPa with mmHg in parentheses.)

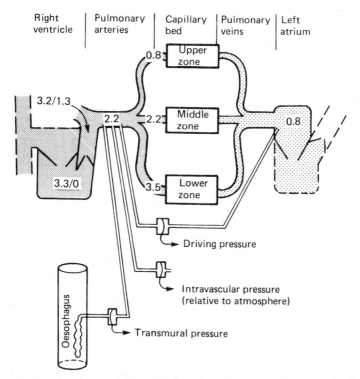

Figure 7.3 Normal values for pressures in the pulmonary circulation relative to atmospheric (kPa). Systolic and diastolic pressures are shown for the right ventricle and pulmonary trunk. Note the effect of gravity on pressures at different levels in the lung fields. Three different manometers are shown connected to indicate driving pressure, intravascular pressure and transmural pressure.

Intravascular pressure is the pressure at any point in the circulation relative to atmosphere. This is the customary way of expressing pressures in the systemic circulation, and is also the commonest method of indicating the pulmonary vascular pressures.

Transmural pressure is the difference in pressure between the inside of a vessel and the tissue surrounding the vessel. In the case of the larger pulmonary vessels, the outside pressure is the intrathoracic pressure (commonly measured as the oesophageal pressure, as shown in Figure 7.3). This method should be used to exclude the physical effect of major changes in intrathoracic pressure.

Driving pressure is the difference in pressure between one point in the circulation and another point downstream. The driving pressure of the pulmonary circulation as a whole is the pressure difference between pulmonary artery and left atrium. This is the pressure that overcomes the flow resistance and should be used for determining vascular resistance.

These differences are far from being solely academic. For example, an increase in intrathoracic pressure due to positive pressure ventilation will increase the pulmonary arterial intravascular pressure but will also similarly increase pulmonary venous intravascular pressure, and therefore driving pressure (and therefore flow) remains unchanged. Similarly, if the primary problem is a raised left atrial pressure, blood will 'back up' through the pulmonary circulation and pulmonary arterial intravascular pressure will also be raised, but again the driving pressure will not be increased. Therefore for assessing pulmonary blood flow (and so resistance), driving pressure is the correct measurement, but this requires pulmonary venous (left atrial) pressure to be recorded, which is difficult to achieve continuously (page 157). Pulmonary arterial intravascular pressure is usually measured and the value must be interpreted with caution.

Typical normal values for pressures in the pulmonary circulation are shown in Figure 7.3. The effect of gravity on the pulmonary vascular pressure may be seen, and it will be clear why pulmonary oedema is most likely to occur in the lower zones of the lungs where the intravascular pressures and the transmural pressure gradients are highest.

Effect of intra-alveolar pressure

Alteration of intra-alveolar pressure causes changes in intrathoracic pressure according to the following relationship:

Intrathoracic pressure = Alveolar pressure – Alveolar transmural pressure

Alveolar transmural pressure is a function of lung volume (see Figure 3.8) and, when the lungs are passively inflated, the intrathoracic pressure will normally increase by rather less than half the inflation pressure. The increase will be even less if the lungs are stiff, and thus a low compliance protects the circulation from inflation pressure (page 613). Intravascular pressures are normally increased directly and instantaneously by the effects of changes in intrathoracic pressure, and this explains the initial rise in systemic arterial pressure during a Valsalva manoeuvre (page 609). It also explains the cyclical changes in pulmonary arterial pressure during spontaneous respiration, with pressures greater during expiration than during inspiration. Such changes would not be seen if transmural pressure were measured (Figure 7.3).

In addition to the immediate physical effect of an increase in intrathoracic pressure on intravascular pressures, there is a secondary physiological effect due to interference with venous filling. This accounts for the secondary decline in systemic pressure seen in the Valsalva manoeuvre.

Pulmonary vascular resistance

Vascular resistance is an expression of the relationship between driving pressure and flow, as in the case of resistance to gas flow. It may be expressed in similar terms as follows:

$$\text{Pulmonary vascular resistance} = \frac{\text{Pulmonary driving pressure}}{\text{Cardiac output}}$$

There are, however, important caveats and the concept of pulmonary vascular resistance is not a simple parallel to Ohm's law, appropriate to laminar flow (page 59). When gases flow through rigid tubes the flow is laminar, or turbulent, or a mixture of the two. In the first case, pressure increases in direct proportion to flow rate and the resistance remains constant (Poiseuille's law). In the second case, pressure increases according to the square of the flow rate, and the resistance increases with flow. When the type of flow is mixed, the pressure rises in proportion to the flow rate raised to a power between one and two.

The circumstances are two stages more complicated in the case of blood. First, the tubes through which the blood flows are not rigid but tend to expand as flow is increased, particularly in the pulmonary circulation with its low vasomotor tone. Consequently the resistance tends to fall as flow increases and the plot of pressure against flow rate is neither linear (see Figure 4.2) nor curved with the concavity upwards (see Figure 4.3) but curved with the concavity downwards. The second complication is that blood is a non-newtonian fluid (owing to the presence of the corpuscles) and its viscosity varies with the shear rate, which is a function of its linear velocity.

Vascular resistance in the lung Although the relationship between flow and pressure in blood vessels is very far removed from simple linearity, there is a widespread convention that pulmonary vascular resistance should be expressed in a form of the equation above. This is directly analogous to electrical resistance, as though there were laminar flow of a newtonian fluid though rigid pipes. It would, of course, be quite impractical in the clinical situation to measure pulmonary driving pressure at different values of cardiac output to determine the true nature of their relationship.

Vascular resistance is expressed in units derived from those used for expression of pressure and flow rate. Using conventional units, vascular resistance is usually expressed in units of $mmHg.litre^{-1}.minute$. In absolute CGS units, vascular resistance is usually expressed in units of dynes/square centimetre per cubic centimetre/second (i.e. $dyn.sec.cm^{-5}$). The appropriate SI units will probably be $kPa.l^{-1}.minute$. Normal values for the pulmonary circulation in the various units are as follows:

	Driving pressure	Pulmonary blood flow	Pulmonary vascular resistance
SI units	1.2 kPa	$5\,l.min^{-1}$	$0.24\,kPa.l^{-1}.min$
Conventional units	9 mmHg	$5\,l.min^{-1}$	$1.8\,mmHg.l^{-1}.min$
Absolute CGS units	$12\,000\,dyn.cm^{-2}$	$83\,cm^3.sec^{-1}$	$144\,dyn.sec.cm^{-5}$

Localization of the pulmonary vascular resistance

By far the greatest part of the systemic resistance is in the arterioles, along which the pressure falls from a mean value of about 12 kPa (90 mmHg) down to about 4 kPa

(30 mmHg) (see Figure 7.2). This pressure drop largely obliterates the pulse pressure wave, and the systemic capillary flow is not pulsatile to any great extent. In the pulmonary circulation, the pressure drop along the arterioles is very much smaller than in the systemic circulation and, as an approximation, the pulmonary vascular resistance is divided equally between arteries, capillaries and veins. Pulmonary arteries and arterioles, with muscular vessel walls, are mostly extra-alveolar and involved in active control of pulmonary vascular resistance by mechanisms such as nervous, humoral or gaseous control. In contrast, pulmonary capillaries are intimately associated with the alveolus (see Figure 2.7), so resistance of these vessels is greatly influenced by alveolar pressure and volume. Thus in the pulmonary circulation, vessels without the power of active vasoconstriction play a major role in governing total vascular resistance and the distribution of the pulmonary blood flow.

Passive changes in pulmonary vascular resistance
Effect of pulmonary blood flow (cardiac output)

The pulmonary circulation can adapt to large changes in cardiac output with only small increases in pulmonary arterial pressure. Thus pulmonary vascular resistance must decrease as flow increases. Reduced resistance implies an increase in the total cross-sectional area of the pulmonary vascular bed and particularly the capillaries. These adaptations to increased flow occur partly by passive dilatation of vessels and partly by recruitment of collapsed vessels, the former now being considered the most important factor.[6]

Recruitment of previously unperfused pulmonary vessels may occur in response to increased pulmonary flow. This is particularly true of the capillary bed, which is devoid of any vasomotor control, so allowing the opening of new passages in the network of capillaries lying in the alveolar septa, and is most likely to occur in the upper part of the lung where capillary pressure is lowest (zone 1, see below). This phenomenon was first described in histological studies involving sections cut in lungs rapidly frozen while perfused with blood, which showed that the number of open capillaries increased with rising pulmonary arterial pressure, particularly in the mid-zone of the lung.[7] Recruitment of capillaries in the intact lung remains poorly understood. Animal studies, using colloidal gold particles in the circulation, have shown that there is perfusion in all pulmonary capillaries, including in zone 1, during normal ventilation.[8] A similar study using fluorescent-labelled albumin but with airway pressure increased above pulmonary capillary pressure showed no flow in almost two-thirds of capillaries in zone 1.[9] It therefore seems that with increased alveolar pressure (e.g. during positive pressure ventilation) unperfused capillaries are available for recruitment but that under normal circumstances, with low airway pressures, there is flow in all capillaries. However, the studies using colloidal particles cannot discriminate between plasma or blood flow and have led to speculation that some, *almost* collapsed, capillaries may contain only plasma ('plasma skimming') or even blood flow from the bronchial circulation.[10]

Distension in the entire pulmonary vasculature occurs in response to increased transmural pressure gradient, and is again most likely to occur in capillaries devoid of muscular control. In one study, capillary diameter increased from 5 to 10 μm as the transmural pressure increased from 0.5 to 2.5 kPa (5 to 25 cmH$_2$O).[11] As described in the previous section, it now seems likely that capillaries never collapse completely and therefore passive distension is clearly the more important adaptation to increased flow.[6]

A striking example of the ability of the pulmonary vasculature to adapt to changing flow occurs after pneumonectomy, when the remaining lung will normally take the entire resting pulmonary blood flow without a rise in pulmonary arterial pressure. There is, inevitably, a limit to the flow that can be accommodated without an increase in pressure, and this will be less if the pulmonary vascular bed is diminished by disease or surgery. The most important pathological cause of increased flow is left-to-right shunting through a patent ductus arteriosus or through atrial or ventricular septal defects. In these circumstances the pulmonary blood flow may be several-fold greater than the systemic flow before pulmonary hypertension develops. Despite this, secondary changes in pulmonary vessels commonly lead to an increase in vascular resistance, causing an earlier and more severe rise in pulmonary arterial pressure.

Effect of lung inflation

Reference has been made above to the effect of alveolar pressure on pulmonary vascular pressures. The effect on pulmonary vascular resistance is complex. Confusion has arisen in the past because of failure to appreciate that pulmonary vascular resistance must be derived from driving pressure and not from pulmonary arterial or transmural pressure (Figure 7.3). This is important because inflation of the lungs normally influences the pressure in the oesophagus, pulmonary artery and left atrium, and so can easily conceal the true effect on vascular resistance.

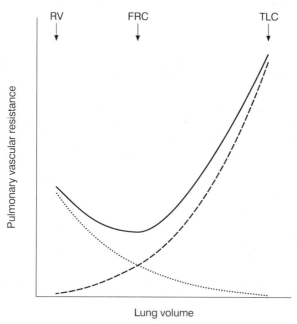

Figure 7.4 Relationship between pulmonary vascular resistance (PVR) and lung volume. The solid line represents total PVR and is minimal at the functional residual capacity (FRC). Compression of alveolar vessels (dashed line) is responsible for the increased PVR as lung volume approaches total lung capacity (TLC). Increasing PVR as lung volume approaches residual volume (RV) may result from either compression of corner vessels or hypoxia-induced vasoconstriction in collapsed lung units (dotted line). It should be noted that this graph is derived from studies mainly involving isolated animal lungs and may not be applicable to the intact subject.

When pulmonary vascular resistance is correctly calculated from the driving pressure, there is reasonable agreement that the pulmonary vascular resistance is minimal at FRC and that changes in lung volume in either direction cause a small increase in resistance, particularly at high lung volumes (Figure 7.4). These observations may be explained by considering pulmonary capillaries as belonging to two distinct groups, discussed below.[12]

Alveolar capillaries are sandwiched between two adjacent alveolar walls, usually bulging into one alveolus (see Figure 2.7) and supported from collapse only by the pressure in the capillary and flimsy septal fibrous tissue. Expansion of the alveolus will therefore compress these capillaries and increase their contribution to pulmonary vascular resistance. If the lung consisted entirely of alveolar capillaries, pulmonary vascular resistance would be directly related to lung volume.

Corner capillaries lie in the junction between three or more alveoli, and are not therefore sandwiched between alveolar walls. In this area, the alveolar wall is believed to form 'pleats' during lung deflation, which are then stretched out longitudinally (rather than expanded outwards) during inspiration and so have little effect on the blood vessels nearby.[12] Indeed, blood vessels in this area are generally uninfluenced by alveolar pressure but may expand at high lung volume and constrict at very small lung volumes possibly secondary to local hypoxia surrounding the collapsed alveoli.[12]

Extra-alveolar vessels. An additional explanation for the increased pulmonary vascular resistance at small lung volumes lies in the extra-alveolar vessels. As long ago as 1968 Hughes and colleagues suggested that compression of larger pulmonary vessels at low lung volumes results in reduced flow in dependent parts of the lung (page 169), and this is likely to contribute to the overall change in pulmonary vascular resistance.

The anatomical difference between these capillaries is undoubted, although the effects of the anatomical features on physiology are unproven. Much of the work has involved mathematical modelling based on animal studies in the open-chested or isolated preparation, and the relevance of these to the intact human is as yet uncertain.

Effect of gravity on alveolar and vascular pressures

The vascular weir. The interplay of alveolar pressure, flow rate and vascular resistance is best considered by dividing the lung field into three zones.[13,14] Figure 7.5 shows behaviour as a Starling resistor and also the analogy of a weir. A Starling, or threshold, resistor can be visualized as a length of compressible tubing in a rigid chamber, such that flow occurs only when the upstream pressure (left gauges in Figure 7.5) exceeds the pressure in the chamber (middle gauges) and a reduction in the downstream pressure (right gauges) cannot initiate flow. In zone 1 of Figure 7.5, the pressure within the arterial end of the collapsible vessels is less than the alveolar pressure, and therefore insufficient to open the vessels, which remain collapsed as in a Starling resistor. The upstream water is below the top of the weir and so there can be no flow. The downstream (venous) pressure is irrelevant. Zone 1 corresponds to conditions that may apply in the uppermost parts of the lungs.

In the mid-zone of the lungs (zone 2 of Figure 7.5), the pressure at the arterial end of the collapsible vessels exceeds the alveolar pressure and, under these conditions, a collapsible vessel, behaving like a Starling resistor, permits flow in such a way that the

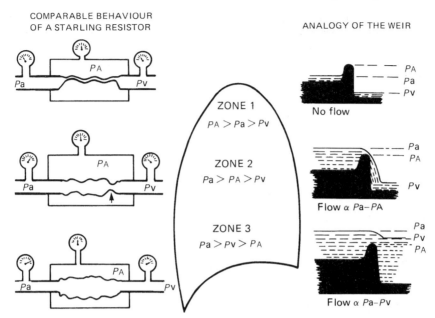

COMPARABLE BEHAVIOUR
OF A STARLING RESISTOR

ANALOGY OF THE WEIR

Figure 7.5 The effect of gravity on pulmonary vascular resistance is shown by comparison with a Starling resistor (left) and with a weir (right). *Pa*, pulmonary artery pressure; *PA*, alveolar pressure; *Pv*, pulmonary venous pressure (all pressures relative to atmosphere). See text for full discussion.

flow rate depends on the arterial/alveolar pressure difference. Resistance in the Starling resistor is concentrated at the point marked with the arrows in Figure 7.5. The greater the difference between arterial and alveolar pressure, the more widely the collapsible vessels will open and the greater will be the flow. Note that the venous pressure is still not a factor that affects flow or vascular resistance. This condition is still analogous to a weir, the upstream depth (head of pressure) corresponding to the arterial pressure and the height of the weir corresponding to alveolar pressure. Flow depends solely on the difference in height between the upstream water level and the top of the weir. The depth of water below the weir (analogous to venous pressure) cannot influence the flow of water over the weir unless it rises above the height of the weir.

In the lower zone of the lungs (zone 3 of Figure 7.5), the pressure in the venous end of the capillaries is above the alveolar pressure, and under these conditions a collapsible vessel behaving like a Starling resistor will be held wide open and the flow rate will, as a first approximation, be governed by the arterial/venous pressure difference (the driving pressure) in the normal manner for the systemic circulation. However, as the intravascular pressure increases in relation to the alveolar pressure, the collapsible vessels will be further distended and their resistance will be correspondingly reduced. Returning to the analogy of the weir, the situation is now one in which the downstream water level has risen until the weir is completely submerged and offers little resistance to the flow of water, which is largely governed by the difference in the water level above and below the weir. However, as the levels rise further, the weir is progressively more and more submerged and what little resistance it offers to water flow is diminished still further.

Active control of pulmonary vascular resistance

In addition to the passive mechanisms described, pulmonary blood vessels are also able to control vascular resistance by active vasoconstriction and vasodilatation, and there is now evidence that the pulmonary vasculature is normally kept in a state of active vasodilatation.[15]

Cellular mechanisms controlling pulmonary vascular tone[16,17,18]

There are many mechanisms by which pulmonary vascular tone may be controlled (Table 7.1), but the role of many of these in the human lung is uncertain. Some of the receptor–agonist systems in Table 7.1 have only been demonstrated *in vitro* using animal tissue, but may eventually emerge as important in humans either for normal maintenance of pulmonary vascular tone or during lung injury (Chapter 30). Activity of some, though not all, of the mechanisms listed in Table 7.1 are dependent on the endothelial lining of the pulmonary blood vessels. It seems likely that many basic control mechanisms act directly on the smooth muscle itself whilst the endothelium acts as a modulator of the response. Some control mechanisms such as the autonomic nervous system and hypoxic pulmonary

Table 7.1 Receptors and agonists involved in active control of pulmonary vascular tone

Receptor group	Subtypes	Principal agonists	Responses	Endothelium dependent?
Adrenergic	α_1	Noradrenaline	Constriction	No
	α_2	Noradrenaline	Dilatation	Yes
	β_2	Adrenaline	Dilatation	Yes
Cholinergic	M_3	Acetylcholine	Dilatation	Yes
Amines	H_1	Histamine	Variable	Yes
	H_2	Histamine	Dilatation	No
	5-HT_1	5-HT	Variable	Variable
Purines	P_{2x}	ATP	Constriction	No
	P_{2y}	ATP	Dilatation	Yes
	A_1	Adenosine	Constriction	No
	A_2	Adenosine	Dilatation	No
Eicosanoids	TP	Thromboxane A_2	Constriction	No
	?	Prostacyclin (PGI_2)	Dilatation	?
Peptides	NK_1	Substance P	Dilatation	Yes
	NK_2	Neurokinin A	Constriction	No
	?	VIP	Relaxation	Variable
	AT	Angiotensin	Constriction	No
	ANP	ANP	Dilatation	No
	B_2	Bradykinin	Dilatation	Yes
	ET_A	Endothelin	Constriction	No
	ET_B	Endothelin	Dilatation	Yes
	?	Adrenomedullin	Dilatation	?
	V_1	Vasopressin	Dilatation	Yes

The existence of many of the substances listed is at present established only in animals, and their physiological or pathological relevance in humans therefore remains uncertain. From references 16 and 17. 5-HT, 5-hydroxytryptamine; ANP, atrial natriuretic peptide; ATP, adenosine triphosphate; VIP, vasoactive intestinal peptide.

vasoconstriction have been investigated extensively in humans, and are described separately below.

Receptors. Endothelial and muscle cells of the pulmonary vasculature each have numerous receptor types, and the agonists for these receptors may originate from nerve endings (e.g. acetylcholine, noradrenaline), be produced locally (e.g. eicosanoids) or arrive via the blood (e.g. peptides). In addition, many similar or identical compounds produce opposing effects by their actions on differing sub-groups of receptors, for example α_1 (vasoconstrictor) and β_2 (vasodilator) adrenergic receptors. There remains a large number of poorly understood systems acting together to bring about control of vascular smooth muscle.

Second messengers. Pulmonary vasodilators that act directly on the smooth muscle such as prostaglandins, VIP and, in some circumstances, β_2-agonists mostly activate adenyl cyclase to produce cyclic adenosine-3',5'-monophosphate (cAMP) as a second messenger. In turn, cAMP causes a host of intracellular activity via activation of protein kinase enzymes, which reduces both the phosphorylation of myosin and intracellular calcium levels to bring about relaxation of the muscle cell.[19]

Receptors that result in contraction of pulmonary vascular smooth muscle are usually G-protein coupled. Activation produces a second messenger, inositol-1,4,5-triphosphate (IP_3), which releases calcium from intracellular stores and activates myosin phosphorylation to produce contraction. Some compounds with vascular activity act by direct effects on potassium and calcium channels.[16] For example, in pulmonary vessels of the rabbit an ATP-sensitive K^+ channel controls membrane potential and, therefore, the degree of contraction of the muscle cell.[20]

Role of the endothelium and nitric oxide.[16,21,22,23] Furchgott and Zawadzki in 1980 were the first to demonstrate that endothelial cells were required for acetylcholine (ACh) -induced relaxation in isolated aortic tissue.[24] The messenger passing between the endothelium and smooth muscle cells was termed endothelium-derived relaxing factor (EDRF),[25] the major part of which was subsequently shown to be nitric oxide (NO).[23] Nitric oxide is not the only form of EDRF, some species showing a quite separate messenger termed endothelium-derived hyperpolarizing factor (EDHF).[26] The chemical nature of EDHF remains uncertain, but studies indicate that it is a cytochrome P-450 monooxygenase (page 227) derived metabolite of arachidonic acid.[27]

Many pulmonary vasodilator mechanisms have been shown to be endothelium dependent (Table 7.1) so it seems likely that NO, possibly in combination with other forms of EDRF, is a common pathway for producing relaxation of vascular smooth muscle from a variety of stimuli.

Nitric oxide synthase[22] produces NO by the conversion of L-arginine to L-citrulline, via a highly reactive hydroxyarginine intermediate (Figure 7.6). NOS is involved in both stages, and requires many cofactors, including calmodulin and NADPH, and probably other flavine-derived factors such as flavine adenine dinucleotide. Control of NOS activity is believed to depend on the availability of the substrate arginine and the concentrations of the various cofactors. Citrulline produced by NOS enters the urea cycle and is converted back into arginine (Figure 7.6). This pathway uses ammonia derived from the conversion of amino acids into energy-producing substrates such as pyruvate, and provides a mechanism by which ammonium ions may be converted into relatively harmless nitrates (via NO). The biological disposal of nitric oxide is described on page 273.

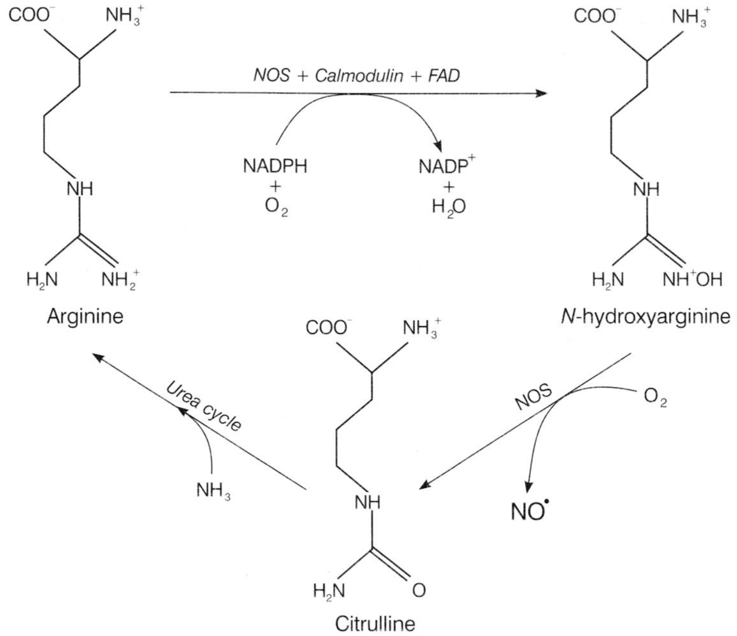

Figure 7.6 Biochemical production of nitric oxide (NO). Nitric oxide synthase (NOS) acts as a catalyst for a two-stage reaction to convert arginine to citrulline. Oxygen is required at both stages, and NADPH, calmodulin and flavine adenine dinucleotide (FAD) are required as cofactors for the first stage and are believed to control the rate of NO production. Citrulline produced in this reaction may then enter the urea cycle and, using ammonia derived from amino acid metabolism, is converted back into arginine.

Nitric oxide synthase exists in two forms known as constitutive and inducible. Inducible NO synthase (iNOS) is produced in many cells but only in response to activation by inflammatory mediators and other cytokines, and once activated can produce large amounts of NO for long periods. Constitutive NO (cNOS) is permanently present in some cells, including pulmonary endothelium, and produces short bursts of low levels of NO in response to changes in calcium and calmodulin levels. In systemic vessels, sheer stress of the blood vessel wall may directly activate calcium-dependent potassium channels to activate cNOS, but in the pulmonary circulation receptor stimulation is the usual source of altered calcium levels and cNOS activation.

The mechanism by which receptor activation leads to muscle relaxation is illustrated in Figure 7.7. Nitric oxide diffuses from the site of production to the smooth muscle cell where it activates guanylate cyclase to produce cyclic guanosine-3′, 5′-monophosphate (cGMP), which in turn activates a protein kinase enzyme (G kinase). This system is similar to the cAMP pathway described above, and causes relaxation by a combination of effects on cytosolic calcium levels and the activity of enzymes controlling myosin activity.

There is now good evidence that basal production of NO occurs in normal human lungs and contributes to the maintenance of low pulmonary vascular resistance.[15,28] Both studies have used N^G-monomethyl-L-arginine (L-NMMA), a NOS inhibitor, to demonstrate reduced global[28] or regional[15] pulmonary blood flow.

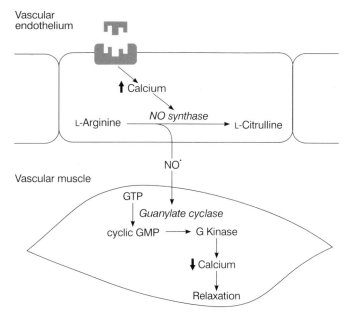

Figure 7.7 Schematic pathway for the activation of constitutive nitric oxide synthase and the action of nitric oxide in the pulmonary vasculature. There are many different receptors thought to act via this mechanism to bring about vasodilatation. See text for details.

Effect of respiratory gases

Hypoxia. When vasoconstriction occurs in response to hypoxia, pulmonary blood vessels are displaying their fundamental difference from all systemic vessels. Hypoxic pulmonary vasoconstriction (HPV) is mediated both by mixed venous (pulmonary arterial) Po_2 and by alveolar Po_2 (Figure 7.8), the greater influence being from the alveolus. The overall response to Po_2 is non-linear. This may be deduced from Figure 7.8 by noting the pressure response for different values of the isobaric Po_2 (the broken line), and it will be seen that the general shape of the response curve resembles an oxyhaemoglobin dissociation curve with a P_{50} of about 4 kPa (30 mmHg). The combined effect of hypoxia in alveolar gas and mixed venous blood may be considered as acting at a single point,[29] which exerts a 'stimulus' Po_2 as follows:

$$P(\text{stimulus})o_2 = P\bar{v}_{O_2}{}^{0.375} \times P_{AO_2}{}^{0.626}$$

In addition to the effect of mixed venous and alveolar Po_2, the bronchial arterial Po_2 influences tone in the larger pulmonary arteries via the vasa vasorum.[30]

Regional hypoxic pulmonary vasoconstriction is beneficial as a means of diverting the pulmonary blood flow away from regions in which the oxygen tension is low, and is an important factor in the optimization of ventilation/perfusion relationships (Chapter 8).[32] It is also important in the fetus to minimize perfusion of the unventilated lung. However, overall chronic or intermittent hypoxic pulmonary vasoconstriction results in pulmonary hypertension, and this response is disadvantageous in a range of clinical conditions (see Chapter 28).

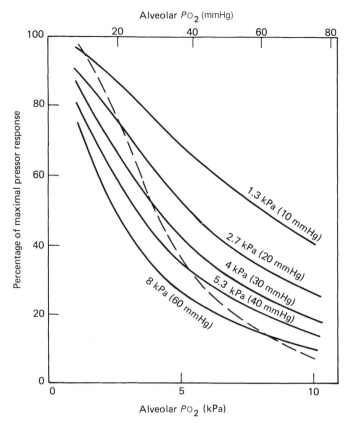

Figure 7.8 Pulmonary vasoconstriction (ordinate) as a function of alveolar P_{O_2} (abscissa) for different values of mixed venous P_{O_2} (indicated for each curve). The broken line shows the response when the alveolar and mixed venous P_{O_2} are identical. (Drawn from data in reference 31.)

Mechanism of HPV. The pressor response to hypoxia results from constriction of small arterioles of 30–200 μm in diameter.[33] Neural connections to the lung are not required, as demonstrated by the observations that HPV occurs in isolated lung preparations and in humans following lung transplantation.[34] There is no evidence for release of a vasoconstrictor substance in response to acute hypoxia, although almost all the vasoconstrictor substances listed in Table 7.1 have at some time been implicated but with no subsequent confirmation.[33] With systemic arterial hypoxaemia some pulmonary vasoconstriction may result from hypoxic stimulation of the peripheral chemoreceptors by way of sympathetic efferent pathways[35] but this is manifestly less important than the local effect.

Animal studies have shown that HPV begins within a few seconds of the P_{O_2} decreasing.[36] In humans, hypoxia in a single lobe of the lung results in a rapid decline in perfusion of the lobe such that after 5 minutes regional blood flow is half that during normoxia.[37] *In vitro* and animal studies have shown that over a longer period HPV is biphasic.[38] The first phase is similar to that seen in the human study already described, being rapid in onset with a maximum vasoconstriction after 5–10 minutes of hypoxia before rapidly returning to almost baseline levels of vascular activity. A second phase then develops, involving a slow and sustained vasoconstriction that reaches a plateau after 40 minutes.

Attempts to elucidate the mechanism of HPV have been hampered by species differences, the multitude of systems affecting pulmonary vascular tone and a lack of appreciation of the biphasic nature of the response. There remain many hypotheses on the cellular mechanism of HPV, based around either the inhibition of a vasodilator mechanism or stimulation of vasoconstriction. First, hypoxia may inhibit endothelial NO production and so induce vasoconstriction. This assumes a high level of normal NO production, and, though basal NO production does occur, its inhibition cannot alone explain HPV. Results of studies of NO and HPV are contradictory[38] and it is likely that NO is involved in modulation of HPV rather than being the underlying mechanism. Furthermore, it has been suggested that NO may be responsible for opposing HPV to maintain some perfusion of hypoxic regions.[39] Secondly, cyclooxygenase activity is inhibited by hypoxia, which may diminish the effects of vasodilator products such as prostacyclin (PGI_2), but again there are contradictory studies implying that this pathway is also involved only in modulation of HPV.[38,40] Thirdly, hypoxia promotes the production of endothelin, a vasoconstrictor peptide, which has a prolonged effect on pulmonary vascular tone such that this mechanism is probably involved in the second slow phase of HPV and is likely to be important in the development of pulmonary hypertension with chronic hypoxia.[38] Finally, there is continuing interest in the possibility of a direct effect of hypoxia on pulmonary vascular smooth muscle cells. Pulmonary blood vessels, unlike systemic ones, have been shown to have oxygen-sensitive K^+ channels, which under hypoxic conditions will alter the membrane potential of the smooth muscle cell and allow voltage-gated calcium channels to open and produce contraction.[16,41,42] Similarly, ATP-sensitive ion channels can control smooth muscle contraction and, in this way, intracellular ATP concentration may be acting as an oxygen sensor.[20] Whether or not these direct ion channel mechanisms alone are sufficient to produce HPV is disputed,[38] but they do show a fundamental difference between pulmonary and systemic vasculature. Hypoxic pulmonary vasoconstriction is therefore almost certainly multifactorial in origin, and likely to result from a combination of direct effects of hypoxia on smooth muscle modulated by endothelium-dependent factors.

Hypercapnia and acidosis. Elevated P_{CO_2} has a slight pressor effect. For example, hypoventilation of one lobe of a dog's lung reduces perfusion of that lobe, although its ventilation/perfusion ratio is still reduced.[43] Both respiratory and metabolic acidosis augment HPV.[12,44]

Hypocapnia and alkalosis. Alkalosis, whether respiratory or metabolic in origin, causes pulmonary vasodilatation[12] and reduces[45] or even abolishes[46] HPV.

Neural control

There are three systems involved in autonomic control of the pulmonary circulation[16,17] which are similar to those controlling airway tone (page 71).

Adrenergic sympathetic nerves originate from the first five thoracic nerves and travel to the pulmonary vessels via the cervical ganglia and a plexus of nerves around the trachea and smaller airways. They act mainly on the smooth muscle of arteries and arterioles down to a diameter of less than 60 μm.[12,16] There are both α_1-receptors which mediate vasoconstriction, usually in response to noradrenaline release, and β_2-receptors which produce vasodilatation mainly in response to circulating adrenaline. Finally, pulmonary blood vessels contain α_2-receptors which cause vasodilatation either presynaptically where they inhibit noradrenaline release or postsynaptically on endothelial cells where they increase NO production (Figure 7.7).[47] Over all, α_1 effects predominate and sympathetic stimulation increases pulmonary vascular resistance.[16] The influence of the sympathetic system is not as strong as in the systemic circulation and seems to have little influence under resting conditions. There is no obvious disadvantage in this respect in patients with lung transplant (Chapter 33). The sympathetic system does, however, have an appreciable effect when there is general activation, as for example under conditions of flight, fright or fight, and is also activated when the peripheral chemoreceptors are stimulated by hypoxia.

Cholinergic nerves of the parasympathetic system travel in the vagus nerve and cause pulmonary vasodilatation by release of ACh following stimulation of M_3 muscarinic receptors.[16] Acetylcholine-mediated vasodilatation is now accepted as being endothelium and NO dependent,[15,24] and in the absence of endothelium ACh is a vasoconstrictor. The significance of cholinergic nerves in humans is less clear than that of adrenergic systems. Infusion of ACh into the pulmonary artery in normal subjects results in vasodilatation,[15] so ACh receptors clearly exist, but cholinergic nerve fibres have not been demonstrated histologically around human pulmonary vessels.[16]

Non-adrenergic, non-cholinergic (NANC)[16] nerves are closely related anatomically to the other autonomic mechanisms but with different neurotransmitters and are similar to the NANC nerves controlling airway smooth muscle (page 71). In the lung, most NANC nerves are inhibitory, causing vasodilatation via release of NO, possibly in conjunction with peptides (Table 7.1). The functional significance of this system is unknown.

Humoral control

Pulmonary vascular endothelium is involved in the metabolism of many circulating substances (Chapter 12), some of which cause changes in vascular tone (Table 7.1). Which of these are involved in the control of normal pulmonary vascular resistance is unclear, and it is quite possible that very few are, but some are undoubtedly involved in pulmonary vascular disease (Chapters 13 and 28).

Catecholamines. Circulating adrenaline following sympathetic stimulation acts on both α- and β-receptors and results in a predominantly vasoconstrictor response. Exogenous adrenaline and related inotropes such as dopamine have a similar effect.

Eicosanoids. Arachidonic acid (AA) metabolism via the cyclooxygenase pathway (to prostaglandins and thromboxane) and the lipoxygenase pathway (to leukotrienes) has been demonstrated in pulmonary vessels in animals. The products of AA metabolism have diverse biological effects in many physiological systems and the pulmonary vasculature is no exception. Arachidonic acid itself, thromboxane A_2, $PGF_{2\alpha}$, PGD_2, PGE_2 and LTB_4 are all vasoconstrictors whilst PGI_2 (prostacyclin) is usually a vasodilator. These pathways are believed to be involved in pathological pulmonary hypertension resulting from sepsis, reperfusion injury or congenital heart disease.[16]

Amines. Histamine relaxes pulmonary vascular smooth muscle during adrenaline-induced constriction but constricts resting smooth muscle. Constriction is in response to H_1 stimulation on smooth muscle cells whilst relaxation occurs either via H_1 receptors on endothelium (NO dependent) or H_2 receptors on smooth muscle cells. 5-Hydroxy-tryptamine (5-HT, serotonin) is liberated from activated platelets and is a potent vasoconstrictor. It may be involved in pulmonary hypertension secondary to emboli (page 551).

Peptides. Numerous peptides that are vasoactive in the pulmonary circulation are shown in Table 7.1. Responses are again diverse, many systems producing vasodilatation via endothelium receptors and vasoconstriction via direct effects on smooth muscle (e.g. substance P and neurokinin A).[16]

Purine nucleosides such as adenosine and ATP are highly vasoactive, again with variable responses according to the amount of tone in the pulmonary blood vessel.[16] Adenosine is a pulmonary vasodilator in normal subjects.[48]

Principles of measurement of the pulmonary circulation

Detailed consideration of haemodynamic measurement techniques lies outside the scope of this book. The following section presents only the broad principles of measurement such as may be required in relation to respiratory physiology.

Pulmonary blood volume

Available methods are based on the technique used for measurement of cardiac output by dye dilution (see below). The flow rate so obtained is multiplied by the interval between the time of the injection of the dye and the mean arrival time of the dye at the sampling point. This product indicates the amount of blood lying between injection and sampling sites, and the volume result obtained therefore depends very much on exactly where sampling occurs. Total pulmonary blood volume may be measured by sampling from the proximal pulmonary artery and the pulmonary vein (or left atrium). Typical values are of the order of 0.5–1 litre or 10–20 per cent of total blood volume in an adult.

Table 2.2 shows the anatomical distribution of the pulmonary blood volume in the pulmonary arterial tree, which has a volume of the order of 150 ml. Pulmonary capillary volume may be calculated from measurements of diffusing capacity (Chapter 9), and this technique yields values of the order of 80 ml. The pulmonary veins therefore contain over half of the pulmonary blood volume owing to much less vasomotor tone than the pulmonary arteries.

Pulmonary vascular pressures

Pressure measurements in the pulmonary circulation are almost always made with electronic differential pressure transducers, which measure pressure in a column of liquid in continuity with a blood vessel compared with atmospheric pressure. If the system is to have the ability to respond to rapid changes of pressure such as a pulsatile artery, damping must be 'critical' – that is, reduced to a minimum required to remove noise from the signal without overdamping and losing the peaks and troughs of the pressure wave. This requires the total exclusion of bubbles of air from the manometer and connecting tubing, and the

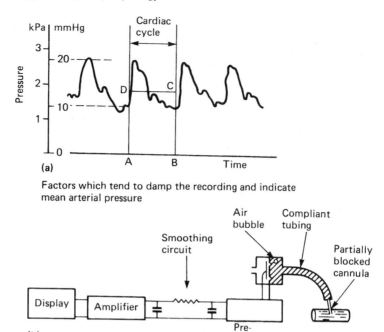

Figure 7.9 Determination of mean pulmonary arterial pressure. (a) An actual trace of instantaneous intravascular pulmonary arterial pressure during four cardiac cycles. For the second cycle, a rectangle has been constructed (ABCD) which has an area equal to that under the curve over the same interval. The height of the rectangle (AD) indicates the effective mean pressure. (b) Factors that tend to over-damp the recording of instantaneous pressure (i.e. lower the indicated systolic pressure and raise the indicated diastolic pressure) tending towards an indication of mean pressure. Some of these factors are accidental (e.g. air bubble or blocked cannula) but others (e.g. smoothing circuit) may be employed deliberately to allow a continuous display of mean pressures.

intravascular cannula must be unobstructed. Electrical manometry then yields a plot of instantaneous pressure against time (Figure 7.9a). Mean pressure (integrated with respect to time) is the height of a rectangle (ABCD in Figure 7.9a) with length equal to one cardiac cycle and area equal to that under the pressure curve over the same interval. In practice, mean pressure is more commonly derived by use of a smoothing circuit in the amplifier (Figure 7.9b), but hydraulic damping in the manometer tubing can achieve the same result.

Figure 7.3 shows the sites at which pressure must be measured to obtain the various forms of pulmonary vascular pressure (page 140). Driving pressure, the most useful of these, requires measurement of pulmonary arterial and pulmonary venous (left atrial) pressures.

Pulmonary arterial pressure may be measured using a balloon flotation catheter. Following insertion into the right atrium via a central vein, a balloon of <1 ml volume is inflated to encourage the catheter tip to follow the flow of blood through the right ventricle and pulmonary valve into the pulmonary artery. The most commonly used catheter is the Swan–Ganz, named after the two cardiologists who devised the catheter after Dr Swan watched sailboats being propelled by the wind in 1967.[49]

Left atrial pressure represents pulmonary venous pressure and is measured by one of five possible techniques, of which only the first three are applicable in humans, and only the first routinely possible though still very invasive.

1. Pulmonary capillary wedge pressure (PCWP). Wedge pressures are obtained by advancing the Swan–Ganz catheter into a branch of the pulmonary artery and inflating the balloon to the point at which the arterial pulsation disappears. There should then be no flow in the column of blood between the tip of the catheter and the left atrium, and the manometer will indicate left atrial pressure.
2. A left atrial catheter may be sited during cardiac surgery and passed through the chest wall for use postoperatively.
3. A catheter may be passed retrogradely from a peripheral systemic artery.
4. The left atrium may be punctured by a needle at bronchoscopy.
5. The atrial septum may be pierced from a catheter in the right atrium.

Pulmonary blood flow

The method used for measuring pulmonary blood flow will affect whether or not the result includes venous admixture such as the bronchial circulation and intrapulmonary shunts shown in Figure 7.1. Though of minimal relevance in normal subjects, in patients with lung disease venous admixture may be highly significant. In general, methods involving uptake of an inert gas from the alveoli will exclude venous admixture, and all other methods include it.

The Fick principle states that the amount of oxygen extracted from the respired gases equals the amount added to the blood that flows through the lungs. Thus the oxygen uptake of the subject must equal the product of pulmonary blood flow and arteriovenous oxygen content difference:

$$\dot{V}_{O_2} = \dot{Q}(Ca_{O_2} - C\bar{v}_{O_2})$$

Therefore:

$$\dot{Q} = \frac{\dot{V}_{O_2}}{(Ca_{O_2} - C\bar{v}_{O_2})}$$

All the quantities on the right-hand side can be measured, although determination of the oxygen content of the mixed venous blood requires catheterization of the right ventricle or, preferably, of the pulmonary artery as described above. Interpretation of the result is less easy. The calculated value includes the intrapulmonary arteriovenous shunt, but the situation is complicated beyond the possibility of easy solution if there is appreciable extrapulmonary admixture of venous blood (see Figure 7.1). The second major problem is that spirometry measures the total oxygen consumption, including that of the lung. The Fick equation excludes the lung (see Figure 11.22) but the difference is negligible with healthy lungs. There is now strong evidence that the oxygen consumption of infected lungs may be very large (page 300) and therefore the Fick method of measurement of cardiac output would seem to be invalid in such circumstances.

Methods based on uptake of inert tracer gases. A modified Fick method of measurement of cardiac output may be employed with any fairly soluble inert gas. The tracer gas is inhaled either continually or for a single breath and the end-tidal partial pressure of tracer gas then measured. Analysis of volume and composition of expired tracer gas permits measurement of gas uptake. Because the duration of the procedure is short and does not permit recirculation, it may be assumed that the mixed venous concentration of the tracer gas is zero. The Fick equation then simplifies to the following:

cardiac output = tracer gas uptake/arterial tracer gas concentration

The arterial tracer gas concentration equals the product of the arterial gas tension (assumed equal to the alveolar [end-tidal] gas tension) and the solubility coefficient of the tracer gas in blood. Thus the need for arterial blood sampling may be avoided, so the method is relatively non-invasive.

All the methods based on the uptake of inert tracer gases have the following characteristics:

1. They measure pulmonary capillary blood flow, excluding any flow through shunts. This is in contrast to the Fick and dye methods.
2. The assumption that the tension of the tracer gas is the same in end-expiratory gas and arterial blood is invalid in the presence of either alveolar dead space or shunt (see Chapter 8).
3. Some of the tracer gas dissolves in the tissues lining the respiratory tract and is carried away by blood perfusing these tissues. The indicated blood flow is therefore greater than the actual pulmonary capillary blood flow.

The tracer gas used has varied through the years, nitrous oxide and acetylene being used early this century. Nitrous oxide is still used today but with a body plethysmograph to measure its uptake. The subject inhales a mixture of about 15% nitrous oxide and then holds his breath with his mouth open inside the body plethysmograph. Nitrous oxide uptake is measured directly from the fall of the pressure within the box, and the arterial nitrous oxide content is again derived as the product of the alveolar nitrous oxide tension and its solubility coefficient in blood to avoid arterial sampling. It is assumed that the mixed venous nitrous oxide concentration is zero and the calculation is as described above. With this technique it is possible to detect phasic changes in uptake, in time with the cardiac cycle and maximal during systole. This is taken as evidence that pulmonary capillary blood flow is pulsatile.

A refined version of the tracer gas technique has been developed, involving automated analysis of expired gas using a mass spectrometer and immediate computation of the results with a simple computer. Freon is the tracer gas used, with argon (highly insoluble gas) also added to the gas mixture to ensure complete mixing of the freon with alveolar gas, and to detect subjects with a large respiratory dead space (Chapter 8) in whom the method is invalid.[50]

Dye or thermal dilution. Currently the most popular technique for measurement of cardiac output is by dye dilution. An indicator substance is introduced as a bolus into a large vein and its concentration is measured continuously at a sampling site in the systemic arterial tree. Figure 7.10a shows the method as it is applied to continuous non-circulating flow, as for example of fluids through a pipeline. The downstream concentration of dye is displayed on the Y axis of the graph against time on the X axis. The dye is injected at time t_1 and is first detected at the sampling point at time t_2. The uppermost curve shows the form of a typical curve. There is a rapid rise to maximum concentration followed by a decay that is an exponential wash-out in form (see Appendix F), reaching insignificant levels at time t_3. The second graph shows the concentration (Y axis) on a logarithmic scale when the exponential part of the decay curve becomes a straight line (see Figure F.5). Between times t_2 and t_3, the mean concentration of dye equals the amount of dye injected, divided by the volume of fluid flowing past the sampling point during the interval t_2-t_3, which is the product of the fluid flow rate and the time interval t_2-t_3. The equation may now be rearranged to indicate the flow rate of the fluid as the following expression:

$$\frac{\text{amount of dye injected}}{\text{mean concentration of dye} \times \text{time interval } t_2-t_3}$$

The amount of dye injected is known and the denominator is the area under the curve.

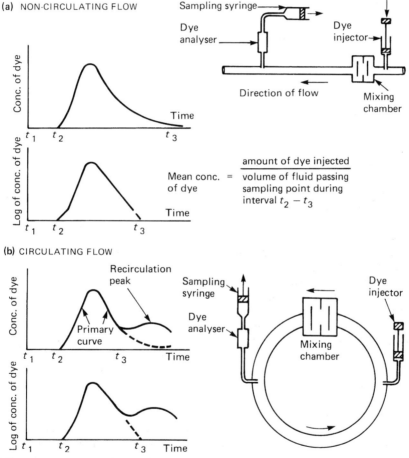

Figure 7.10 Measurement of flow by dye dilution. (a) The measurement of continuous non-circulating flow rate of fluid in a pipeline. The bolus of dye is injected upstream and its concentration is continuously monitored downstream. The relationship of the relevant quantities is shown in the equation. Mean concentration of dye is determined from the area under the curve as shown in Figure 7.9. (b) The more complicated situation when recirculation occurs and the front of the circulating dye laps its own tail, giving a recirculation peak. Reconstruction of the primary curve is based on extrapolation of the primary curve before recirculation occurs. This is facilitated by the fact that the down curve is exponential and therefore a straight line on a logarithmic plot.

Figure 7.10b shows the more complicated situation when fluid is flowing round a circuit. Under these conditions, the front of the dye-laden fluid may lap its own tail such that a recirculation peak appears on the graph before the primary peak has decayed to insignificant levels. This commonly occurs when cardiac output is determined in humans, and steps must be taken to reconstruct the tail of the primary curve as it would have been had recirculation not taken place. This is done by extrapolating the exponential wash-out, which is usually established before the recirculation peak appears. This is shown as the broken lines in the graphs of Figure 7.10b. The calculation of cardiac output then proceeds as described above for non-recirculating flow. This previously laborious procedure is now performed electronically as an integral part of the apparatus for measuring cardiac output.

Many different indicators have been used for the dye dilution technique, but currently the most satisfactory appears to be 'coolth'. A bolus of cold saline is injected and the dip in temperature is recorded downstream with the temperature record corresponding to the dye curve. No blood sampling is required and temperature is measured directly with a thermometer mounted on the catheter. The 'coolth' is dispersed in the systemic circulation and therefore there is no recirculation peak to complicate the calculation. The thermal method is particularly suitable for repeated measurements.

Methods of measurement of regional distribution of pulmonary blood flow are considered in Chapter 8.

References

1. Harris P. The evolution of the pulmonary circulation. *Thorax* 1995; **49**: S5–8.
2. Servetus M. *Christianismi restitutio.* Vienne, 1553.
3. Deffebach ME, Charan NB, Lakshminarayan S, Butler J. The bronchial circulation: small but a vital attribute to the lung. *Am Rev Respir Dis* 1987; **135**: 463–81.
4. Verloop MC. The arteriae bronchiales and their anastomoses with the arteriae pulmonalis in the human lung: a micro-anatomical study. *Acta Anat* 1948; **5**: 171–205.
5. Harris P, Heath D. *The human pulmonary circulation.* Edinburgh & London: Churchill Livingstone, 1962.
6. Marshall BE, Marshall C. Pulmonary circulation during anaesthesia. In: Stanley TH, Sperry RJ, eds. *Anesthesia and the lung.* Dordrecht: Kluwer, 1992: 31–43.
7. Warrell DA, Evans JW, Clarke RO, Kingaby GP, West JB. Pattern of filling in the pulmonary capillary bed. *J Appl Physiol* 1972; **32**: 346–56.
8. König MF, Lucocq JM, Weibel ER. Demonstration of pulmonary vascular perfusion by electron and light microscopy. *J Appl Physiol* 1993; **75**: 1877–83.
9. Conhaim RL, Harms BA. Perfusion of alveolar septa in isolated rat lungs in zone 1. *J Appl Physiol* 1993; **75**: 704–11.
10. Johnson RL, Hsai CCW. Functional recruitment of pulmonary capillaries. *J Appl Physiol* 1994; **76**: 1405–7.
11. Sobin SS, Fung YC, Tremer HM, Rosenquist TH. Elasticity of the pulmonary alveolar microvascular sheet in the cat. *Circ Res* 1972; **30**: 440–50.
12. Fishman AP. Pulmonary circulation. In: Fishman AP, Fisher AB, Geiger SR, eds. *Handbook of Physiology, Section 3 – The respiratory system.* Bethesda MD: American Physiological Society, 1987; 93–7.
13. West JB, Dollery CT, Naimark A. Distribution of blood flow in isolated lung; relation to vascular and alveolar pressures. *J Appl Physiol* 1964; **19**: 713–24.
14. West JB, Dollery CT. Distribution of blood flow and the pressure–flow relations of the whole lung. *J Appl Physiol* 1965; **20**: 175–83.
15. Cooper CJ, Landzberg MJ, Anderson TJ, Charbonneau F, Craeger MA, Ganz P, Selwyn AP. Role of nitric oxide in the local regulation of pulmonary vascular resistance in humans. *Circulation* 1996; **93**: 266–71.
16. Barnes PJ, Liu SF. Regulation of pulmonary vascular tone. *Pharmacol Rev* 1995; **47**: 87–131.

17. Kobayashi Y, Amenta F. Neurotransmitter receptors in the pulmonary circulation with particular emphasis on pulmonary endothelium. *J Auton Pharmacol* 1994; **14**: 137–64.

18. Wilkins MR, Zhao L, Al-Tubuly R. The regulation of pulmonary vascular tone. *Br J Clin Pharmacol* 1996; **42**: 127–31.

19. Murray KJ. Cyclic AMP and mechanisms of vasodilatation. *Pharmacol Ther* 1990; **47**: 329–45.

20. Clapp LH, Gurney AM. ATP-sensitive K^+ channels regulate resting potential of pulmonary arterial smooth muscle cells. *Am J Physiol* 1992; **262**: H916–20.

21. Adnot S, Raffestin B, Eddahibi S. NO in the lung. *Respir Physiol* 1995; **101**: 109–20.

22. Anggard E. Nitric oxide: mediator, murderer, and medicine. *Lancet* 1994; **343**: 1199–206.

23. Moncada S, Palmer R, Higgs E. Nitric oxide: physiology, pathophysiology and pharmacology. *Pharmacol Rev* 1991; **43**: 109–42.

24. Furchgott RF, Zawadzki JV. The obligatory role of endothelial cells in the relaxation of arterial smooth muscle by acetylcholine. *Nature* 1980; **288**: 373–6.

25. Cherry PD, Furchgott RF, Zawadzki JV, Jothianandan D. Role of endothelial cells in relaxation of isolated arteries by bradykinin. *Proc Natl Acad Sci USA* 1982; **79**: 2106–10.

26. Nagao T, Vanhoute PM. Endothelium-derived hyperpolarizing factor and endothelium-dependent relaxations. *Am J Respir Cell Mol Biol* 1993; **8**: 1–6.

27. Miura H, Gutterman DD. Human coronary arteriolar dilation to arachidonic acid depends on cytochrome P-450 monooxygenase and Ca^{2+}-activated K^+ channels. *Circ Res* 1998; **83**: 501–7.

28. Stamler JS, Loh E, Roddy M-A, Currie KE, Craeger MA. Nitric oxide regulated basal systemic and pulmonary vascular resistance in healthy humans. *Circulation* 1994; **89**: 2035–40.

29. Marshall BE, Marshall C, Frasch HF. Control of the pulmonary circulation. In: Stanley TH, Sperry RJ, eds. *Anesthesia and the lung.* Dordrecht: Kluwer, 1992: 9–18.

30. Marshall BE, Marshall C, Magno M, Lilagan P, Pietra GG. Influence of bronchial artery Po_2 on pulmonary vascular resistance. *J Appl Physiol* 1991; **70**: 405–15.

31. Marshall BE, Marshall C. Anesthesia and the pulmonary circulation. In: Covino BG, Fozzard HA, Rehder K, Strichartz G, eds. *Effects of anesthesia.* Bethesda MD: American Physiological Society, 1983.

32. Marshall BE. Pulmonary vasoconstriction. *Acta Anesthesiol Scand* 1990; **34** (Supp 94): 37–41.

33. Anand IS. Hypoxia and the pulmonary circulation. *Thorax* 1994; **49**: S19–S24.

34. Robin ED, Theodore J, Burke CM, Oesterle SN, Fowler MB, Jamieson SW et al. Hypoxic pulmonary vasoconstriction persists in the human transplanted lung. *Clin Sci* 1987; **72**: 283–7.

35. Daly I de B, Daly M de B. The effects of stimulation of the carotid body chemoreceptors on the pulmonary vascular bed in the dog. *J Physiol* 1959; **148**: 201–19.

36. Jensen KS, Micco AJ, Czartolomna J, Latham L, Voelkel NF. Rapid onset of hypoxic vasoconstriction in isolated lungs. *J Appl Physiol* 1992; **72**: 2018–23.

37. Morrell NW, Nijran KS, Biggs T, Seed WA. Magnitude and time course of acute hypoxic pulmonary vasoconstriction in man. *Respir Physiol* 1995; **100**: 271–81.

38. Ward JPT, Robertson TP. The role of endothelium in hypoxic pulmonary vasoconstriction. *Exp Physiol* 1995; **80**: 793–801.

39. Sprague RS, Thiemermann C, Vane JR. Endogenous endothelium-derived relaxing factor opposes hypoxic pulmonary vasoconstriction and supports blood flow to hypoxic alveoli in anaesthetized rabbits. *Proc Natl Acad Sci USA* 1992; **89**: 8711–15.

40. Demiryurek AT, Wadsworth RM, Kane KA, Peacock AJ. The role of endothelium in hypoxic constriction of human pulmonary artery rings. *Am Rev Respir Dis* 1993; **147**: 283–90.

41. Post JM, Hume JR, Archer SL, Weir EK. Direct role for potassium channel inhibition in hypoxic pulmonary vasoconstriction. *Am J Physiol* 1992; **262**: C882–90.

42. Cornfield DN, Stevens T, McMurtry IF, Abman SH, Rodman DM. Acute hypoxia causes membrane depolarization and calcium influx in fetal pulmonary artery smooth muscle cells. *Am J Physiol* 1992; **266**: L469–75.

43. Suggett AJ, Barer GR, Mohammed FH, Gill GW. The effects of localised hyperventilation on ventilation/perfusion ($\dot{V}/\dot{Q}$) ratios and gas exchange in the dog lung. *Clin Sci* 1982; **63**: 497–503.

44. Rudolph AM, Yuan S. Response of the pulmonary vasculature to hypoxia and H^+ ion concentration changes. *J Clin Invest* 1966; **45**: 399–411.

45. Benumof JL, Wahrenbrock EA. Blunted hypoxic pulmonary vasoconstriction by increased lung vascular pressures. *J Appl Physiol* 1975; **38**: 846–50.

46. Lloyd TC. Influence of blood pH on hypoxic pulmonary vasoconstriction. *J Appl Physiol* 1966; **21**: 358–64.
47. Pepke-Zaba J, Higgenbottam T, Dinh-Xuan AT, Ridden C, Kealey T. α-Adrenoceptor stimulation of porcine pulmonary arteries. *Eur J Pharmacol* 1993; **235**: 169–75.
48. Reid PG, Fraser A, Watt A, Henderson A, Routledge P. Acute haemodynamic effects of adenosine in conscious man. *Eur Heart J* 1990; **11**: 1018–28.
49. Swan HJC, Ganz W. Hemodynamic monitoring: a personal and historical perspective. *Can Med Assoc J* 1979; **121**: 868–71.
50. Winter SM. Clinical non-invasive measurement of effective pulmonary blood flow. *Int J Clin Monit Comput* 1995; **12**: 121–40.

Chapter 8

Distribution of pulmonary ventilation and perfusion

The lung may be considered as a simple exchanger with a gas inflow and outflow, and a blood inflow and outflow (Figure 8.1). There is near-equilibrium of oxygen and carbon dioxide tensions between the two outflow streams from the exchanger itself. This theoretical model assumes that gas flow in and out of the alveolus and blood flow through the pulmonary capillary are both continuous. This assumption may be true within alveoli where at normal tidal volumes gas movement is by diffusion (page 23) but pulmonary capillary blood flow is pulsatile (page 158). This model has been deliberately drawn without countercurrent flow, which would be far more efficient. Such a system operates in the gills of fishes, and brings the Po_2 of arterial blood close to the Po_2 of the environment.

Gas exchange will clearly be optimal if ventilation and perfusion are distributed in the same proportion to one another throughout the lung. Conversely, to take an extreme example, if ventilation were distributed entirely to one lung and perfusion to the other, there could be no gas exchange, although total ventilation and perfusion might each be normal. This chapter begins with consideration of the spatial and temporal distribution of ventilation, followed by similar treatment for the pulmonary circulation. Distribution of ventilation and perfusion are then considered in relation to one another. Finally, the concepts of dead space and shunt are presented.

Distribution of ventilation

Spatial and anatomical distribution of inspired gas

Distribution between the two lungs in the normal subject is influenced by posture and by the manner of ventilation. By virtue of its larger size, the right lung normally enjoys a ventilation slightly greater than the left lung in both the upright and the supine position (Table 8.1). In the lateral position, the lower lung is always better ventilated regardless of the side on which the subject is lying, although there still remains a bias in favour of the right side.[1] The preferential ventilation of the dependent lung is due to the lower diaphragm lying higher in the chest, and with increased length of muscle fibres it will therefore contract more effectively during inspiration (page 121). Fortunately, the preferential ventilation of the lower lung accords with increased perfusion of the same lung, so the ventilation/perfusion ratios of the two lungs are not greatly altered on assuming the lateral position. However, the upper lung tends to be better ventilated in the

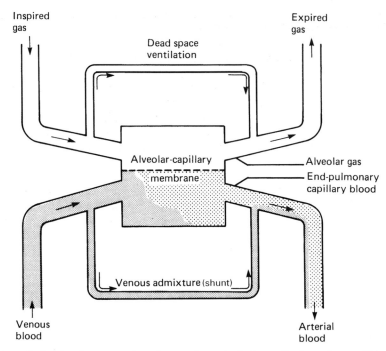

Figure 8.1 In this functional representation of gas exchange in the lungs, the flow of gas and blood is considered as a continuous process with movement from left to right. In most circumstances, equilibrium is obtained between alveolar gas and end-pulmonary capillary blood, the gas tensions in the two phases being almost identical. However, alveolar gas is mixed with dead space gas to give expired gas. Meanwhile, end-pulmonary capillary blood is mixed with shunted venous blood to give arterial blood. Thus both expired gas and arterial blood have tensions that differ from those in alveolar gas and end-pulmonary capillary blood.

Table 8.1 Distribution of resting lung volume (FRC) and ventilation between the two lungs in man

	Supine		Right lateral (left side up)		Left lateral (right side up)	
	Right lung	*Left lung*	*Right lung*	*Left lung*	*Right lung*	*Left lung*
Conscious man[1]	1.69	1.39	1.68	2.07	2.19	1.38
	53%	47%	61%	39%	47%	53%
Anaesthetized man – spontaneous breathing[2]	1.18	0.91	1.03	1.32	1.71	0.79
	52%	48%	45%	55%	56%	44%
Anaesthetized man – artificial ventilation[3]	1.36	1.16	1.33	2.21	2.29	1.12
	52%	48%	44%	56%	60%	40%
Anaesthetized man – thoracotomy[4]					–	–
					83%	17%

The first figure is the unilateral FRC (litres) and the second the percentage partition of ventilation. Each study refers to separate subjects or patients.

anaesthetized patient in the lateral position, regardless of the mode of ventilation and particularly with an open chest (Table 8.1).

Distribution to horizontal slices of lung was first studied by West in 1962 using a radioactive isotope of oxygen.[5] He found the ventilation of the uppermost slices to be one-third that of slices at the bases of the lungs in the upright position (Figure 8.2). However, these studies were carried out with slow vital capacity inspirations starting from residual volume, circumstances that differ greatly from normal breathing. A slow inspiration from functional residual capacity (FRC), as occurs during normal resting ventilation, does result in a small vertical gradient down the lung with the ratio of basal to apical ventilation being about 1.5:1.[6] Starting from FRC, preferential ventilation of the dependent parts of the lung is only present at inspiratory flow rates below $1.5\,l.s^{-1}$. At higher flow rates, distribution becomes approximately uniform. Fast inspirations from FRC reverse the distribution of ventilation, with preferential ventilation of the upper parts of the lungs (Figure 8.2), which is contrary to the distribution of pulmonary blood flow (see below). Normal inspiratory flow rate is, however, much less than $1.5\,l.s^{-1}$ (approx. $0.5\,l.s^{-1}$), so there will be a small vertical gradient of ventilation during normal breathing.

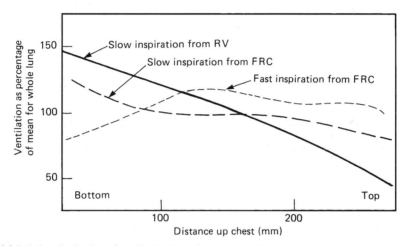

Figure 8.2 Relative distribution of ventilation in horizontal strata of the lungs in the upright position. (Data from references 5 and 6)

Posture affects distribution because *inter alia* the vertical height of the lung is reduced by about 30 per cent in the supine position. Therefore the gravitational force generating maldistribution is much less. Normal tidal breathing in the supine position results in preferential ventilation of the posterior slices of the lungs compared with the anterior slices.[7,8] Over all, the effect of gravity on ventilation seems to be of minor importance in comparison with its effect on perfusion, which is considered below.

Distribution of inspired gas in relation to the rate of alveolar filling

The rate of inflation of the lung as a whole is a function of inflation pressure, compliance and airway resistance. It is convenient to think in terms of the time constant (explained in Appendix F), which is the product of the compliance and resistance and is:

1. The time required for inflation to 63 per cent of the final volume attained if inflation is prolonged indefinitely.
   or
2. The time that would be required for inflation of the lungs if the initial gas flow rate were maintained throughout inflation (see Appendix F, Figure F.6).

These considerations apply equally to large and small areas of the lungs; Figure 3.6 shows fast and slow alveoli, the former with a short time constant and the latter with a long time constant. Figure 8.3 shows some of the consequences of different *functional units* of the lung having different time constants. For simplicity, Figure 8.3 describes the response to passive inflation of the lungs by development of a constant mouth pressure but the considerations are fundamentally similar for both spontaneous respiration and artificial ventilation.

Figure 8.3a shows two functional units of identical compliance and resistance. If the mouth pressure is increased to a constant level, there will be an increase in volume of each unit equal to the mouth pressure multiplied by the compliance of the unit. The time course of inflation will follow the wash-in type of exponential function (Appendix F), and the time constants will be equal to the product of compliance and resistance of each unit and therefore identical. If the inspiratory phase is terminated at any instant, the pressure and volume of each unit will be identical and no redistribution of gas will occur between the two units.

Figure 8.3b shows two functional units, one of which has half the compliance but twice the resistance of the other. The time constants of the two will thus be equal. If a constant inflation pressure is maintained, the one with the lower compliance will increase in volume by half the volume change of the other. Nevertheless, the pressure build-up within each unit will be identical. Thus, as in the previous example, the relative distribution of gas between the two functional units will be independent of the rate or duration of inflation. If the inspiratory phase is terminated at any point, the pressure in each unit will be identical and no redistribution will occur between the different units.

In Figure 8.3c, the compliances of the two units are identical but the resistance of one is twice that of the other. Therefore, its time constant is double that of its fellow and it will fill more slowly, although the volume increase in both units will be the same if inflation is prolonged indefinitely. Relative distribution between the units is thus dependent on the rate and duration of inflation. If inspiration is checked by closure of the upper airway after 2 seconds (for example), the pressure will be higher in the unit with the lower resistance. Gas will then be redistributed from one unit to the other as shown by the arrow in the diagram.

Figure 8.3d shows a pair of units with identical resistances but the compliance of one being half that of the other. Its time constant is thus half that of its fellow and has a faster time course of inflation. However, because its compliance is half that of the other, the ultimate volume increase will only be half that of the other unit when the inflation is prolonged indefinitely. The relative distribution of gas between the two units is dependent on the rate and duration of inflation. Pressure rises more rapidly in the unit with the lower compliance, and if inspiration is checked by closure of the upper airway at 2 seconds (for example), gas will be redistributed from one unit to the other as shown by the arrow.

An interesting and complex situation occurs when one unit has an increased resistance and the other a reduced compliance (Figure 8.3e). This combination also features in the presentation of the concept of fast and slow alveoli in Figure 3.6. In the present example the time constant of one unit is four times that of the other, while the ultimate volume changes are determined by the compliance as in Figure 8.3d. When the inflation pressure

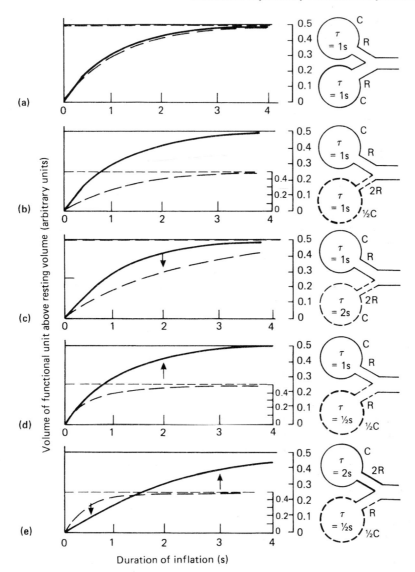

Figure 8.3 The effect of mechanical characteristics on the time course of inflation of different functional units of the lung when exposed to a sustained constant inflation pressure. The Y coordinate is volume change, but a scale showing intra-alveolar pressure is shown on the right. Separate pressure scales are necessary when the compliances are different. In each case the continuous curve relates to the upper unit and the broken curve to the lower unit. Arrows show the direction of gas redistribution if inflow is checked by closure of the upper airway at the times indicated. See text for explanation of the changes. τ = time constant.

is sustained, the unit with the lower resistance (the 'fast alveolus') shows the greater volume change at first, but rapidly approaches its equilibrium volume. Thereafter the other unit (the 'slow alveolus') undergoes the major volume changes, the inflation of the two units being out of phase with one another. Throughout inspiration, the pressure build-up in the unit with the shorter time constant is always greater and, if inspiration is checked by closure of the upper airway, gas will be redistributed from one unit to the other as shown by the arrows in Figure 8.3e.

These complex relationships may be summarized as follows. If the inflation pressure is sustained indefinitely, the volume change in different units of the lungs will depend solely upon their regional compliances. *If their time constants are equal*, the build-up of pressure in the different units will be identical at all times during inflation and therefore:

1. Distribution of inspired gas will be independent of the rate, duration or frequency of inspiration.
2. Dynamic compliance (so far as it is influenced by considerations discussed in relation to Figure 3.6) will not be affected by changes in frequency and should not differ greatly from static compliance.
3. If inspiration is checked by closure of the upper airway, there will be no redistribution of gas in the lungs.

If, however, *the time constants of different units are different*, for whatever cause, it follows that:

1. Distribution of inspired gas will be dependent on the rate, duration and frequency of inspiration.
2. Dynamic compliance will be decreased as respiratory frequency is increased and should differ significantly from static compliance.
3. If inspiration is checked by closure of the upper airway, gas will be redistributed in the lungs.

Effect of maldistribution on the alveolar 'plateau'

If different functional units of the lung empty synchronously during expiration, the composition of the expired air will be approximately constant after the anatomical dead space has been flushed out. However, this will not occur when there is maldistribution with fast and slow units as shown in Figure 3.6. The slow units are slow both to fill and to empty, and thus are hypoventilated for their volume; therefore they tend to have a high P_{CO_2} and low P_{O_2} and are slow to respond to a change in the inspired gas composition. This forms the basis of the single-breath test of maldistribution in which a single breath of 100% oxygen is used to increase alveolar P_{O_2} and decrease alveolar P_{N_2}. The greatest increase of P_{O_2} will clearly occur in the functional units with the best ventilation per unit volume, which will usually have the shortest time constants. The *slow* units will make the predominant contribution to the *latter* part of exhalation, when the mixed exhaled P_{O_2} will decline and the P_{N_2} will increase. Thus the expired alveolar plateau of nitrogen will be sloping upwards in patients with maldistribution. It should, however, be stressed that this test will be positive only if maldistribution is accompanied by sequential emptying of units due to differing time constants. For example, Figure 8.3b shows definite maldistribution, due to the different regional compliances that directly influence the regional ventilation. However, because time constants are equal, there will be a constant mix of gas from both units during the course of expiration (i.e. no sequential emptying) and therefore the alveolar plateau would remain flat in spite of P_{O_2} and P_{N_2} being different for the two units. However, maldistribution due to the more common forms of lung disease is usually associated with different time constants and sequential emptying. Routine continuous monitoring of expired carbon dioxide concentration during anaesthesia now allows some assessment of maldistribution of ventilation. As for the single-breath nitrogen test, an upward-sloping expiratory plateau of carbon dioxide indicates sequential emptying of alveoli with different time constants (page 243), but a level plateau does not indicate normal distribution of ventilation, just equal time constants of lung units.

Distribution of perfusion

Because the pulmonary circulation operates at low pressure, it is rarely distributed evenly to all parts of the lung and the degree of non-uniformity is usually greater than for gas. Maldistribution of pulmonary blood flow is the commonest cause of impaired oxygenation of the arterial blood. Uneven distribution may be present between the two lungs and between different lobes but is always seen between successive horizontal slices of the lungs, except at zero gravity (page 395).[9]

Distribution between the two lungs

There are considerable difficulties in measuring unilateral pulmonary blood flow in humans. However, Defares et al. in 1960 studied supine subjects using an indirect method based on the Fick principle for carbon dioxide,[10] and obtained values for unilateral flow that agree closely with the distribution of ventilation observed in the supine position (Table 8.1).[1]

The lateral position. In humans the lateral diameter of the thorax is of the order of 30 cm and so, in the lateral position, the column of blood in the pulmonary circulation exerts a hydrostatic pressure that is high in relation to the mean pulmonary arterial pressure. A fairly gross maldistribution is therefore to be expected with much of the upper lung comprising zone 2 and much of the lower lung comprising zone 3 (see Figure 7.5). This was first confirmed in 1966 using ^{133}Xe, which showed uniform high perfusion of the dependent lung (apparently in zone 3) with reduced perfusion of the upper lung (which seemed to be mainly in zone 2).[11]

Distribution in horizontal slices of the lung

In the previous chapter, it was shown that pulmonary vascular resistance is mainly in the capillary bed and is governed by the relationship between alveolar, pulmonary arterial and pulmonary venous pressures. Figure 7.5 presented the concept of the vascular weir with pulmonary vascular resistance decreasing and pulmonary blood flow increasing with distance down the lung. The first studies with radioactive tracers in the blood took place at total lung capacity and showed flow increasing progressively down the lung in the upright position.[12] However, Hughes et al. later found that there was a significant reduction of flow in the most dependent parts of the lung, which was termed zone 4, where the reduction in flow seems to be due to compression of larger blood vessels by increased interstitial pressure.[13] This effect becomes progressively more important as lung volume is reduced from total lung capacity towards the residual volume. Figure 8.4 is redrawn from the work of Hughes' group, and shows that pulmonary perfusion *per alveolus* is, in fact, reasonably uniform at the lung volumes relevant to normal tidal exchange. However, the dependent parts of the lung contain larger numbers of smaller alveoli than the apices at FRC, and the perfusion *per unit lung volume* is therefore increased at the bases.[11]

In the supine position the differences in blood flow between apices and bases are replaced by differences between anterior and posterior aspects.[7,14] Supine subjects can be studied using positron emission tomography (PET) scans, which show gradients in

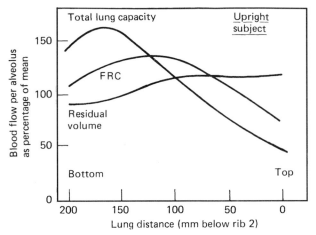

Figure 8.4 Pulmonary perfusion per alveolus as a percentage of that expected if all alveoli were equally perfused. At total lung capacity, perfusion increases down to 150 mm, below which perfusion is slightly decreased (zone 4). At FRC, zone 4 conditions apply below 100 mm, and at residual volume the perfusion gradient is actually reversed. It should be noted that perfusion has been calculated *per alveolus*. If shown as perfusion *per unit lung volume*, the non-uniformity at total lung capacity would be the same because alveoli are all the same size at total lung capacity. At FRC there are more but smaller alveoli at the bases and the non-uniformity would be greater. (Data are redrawn from reference 13.)

alveolar size, ventilation and perfusion that are similar to earlier observations in upright subjects. Blood flow *per unit lung volume* increases by 11 per cent per centimetre of descent through the lung,[15] whilst ventilation increases but less dramatically (Figure 8.5),[8] resulting in a smaller ventilation to perfusion ratio in dependent areas.[15] These studies also showed that the number of alveoli per cubic centimetre of lung was about 30 per cent greater in the posterior than the anterior lung (Figure 8.5).[8] Thus the increased perfusion in dependent areas of lung is again caused mainly by an increase in the number of (relatively small) alveoli. Smaller more numerous alveoli in dependent areas result from the weight of lung tissue above, and as blood accounts for two-thirds of the weight of lung tissue this provides an automatic matching of ventilation and perfusion. This is confirmed in PET scanning of prone patients, in whom there is a rapid reversal of the gradients described in the supine position.[8,15]

Ventilation in relation to perfusion[16]

Inspired gas distributed to regions that have no pulmonary capillary blood flow cannot take part in gas exchange and, conversely, pulmonary blood flow distributed to regions without ventilation cannot become oxygenated. This principle was appreciated by John Hunter who, in the eighteenth century, wrote:

> 'In animals where there is no circulation, there can be no lungs: for lungs are an apparatus for the air and blood to meet, and can only accord with motion of blood in vessels . . . As the lungs are to expose the blood to the air, they are so constructed as to answer this purpose exactly with the blood brought to them, and so disposed in them as to go hand in hand.'

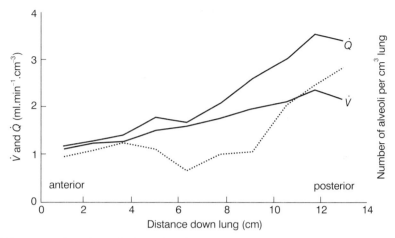

Figure 8.5 Vertical gradients in ventilation and perfusion in the supine position. Data are mean results from PET scans of 8 subjects during normal breathing, and for each vertical level represent the average value for a horizontal slice of lung. The solid lines relate to the left ordinate and are ventilation ($\dot{V}$) and perfusion ($\dot{Q}$) per cubic centimetre of lung tissue. Both ventilation and perfusion increase on descending through the lung. The dotted line relates to the right ordinate and represents the number of alveoli per unit lung volume, which increases in dependent areas such that the blood flow *per alveolus* remains fairly constant. (Redrawn from references 8 and 15.)

It is convenient to consider the relationship between ventilation and perfusion in terms of the ventilation/perfusion ratio (abbreviated to $\dot{V}/\dot{Q}$). Each quantity is measured in litres per minute and, taking the lungs as a whole, typical resting values might be $4\,l.min^{-1}$ for alveolar ventilation and $5\,l.min^{-1}$ for pulmonary blood flow. Thus the overall ventilation perfusion ratio would be 0.8 (which happens to be close to the respiratory exchange ratio but this is coincidental). If ventilation and perfusion of all alveoli were uniform, each alveolus would have an individual $\dot{V}/\dot{Q}$ ratio of 0.8.

In fact, ventilation and perfusion are not uniformly distributed but may range all the way from unventilated alveoli to unperfused alveoli, with every gradation in between. Unventilated alveoli will have a $\dot{V}/\dot{Q}$ ratio of zero and the unperfused alveoli a $\dot{V}/\dot{Q}$ ratio of infinity.

Alveoli with no ventilation ($\dot{V}/\dot{Q}$ ratio of zero) will have Po_2 and Pco_2 values that are the same as those of mixed venous blood, because the trapped air in the unventilated alveoli will equilibrate with mixed venous blood. Alveoli with no perfusion ($\dot{V}/\dot{Q}$ ratio of infinity) will have Po_2 and Pco_2 values that are the same as those of the inspired gas, because there is no gas exchange to alter the composition of the inspired gas that is drawn into these alveoli. Alveoli with intermediate values of $\dot{V}/\dot{Q}$ ratio will thus have Po_2 and Pco_2 values that are intermediate between those of mixed venous blood and inspired gas. Figure 8.6 is a Po_2/Pco_2 plot with the thick line joining the mixed venous point to the inspired gas point. This line covers all possible combinations of alveolar Po_2 and Pco_2, with an indication of the $\dot{V}/\dot{Q}$ ratios that determine them.

The inhalation of higher than normal partial pressures of oxygen moves the inspired point of the curve to the right. The mixed venous point also moves to the right but only by a small amount, for reasons that are explained on page 492. A new curve must be prepared for each combination of values for mixed venous blood and inspired gas.[17] The

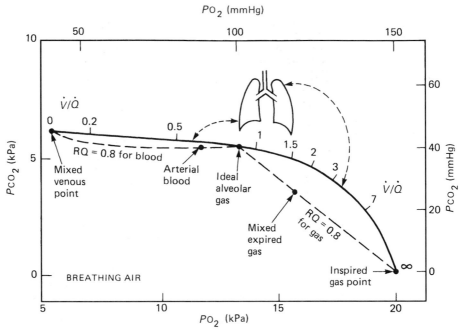

Figure 8.6 The heavy line indicates all possible values for Po_2 and Pco_2 of alveoli with ventilation/perfusion ($\dot{V}/\dot{Q}$) ratios ranging from zero to infinity (subject breathing air). Values for normal alveoli are distributed as shown in accord with their vertical distance up the lung field. Mixed expired gas may be considered as a mixture of 'ideal' alveolar and inspired gas (dead space). Arterial blood may be considered as a mixture of blood with the same gas tensions as 'ideal' alveolar gas and mixed venous blood (the shunt).

curve can then be used to demonstrate the gas tensions in the horizontal strata of the lung according to their different $\dot{V}/\dot{Q}$ ratios (Figure 8.6).

The use of collimated counters with ^{133}Xe to measure ventilation and perfusion in horizontal strata of the lung can discriminate only rather thick slices of the lung and is unable to detect changes in small areas of lung in the slices. This limitation has been overcome by the multiple inert gas elimination technique (MIGET).[18] The methodology, which is outlined on page 191, permits the plotting of the distribution of pulmonary ventilation and perfusion, not in relation to anatomical location but in a large number of compartments defined by their $\dot{V}/\dot{Q}$ ratios, expressed on a logarithmic scale.

Figure 8.7 shows typical plots for healthy subjects.[19] For the young adult, both ventilation and perfusion are mainly confined to alveoli with $\dot{V}/\dot{Q}$ ratios in the range 0.5–2.0. There is no measurable distribution to areas of infinite $\dot{V}/\dot{Q}$ (i.e. alveolar dead space) or zero $\dot{V}/\dot{Q}$ ratio (i.e. shunt), but the method does not detect extrapulmonary shunt, which must be present to a small extent (page 181). For the older subject (Figure 8.7b) there is a widening of the distribution of $\dot{V}/\dot{Q}$ ratios, with the main part of the curve now in the range of $\dot{V}/\dot{Q}$ ratios 0.3–5.0. In addition, there is the appearance of a 'shelf' of distribution of blood flow to areas of low $\dot{V}/\dot{Q}$ ratio in the range 0.01–0.3. This probably represents gross underventilation of dependent areas of the lung due to airway closure when the closing capacity exceeds the FRC (see Figure 3.11). The effect of increased spread of $\dot{V}/\dot{Q}$ ratios on gas exchange is considered below (page 187).

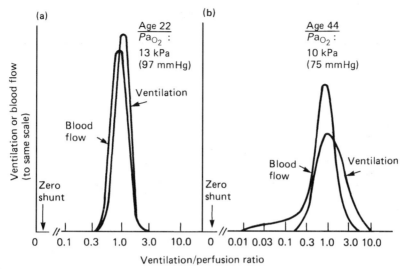

Figure 8.7 The distribution of ventilation and blood flow in relation to ventilation/perfusion ratios in two normal subjects. (a) A male aged 22 years with typical narrow spread and no measurable intrapulmonary shunt or alveolar dead space. This accords with high arterial Po_2 while breathing air. (b) The wider spread in a male aged 44 years. Note in particular the 'shelf' of blood flow distributed to alveoli with $\dot{V}/\dot{Q}$ ratios in the range 0.01–0.3. There is still no measurable intrapulmonary shunt or alveolar dead space. However, the appreciable distribution of blood flow to underperfused alveoli is sufficient to reduce the arterial Po_2 to 10 kPa (75 mmHg) while breathing air. (Redrawn from reference 19 by permission of the authors and copyright permission of the American Society for Clinical Investigation.)

The pattern of distribution of $\dot{V}/\dot{Q}$ ratios reveals characteristic changes in a number of pathological conditions such as pulmonary oedema and pulmonary embolus.[14,17] Some examples are shown in Figure 8.8.

Quantification of spread of $\dot{V}/\dot{Q}$ ratios as if it were due to dead space and shunt

The MIGET method of analysis illustrated in Figures 8.7 and 8.8 is technically complex. A less precise but highly practical approach was described in the 1940s by both Fenn and colleagues[20] and Riley and Cournand.[21] The essence of what has generally become known as the Riley approach is to consider the lung as if it were a three-compartment model (Figure 8.9) comprising:

1. Ventilated but unperfused alveoli.
2. Perfused but unventilated alveoli.
3. Ideally perfused and ventilated alveoli.

The ventilated but unperfused alveoli comprise alveolar dead space (described below). The perfused but unventilated alveoli are here represented as an intrapulmonary shunt. Gas exchange can occur only in the 'ideal' alveolus. There is no suggestion that this is an accurate description of the actual state of affairs, which is better depicted by the type of plot shown in Figure 8.7, where the analysis would comprise some 50 compartments in contrast to the three compartments of the Riley model. However, the parameters of the three-compartment model may be easily determined with equipment to be found in any department that is concerned with respiratory problems. Furthermore, the values obtained

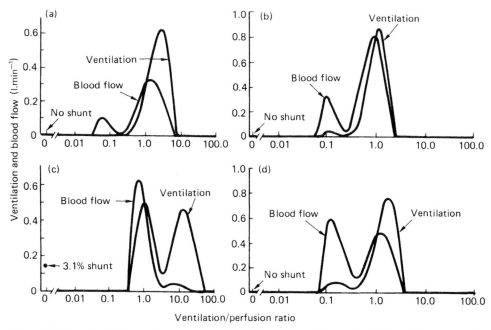

Figure 8.8 Examples of abnormal patterns of maldistribution of ventilation and perfusion, to be compared with the normal curves in Figure 8.7. (a) Chronic obstructive pulmonary disease. The blood flow to units of very low $\dot{V}/\dot{Q}$ ratio would cause arterial hypoxaemia and simulate a shunt. (b) Asthma with a more pronounced bimodal distribution of blood flow than the patient shown in (a). (c) Bimodal distribution of ventilation in a 60-year-old patient with chronic obstructive pulmonary disease, predominantly emphysema. A similar pattern is seen after pulmonary embolism. (d) Pronounced bimodal distribution of perfusion after a bronchodilator was administered to the patient shown in (b). (Redrawn from reference 17 by permission of the author and publishers.)

are of direct relevance to therapy. Thus an increased dead space can usually be offset by an increased minute volume, and arterial P_{O_2} can be restored to normal with shunts up to about 30 per cent by an appropriate increase in the inspired oxygen concentration (see Figure 8.12, below).

Methods for calculating dead space and shunt for the three-compartment model are described at the end of the chapter, but no analytical techniques are required beyond measurement of blood and gas P_{CO_2} and P_{O_2}. It is then possible to determine what fraction of the inspired tidal volume does not participate in gas exchange and what fraction of the cardiac output constitutes a shunt or venous admixture. However, it is most important to remember that the measured value for 'dead space' will include a fraction representing ventilation of *relatively* underperfused alveoli, and the measured value for 'shunt' will include a fraction representing perfusion of *relatively* underventilated alveoli. Furthermore, although perfusion of relatively underventilated alveoli will reduce arterial P_{O_2}, the pattern of change, in relation to the inspired oxygen concentration, is quite different from that of a true shunt (see Figure 8.13, below).

The concept of ideal alveolar gas is considered below (page 192), but it will be clear from Figure 8.9 that ideal alveolar gas cannot be sampled for analysis. There is a convention that ideal alveolar P_{CO_2} is assumed to be equal to the arterial P_{CO_2} and that the respiratory exchange ratio of ideal alveolar gas is the same as that of expired air.

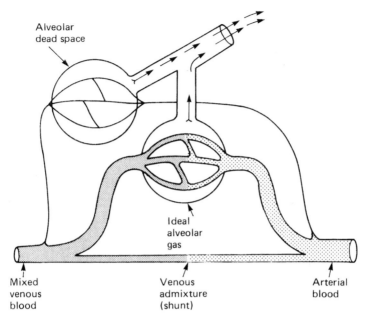

Figure 8.9 Three-compartment (Riley) model of gas exchange. The lung is imagined to consist of three functional units comprising alveolar dead space, 'ideal' alveoli and venous admixture (shunt). Gas exchange occurs only in the 'ideal' alveoli. The measured alveolar dead space consists of true alveolar dead space together with a component caused by $\dot{V}/\dot{Q}$ scatter. The measured venous admixture consists of true venous admixture (shunt) together with a component caused by $V/\dot{Q}$ scatter. Note that 'ideal' alveolar gas is exhaled contaminated with alveolar dead space gas, so it is not possible to sample 'ideal' alveolar gas.

Dead space

It was realized in the nineteenth century that an appreciable part of each inspiration did not penetrate to the regions of the lungs in which gas exchange occurred and was therefore exhaled unchanged. This fraction of the tidal volume has long been known as the dead space, while the effective part of the minute volume of respiration is known as the alveolar ventilation. The relationship is as follows:

alveolar ventilation = respiratory frequency (tidal volume − dead space)

$$\dot{V}_A = f\,(V_T - V_D)$$

It is often useful to think of two ratios. The first is the dead space/tidal volume ratio (often abbreviated to V_D/V_T and expressed as a percentage). The second useful ratio is the alveolar ventilation/minute volume ratio. The first ratio indicates the wasted part of the breath, and the second gives the used portion of the minute volume. The sum of the two ratios is unity, so one may easily be calculated from the other.

Components of the dead space

The preceding section considered dead space as though it were a single homogeneous component of expired air. The situation is actually more complicated, and Figure 8.10 shows in diagrammatic form the various components of a single expirate.

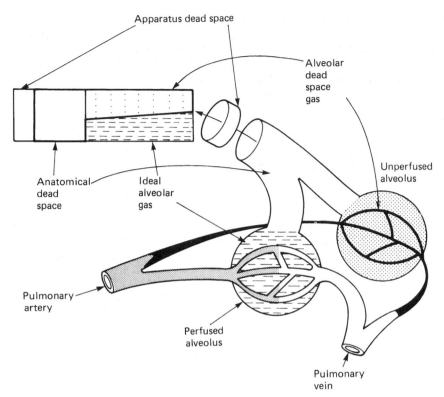

Figure 8.10 Components of a single breath of expired gas. The rectangle is an idealized representation of a single expirate. The physiological dead space equals the sum of the anatomical and alveolar dead spaces and is outlined in the heavy black line. The alveolar dead space does not equal the volume of unperfused spaces at alveolar level but only the part of their contents that is exhaled. This varies with tidal volume.

The first part to be exhaled will be the *apparatus dead space* if the subject is employing any form of external breathing apparatus. The next component will be from the *anatomical dead space*, which is related to the volume of the conducting air passages. Thereafter gas is exhaled from the alveolar level, and the diagram shows two representative alveoli corresponding to the two ventilated compartments of the three-compartment lung model shown in Figure 8.9. One alveolus is perfused and, from this, '*ideal*' alveolar gas is exhaled. The other alveolus is unperfused and so without gas exchange. From this alveolus is exhaled gas approximating in composition to inspired gas. This component of the expirate is known as *alveolar dead space* gas, which is important in many pathological conditions. The *physiological dead space* is the sum of the anatomical and alveolar dead spaces and is defined as the sum of all parts of the tidal volume that do not participate in gas exchange, as defined by the appropriate Bohr equation (see below).

In Figure 8.10, the final part of the expirate is called an end-tidal or, preferably, an end-expiratory sample and consists of a mixture of 'ideal' alveolar gas and alveolar dead space gas. The proportion of alveolar dead space gas in an end-expiratory sample is variable. In a healthy resting subject the composition of such a sample will be close to that of 'ideal' alveolar gas. However, in many pathological states (and during anaesthesia), an end-expiratory sample may contain a substantial proportion of alveolar dead space gas and thus be unrepresentative of the alveolar (and therefore arterial) gas tensions. For symbols, the small capital A relates to 'ideal' alveolar gas as in Pa_{CO_2}, while end-expiratory gas is distinguished by a small capital E, suffixed with a prime (e.g. Pe'_{CO_2}) and mixed expired gas a small capital E with a bar ($P\bar{e}_{CO_2}$). The term 'alveolar/arterial Po_2 difference' always refers to 'ideal' alveolar gas. Unqualified, the term 'alveolar' may mean either end-tidal or 'ideal' alveolar, depending on the context. This is a perennial source of confusion and it is better to specify either 'ideal' alveolar gas or end-expiratory gas.

It must again be stressed that Figure 8.10 is only a model to simplify quantification and there may be an infinite gradation between $\dot{V}/\dot{Q}$ ratios of zero and infinity. However, it is often helpful from the quantitative standpoint, particularly in the clinical field, to consider alveoli *as if* they fell into the three categories shown in Figure 8.9.

The Bohr equation

Bohr introduced his equation in 1891,[22] when the dead space was considered simply as gas exhaled from the conducting airways (i.e. anatomical dead space only). It may be simply derived as follows. During expiration all the CO_2 eliminated is contained in the alveolar gas. Therefore:

$$\begin{array}{c} \text{The quantity of } CO_2 \text{ eliminated} \\ \text{in the alveolar gas} \end{array} = \begin{array}{c} \text{quantity of } CO_2 \text{ eliminated} \\ \text{in the mixed expired gas} \end{array}$$

that is to say:

$$\begin{array}{c} \text{alveolar } CO_2 \text{ concentration} \\ \times \text{ alveolar ventilation} \end{array} = \begin{array}{c} \text{mixed-expired } CO_2 \text{ concentration} \\ \times \text{ minute volume} \end{array}$$

or, for a single breath:

$$\begin{array}{c} \text{alveolar } CO_2 \text{ concentration} \\ \times \text{ (tidal volume } - \text{ dead space)} \end{array} = \begin{array}{c} \text{mixed-expired } CO_2 \text{ concentration} \\ \times \text{ tidal volume} \end{array}$$

There are four terms in this equation. There is no serious difficulty in measuring two of them – the tidal volume and the mixed-expired CO_2 concentration. This leaves the alveolar CO_2 concentration and the dead space. Therefore, the alveolar CO_2 concentration may be derived if the dead space is known or, alternatively, the dead space may be derived if the alveolar CO_2 concentration is known. In the nineteenth century it was not realized that alveolar gas could be sampled and the Bohr equation was used to calculate the alveolar CO_2 concentration, substituting an assumed value for the dead space. After the historic discovery of the constancy of the alveolar gas by Haldane and Priestley in 1905,[23] the position was reversed and the alveolar CO_2 concentration was measured directly and the Bohr equation used to calculate the dead space.

More recently the use of this equation has been expanded to measure various components of the dead space by varying the interpretation of the term 'alveolar'. In the paragraph above, the word 'alveolar' means end-expiratory gas, and therefore this use of the Bohr equation indicates the anatomical dead space. If the 'ideal' alveolar CO_2 concentration were used, the equation would indicate the physiological dead space comprising the sum of the anatomical and alveolar dead spaces (Figure 8.10). 'Ideal' alveolar gas cannot be sampled but arterial Pco_2 may be substituted for alveolar Pco_2 in the Bohr equation, and the value so derived is now widely accepted as the definition of the physiological dead space:

$$V_D/V_T = (Pa_{CO_2} - P\bar{e}_{CO_2})/Pa_{CO_2}$$

In the healthy conscious resting subject, there is no significant difference between Pco_2 of end-expiratory gas and arterial blood. The former may therefore be used as a substitute for the latter, because the anatomical and physiological dead spaces should be the same (the normal alveolar dead space being too small to measure). However, the use of the end-expiratory Pco_2 in the Bohr equation may cause difficulties in certain situations. In exercise, in acute hyperventilation or if there is maldistribution of inspired gas with sequential emptying, the alveolar Pco_2 rises, often steeply, during expiration of the alveolar gas, and the end-tidal Pco_2 will depend on the duration of expiration. The dead space so derived will not necessarily correspond to any of the compartments of the dead space shown in Figure 8.10.

Anatomical dead space

The gills of fishes are perfused by a stream of water that enters by the mouth and leaves by the gill slits. All of the water is available for gaseous exchange. Mammals, however, employ tidal ventilation, which suffers from the disadvantage that a considerable part of the inspired gas comes to rest in the conducting air passages and is thus not available for gaseous exchange. The anatomical dead space is, in effect, the volume of the conducting air passages with the qualifications considered below.

This imperfection in mammalian ventilation was understood in the nineteenth century when the volume of the anatomical dead space was calculated from *post mortem* casts of the respiratory tract.[24] The value so obtained was used in calculating the composition of the alveolar gas according to the Bohr equation[22] as described above. The anatomical dead space is now generally defined as the volume of gas exhaled before the CO_2 concentration rises to its alveolar plateau, according to the technique of Fowler[25] outlined at the end of this chapter (see Figure 8.17).

The volume of the anatomical dead space, in spite of its name, is not constant and is influenced by many factors, some of which are of considerable clinical importance. Most of these factors influence the anatomical dead space by changing the volume of the conducting airways, except for changes in tidal volume and respiratory rate which affect the flow pattern of gas passing along the airways.

The following factors influence anatomical dead space.

Size of the subject must clearly influence the dimensions of the conducting air passages, and anatomical dead space increases with body size.

Age. In early infancy, anatomical dead space is normally 3.3 ml.kg^{-1}, and by the age of 6 years this has decreased to the adult value of approximately 2 ml.kg^{-1}. Throughout this period of development, intrathoracic anatomical dead space remains constant at 1 ml.kg^{-1} whilst the volume of the nose, mouth and pharynx change relative to body weight.[26]

Posture influences many lung volumes, including the anatomical dead space, with typical mean values for healthy subjects of:[27]

sitting	147 ml
semi-reclining	124 ml
supine	101 ml

Position of the neck and jaw has a pronounced effect on the anatomical dead space, with mean values in conscious subjects of:[28]

neck extended, jaw protruded   143 ml
normal position   119 ml
neck flexed, chin depressed   73 ml

It is noteworthy that the first position is the one used by resuscitators and anaesthetists to procure the least possible airway resistance. Unfortunately, it also results in the maximum dead space.

Lung volume at the end of inspiration affects the anatomical dead space, because the volume of the air passages changes in proportion to the lung volume. The increase is of the order of 20 ml additional anatomical dead space for each litre increase in lung volume.[29]

Tracheal intubation or tracheostomy will bypass the extrathoracic anatomical dead space, which is normally about 70 ml. Thus tracheal intubation or tracheostomy will bypass about half the total anatomical dead space,[28,30] although this advantage will clearly be lost if a corresponding volume of apparatus dead space is added to the circuit.

Tidal volume and respiratory rate. A reduction in tidal volume results in a marked reduction of the anatomical dead space as measured by Fowler's method, and this limits the fall of alveolar ventilation resulting from small tidal volumes. This is important in the case of comatose or anaesthetized patients who are left to breathe for themselves, often with tidal volumes smaller than the normal anatomical dead space of 140 ml.[31]

Reduced anatomical dead space as a result of small tidal volumes are unlikely to result from changes in the physical dimensions of the airways, and result mostly from changes in the flow patterns and mixing of gases within the airways. First, at low flow rates there is a greater tendency towards laminar flow of gas through the air passages (page 58). Inspired gas advances with a cone front and the tip of the cone penetrates the alveoli before all the gas in the conducting passages has been washed out. In conscious subjects some inspired gas may be detected in the alveoli with tidal volumes as small as 60 ml.[32] Secondly, with a slow respiratory rate and/or a prolonged inspiratory time, there is more time for mixing of gases between the alveoli and the smaller airways. Mixing will occur by simple diffusion, possibly aided by a mixing effect of the heartbeat, which tends to mix all gas lying below the carina. This effect is negligible at normal rates of ventilation, but becomes more marked during hypoventilation. For example, in one hypoventilating patient, Nunn and Hill found alveolar gas at the carina at the beginning of expiration.[30] A similar effect occurs during breath holding when alveolar gas mixes with dead space gas as far up as the glottis.

Drugs acting on the bronchiolar musculature will affect the anatomical dead space. All bronchodilator drugs will increase dead space; for example, atropine causes an increase of 20–45 ml,[33,34] whilst the bronchoconstrictor histamine causes a small decrease in anatomical dead space.

Alveolar dead space

Alveolar dead space may be defined as the part of the inspired gas that passes through the anatomical dead space to mix with gas at the alveolar level, but which does not take part in gas exchange. The cause of the failure of gas exchange is lack of effective perfusion of the spaces to which the gas is distributed at the alveolar level. Measured alveolar dead space must sometimes contain a component due to the ventilation of *relatively* underperfused alveoli which have a very high (but not infinite) $\dot{V}/\dot{Q}$ ratio (Figure 8.8). The alveolar dead space is too small to be measured with confidence in healthy supine humans, but becomes appreciable in some circumstances:

Low cardiac output, regardless of the cause, results in pulmonary hypotension and failure of perfusion of the uppermost parts of the lungs (zone 1, see page 146). During anaesthesia with controlled ventilation, sudden changes in end-expiratory CO_2 therefore usually indicate changing alveolar dead space secondary to abrupt variations in cardiac output (page 239).

Pulmonary embolism is considered separately in Chapter 28. Apart from its effect on cardiac output, pulmonary embolism is a direct cause of alveolar dead space, which may reach massive proportions.

Posture. Changes in position have a significant effect on pulmonary blood flow (page 169). Fortunately, during normal breathing there are similar changes in the distribution of ventilation so that $\dot{V}/\dot{Q}$ mismatch is uncommon and there are no significant changes in alveolar dead space. However, if a patient is ventilated artificially in the lateral position, ventilation is distributed in favour of the upper lung (Table 8.1), particularly in the presence of an open pneumothorax;[4] under these conditions, part of the ventilation of the upper lung will constitute alveolar dead space.

Physiological dead space

The physiological dead space is the sum of all parts of the tidal volume that do not participate in gaseous exchange and is usually described by the term V_D. Nowadays it is universally defined by the Bohr mixing equation with substitution of arterial P_{CO_2} for alveolar P_{CO_2} as described above.

Enghoff in 1931 was the first to demonstrate that the physiological dead space remained a fairly constant fraction of the tidal volume over a wide range of tidal volumes.[35] It is, therefore, generally more useful to use the V_D/V_T ratio: the alveolar ventilation will then be $(1 - V_D/V_T) \times$ the respiratory minute volume. Thus if the physiological dead space is 30 per cent of the tidal volume (i.e. $V_D/V_T = 0.3$), the alveolar ventilation will be 70 per cent of the minute volume. This approach is radically different from the assumption of a constant 'dead space' that is subtracted from the tidal volume, the difference then being multiplied by the respiratory frequency to indicate the alveolar ventilation.

Factors influencing the physiological dead space

This section summarizes information on the value of the total physiological dead space in normal subjects, but reasons for the changes have been considered above in the sections on the anatomical and alveolar dead space.

Age and gender.[36] There is a tendency for V_D and also the V_D/V_T ratio to increase with age, the anatomical component of V_D increasing by slightly less than 1 ml per year. V_D in men is around 50 ml greater than in women but the former group has larger tidal volumes and there is little difference in the V_D/V_T ratios between men and women.

Body size. As described above, it is evident that anatomical dead space and therefore V_D, in common with other pulmonary volumes, will be larger in larger people. In 1955

Radford showed that the volume of the air passages (in millilitres) approximates to the weight of the subject in pounds (1 pound = 0.45 kg).[37] Later, Harris' group recommended correlation with height, and reported that V_D increased by 17 ml for every 10 cm increase in height.[36]

Posture. The V_D/V_T ratio decreases from a mean value of 34 per cent in the upright position to 30 per cent in the supine position.[38] This is largely explained by the change in anatomical dead space (see above).

Pathology. Changes in dead space are important features of many causes of lung dysfunction such as pulmonary embolism, smoking, anaesthesia, artificial ventilation, etc. These topics are discussed in later chapters of this book.

Effects of an increased physiological dead space

Regardless of whether an increase in physiological dead space is in the anatomical or the alveolar component, alveolar ventilation is reduced unless there is a compensatory increase in minute volume. Reduction of alveolar ventilation due to an increase in physiological dead space produces changes in the 'ideal' alveolar gas tensions that are identical to those produced when alveolar ventilation is decreased by reduction in respiratory minute volume (see Figure 6.12).

It is usually possible to counteract the effects of an increase in physiological dead space by a corresponding increase in the respiratory minute volume. If, for example, the minute volume is $10\,l.min^{-1}$ and the V_D/V_T ratio 30 per cent, the alveolar ventilation will be $7\,l.min^{-1}$. If the patient were then subjected to pulmonary embolism resulting in an increase of the V_D/V_T ratio to 50 per cent, the minute volume would need to be increased to $14\,l.min^{-1}$ to maintain an alveolar ventilation of $7\,l.min^{-1}$. However, should the V_D/V_T increase to 80 per cent, the minute volume would need to be increased to $35\,l.min^{-1}$. Ventilatory capacity may be a limiting factor with massive increases in dead space, and this is a rare cause of ventilatory failure (Chapter 26).

Venous admixture or shunt

Admixture of arterial blood with poorly oxygenated or mixed venous blood is a most important cause of arterial hypoxaemia.

Nomenclature of venous admixture

Venous admixture refers to the degree of admixture of mixed venous blood with pulmonary end-capillary blood that would be required to produce the observed difference between the arterial and the pulmonary end-capillary P_{O_2} (usually taken to equal ideal alveolar P_{O_2}), the principles of the calculation being shown in Figure 8.11. Note that the venous admixture is not the *actual* amount of venous blood that mingles with the arterial blood, but the *calculated* amount that would be required to produce the observed value for the arterial P_{O_2}. Calculated venous admixture and the actual volume of blood mixing differ because of two factors. First, the thebesian and bronchial venous drainage does not necessarily have the same P_{O_2} as mixed venous blood. Secondly, venous admixture includes the contribution to the arterial blood from alveoli having a $\dot{V}/\dot{Q}$ ratio of more than zero but less than the normal value (Figure 8.7), when, again, P_{O_2} will differ from that of

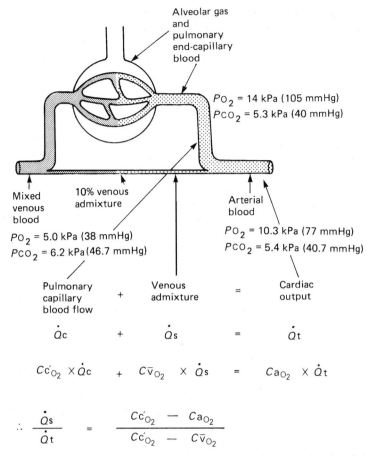

Figure 8.11 A schematic representation of venous admixture. It makes the assumption that all the arterial blood has come either from alveoli with normal $\dot{V}/\dot{Q}$ ratios or from a shunt carrying only mixed venous blood. This is never true but it forms a convenient method of quantifying venous admixture from whatever cause. The shunt equation is similar to the Bohr equation and is based on the axiomatic relationship that the total amount of oxygen in 1 minute's flow of arterial blood equals the sum of the amount of oxygen in 1 minute's flow through both the pulmonary capillaries and the shunt. Amount of oxygen in 1 minute's flow of blood equals the product of blood flow rate and the concentration of oxygen in the blood. Ca_{O_2}, oxygen content of arterial blood; Cc'_{O_2}, oxygen content of pulmonary end-capillary blood; $C\bar{v}_{O_2}$, oxygen content of mixed venous blood $\dot{Q}c$, pulmonary capillary blood flow; $\dot{Q}s$, blood flow through shunt; $\dot{Q}t$, total cardiac output.

mixed venous blood. Venous admixture is thus a convenient index but defines neither the precise volume nor the anatomical pathway of the shunt. Nevertheless, it is often loosely termed 'shunt'.

Anatomical (extra-pulmonary) shunt refers to the amount of venous blood that mixes with the pulmonary end-capillary blood on the arterial side of the circulation. The term embraces bronchial and thebesian venous blood flow and also admixture of mixed venous blood caused by atelectasis, bronchial obstruction, congenital heart disease with right-to-left shunting, etc. Clearly, different components may have different oxygen contents that will not necessarily equal the mixed venous oxygen content. Anatomical shunt excludes blood draining any alveoli with a $\dot{V}/\dot{Q}$ ratio of more than zero.

Virtual shunt refers to shunt values derived from calculations in which the arterial to mixed-venous oxygen difference is assumed rather than actually measured (see below).

Pathological shunt is sometimes used to describe the forms of anatomical shunt that do not occur in the normal subject.

Physiological shunt. This term is, unfortunately, used in two senses. In the first sense it is used to describe the degree of venous admixture that occurs in a normal healthy subject. Differences between the actual measured venous admixture and the normal value for the 'physiological shunt' thus indicate the amount of venous admixture that results from the disease process. In its alternative sense, physiological shunt is synonymous with venous admixture as derived from the mixing equation (Figure 8.11). The term is probably best avoided.

Forms of venous admixture

The contribution of $\dot{V}/\dot{Q}$ mismatch to venous admixture is discussed in detail below. Other important sources of venous admixture, both normal and pathological, include the following.

Venae cordis minimae (thebesian veins). Some small veins of the left heart drain directly into the chambers of the left heart and so mingle with the pulmonary venous blood. The oxygen content of this blood is probably very low, and therefore the flow (believed to be about 0.3 per cent of cardiac output[39]) causes an appreciable fall in the mixed arterial oxygen tension.

Bronchial veins. Figure 7.1 shows that part of the venous drainage of the bronchial circulation passes by way of the deep true bronchial veins to reach the pulmonary veins. It is uncertain how large this component is in the healthy subject but is probably less than 1 per cent of cardiac output. In bronchial disease and coarctation of the aorta the flow through this channel may be greatly increased, and in bronchiectasis and emphysema may be as large as 10 per cent of cardiac output. In these circumstances it becomes a major cause of arterial desaturation.

Congenital heart disease. Right-to-left shunting in congenital heart disease is the cause of the worst examples of venous admixture. When there are abnormal communications between right and left hearts, shunting will usually be from left to right unless the pressures in the right heart are raised above those of the left heart. This occurs in conditions involving obstruction to the right ventricular outflow tract (e.g. Fallot's tetralogy) or in prolonged left-to-right shunt when the increased pulmonary blood flow causes pulmonary hypertension and eventually a reversal of the shunt (Eisenmenger's syndrome).

Pulmonary pathology often results in increased venous admixture, thus causing hypoxaemia. Venous drainage from lung tumours constitutes a pathological shunt, but more commonly venous admixture results from pulmonary blood flow past non-ventilated alveoli in conditions such as lobar and bronchopneumonia, pulmonary collapse and acute lung injury. The degree of venous admixture that occurs with lung disease is variable, depending on the balance between hypoxic pulmonary vasoconstriction (page 151) and pathological vasodilatation of the pulmonary vessels by sepsis or inflammatory mediators. For a detailed description of venous admixture and lung pathology see Part 3 of this book.

Effect of venous admixture on arterial P_{CO_2} and P_{O_2}

Qualitatively, it will be clear that venous admixture reduces the overall efficiency of gas exchange and results in arterial blood gas tensions that are closer to those of mixed venous blood than would otherwise be the case. Quantitatively, the effect is simple provided that we consider the *contents* of gases in blood. In the case of the anatomical shunt in Figure 8.11, conservation of mass (oxygen) is the basis of the equations, which simply state that the amount of oxygen flowing in the arterial system equals the sum of the amount of oxygen leaving the pulmonary capillaries and the amount of oxygen flowing through the shunt. For each term in this equation the amount of oxygen flowing may be expressed as the product of the blood flow rate and the oxygen content of blood flowing in the vessel (the symbols are explained in Figure 8.11 and Appendix D). Figure 8.11 shows how the equation may be cleared and solved for the ratio of the venous admixture to the cardiac output. The final equation has a form that is rather similar to that of the Bohr equation for the physiological dead space.

In terms of *content*, the shunt equation is very simple to solve for the effect of venous admixture on arterial oxygen content. If, for example, pulmonary end-capillary oxygen content is $20\,ml.dl^{-1}$ and mixed venous blood oxygen content is $10\,ml.dl^{-1}$, a 50 per cent venous admixture will result in an arterial oxygen content of $15\,ml.dl^{-1}$, a 25 per cent venous admixture will result in an arterial oxygen content of $17.5\,ml.dl^{-1}$, and so on. It is then necessary to convert arterial oxygen content to P_{O_2} by reference to the haemoglobin dissociation curve (see page 266). Because arterial P_{O_2} is usually on the flat part of the haemoglobin dissociation curve, small changes in content tend to have a very large effect on P_{O_2}, though this effect diminishes at lower arterial P_{O_2} when the dissociation curve becomes steeper.

The effect of venous admixture on arterial CO_2 *content* is roughly similar in magnitude to that of oxygen content. However, due to the steepness of the CO_2 dissociation curve near the arterial point (see Figure 10.2), the effect on arterial P_{CO_2} is very small and far less than the change in arterial P_{O_2} (Table 8.2).

Two conclusions may be drawn:

1. Arterial P_{O_2} is the most useful blood gas measurement for the detection of venous admixture.
2. Venous admixture reduces the arterial P_{O_2} markedly, but has relatively little effect on arterial P_{CO_2} or on the content of either CO_2 or O_2 unless the venous admixture is large.

Elevations of arterial P_{CO_2} are seldom caused by venous admixture, and it is customary to ignore the effect of moderate shunts on P_{CO_2}. In the clinical situation, it is more usual for venous admixture to lower the P_{CO_2} indirectly, because the decreased P_{O_2} commonly causes hyperventilation, which more than compensates for the very slight elevation of P_{CO_2} that would otherwise result from the venous admixture (see Figure 26.1).

Table 8.2 Effect of 5% venous admixture on the difference between arterial and pulmonary end-capillary blood levels of carbon dioxide and oxygen

	Pulmonary end-capillary blood	Arterial blood
CO_2 content (ml.dl^{-1})	49.7	50.0
P_{CO_2} (kPa)	5.29	5.33
(mmHg)	39.7	40.0
O_2 content (ml.dl^{-1})	19.9	19.6
O_2 saturation (%)	97.8	96.8
P_{O_2} (kPa)	14.0	12.0
(mmHg)	105	90

It has been assumed that the arterial/venous oxygen content difference is 4.5 ml.dl^{-1} and that the haemoglobin concentration is 14.9 g.dl^{-1}. Typical changes in P_{O_2} and P_{CO_2} have been shown for a 10% venous admixture as in Figure 8.11.

Effect of cardiac output on shunt

Cardiac output influences venous admixture and its consequences in two opposing ways. First, a reduction of cardiac output causes a decrease in mixed venous oxygen content, with the result that a given shunt causes a greater reduction in arterial P_{O_2} *provided the shunt fraction is unaltered*, a relationship that is illustrated in Figure 11.5. Secondly, it has been observed that, in a very wide range of pathological and physiological circumstances, a reduction in cardiac output causes an approximately proportional reduction in the shunt fraction,[40,41] the only apparent exception being a shunt through regional pulmonary atelectasis.[42] One possible explanation for the observed change in shunt fraction is that the reduction in shunt is due to pulmonary vasoconstriction in consequence of the reduction in P_{O_2} of the mixed venous blood flowing through the shunt.[43] It is remarkable that these two effects tend to have approximately equal and opposite effects on arterial P_{O_2}. Thus with a decreased cardiac output there is usually a reduced shunt of a more desaturated mixed venous blood, with the result that the arterial P_{O_2} is scarcely changed.

The iso-shunt diagram

If we assume normal values for arterial P_{CO_2}, haemoglobin and arterial/mixed venous oxygen content difference, the arterial P_{O_2} is determined mainly by the inspired oxygen concentration and venous admixture considered in the context of the three-compartment model (Figure 8.9). The relationship between inspired oxygen concentration and arterial P_{O_2} is a matter for constant attention in such situations as intensive therapy, and it has been found a matter of practical convenience to prepare a graph of the relationship at different levels of venous admixture (Figure 8.12). The arterial/mixed venous oxygen content difference is often unknown in the clinical situation and therefore the diagram has been prepared for an assumed content difference of 5 ml oxygen per 100 ml of blood. Iso-shunt bands have then been drawn on a plot of arterial P_{O_2} against inspired oxygen concentration. The bands are sufficiently wide to encompass all values of P_{CO_2} between 3.3 and 5.3 kPa (25–40 mmHg) and haemoglobin levels between 10 and 14 g.dl^{-1}. Normal barometric pressure is assumed. Because calculation of the venous admixture requires knowledge of the actual arterial/mixed venous oxygen content difference, the iso-shunt lines in Figure 8.12 refer to the *virtual shunt*, which is defined as the calculated shunt on the basis of an assumed value of the arterial/mixed venous oxygen content difference of 5 ml.dl^{-1}.

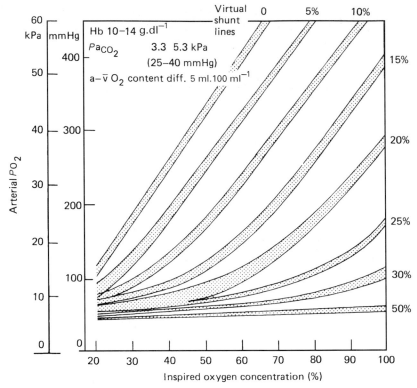

Figure 8.12 Iso-shunt diagram. On coordinates of inspired oxygen concentration (abscissa) and arterial Po_2 (ordinate), iso-shunt bands have been drawn to include all values of Hb, Pa_{CO_2} and arterial/venous oxygen content difference shown above. (Redrawn from reference 44 by permission of the Editor of the *British Journal of Anaesthesia*.)

In practice, the iso-shunt diagram is useful for adjusting the inspired oxygen concentration to obtain a required level of arterial Po_2. Under static pathological conditions, changing the inspired oxygen concentration results in changes in arterial Po_2 that are reasonably well predicted by the iso-shunt diagram.[45] In intensive care, the iso-shunt graph may therefore be used to determine the optimal inspired oxygen concentration to prevent hypoxaemia while avoiding the administration of an unnecessarily high concentration of oxygen.[44] For example, if a patient is found to have an arterial Po_2 of 30 kPa (225 mmHg) while breathing 90% oxygen, he has a virtual shunt of 20%; if it is required to attain an arterial Po_2 of 10 kPa (75 mmHg), this should be achieved by reducing the inspired oxygen concentration to 45%. Calculation of virtual shunt from the iso-shunt graph may also be used as an indication of progress in patients with lung injury.

With inspired oxygen concentrations in excess of 35%, perfusion of alveoli with low (but not zero) $\dot{V}/\dot{Q}$ ratios has relatively little effect on arterial Po_2. However, with inspired oxygen concentrations in the range 21–35%, increased scatter of $\dot{V}/\dot{Q}$ ratios has an appreciable effect on arterial Po_2 for reasons that are explained below. Therefore in these circumstances, the standard iso-shunt diagram is not applicable, because arterial Po_2 is less than predicted as the inspired oxygen concentration is reduced towards 21%. A new diagram, which provides a reasonable simulation of scatter of $\dot{V}/\dot{Q}$ ratios *plus* a shunt, is explained below, and this diagram (see Figure E.4) seems to be a satisfactory model for a wide range of patients requiring the administration of oxygen in this range.[46]

The effect of scatter of $\dot{V}/\dot{Q}$ ratios on arterial P_{O_2}

It is usually extremely difficult to say whether reduction of arterial P_{O_2} is due to true shunt (areas of zero $\dot{V}/\dot{Q}$) ratio, or increased scatter of $\dot{V}/\dot{Q}$ ratios with an appreciable contribution to arterial blood from alveoli with very low (but not zero) $\dot{V}/\dot{Q}$ ratio. In the

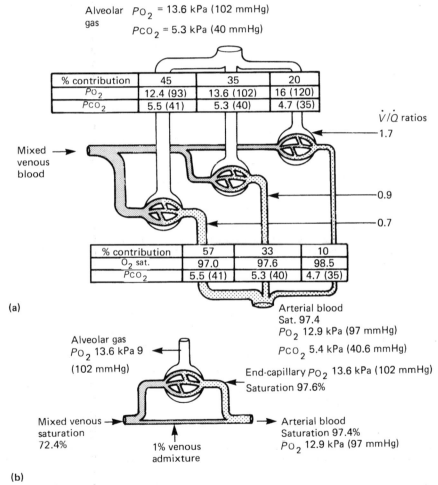

Figure 8.13 Alveolar to arterial P_{O_2} difference caused by scatter of $\dot{V}/\dot{Q}$ ratios and its representation by an equivalent degree of venous admixture. (a) Scatter of $\dot{V}/\dot{Q}$ ratios corresponding roughly to the three zones of the lung in the normal upright subject. Mixed alveolar gas P_{O_2} is calculated with allowance for the volume contribution of gas from the three zones. Arterial saturation is similarly determined and the P_{O_2} derived. There is an alveolar/arterial P_{O_2} difference of 0.7 kPa (5 mmHg). (b) An entirely imaginary situation that would account for the difference. This is a useful method of quantifying the functional effect of $\dot{V}/\dot{Q}$ ratios but should be carefully distinguished from the actual situation.

clinical field, it is quite usual to ignore scatter of $\dot{V}/\dot{Q}$ ratios (which are difficult to quantify) and treat blood-gas results *as if* the alveolar/arterial Po_2 difference was caused entirely by true shunt. In the example shown in Figure 8.13, it is quite impossible to distinguish between scatter of $\dot{V}/\dot{Q}$ ratios and a shunt on the basis of a single measurement of arterial Po_2. However, the two conditions are quite different in the effect of different inspired oxygen concentrations on the alveolar/arterial Po_2 difference and therefore the apparent shunt.

Figure 8.12 shows that, for a true shunt, with increasing inspired oxygen concentration, the effect on arterial Po_2 increases to reach a plateau value of 2–3 kPa (15–22 mmHg) for each 1 per cent of shunt. This is shown more precisely in terms of alveolar/arterial Po_2 difference, plotted as a function of alveolar Po_2 in Figure 11.4.

It is not intuitively obvious why an increased spread of $\dot{V}/\dot{Q}$ ratios should increase the alveolar/arterial Po_2 difference. There are essentially two reasons. First, there tends to be more blood from the alveoli with low $\dot{V}/\dot{Q}$ ratio. For example, in Figure 8.13, 57 per cent of the arterial blood comes from the alveoli with low $\dot{V}/\dot{Q}$ ratio and low Po_2, while only

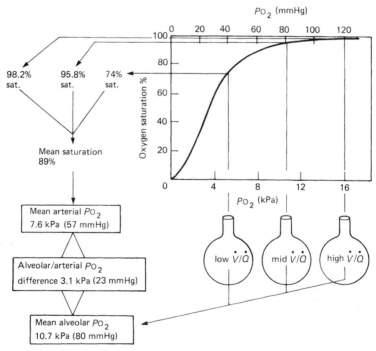

Figure 8.14 Alveolar to arterial Po_2 difference caused by scatter of $\dot{V}/\dot{Q}$ ratios resulting in oxygen tensions along the upper inflexion of the oxygen dissociation curve. The diagram shows the effect of three groups of alveoli with Po_2 values of 5.3, 10.7 and 16.0 kPa (40, 80 and 120 mmHg). Ignoring the effect of the different volumes of gas and blood contributed by the three groups, the mean alveolar Po_2 is 10.7 kPa. However, due to the bend of the dissociation curve, the saturations of the blood leaving the three groups are not proportional to their Po_2. The mean arterial saturation is, in fact, 89% and the Po_2 therefore is 7.6 kPa. The alveolar/arterial Po_2 difference is thus 3.1 kPa. The actual difference would be somewhat greater, because gas with a high Po_2 would make a relatively greater contribution to the alveolar gas, and blood with a low Po_2 would make a relatively greater contribution to the arterial blood. In this example, a calculated venous admixture of 27% would be required to account for the scatter of $\dot{V}/\dot{Q}$ ratios in terms of the measured alveolar/arterial Po_2 difference, at an alveolar Po_2 of 10.7 kPa.

10 per cent is contributed by the alveoli with high $\dot{V}/\dot{Q}$ ratio and high P_{O_2}. Therefore, the latter cannot compensate for the former, when arterial oxygen levels are determined with due allowance for volume contribution. The second reason is illustrated in Figure 8.14. Alveoli with high $\dot{V}/\dot{Q}$ ratios are on a flatter part of the haemoglobin dissociation curve than are alveoli with low $\dot{V}/\dot{Q}$ ratios. Therefore, the adverse effect on oxygen *content* is greater for alveoli with a low $\dot{V}/\dot{Q}$ and therefore low P_{O_2} than is the beneficial effect of alveoli with a high $\dot{V}/\dot{Q}$ and therefore high P_{O_2}. Therefore, the greater the spread of $\dot{V}/\dot{Q}$ ratios, the larger the alveolar/arterial P_{O_2} difference.

Modification of the iso-shunt diagram to include $\dot{V}/\dot{Q}$ scatter. The iso-shunt diagram described above does not take into account $\dot{V}/\dot{Q}$ scatter, so has bands too wide for practical use below an inspired oxygen concentration of 40% (Figure 8.12). This problem has been overcome by the development of a two-compartment model including both true shunt and $\dot{V}/\dot{Q}$ scatter components,[46] which for the latter factor assumes a bimodal distribution of $\dot{V}/\dot{Q}$ scatter and uses five grades of $\dot{V}/\dot{Q}$ mismatch 'severity' (Table 8.3). Figure 8.15

Table 8.3 Ventilation/perfusion ratios for the bimodal two-compartment model of maldistribution[46] of $\dot{V}/\dot{Q}$ ratios used in the construction of Figure 8.15

	Compartment with high $\dot{V}/\dot{Q}$ ratio	Compartment with low $\dot{V}/\dot{Q}$ ratio
Perfect match (grade 0)	0.86	0.86
Mismatch grade 1	1.18	0.55
Mismatch grade 2	1.56	0.38
Mismatch grade 3	2.15	0.30
Mismatch grade 4	3.34	0.16

It is assumed that the ratio of actual perfusions is inversely related to the square root of the $\dot{V}/\dot{Q}$ ratios.

shows the effect of $\dot{V}/\dot{Q}$ mismatch on the 0 per cent iso-shunt line, clearly displaying the variation in arterial P_{O_2} with $\dot{V}/\dot{Q}$ scatter at lower inspired oxygen concentrations. Figure E.4 shows further examples of the effect of $\dot{V}/\dot{Q}$ scatter on the inspired to arterial oxygen gradients. This model is clearly an oversimplification of such situations as those shown in Figure 8.8. Nevertheless, the second grade of $\dot{V}/\dot{Q}$ mismatch, when combined with a range of shunt values, was found to provide a close simulation of the relationship between arterial P_{O_2} and inspired oxygen concentration for a wide variety of patients with moderate respiratory dysfunction requiring oxygen therapy in the range 25–35% inspired oxygen concentration.[46,47] The modified iso-shunt diagram (Figure E.4) is not appreciably different from the standard iso-shunt diagram at higher concentrations of inspired oxygen.

Principles of assessment of distribution of ventilation and pulmonary blood flow

Distribution of inspired gas

Radioactive tracer methods allow the regional distribution of ventilation to be conveniently studied with a gamma camera following inhalation of a suitable radioactive

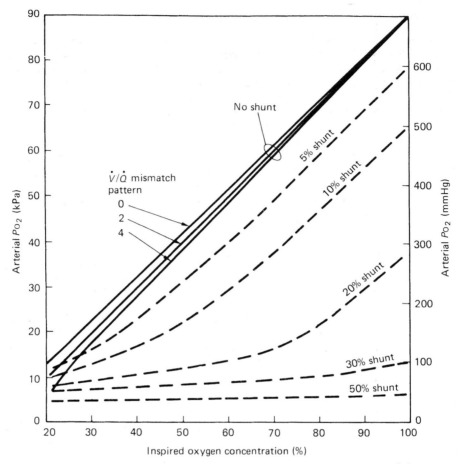

Figure 8.15 The continuous curves show the effect on arterial Po_2 of increasing degrees of $\dot{V}/\dot{Q}$ mismatch (using the bimodal two-compartment model of maldistribution specified in Table 8.3) for different values of inspired oxygen concentration in the absence of a true shunt. At lower inspired oxygen the arterial Po_2 is progressively decreased below normal for the reasons shown in Figures 8.13 and 8.14. These concave-downward curves may be compared with the concave-upward iso-shunt curves shown as broken lines. $\dot{V}/\dot{Q}$ mismatch patterns 1–4 are combined with the iso-shunt curves in Appendix Figure E.4.

gas that is not too soluble in blood. Both ^{133}Xe and [81]Kr are suitable for this purpose and the technique has become a routine clinical investigation, usually using [81]Kr because its short half-life (13 s) reduces uptake by the pulmonary circulation. The technique defines zones of the lung that can be related to anatomical subdivisions by comparing anteroposterior and lateral scans. The technique is useful for defining pathological causes of failure of regional ventilation and is usually related to scans that indicate perfusion.

PET scanning is used for research purposes and allows more precise definition of regional ventilation, though only in horizontal positions.[47] Once again, radioactive isotopes are inhaled, in this case [19]Ne, and the radioisotopic concentration in a three-dimensional field measured during normal breathing.

Measurement of distribution of pulmonary blood flow

Single lung and lobar blood flow. There is no simple method to estimate the partitioning of the pulmonary blood flow in humans. Unilateral oxygen consumption can be measured during single lung ventilation and this gives an approximate indication of the relative perfusion of the two lungs. However, the Fick equation cannot be solved separately for the two lungs, because the anatomical arrangement of the pulmonary veins makes it impossible to sample representative pulmonary venous blood from the two lungs. It is, however, possible to make a very approximate estimate of the pulmonary venous oxygen content from the unilateral end-expiratory Po_2.

For lobar blood flow, end-expiratory gases sampled from different lobes at bronchoscopy will give some qualitative indication of blood flow, although precise calculation of flow is, again, not possible. A more complete assessment has been made by the simultaneous analysis of a number of gases exhaled from various bronchi, using a mass spectrometer at bronchoscopy.[48]

Distribution to zones of the lung. The techniques most widely used in the clinical field are analogous to the methods for studying the zonal distribution of ventilation outlined above. A relatively insoluble gas such as ^{133}Xe or ^{99}Tc may be dissolved in saline and administered intravenously and its distribution within the lung recorded with a gamma camera.

PET scanning may also be used to measure regional perfusion as for ventilation. In this case, inhalation of small concentrations of ^{11}CO allows non-invasive labelling of the haemoglobin, after which, radioisotopic concentration in the lung will equate to blood flow.[47]

Measurement of ventilation and perfusion as a function of $\dot{V}/\dot{Q}$ ratio

The information of the type displayed in Figures 8.7 and 8.8 is obtained by MIGET studies, a technique first developed in the 1970s[49] and reviewed more recently.[17,18] It employs six tracer gases with different blood solubility ranging from very soluble (acetone) to very insoluble (sulphur hexafluoride). Saline is equilibrated with these gases and infused intravenously at a constant rate. After about 20 minutes a steady state is achieved and samples of arterial blood and mixed expired gas are collected. Levels of the tracer gases in the arterial blood are then measured by gas chromatography, and levels in the mixed venous blood are derived by use of the Fick principle. It is then possible to calculate the retention of each tracer in the blood passing through the lung and the elimination of each in the expired gas. Retention and elimination are related to the solubility coefficient of each tracer in blood and then, by numerical analysis, it is possible to compute a distribution curve for pulmonary blood flow and alveolar ventilation respectively in relation to the spectrum of $\dot{V}/\dot{Q}$ ratios (Figure 8.7).

The technique is technically demanding and laborious. It has not become widely used, but studies using the technique from a small number of laboratories have made major contributions to our understanding of gas exchange in a wide variety of circumstances.

Measurement of venous admixture

Venous admixture, according to the Riley three-compartment model (Figure 8.9) is calculated by solution of the equation shown in Figure 8.11. When the alveolar Po_2 is less than about 30 kPa (225 mmHg), scatter of $\dot{V}/\dot{Q}$ ratios contributes appreciably to the total calculated venous admixture (Figure 8.15). When the subject breathes 100% oxygen, the component due to scatter of $\dot{V}/\dot{Q}$ ratios is minimal. Nevertheless, the calculated quantity still does not indicate the precise value of shunted blood because some of the shunt consists of blood of which the oxygen content is unknown (e.g. from bronchial veins and venae cordis minimae). The calculated venous admixture is thus at best an index rather than a precise measurement of contamination of arterial blood with venous blood.

To solve the equation shown in Figure 8.11, three quantities are required:

1. *Arterial oxygen content*. Arterial Po_2 may be measured on blood drawn from any convenient systemic artery. The resulting oxygen partial pressure must then be converted to oxygen content – the relevant calculations are described in Chapter 11 (page 266 *et seq.*). This requires knowledge of haemoglobin concentration, shift of the haemoglobin dissociation curve and haemoglobin saturation. The last of these may be determined from the nomogram shown in Figure 11.11, measured directly or calculated from the following equation which, though highly convenient, is valid only for Po_2 values above 4 kPa (30 mmHg):[50]

$$So_2 = \frac{100(Po_2^3 + 2.667 \times Po_2)}{Po_2^3 + 2.667 \times Po_2 + 55.47}$$

(Po_2 is in kPa; So_2 in %)
2. *Mixed venous oxygen content*. Mixed venous blood must be sampled from the right ventricle or pulmonary artery. Blood from inferior and superior venae cavae and coronary sinus, each with quite different oxygen contents, remain separate in the right atrium. Oxygen content may then be calculated from measured Po_2 as for the arterial sample. An assumed value for arterial/mixed venous blood oxygen content difference is often made if it is not feasible to sample mixed venous blood, and this is inherent in the iso-shunt diagram (Figure 8.12).
3. *Pulmonary end-capillary oxygen content*. This cannot be measured directly, and is assumed equal to the alveolar Po_2 (page 207). If Figure 8.9 is studied in conjunction with Figure 8.11, it will be seen that the 'alveolar' Po_2 required is the 'ideal' alveolar Po_2 and not the end-expiratory Po_2, which may be contaminated with alveolar dead space gas. The 'ideal' alveolar Po_2 is derived by solution of one of the alveolar air equations (see below), and again converted to oxygen content.

Non-invasive estimation of venous admixture may be performed without sampling arterial or mixed venous blood, using only measurement of haemoglobin concentration (Hb), end-tidal Pco_2, inspired oxygen concentration and peripheral oxygen saturation (Spo_2).[51] Arterial oxygen content is calculated from Hb and Spo_2 and alveolar Po_2 from the alveolar air equation described below using inspired oxygen concentration and end-tidal Pco_2 (therefore assuming a normal end-tidal to arterial Pco_2 difference). In a similar fashion to the iso-shunt lines, mixed venous oxygen content is derived from arterial oxygen content and an assumed value for arterial/venous oxygen difference. Shunt estimated in this way gives results that are ±16 per cent shunt compared with invasive measurements, but the value of this method in the clinical setting is as yet uncertain.[51]

The alveolar air equation

The Po_2 of 'ideal' alveolar gas (Figure 8.9) must be derived by indirect means and was first formulated with some precision by Riley et al. in 1946.[52] It exists in several forms that seem very different but give the same result.

Derivation of the 'ideal' alveolar Po_2 is based on the following assumptions:

1. Quite large degrees of venous admixture or $\dot{V}/\dot{Q}$ scatter cause relatively little difference between the Pco_2 of 'ideal' alveolar gas (or pulmonary end-capillary blood) and arterial blood (Table 8.2). Therefore, 'ideal' alveolar Pco_2 is approximately equal to arterial Pco_2.
2. The respiratory exchange ratio of ideal alveolar gas (in relation to inspired gas) equals the respiratory exchange ratio of mixed expired gas (again in relation to inspired gas).

From these assumptions it is possible to derive an equation that indicates the 'ideal' alveolar Po_2 in terms of arterial Pco_2 and inspired gas Po_2. As a very rough approximation, the oxygen and carbon dioxide in the alveolar gas replace the oxygen in the inspired gas. Therefore, very approximately:

$$\text{alveolar } Po_2 \approx \text{inspired } Po_2 - \text{arterial } Pco_2$$

This equation is not sufficiently accurate for use, except in the special case when 100% oxygen is breathed. In other situations, three corrections are required to overcome errors due to the following factors:

1. Usually, less carbon dioxide is produced than oxygen is consumed (effect of the respiratory exchange ratio, RQ).
2. The respiratory exchange ratio produces a secondary effect due to the fact that the expired volume does not equal the inspired volume.
3. The inspired and expired gas volumes may also differ because of inert gas exchange.

The simplest practicable form of the equation makes correction for the principal effect of the respiratory exchange ratio (1), but not the small supplementary error due to the difference between the inspired and expired gas volumes (2):

$$\text{alveolar } Po_2 \approx \text{inspired } Po_2 - \text{arterial } Pco_2/RQ$$

This form is suitable for rapid bedside calculations of alveolar Po_2, when great accuracy is not required.

One stage more complicated is an equation that allows for differences in the volume of inspired and expired gas due to the respiratory exchange ratio, but still does not allow for differences due to the exchange of inert gases. This equation exists in various forms, all algebraically identical:

$$\text{alveolar } Po_2 = P_{I_{O_2}} - \frac{Pa_{CO_2}}{RQ}(1 - F_{I_{O_2}}(1 - RQ))$$

(derived from reference 52).

This equation is suitable for use whenever the subject has been breathing the inspired gas mixture long enough for the inert gas to be in equilibrium. It is unsuitable when the inspired oxygen concentration has recently been changed, when the ambient pressure has recently been changed (e.g. during hyperbaric oxygen therapy) or when the inert gas concentration has recently been changed (e.g. soon after the start or finish of a period of inhaling nitrous oxide).

Perhaps the most satisfactory form of the alveolar air equation is the one that was advanced by Filley, MacIntosh and Wright in 1954.[53] This equation makes no assumption that inert gases are in equilibrium and allows for the difference between inspired and expired gas from whatever cause. It also proves to be very simple in use and does not require the calculation of the respiratory exchange ratio:

$$\text{alveolar } P_{O_2} = P_{I_{O_2}} - P_{a_{CO_2}} \left(\frac{P_{I_{O_2}} - P_{\bar{E}_{O_2}}}{P_{\bar{E}_{CO_2}}} \right)$$

If the alveolar P_{O_2} is calculated separately according to the last two equations, the difference (if any) will be that due to inert gas exchange.

When using these equations in practice, it is important to take water vapour into account, as alveolar gas will be saturated with water at body temperature, such that:

$$P_{I_{O_2}} = F_{I_{O_2}} \times (P_B - P_{H_2O})$$

Where $F_{I_{O_2}}$ is the fractional inspired oxygen concentration, P_B is barometric pressure, and P_{H_2O} is saturated vapour pressure of water at 37°C (6.3 kPa, 47 mmHg).

Distinction between shunt and the effect of $\dot{V}/\dot{Q}$ scatter

Shunt and scatter of $\dot{V}/\dot{Q}$ ratios will each produce an alveolar/arterial P_{O_2} difference from which a value for venous admixture may be calculated. It is usually impossible to say to what extent the calculated venous admixture is due to a true shunt or to perfusion of alveoli with low $\dot{V}/\dot{Q}$ ratio. Three methods are available for distinction between the two conditions.

If the inspired oxygen concentration is altered, the effect on the arterial P_{O_2} will depend on the nature of the disorder. If oxygenation is impaired by a shunt, the arterial P_{O_2} will increase as shown in the iso-shunt diagram (Figure 8.12). If, however, the disorder is due to scatter of $\dot{V}/\dot{Q}$ ratios, the arterial P_{O_2} will approach the normal value for the inspired oxygen concentration as the inspired oxygen concentration is increased (Figure 8.15). $\dot{V}/\dot{Q}$ scatter has virtually no effect when the subject breathes 100% oxygen. This difference between shunt and $\dot{V}/\dot{Q}$ scatter forms the basis of a recently described non-invasive method for investigating the mechanism of impaired gas exchange,[54] which is similar to the method already described for assessing venous admixture (page 192). In ventilated patients Sp_{O_2} is measured at several different inspired oxygen concentrations and an Sp_{O_2} versus $P_{I_{O_2}}$ curve drawn. Mathematical modelling, again using an assumed value for arterial/venous oxygen difference, and studies during one-lung anaesthesia have shown that shunt depresses the curve downwards whilst increasing $\dot{V}/\dot{Q}$ mismatch moves the curve to the right (Figure 8.16).[54]

Measurement of the alveolar/arterial P_{N_2} difference is a specific method for quantification of $\dot{V}/\dot{Q}$ scatter, because the P_{N_2} difference is entirely uninfluenced by true shunt.[55] Subjects must be in a state of complete nitrogen equilibrium, which may be difficult to achieve in the clinical environment. The method has not come into general use owing to difficulties in measuring P_{N_2} with adequate precision.

The multiple inert gas elimination technique for analysis of distribution of blood flow in relation to $\dot{V}/\dot{Q}$ ratio is the best method of distinction between shunt and areas of low $\dot{V}/\dot{Q}$ ratio (see above).

Measurement of dead space

Anatomical dead space is most conveniently measured by the technique illustrated in Figure 8.17, originally developed for use with a nitrogen analyser by Fowler in 1948.[25] The CO_2 concentration at the lips is measured continuously with a rapid gas analyser, and

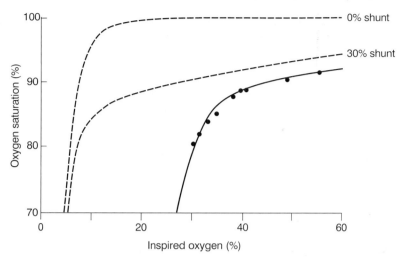

Figure 8.16 Non-invasive evaluation of impaired gas exchange during one-lung anaesthesia and thoracotomy. Oxygen saturation has been measured at nine different inspired oxygen concentrations (circles) and a curve fitted to the points (solid line). Mathematical modelling (broken lines) shows that shunt displaces the curve downwards (0% and 30% shunt shown) whilst $\dot{V}/\dot{Q}$ mismatch displaces the curve to the right. A computer algorithm, using an assumed value for arterial/venous oxygen difference, can compute the virtual shunt and the shift due to $\dot{V}/\dot{Q}$ mismatch from the actual curve obtained from the patient, in this case 30% shunt *and* marked $\dot{V}/\dot{Q}$ mismatch in the patient during one-lung ventilation (page 451). (After reference 54 by permission of the authors and the Editor of *Anaesthesia*)

then displayed against the volume actually expired. The 'alveolar plateau' of CO_2 concentration is not flat but slopes gently. Anatomical dead space is easily derived by the graphical solution shown in the Figure.

Physiological dead space. Mixed expired air is collected over a period of two or three minutes, during which time an arterial blood sample is collected, and the P_{CO_2} of blood and gas are then determined. Provided that the inspired gas is free from carbon dioxide, physiological dead space is indicated by the following form of the Bohr equation:

Physiological dead space

$$= \text{tidal volume} \left(\frac{\text{arterial } P_{CO_2} - \text{mixed expired gas } P_{CO_2}}{\text{arterial } P_{CO_2}} \right) - \text{apparatus dead space}$$

Apparatus dead space includes such items as the facemask and unidirectional valve box, and is usually measured by water displacement. The result is often most conveniently expressed as the ratio of the physiological dead space to the tidal volume.

Alveolar dead space is measured as the difference between the physiological and anatomical dead space, determined separately but at the same time. When only the physiological dead space is measured, it is often possible to attribute a large increase in physiological dead space to an increase in the alveolar component, because there are few circumstances in which the anatomical dead space is greatly enlarged.

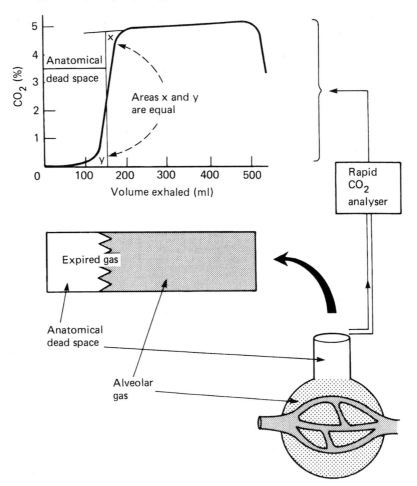

Figure 8.17 Measurement of anatomical dead space using CO_2 as the tracer gas. If the gas passing the patient's lips is continuously analysed for CO_2 concentration, there is a sudden rise to the alveolar plateau level, after the expiration of gas from the anatomical dead space. If the instantaneous CO_2 concentration is plotted against the volume exhaled (allowing for delay in the CO_2 analyser), a graph similar to that shown is obtained. A vertical line is constructed so that the two areas x and y are equal. This line will indicate the volume of the anatomical dead space. Note that the abscissa records *volume* rather than *time* as seen with capnography performed in clinical situations.

The arterial/end-expiratory P_{CO_2} *difference* is a convenient and relatively simple method of assessing the magnitude of the alveolar dead space. In Figure 8.10, end-expiratory gas is shown to consist of a mixture of 'ideal' alveolar gas and alveolar dead space gas. If the patient has an appreciable alveolar dead space, the end-expiratory P_{CO_2} will be less than the arterial P_{CO_2}, which is assumed equal to the 'ideal' alveolar P_{CO_2}.

If, for example, 'ideal' alveolar gas has a P_{CO_2} of 5.3 kPa (40 mmHg) and the end-expiratory P_{CO_2} is found to be 2.65 kPa (20 mmHg), it follows that the end-expiratory gas consists of equal parts of 'ideal' alveolar gas and alveolar dead space gas. Thus if the tidal volume is 500 ml and the anatomical dead space 100 ml, the components of the tidal volume would be as follows:

anatomical dead space   100 ml
alveolar dead space   200 ml
'ideal' alveolar gas   200 ml

The physiological dead space would be $100 + 200 = 300$ ml and the V_D/V_T ratio 60 per cent.

References

1. Svanberg L. Influence of posture on lung volumes, ventilation and circulation in normals. *Scand J Clin Lab Invest* 1957; **9**: Supp 25.
2. Rehder K, Sessler AD. Function of each lung in spontaneously breathing man anesthetized with thiopental-meperidine. *Anesthesiology* 1973; **38**: 320–7.
3. Rehder K, Hatch DJ, Sessler AD, Fowler WS. The function of each lung of anesthetized and paralyzed man during mechanical ventilation. *Anesthesiology* 1972; **37**: 16–26.
4. Nunn JF. The distribution of inspired gas during thoracic surgery. *Ann R Coll Surg Eng* 1961; **28**: 223–37.
5. West JB. Regional differences in gas exchange in the lung of erect man. *J Appl Physiol* 1962; **17**: 893–8.
6. Hughes JMB, Grant BJB, Greene RE, Iliff LD, Milic-Emili J. Inspiratory flow rate and ventilation distribution in normal subjects and in patients with simple chronic bronchitis. *Clin Sci* 1972; **43**: 583–95.
7. Hulands GH, Green R, Iliff LD, Nunn JF. Influence of anaesthesia on the regional distribution of perfusion and ventilation in the lung. *Clin Sci* 1970; **38**: 451–60.
8. Brudin LH, Rhodes CG, Valind SO, Jones T, Jonson B, Hughes JB. Relationship between regional ventilation and vascular and extravascular volume in supine humans. *J Appl Physiol* 1994; **76**: 1195–204.
9. Michels DB, West JB. Distribution of pulmonary ventilation and perfusion during short periods of weightlessness. *J Appl Physiol* 1978; **45**: 987–98.
10. Defares JG, Lundin G, Arborelius M, Stromblad R, Svanberg L. Effect of 'unilateral hypoxia' on pulmonary blood flow distribution in normal subjects. *J Appl Physiol* 1960; **15**: 169–74.
11. Kaneko K, Milic-Emili ME, Dolovich MB, Dawson A, Bates DV. Regional distribution of ventilation and perfusion as a function of body position. *J Appl Physiol* 1966; **21**: 767–77.
12. West JB. Distribution of gas and blood in the normal lung. *Br Med Bull* 1963; **19**: 53–8.
13. Hughes JMB, Glazier JB, Maloney JE, West JB. Effect of lung volume on the distribution of pulmonary blood flow in man. *Respir Physiol* 1968; **4**: 58–72.
14. Wagner PD, Laravuso RB, Goldzimmer E, Nauman PF, West JB. Distribution of ventilation–perfusion ratios in dogs in normal and abnormal lungs. *J Appl Physiol* 1975; **38**: 1099–109.
15. Brudin LH, Rhodes CG, Valind SO, Jones T, Hughes JB. Interrelationship between regional blood flow, blood volume, and ventilation in supine humans. *J Appl Physiol* 1994; **76**: 1205–10.
16. Hlastala MP. Ventilation/perfusion: from the bench to the patient. *Cardiologia* 1996; **41**: 405–15.
17. West JB. *Ventilation: blood flow and gas exchange*. Oxford: Blackwell Scientific, 1990.
18. Roca J, Wagner PD. Principles and information content of the multiple inert gas elimination technique. *Thorax* 1993; **49**: 815–24.
19. Wagner PD, Laravuso RB, Uhl RR, West JB. Continuous distributions of ventilation–perfusion ratios in normal subjects breathing air and 100% O_2. *J Clin Invest* 1974; **54**: 54–68.
20. Fenn WO, Rahn H, Otis AB. A theoretical analysis of the composition of alveolar air at altitude. *Am J Physiol* 1946; **146**: 637–53.
21. Riley RL, Cournard A. 'Ideal' alveolar air and the analysis of ventilation perfusion relationships in the lung. *J Appl Physiol* 1949; **1**: 825–49.

22. Bohr C. Über die Lungenathmung. *Skand Arch Physiol* 1891; **2**: 236.

23. Haldane JS, Priestley JG. The regulation of the lung ventilation. *J Physiol* 1905; **32**: 225–66.

24. Zuntz N. Physiologie der Blutgase und des respiratorischen Gaswechels. *Hermann's Handbuch Physiol* 1882; **4**: 1.

25. Fowler WS. Lung function studies. II. The respiratory dead space. *Am J Physiol* 1948; **154**: 405–16.

26. Numa AH, Newth CJL. Anatomic dead space in infants and children. *J Appl Physiol* 1996; **80**: 1485–9.

27. Fowler WS. Lung function studies. IV. Postural changes in respiratory dead space and functional residual capacity. *J Clin Invest* 1950; **29**: 1437–8.

28. Nunn JF, Campbell EJM, Peckett BW. Anatomical subdivisions of the volume of respiratory dead space and effect of position of the jaw. *J Appl Physiol* 1959; **14**: 174–6.

29. Lifshay A, Fast CW, Glazier JB. Effects of changes in respiratory pattern on physiological dead space. *J Appl Physiol* 1971; **31**: 478–83.

30. Nunn JF, Hill DW. Respiratory dead space and arterial to end-tidal CO_2 tension difference in anesthetized man. *J Appl Physiol* 1960; **15**: 383–9.

31. Nunn JF. Ventilation and end-tidal carbon dioxide tension. *Anaesthesia* 1958; **13**: 124–37.

32. Briscoe WA, Forster RE, Comroe JH. Alveolar ventilation at very low tidal volumes. *J Appl Physiol* 1954; **7**: 27–30.

33. Severinghaus JW, Stupfel M. Respiratory dead space increases following atropine in man, and atropine, vagal or ganglionic blockade and hypothermia in dogs. *J Appl Physiol* 1955; **8**: 81–7.

34. Nunn JF, Bergman NA. The effect of atropine on pulmonary gas exchange. *Br J Anaesth* 1964; **36**: 68–72.

35. Enghoff H. Zur frage des schädlichen raumes bei der atmung. *Skand Arch Physiol* 1931; **63**: 15.

36. Harris EA, Hunter ME, Seelye ER, Vedder M, Whitlock RML. Prediction of the physiological dead-space in resting normal subjects. *Clin Sci* 1973; **45**: 375–86.

37. Radford EP. Ventilation standards for use in artificial respiration. *J Appl Physiol* 1955; **7**: 451–63.

38. Craig DB, Wahba WM, Don HF, Couture JG, Becklake MR. 'Closing volume' and its relationship to gas exchange in seated and supine positions. *J Appl Physiol* 1971; **31**: 717–21.

39. Ravin MG, Epstein RM, Malm JR. Contribution of thebesian veins to the physiologic shunt in anesthetized man. *J Appl Physiol* 1965; **20**: 1148–52.

40. Dantzker DR, Lynch JP, Weg JG. Depression of cardiac output is a mechanism of shunt reduction in the therapy of acute respiratory failure. *Chest* 1980; **77**: 636–47.

41. Lynch JP, Mhyre JG, Dantzker DR. Influence of cardiac output on intrapulmonary shunt. *J Appl Physiol* 1979; **46**: 315–21.

42. Cheney FW, Colley PS. The effect of cardiac output on arterial blood oxygenation. *Anesthesiology* 1980; **52**: 496–503.

43. Marshall BE, Marshall C. Anesthesia and the pulmonary circulation. In: Covino BG, Fozzard HA, Rehder K, Strichartz G, eds. *Effects of anesthesia*. Bethesda MD: American Physiological Society, 1985.

44. Benator SR, Hewlett AM, Nunn JF. The use of iso-shunt lines for control of oxygen therapy. *Br J Anaesth* 1973; **45**: 711–18.

45. Lawler PGP, Nunn JF. A reassessment of the validity of the iso-shunt graph. *Br J Anaesth* 1984; **56**: 1325–35.

46. Petros AJ, Doré CJ, Nunn JF. Modification of the iso-shunt lines for low inspired oxygen concentrations. *Br J Anaesth* 1994; **72**: 515–22.

47. Drummond GB, Wright DJ. Oxygen therapy after abdominal surgery. *Br J Anaesth* 1977; **49**: 789–97.

48. Hugh-Jones P, West JB. Detection of bronchial and arterial obstruction by continuous gas analysis from individual lobes and segments of the lung. *Thorax* 1960; **15**: 154–64.

49. Wagner PD, Saltzman HA, West JB. Measurement of continuous distribution of ventilation–perfusion ratios: theory. *J Appl Physiol* 1974; **36**: 588–99.

50. Severinghaus JW, Stafford M, Thunstron AM. Estimation of skin metabolism and blood flow with $tcPO_2$ and $tcPCO_2$ electrodes by cuff occlusion of the circulation. *Acta Anaesthesiol Scand Suppl* 1978; **68**: 9–15.

51. Hope DA, Jenkins BJ, Willis N, Maddock H, Mapleson WW. Non-invasive estimation of venous admixture: validation of a new formula. *Br J Anaesth* 1995; **74**: 538–43.

52. Riley RL, Lilienthal JL, Proemmel DD, Franke RE. On the determination of the physiologically effective pressures of oxygen and carbon dioxide in alveolar air. *Am J Physiol* 1946; **147**: 191–8.
53. Filley GF, MacIntosh DJ, Wright GW. Carbon monoxide uptake and pulmonary diffusing capacity in normal subject at rest and during exercise. *J Clin Invest* 1954; **33**: 530–9.
54. de Gray L, Rush EM, Jones JG. A noninvasive method for evaluating the effect of thoracotomy on shunt and ventilation perfusion inequality. *Anaesthesia* 1997; **52**: 630–5.
55. Rahn H, Farhi LE. Ventilation, perfusion, and gas exchange – V$_A$/Q concept. *Handbook of Physiology, Section 3* 1964; **1**: 735.

Chapter 9

Diffusion of respiratory gases

The previous chapters have described in detail how alveolar gases and pulmonary capillary blood are delivered to their respective sides of the alveolar wall. This chapter deals with the final step of lung function by discussing the transfer of respiratory gases between the alveolus and blood.

Nomenclature in this field is confusing. In Europe, measurements of the passage of gases between the alveoli and pulmonary capillaries is referred to as lung 'transfer factor' (e.g. $T_{L_{CO}}$ represents lung transfer factor for carbon monoxide). However, the older term 'diffusing capacity' (e.g. $D_{L_{CO}}$ for lung diffusing capacity for carbon monoxide) remains in more common usage, particularly in the USA,[1] in spite of the finding that some of the barrier to oxygen transfer is unrelated to diffusion (see below).

Fundamentals of the diffusion process

Diffusion of a gas is a process by which a net transfer of molecules takes place from a zone in which the gas exerts a high partial pressure to a zone in which it exerts a lower partial pressure. The mechanism of transfer is the random movement of molecules and the term excludes both active biological transport and transfer by mass movement of gas in response to a *total* pressure difference (i.e. gas flow as occurs during tidal ventilation). The partial pressure (or tension) of a gas in a gas mixture is the pressure which it would exert if it occupied the space alone (equal to total pressure multiplied by fractional concentration). Gas molecules pass in each direction but at a rate proportional to the partial pressure of the gas in the zone which they are leaving. The net transfer of the gas is the difference in the number of molecules passing in each direction, and is thus proportional to the difference in partial pressure between the two zones. Typical examples of diffusion are shown in Figure 9.1.

In each of the examples shown in Figure 9.1 there is a finite resistance to the transfer of the gas molecules. In Figure 9.1a the resistance is concentrated at the restriction in the neck of the bottle. Clearly, the narrower the neck, the slower will be the process of equilibration with the outside air. In Figure 9.1b the site of the resistance to diffusion is less circumscribed but includes gas diffusion in the alveolus, the alveolar/capillary membrane, the diffusion path through the plasma, and the delay in combination of oxygen with the reduced haemoglobin in the red blood cell (RBC). In Figure 9.1c the resistance commences with the delay in the release of oxygen by haemoglobin, and includes all the

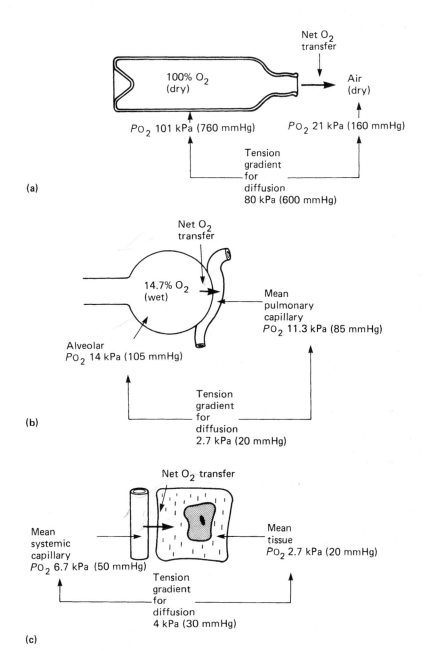

Figure 9.1 Three examples of diffusion of oxygen. In each case there is a net transfer of oxygen from left to right in accord with the tension gradient. (a) Oxygen passes from one gaseous phase to another. (b) Oxygen passes from a gaseous phase to a liquid phase. (c) Oxygen passes from one liquid to another.

interfaces between the RBC membrane and the site of oxygen consumption in the mitochondria. There may then be an additional component in the rate at which oxygen enters into chemical combination.

In the living body oxygen is constantly being consumed, while carbon dioxide is being produced, so equilibrium cannot be attained as in the case of the open bottle of oxygen in Figure 9.1a. Instead, a dynamic equilibrium is attained with diffusion down a gradient between the alveolus and the mitochondria for oxygen and the reverse for carbon dioxide. The maintenance of these tension gradients is, in fact, a characteristic of life.

In the case of gases that are not metabolized to any great extent, such as nitrogen and most inhalational anaesthetic agents, there is always a tendency towards a static equilibrium at which all tissue partial pressures become equal to the partial pressure of the particular gas in the inspired air. This occurs with nitrogen (apart from the small effect of the respiratory exchange ratio), and would also be attained with an inhalational anaesthetic agent if it were administered for a very long time.

Quantification of resistance to diffusion

The propensity of a gas to diffuse as a result of a given pressure gradient is known as its diffusing capacity according to the equation:

$$\text{diffusing capacity} = \frac{\text{net rate of gas transfer}}{\text{partial pressure gradient}}$$

The usual biological unit of diffusing capacity is $ml.min^{-1}.mmHg^{-1}$ or, in SI units, $ml.min^{-1}.kPa^{-1}$.

Small molecules diffuse more easily than large molecules. Graham's law states that the rate of diffusion of a gas is inversely proportional to the square root of its density. In addition, gases also diffuse more readily at higher temperatures.

Apart from these factors, inherent in the gas, the resistance to diffusion is related directly to the length of the diffusion path and inversely to the area of interface that is available for diffusion.

Diffusion of gases in solution

The partial pressure of a gas in solution in a liquid is defined as being equal to the partial pressure of the same gas in a gas mixture that is in equilibrium with the liquid. When a gas is diffusing into or through an aqueous phase, the solubility of the gas in water becomes an important factor, and the diffusing capacity in these circumstances is considered to be directly proportional to the solubility. Nitrous oxide would thus be expected to have about 20 times the diffusing capacity of oxygen in crossing a gas/water interface. High solubility does not confer an increased 'agility' of the gas in its negotiation of an aqueous barrier, but simply means that, for a given partial pressure, more molecules of the gas are present in the liquid.

Tension versus concentration gradients. Non-gaseous substances in solution diffuse in response to concentration gradients. This is also true for gas mixtures at the same total pressure, when the partial pressure of any component gas is directly proportional to its concentration. This is not the case when a gas in solution in one liquid diffuses into a different liquid in which it has a different solubility coefficient. When gases are in solution, the partial pressure they exert is directly proportional to their concentration in the solvent but inversely to the solubility of the gas in the solvent. Thus, if water and oil have the same concentration of nitrous oxide dissolved in each, the partial pressure of nitrous oxide in the oil will be only one-third of the partial pressure in the water because the oil/water solubility ratio is about 3:1. If the two liquids are shaken up together, there will be a net transfer of nitrous oxide from the water to the oil until the tension in each phase is the same. At that time the concentration of nitrous oxide in the oil will be about three times the concentration in the water. There is thus a net transfer of nitrous oxide against the concentration gradient, but always with the partial pressure gradient. Thus, it is useful to consider partial pressure rather than concentrations in relation to movement of gases and vapours from one compartment of the body to another. The same units of pressure may be used in gas, aqueous and lipid phases.

Diffusion of oxygen in the lungs

It is now widely accepted that oxygen passes from the alveoli into the pulmonary capillary blood by a passive process of diffusion according to physical laws. For a long time this view was contested by a school of thought that believed that oxygen was actively secreted into the blood.[2] A similar process was known to occur in the swim-bladders of certain fish, so the postulated mechanism was certainly feasible, but proof of secretion depended on the demonstration of an arterial Po_2 that was higher than the alveolar Po_2. In the early 1900s, a great controversy raged, with active secretion being upheld by Bohr and Haldane while the Kroghs and Barcroft took the opposite view.[2]

There is now strong evidence for believing that diffusion equilibrium is very nearly achieved for oxygen during the normal pulmonary capillary transit time in the resting subject. Therefore, in these circumstances, the uptake of oxygen is limited by pulmonary blood flow and not by diffusing capacity. However, under conditions of exercise, while breathing gas mixtures deficient in oxygen or at reduced barometric pressure, the diffusing capacity becomes important and may limit the oxygen uptake.

Components of the alveolar/capillary diffusion pathway

The gas space in the alveolus. At FRC, the diameter of the average human alveolus is of the order of 200 µm (page 27), and it is likely that mixing of normal alveolar gas is almost instantaneous over the very small distance from the centre to the periphery. Precise calculations are impossible on account of the complex geometry of the alveolus, but the overall efficiency of gas exchange in the lungs suggests that mixing must be complete within less than 10 ms. Therefore, in practice it is usual to consider alveolar gas of normal composition as uniformly mixed.

This generalization does not seem to hold when subjects inhale gases of widely different molecular weights. This was first demonstrated in 1965 in normal subjects inhaling mixtures of sulphur hexafluoride (SF_6) and helium when the SF_6 concentration was found to be higher (relative to helium) earlier in the breath.[3] According to Graham's law, SF_6 (molecular weight 146) would diffuse six times less readily than helium (molecular weight 4) and would therefore tend to remain concentrated at the core of the alveolus. More recently, Landon et al. found that a large proportion of the end-expiratory/arterial partial pressure gradient for the anaesthetic isoflurane (molecular weight 184.5) could not be explained by alveolar dead space or shunt and seemed to be due to failure to achieve uniformity within the alveolus.[4] Nevertheless, it seems unlikely that non-uniformity within a single alveolus is an important factor limiting diffusing capacity under normal conditions with gases such as oxygen, nitrogen and carbon dioxide, which have molecular weights that are not greatly different.

Alveolar lining fluid.[5] Alveoli contain a thin layer of surfactant-rich fluid through which respiratory gases must diffuse. The depth of this fluid layer, and therefore its impediment to diffusion, is very variable. There are believed to be 'pools' of fluid in alveolar corners and in the depressions between where the capillaries bulge into the alveolus, with only a very thin layer on the surface of the capillary bulges, thus providing the minimal diffusion barrier in the most vital area.[6]

Tissue barrier.[5] Electron microscopy has revealed details of the actual path between alveolar gas and pulmonary capillary blood, shown in Figure 2.8. Each alveolus is lined with epithelium which, with its basement membrane, is about 0.2 μm thick except where its nuclei bulge into the alveolar lumen. Beyond the basement membrane is the interstitial space, which is very thin where it overlies the capillaries, particularly on the active side; elsewhere it is thicker and contains collagen and elastic fibres. The pulmonary capillaries are lined with endothelium, also with its own basement membrane, which is approximately the same thickness as the alveolar epithelium except where it is expanded to enclose the endothelial nuclei. The total thickness of the active part of the tissue barrier is thus about 0.5 μm, containing two pairs of lipid bilayers separated by the interstitial space. This arrangement is shown in Figure 2.8.

Plasma layer. Human pulmonary capillaries are estimated to have a mean diameter of 7 μm,[7] similar to the diameter of a red blood cell (RBC), part of which is therefore forced into contact with the endothelial cell surface (Figure 2.8). The diffusion path through plasma may therefore be very short indeed, but only a small proportion of the RBC surface will be in such close proximity with the endothelium, much of the RBC passing through the middle of the capillary, up to 3.5 μm from the endothelial cell. Furthermore, because the diameter of the capillary is about 14 times the thickness of the tissue barrier, it is clear that the diffusion path within the capillary is likely to be much longer than the path through the alveolar/capillary membrane. A complex pattern of diffusion gradients is therefore established in the plasma, depending on the oxygen tension in the alveolus and the number of RBCs present (haematocrit or packed cell volume).[8] This is discussed in more detail below with respect to carbon monoxide.

Diffusion into and within the RBC.[9] Confining haemoglobin within the RBC reduces the oxygen-diffusing capacity by 40 per cent in comparison with free haemoglobin solution.[10] There are three possible explanations for this observation. First, there is now good evidence that the rapid uptake of oxygen and carbon monoxide by RBCs causes depletion of gas in the plasma layer immediately surrounding the RBC.[11] Often referred to as the 'unstirred layer', this phenomenon is most likely to occur at low haematocrit (packed cell volume, PCV) when adjacent RBCs in the pulmonary capillary have more plasma between them.[12] Secondly, oxygen must diffuse across the RBC membrane, though this is not likely to be a significant diffusion barrier. Thirdly, once in the cell, oxygen must diffuse through a varying amount of intracellular fluid before combining with haemoglobin, a process that is aided by mass movement of the haemoglobin molecules caused by the deformation of the erythrocyte as it passes through the capillary bed, in effect 'mixing' the oxygen with the haemoglobin.

RBCs change shape as they pass through capillaries (both pulmonary and systemic), and this seems to play an important role in the uptake and unloading of oxygen.[9] This has led to further work in which the deformability of RBCs is reduced (using chlorpromazine) or increased (using sodium salicylate), which results in increasing diffusing capacity for oxygen with greater deformability.[12] The dependence of diffusing capacity on RBC deformability and shape changes may result from reducing the unstirred layer by 'mixing' the plasma around the RBC, from changes in the cell membrane surface area to RBC volume ratio or from assisting the mass movement of haemoglobin within the cell.

Uptake of oxygen by haemoglobin. The greater part of the oxygen that is taken up in the lungs enters into chemical combination with haemoglobin. This chemical reaction takes a finite time and forms an appreciable part of the total resistance to the transfer of oxygen.[13] This important discovery resulted in an extensive reappraisal of the whole concept of diffusing capacity. In particular, it became clear that measurements of 'diffusing capacity' did not necessarily give an indication of the degree of permeability of the alveolar/capillary membrane.

Quantification of the diffusing capacity for oxygen[14]

The diffusing capacity of oxygen is simply the oxygen uptake (easily measured) divided by the tension gradient from alveolar gas to pulmonary capillary blood where the relevant tension is the mean pulmonary capillary Po_2:

$$\text{oxygen diffusing capacity} = \frac{\text{oxygen uptake}}{\text{alveolar } Po_2 - \text{mean pulmonary capillary } Po_2}$$

The alveolar Po_2 can be derived with some degree of accuracy (page 193) but there are very serious problems in estimating the mean capillary Po_2.

The mean pulmonary capillary Po_2. It is clearly impossible to make a direct measurement of the mean Po_2 of the pulmonary capillary blood, so attempts have been made to derive this quantity indirectly from the presumed changes of Po_2 that occur as blood passes through the pulmonary capillaries.

The earliest analysis of the problem was made by Bohr in 1909.[15] He made the assumption that, at any point along the pulmonary capillary, the rate of diffusion of oxygen was proportional to the Po_2 difference between the alveolar gas and the pulmonary capillary blood at that point. Using this approach, and *assuming a value for the alveolar/pulmonary end-capillary Po_2* gradient, it seemed possible to construct a graph of capillary Po_2, plotted against the time the blood had been in the pulmonary capillary. A typical curve drawn on this basis is shown as the broken line in Figure 9.2a. Once the curve has been drawn, it is relatively easy to derive the mean pulmonary capillary Po_2, which then permits calculation of the oxygen-diffusing capacity. The validity of the assumption of the alveolar/pulmonary end-capillary Po_2 gradient is considered below.

Unfortunately this approach, known as the Bohr integration procedure, was shown to be invalid when it was found that the fundamental assumption was untrue. The rate of transfer of oxygen is not proportional to the alveolar/capillary Po_2 gradient at any point along the capillary. It would no doubt be true if the transfer of oxygen were a purely physical process but the rate of transfer is actually limited by the chemical combination of oxygen with haemoglobin, which is sufficiently slow to comprise a major part of the total resistance to transfer of oxygen.

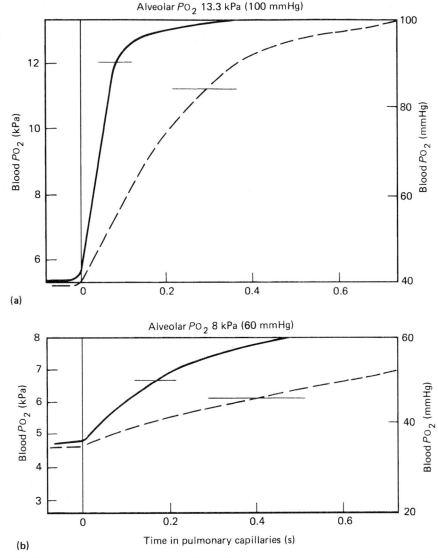

Figure 9.2 Each graph shows the rise in blood Po_2 as blood passes along the pulmonary capillaries. The horizontal line at the top of the graph indicates the alveolar Po_2 that the blood Po_2 is approaching. In (a) the subject is breathing air, while in (b) the subject is breathing about 14% oxygen. The broken curve shows the rise in Po_2 calculated according to the Bohr procedure on an assumed value for the alveolar/end-capillary Po_2 gradient. The continuous curve shows the values obtained by forward integration.[16] Horizontal bars indicate mean pulmonary capillary Po_2 calculated from each curve.

Studies *in vitro* of the rate of combination of oxygen with haemoglobin have shown that this is not directly proportional to the Po_2 gradient, for two distinct reasons:

1. The combination of the fourth molecule of oxygen with the haemoglobin molecule $(Hb_4(O_2)_3 + O_2 \rightleftharpoons Hb_4(O_2)_4)$ has a much higher velocity constant than that of the combination of the other three molecules. This is discussed further on page 264.

2. As the capillary oxygen saturation rises, the number of molecules of reduced haemoglobin diminishes and the velocity of the forward reaction must therefore diminish by the law of mass action. This depends on the haemoglobin dissociation curve and is therefore not a simple exponential function of the actual Po_2 of the blood.

When these two factors are combined it is found that the resistance to 'diffusion' due to chemical combination of oxygen within the RBC is fairly constant up to a saturation of about 80% (Po_2 = 6 kPa or 45 mmHg). Thereafter, it falls very rapidly to become zero at full saturation.[17] In view of these findings the Bohr integration procedure was elaborated to allow for changes in the rate of combination of haemoglobin with oxygen.[17] Assuming traditional values for the alveolar/end-capillary Po_2 difference, the resulting curve lies well to the left of the original Bohr curve, as shown by the continuous curve in Figure 9.2a. This indicated a mean pulmonary capillary Po_2 greater than had previously been believed, and therefore an oxygen-diffusing capacity that was substantially greater than the accepted value. The situation is actually more complicated still, as quick-frozen sections of lung show that the colour of haemoglobin begins to alter to the red colour of oxyhaemoglobin in the pulmonary arterioles before the blood has even entered the pulmonary capillaries. Furthermore, pulmonary capillaries do not cross a single alveolus but may pass over three or more.

Both the classic and the modified Bohr integration procedures for calculation of mean capillary Po_2 depended critically on the precise value of the pulmonary end-capillary Po_2. The constructed curve (Figure 9.2a) and therefore the derived mean capillary Po_2 were considerably influenced by very small variations in the value that was assumed. The 'ideal' alveolar/arterial Po_2 difference could be measured, but the problem was to separate this into its two components – the 'ideal' alveolar/pulmonary end-capillary Po_2 difference (due to diffusion block) and the pulmonary end-capillary/arterial Po_2 difference (due to venous admixture). Figure 8.9 will make this clear. Ingenious attempts were made to resolve the alveolar/arterial Po_2 gradient into its two components[18] but these failed to produce results that were compatible with observed diffusing capacity, mainly because of the lack of appreciation of the part played by the reaction times of oxygen with haemoglobin.

Forward integration. A new and entirely opposite approach was made by Staub in a most important paper in 1963.[16] His approach was based on the new understanding of the kinetics of the combination of oxygen with haemoglobin (see above) and the pattern of blood flow through the pulmonary capillaries. Starting at the arterial end of the pulmonary capillaries, he calculated the Po_2 of the capillary blood progressively along the capillary until he was able to give an estimate of the remaining alveolar/capillary Po_2 gradient at the end of the capillary. This procedure of forward integration was thus the reverse of the classic approach which, starting from the alveolar/end-capillary Po_2 gradient, worked backwards to see what was happening along the capillary.

Staub's forward integrations gave important results (Table 9.1). They suggested that alveolar/end-capillary Po_2 gradients were very much smaller than had previously been thought, although earlier papers had anticipated much of Staub's conclusion.[19]

Capillary transit time[20]

Capillary transit time is a most important factor determining both the pulmonary end-capillary Po_2 and the diffusing capacity. It will be seen from Figure 9.2a that, if the capillary transit time is reduced below 0.25 second, there will be an appreciable gradient

Table 9.1 Values for the alveolar/end capillary Po_2 gradient suggested by the forward integration procedure[16]

Conditions	Capillary transit time (s)	Alveolar/end-capillary Po_2 gradient	
		kPa	mmHg
Resting subject ($\dot{V}o_2 = 270$ ml.min^{-1})			
Breathing air	0.760	0.000 000 001	0.000 000 01
($P_{Ao_2} = 13.3$ kPa = 100 mmHg)			
Breathing low oxygen	0.636	0.03	0.2
($P_{Ao_2} = 6.3$ kPa = 47 mmHg)			
Moderate exercise ($\dot{V}o_2 = 1500$ ml.min^{-1})			
Breathing low oxygen	0.476	0.5	4.0
($P_{Ao_2} = 7.3$ kPa = 55 mmHg)			
Heavy exercise ($\dot{V}o_2 = 3000$ ml.min^{-1})			
Breathing air	0.496	<0.000 1	<0.001
($P_{Ao_2} = 16$ kPa = 120 mmHg)			
Breathing low oxygen	0.304	2.1	16.0
($P_{Ao_2} = 7.9$ kPa = 59 mmHg)			

P_{Ao_2}, alveolar Po_2; $\dot{V}o_2$, oxygen consumption.

between the alveolar and end-capillary Po_2. Because the diffusion gradient from alveolar gas to mean pulmonary capillary blood will be increased, the oxygen diffusing capacity must be decreased.

The mean pulmonary capillary transit time equals the pulmonary capillary blood volume divided by the pulmonary blood flow (approximately equal to cardiac output). This gives a normal time of the order of 0.8 second with a subject at rest. However, because of difficulties measuring pulmonary capillary blood volume and many other methodological problems, there seems to be a wide range of values on either side of the mean, and times as short as 0.1 second[21] or as long as 3 seconds[20] have been suggested. It is therefore likely that, in a similar fashion to ventilation and perfusion, there is a wide range of normal capillary transit times affected by many factors such as posture, lung volume, cardiac output, etc. Blood from capillaries with the shortest time will yield desaturated blood and this will not be compensated by blood from capillaries with longer than average transit times, for the reason shown in Figure 8.14.

Diffusion of carbon dioxide in the lungs

Carbon dioxide has a much higher water solubility than oxygen and, although its vapour density is greater, it may be calculated to penetrate an aqueous membrane about 20 times as rapidly as oxygen (Table 9.2). Therefore it was formerly believed that diffusion problems could not exist for carbon dioxide because the patient would have succumbed from hypoxia before hypercapnia could attain measurable proportions. All of this ignored the fact that chemical reactions of the respiratory gases were sufficiently slow

Table 9.2 The influence of physical properties on the diffusion of gases through a gas/liquid interface

Gas	Density relative to oxygen	Water solubility relative to oxygen	Diffusing capacity relative to oxygen
Oxygen	1.00	1.00	1.00
Carbon dioxide	1.37	24.0	20.5
Carbon monoxide	0.88	0.75	0.80
Ether	2.3	580	380
Helium	0.125	0.37	1.05
Nitric oxide	0.94	1.70	1.71
Nitrogen	0.88	0.515	0.55
Nitrous oxide	1.37	16.3	14.0

to affect the measured 'diffusing capacity', and in fact were generally the limiting factor in gas transfer. The carriage of carbon dioxide in the blood is discussed in Chapter 10, but for the moment it is sufficient to note the essential reactions in the release of chemically combined carbon dioxide:

1. Release of some carbon dioxide from carbamino carriage.
2. Conversion of bicarbonate ions to carbonic acid followed by dehydration to release molecular carbon dioxide.

The latter reaction involves the movement of bicarbonate ions across the RBC membrane, but its rate is probably limited by the dehydration of carbonic acid. This reaction would be very slow indeed if it were not catalysed by carbonic anhydrase, which is present in abundance in the RBC and also on the endothelium. In 1961 the important limiting role of the rate of this reaction was elegantly shown in a study of the effect of inhibition of carbonic anhydrase on carbon dioxide transport. This resulted in a large increase in the arterial/alveolar P_{CO_2} gradient, corresponding to a gross decrease in the apparent 'diffusing capacity' of carbon dioxide.[22]

Equilibrium of carbon dioxide is probably very nearly complete within the normal pulmonary capillary transit time. However, even if it were not so, it would be of little significance because the mixed venous/alveolar P_{CO_2} difference is itself quite small (about 0.8 kPa or 6 mmHg). Therefore an end-capillary gradient as large as 20 per cent of the initial difference would still be too small to be of any importance and, indeed, could hardly be measured by modern analytical methods.

Hypercapnia is, in fact, never caused by decreased 'diffusing capacity' except when carbonic anhydrase is inhibited by drugs such as acetazolamide. Pathological hypercapnia may always be explained by other causes, usually an alveolar ventilation that is inadequate for the metabolic rate of the patient.

The assumption that there is no measurable difference between the P_{CO_2} of the alveolar gas and the pulmonary end-capillary blood is used when the alveolar P_{CO_2} is assumed equal to the arterial P_{CO_2} for the purpose of derivation of the 'ideal' alveolar P_{O_2} (page 193). The assumption is also made that there is no measurable difference between end-capillary and arterial P_{CO_2}. We have seen in the previous chapter (Table 8.2) that this is not strictly true and a large shunt of 50% will cause an arterial/end-capillary P_{CO_2} gradient of about 0.4 kPa.

Diffusion of carbon monoxide in the lungs

Diffusing capacity is usually measured for carbon monoxide, for the very practical reason that affinity of carbon monoxide for haemoglobin is so high that the tension of the gas in the pulmonary capillary blood remains effectively zero. The formula for calculation of this quantity then simplifies to the following:

$$\text{diffusing capacity for carbon monoxide} = \frac{\text{carbon monoxide uptake}}{\text{alveolar } P\text{co}}$$

(compare with corresponding equation for oxygen, page 205).

There are no insuperable difficulties in the measurement of either of the remaining quantities on the right-hand side of the equation, and the methods are outlined at the end of this chapter.

Measurement of the carbon monoxide-diffusing capacity is firmly established as a valuable routine pulmonary function test, which may show changes in a range of conditions in which other pulmonary function tests yield normal values. It does in fact provide an index that shows that something is wrong, and changes in the index provide a useful indication of progress of the disease. It is also used as an epidemiological tool for assessing lung function in seemingly healthy subjects.[23] However, it is much more difficult to explain a reduced diffusing capacity for carbon monoxide in terms of the underlying pathophysiology (see below).

The diffusion path for carbon monoxide

Diffusion of carbon monoxide in the alveolus, through the alveolar/capillary membrane and through the plasma into the RBC, is governed by the same factors that apply to oxygen, and have been outlined above. The quantitative difference is due to the different vapour density and water solubility of the two gases (Table 9.2). These factors indicate that the rate of diffusion of oxygen up to the point of entry into the erythrocyte is 1.25 times the corresponding rate for carbon monoxide.

Diffusion of CO in plasma. The frequent use of carbon monoxide for measurement of lung diffusing capacity has focused attention on the diffusion pathway for CO, which, in spite of the slight differences in the physical properties of CO and oxygen, are likely to be very similar *in vivo*. Clearly, direct measurement of diffusion gradients in a pulmonary capillary is not possible, so attempts to elucidate the diffusion pattern of gases in capillary plasma are based on mathematical models. The first model is known as the morphometric method in which anatomical sections of rapidly fixed lung tissue were examined microscopically. Capillary dimensions were analysed to calculate the mean distance for gases to diffuse between the endothelial cell and erythrocyte,[5,24] assuming a linear diffusion path between the two points – that is, respiratory gases take the shortest possible route between the endothelial cell and erythrocyte. A more recent analysis has assumed that there is a gradient of CO concentration in the capillary, with minimal CO in the centre, and using a 'finite element analysis' shown that diffusion paths for CO are likely to be non-linear.[8] Figure 9.3 is a theoretical drawing of the CO flux within the capillary at both high and low haematocrit (PCV), showing clearly that, except in severe anaemia, CO uptake is achieved long before diffusion to the centre of the capillary is able to take place. In spite of these detailed models, agreement with observed Dm_{CO} (page 212) remains poor under most situations.[8]

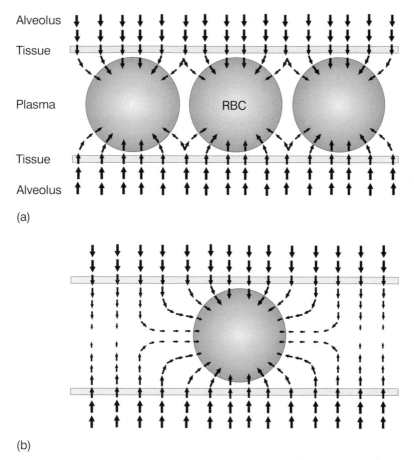

Alveolus

Tissue

Plasma   RBC

Tissue

Alveolus

(a)

(b)

Figure 9.3 Mathematical model of diffusion paths for CO between the alveolus and the erythrocyte (RBC). The size and direction of the arrows indicate the magnitude and direction of the CO flux respectively. The RBC is assumed to be an infinite 'sink' for CO. (a) Normal. Haematocrit 66% under which conditions CO is absorbed by the RBC mainly at the periphery of the capillary. (b) Severe anaemia. Haematocrit 12% when diffusion occurs into the centre of the plasma and follows a non-linear path into the RBC. The thickness of the tissue barrier relative to capillary diameter is drawn to scale, showing the relatively small contribution that the alveolar/capillary membrane makes to the diffusion barrier in total. (Redrawn from reference 8.)

Uptake of carbon monoxide by haemoglobin[25]

The affinity of haemoglobin for carbon monoxide is about 250 times as great as for oxygen. Nevertheless, it does not follow that the *rate* of combination of carbon monoxide with haemoglobin is faster than the *rate* of combination of oxygen with haemoglobin: it is, in fact, rather slower.[26] The reaction is slower still when oxygen must first be displaced from haemoglobin according to the equation:

$$CO + HbO_2 \rightarrow O_2 + HbCO$$

Therefore the reaction rate of carbon monoxide with haemoglobin is reduced when the oxygen saturation of the haemoglobin is high. The inhalation of different concentrations of oxygen thus causes changes in the reaction rate of carbon monoxide with the haemoglobin of a patient, an observation that has been used to study different components of the resistance to diffusion of carbon monoxide in humans.[14]

Quantification of the components of the resistance to diffusion of carbon monoxide

When two resistances are arranged in series, the total resistance of the pair is equal to the sum of the two individual resistances. Diffusing capacity is analogous to conductance, which is the reciprocal of resistance. Therefore, the reciprocal of the diffusing capacity of the total system equals the sum of the reciprocals of the diffusing capacities of the two components.

$$\frac{1}{\text{total diffusing capacity for CO}} = \frac{1}{\begin{array}{c}\text{diffusing capacity of CO}\\\text{for the alveolar-}\\\text{capillary membrane}\end{array}} + \frac{1}{\begin{array}{c}\text{diffusing capacity of CO}\\\text{in the blood}\end{array}}$$

In theory, diffusing capacity of carbon monoxide in the blood includes diffusion across the plasma, red cell membrane, diffusion within the red cell, and the chemical combination of carbon monoxide with haemoglobin. However, *in vivo*, as in the case of oxygen, the reaction rate of carbon monoxide with haemoglobin is a significant factor.[25] This 'diffusing capacity' for blood is equal to the product of the pulmonary capillary blood volume (*Vc*) and the rate of reaction of carbon monoxide with haemoglobin (θ_{CO}), a parameter that varies with the oxygen saturation of the haemoglobin. The equation may now be rewritten:

$$\frac{1}{\text{total diffusing capacity for CO}} = \frac{1}{\begin{array}{c}\text{diffusing capacity of CO}\\\text{for the alveolar-capillary}\\\text{membrane}\end{array}} + \frac{1}{\begin{array}{c}\text{pulmonary capillary blood volume}\\\times \text{ reaction rate of CO with blood}\end{array}}$$

The usual symbols for representation of this equation are:

$$\frac{1}{D_{L_{CO}}} = \frac{1}{Dm_{CO}} = \frac{1}{Vc \times \theta_{CO}}$$

The term *Dm* is often described simply as membrane diffusing capacity. Dm_{CO} equals $0.8\,Dm_{O_2}$ under similar conditions (see Table 9.2).

The total diffusing capacity for carbon monoxide is a routine clinical measurement (see the methods section at the end of this chapter): θ_{CO} may be determined, at different values of oxygen saturation, by studies *in vitro*.[25] This leaves two unknowns – the diffusing capacity through the alveolar/capillary membrane and the pulmonary capillary blood volume. By repeating the measurement of total diffusing capacity at different arterial oxygen saturations (obtained by inhaling different concentrations of oxygen) it is possible to obtain two simultaneous equations with two unknowns that may then be solved to obtain values for Dm_{CO} and pulmonary capillary blood volume.

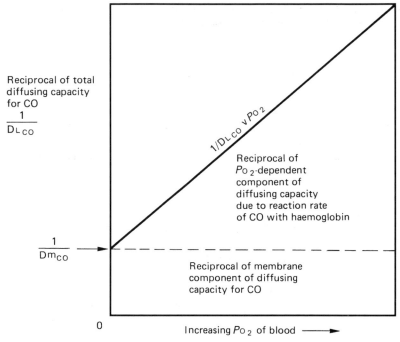

Figure 9.4 The reciprocal of the total diffusing capacity for carbon monoxide (i.e. resistance to diffusion) decreases with decreasing Po_2 of the blood in the pulmonary capillaries. The reciprocal of the component due to the reaction rate of carbon monoxide with haemoglobin depends on displacing oxygen from haemoglobin, and so decreases with decreasing Po_2. Extrapolation to zero Po_2 removes this component entirely, and so indicates the reciprocal of the true membrane component which is independent of Po_2 (see reference 14).

This elegant approach was introduced in 1957 by Roughton and Forster.[27] Although the original data seemed to undergo an unreasonable amount of manipulation, confidence in the whole operation is engendered by the observed fact that the total diffusing capacity of carbon monoxide is undoubtedly reduced by the inhalation of high concentrations of oxygen (Figure 9.4). The change occurs too quickly to be caused by changes in the alveolar/capillary membrane. Measurement of pulmonary capillary blood volume by this technique yields normal values between 60 and 110 ml (depending on subject height),[28]

Table 9.3 Values obtained for diffusing capacity of carbon monoxide by various methods of measurement

Technique of measurement	Total diffusing capacity for CO		Membrane component of diffusing capacity		Pulmonary capillary blood volume (ml)
	$ml.min^{-1}.kPa^{-1}$	$ml.min^{-1}.mmHg^{-1}$	$ml.min^{-1}.kPa^{-1}$	$ml.min^{-1}.mmHg^{-1}$	
Steady state	113	15	195	26	73
Single breath	225	30	428	57	79
Rebreathing	203	27	300	40	110

which agrees well with a morphometric estimate of about 100 ml. Normal values are shown in Table 9.3, including the technique of measurement used, which has some influence on the value obtained – probably because of differing lung volumes during the measurement.[28]

Factors affecting 'diffusing capacity'

The basic principles of pulmonary diffusion described so far indicate that there are three major mechanisms by which diffusing capacity may alter: changes in the effective surface area of the gas exchange membrane, a change in the physical properties of the membrane, or changes related to the uptake of gases by the RBC. Each of these mechanisms will be discussed individually, and then other factors affecting diffusion capacity by either multiple or unknown mechanisms will be described.

Most of the factors outlined in this section apply equally to oxygen and carbon monoxide diffusion, though the majority have been studied using carbon monoxide, for the reasons described in the previous section.

Factors influencing diffusing capacity by changes in membrane surface area

Total lung volume, and therefore the number of alveoli available for gas exchange, will clearly affect diffusing capacity. However, only alveoli that are adequately ventilated and perfused will contribute to gas exchange, and the scatter of $\dot{V}/\dot{Q}$ ratios therefore has an important influence on the diffusing capacity.

Body size. Stature influences diffusing capacity directly because of the relationship between height and lung volume. Normal values for total diffusing capacity may be calculated from the formula:

$$D_{L_{CO}} = 10.9 \times \text{height (m)} - 0.067 \times \text{age (years)} - 5.89$$

A healthy 30-year-old male 1.78 m tall would therefore have a CO diffusing capacity of 11.5 mmol.min^{-1}.kPa^{-1} (34.4 ml.min.$^{-1}$.mmHg^{-1}).[28]

Lung volume.[29] Diffusing capacity is directly related to lung volume and therefore maximal at total lung capacity.[30] Different techniques for the measurement of diffusing capacity use different lung volumes, so it is now standard practice to simultaneously measure 'alveolar volume' (lung volume at which diffusing capacity was measured) by helium dilution.[1] Diffusing capacity can then measured as diffusing capacity per litre alveolar volume with units of mmol.min^{-1}.kPa^{-1}.l^{-1} (ml.min.$^{-1}$.mmHg^{-1}.l^{-1}).

Ventilation/perfusion mismatch results in a physiological dysfunction that presents many of the features of a reduction in diffusing capacity. If, for example, most of the ventilation is distributed to the left lung and most of the pulmonary blood flow to the right lung, the effective interface must be reduced. Minor degrees of maldistribution greatly complicate the interpretation of a reduced diffusing capacity. Both maldistribution and impaired diffusing capacity have a similar effect on the alveolar/arterial P_{O_2} gradient in relation to inspired oxygen concentration (Figure 8.15), and a distinction cannot be made by simple means.

Posture. Diffusing capacity is substantially increased when the subject is supine rather than standing or sitting, in spite of the fact that lung volume is reduced.[28] This change is probably explained by the increase in pulmonary blood volume, and the more uniform distribution of perfusion of the lungs in the supine position.

Pathology. The total area of the alveolar/capillary membrane may be reduced by any disease process or surgery that removes a substantial number of alveoli. For example, emphysema reduces the diffusing capacity mainly by destruction of alveolar septa such that Dl_{CO} correlates with the anatomical degree of emphysematous changes in the lung.[31]

Factors influencing the membrane diffusion barrier

'Alveolar/capillary block' is a term used in the past to describe a syndrome characterized by reduced lung volume, reasonably normal ventilatory capacity, hyperventilation and normal arterial Po_2 at rest, but with desaturation on exercise. These patients had reduced diffusing capacity that was believed to be due to an impediment at the alveolar/capillary membrane itself, which might either be thickened or else have its permeability to gas transfer reduced by some chemical abnormality. Impermeability of the alveolar/capillary membrane was supported by the light microscopy appearance in such conditions as scleroderma, sarcoidosis, asbestosis and pulmonary fibrosis. Evidence for such a condition at the magnification offered by electron microscopy has proved elusive. In retrospect, it seems likely that most of the patients thought to have alveolar/capillary block actually had hypoxaemia as a result of disturbances in distribution of ventilation and/or perfusion.

It will be clear that the oxygen-diffusing capacity may be influenced by many factors that are really nothing at all to do with diffusion *per se*. In fact, there is considerable doubt as to whether a true defect of alveolar/capillary membrane diffusion is ever the limiting factor in transfer of oxygen from the inspired gas to the arterial blood.

Chronic heart failure and pulmonary oedema remain the only likely causes of a membrane diffusion barrier. This may occur via pulmonary capillary congestion increasing the length of the diffusion pathway for oxygen through plasma, by interstitial oedema increasing the thickness of the membrane, or by raised capillary pressure damaging the endothelial and epithelial cells leading to proliferation of type II alveolar cells and thickening of the membrane.[32] Previous work with electron microscopy showed that oedema fluid tends to accumulate on the inactive side of the pulmonary capillary, leaving the active side, and therefore gaseous diffusion, relatively normal. However, the membrane component of diffusing capacity (*Dm*) is reduced in chronic heart failure, and the reduction correlates with symptom severity, whilst capillary volume increases only in severe heart failure.[33] It is therefore possible that, despite the negative findings with electron microscopy, heart failure of a suitable severity over a prolonged period does induce a form of 'alveolar/capillary block' described previously.

Factors related to uptake of gases by haemoglobin

Haemoglobin concentration affects diffusing capacity by influencing the rate and amount of oxygen or carbon monoxide uptake by blood flowing through the pulmonary capillary. Measurements of diffusing capacity are therefore usually mathematically corrected to account for abnormalities in the patient's haemoglobin concentration.[1]

Decreased capillary transit time. In the section above it was explained how a reduction in capillary transit time may reduce the diffusing capacity. The mean transit time is reduced when the cardiac output is raised (as in anaemia or exercise), and the scatter of transit times may be increased in a number of diseases of the lungs.

Other determinants of diffusing capacity

Age. Even when corrected for changes in lung volume, $D_{L_{CO}}$ declines in a linear fashion with increasing age.[29]

Gender. Women have a reduced total pulmonary diffusing capacity in comparison with men. This difference is almost totally explained by differences in stature and haemoglobin concentration.[23] $D_{L_{CO}}$ in women varies throughout the menstrual cycle, reaching a peak prior to menstruation, and seems to result from changes in θ, the reaction rate of CO with blood. The finding may, however, represent a technical problem with measuring $D_{L_{CO}}$ in that the low value during menstruation could result from a high *endogenous* production of carboxyhaemoglobin during the catabolism of haem compounds.[34]

Exercise results in an increase in diffusing capacity, possibly via a significant reduction in capillary transit time. Paradoxically, hypoxaemia from diffusion limitation during exercise is more common among elite, trained athletes than the average individual.[20] Physiological changes in exercise are discussed in Chapter 14.

Racial origin. In a study in the USA of over 4000 healthy individuals, $D_{L_{CO}}$ was significantly lower in black subjects compared with white.[23] The reasons for this are not clear.

Smoking history affects diffusing capacity even when most of the other determinants listed in this section are taken into account. $D_{L_{CO}}$ is reduced in proportion to the number of cigarettes per day currently smoked and the total lifetime number of cigarettes ever smoked.[23] The causes of this decline in lung function with smoking are discussed in Chapter 20.

Diffusion of gases in the tissues
Oxygen

Oxygen leaves the systemic capillaries by the reverse of the process by which it entered the pulmonary capillaries. Chemical release from haemoglobin is followed by diffusion through the endothelium and thence through the tissues to its site of utilization in the mitochondria. Diffusion may possibly be aided by protoplasmic streaming. Diffusion paths are much longer in tissues than in the lung. In well-vascularized tissue, such as brain, each capillary serves a zone of radius about 20 μm, but the corresponding distance is about 200 μm in skeletal muscle and greater still in fat and cartilage.

It is impracticable to talk about mean tissue P_{O_2} because this varies from one organ to another and must also depend on perfusion in relation to metabolic activity. Furthermore, within a tissue there must be some cells occupying more favourable sites towards the arterial ends of capillaries, while others must accept oxygen from the venous ends of the

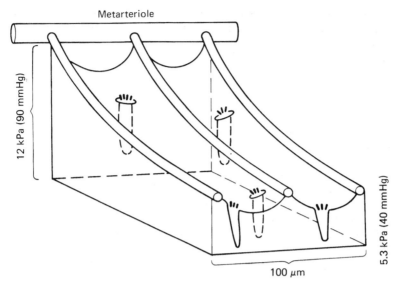

Figure 9.5 Diagrammatic representation of Po_2 within the tissues. The vertical axis represents the actual Po_2; in the horizontal plane is represented the course of three parallel capillaries from the metarteriole to the point of entry into the venule (not shown). The Po_2 falls exponentially along the course of each capillary with a trough of Po_2 between the capillaries. The pits represent the low spots of Po_2 from about 12 kPa (90 mmHg) in the tissue close to the arterial end of the capillaries down to less than 1 kPa at the mitochondria near the venous end of the capillaries. This is the simplest of many possible models of tissue perfusion.

capillaries, where the Po_2 is lower. This is well demonstrated in the liver, where the centrilobular cells must exist at a lower Po_2 than those at the periphery of the lobule. Even in a single cell, there can be no uniformity of Po_2. Not only are there 'low spots' around the mitochondria, but those mitochondria nearest to the capillaries presumably enjoy a higher Po_2 than those lying further away.

Figure 9.5 shows a model in which an area of tissue is perfused by three parallel capillaries. Vertical height indicates Po_2, which falls exponentially along the line of the capillaries, with troughs lying in between the capillaries. Five 'low spots' corresponding to mitochondria are shown. This diagram makes no pretence to histological accuracy but merely illustrates the difficulty of talking about the 'mean tissue Po_2', which is not an entity like the arterial or mixed venous Po_2.

Carbon dioxide

Little is known about the magnitude of carbon dioxide gradients between the mitochondria and the tissue capillaries. It is, however, thought that the tissue/venous Pco_2 gradient can be increased by two methods. The first is by inhibition of carbonic anhydrase, which blocks the uptake of carbon dioxide by the blood. The second is by hyperoxygenation of the arterial blood, caused by breathing 100% oxygen at high pressures. If the Po_2 of the arterial blood exceeds about 300 kPa (2250 mmHg), the dissolved oxygen will be sufficient for the usual tissue requirements. Therefore, there will be no significant amount of reduced haemoglobin, which is more effective than oxyhaemoglobin for carbamino carriage of carbon dioxide. The effect of this on tissue Pco_2 is likely to be too small to be clinically significant, and the alternative method of carbon dioxide carriage as bicarbonate seems to be adequate.

Alveolar/capillary permeability to non-volatile substances

The alveolar epithelium and the capillary endothelium have a very high permeability to water, to most gases and to lipophilic substances such as alcohol. However, for many hydrophilic substances of larger molecular diameter and for molecules carrying a charge, there is normally a very effective barrier. Passage of these substances is mainly through the gaps between the cells and must be considered separately for epithelium and endothelium. It was explained in Chapter 2 that the alveolar epithelial type I cells have very tight junctions, effectively limiting the molecular radius to about 0.6 nm. Endothelial junctions are much larger, with gaps of the order of 4–6 nm.

Passage of solutes across the alveolar/capillary membrane is usually described by the clearance of a molecule from the alveoli (i.e. across the epithelium) into the blood and quantified as the half-time of clearance or, alternatively, as the fractional clearance per minute. Clearance bears an approximate inverse relationship to the molecular weight.[35] Urea (60 daltons) has a fractional clearance of the order of 0.07 per minute, while for sucrose (342 daltons) the corresponding figure is 0.003 per minute and for albumin (64 000 daltons) is of the order of 0.0001 per minute. All of these clearances may be greatly increased if the alveolar epithelium is damaged, as in the permeability type of pulmonary oedema (page 546).

A useful tracer molecule for the assessment of permeability is ^{99m}Tc-DTPA (diethylene triamine penta-acetate) with a molecular weight of 492 daltons.[36] After being aerosolized into the lungs, its concentration can be continuously measured over the lung fields *in vivo* by detection of its gamma emission. In the healthy non-smoker, the clearance is very slow, about 0.01 per minute (half-time about 1 hour), but clearance is dramatically increased in many different types of pulmonary damage – including, for example, smoking, in which there is a threefold increase.

Electrolytes such as sodium ions can cross the epithelial barrier fairly freely, but the rate of passage is governed by concentration gradients. Thus, isotonic sodium solutions are cleared from the alveoli more quickly than hypertonic solutions.[35] The normal alveolar epithelium is almost totally impermeable to protein, the half-time for turnover of albumin between plasma and the alveolar compartment being of the order of 36 hours.[37]

The microvascular endothelium, with its larger intercellular gaps, is far more permeable for all molecular sizes and there is normally an appreciable leak of protein. Thus the concentration of albumin in pulmonary lymph is about half the concentration in plasma and may increase to approximate the plasma concentration in conditions of damaged alveolar/capillary permeability. This problem is discussed further in relation to pulmonary oedema in Chapter 28.

Principles of methods of measurement of carbon monoxide diffusing capacity

All the methods are based on the general equation:

$$D_{CO} = \frac{\dot{V}_{CO}}{P_{A_{CO}} - P\bar{c}_{CO}}$$

In each case it is usual to assume that the mean tension of carbon monoxide in the pulmonary capillary blood ($P\bar{c}_{CO}$) is effectively zero. It is, therefore, only necessary to measure the carbon monoxide uptake ($\dot{V}_{CO}$), and the alveolar carbon monoxide tension ($P_{A_{CO}}$). The diffusing capacity so measured (D_{CO}) is the total diffusing capacity, including that of the alveolar capillary membrane, plasma and the component due to the reaction time of carbon monoxide with haemoglobin.

The steady state method

The subject breathes a gas mixture containing about 0.3% carbon monoxide for about a minute. After this time, expired gas is collected when the alveolar P_{CO} is steady but the mixed venous P_{CO} has not yet reached a level high enough to require consideration in the calculation.

The carbon monoxide uptake ($\dot{V}_{CO}$) is measured in exactly the same way as oxygen consumption by the open method (page 290): the amount of carbon monoxide expired (expired minute volume × mixed expired CO concentration) is subtracted from the amount of carbon monoxide inspired (inspired minute volume × inspired CO concentration). The alveolar P_{CO} is calculated from the Filley version of the alveolar air equation (page 194), using carbon monoxide in place of oxygen.

Measurement of inspiratory and expiratory carbon monoxide and expiratory carbon dioxide concentrations presents no serious difficulty, and infrared analysis has proved satisfactory, though care must be taken following general anaesthesia, when expired nitrous oxide may affect the measurement of carbon dioxide.[38] Alveolar P_{CO_2} for entry into the alveolar air equation may be determined by sampling arterial blood and assuming that the alveolar P_{CO_2} is equal to the arterial P_{CO_2}. This is not strictly true in the presence of maldistribution. As an alternative, some workers measure the end-expiratory P_{CO_2} but neither does this equal the arterial P_{CO_2} in the presence of alveolar dead space (see Figure 8.10).

The steady state method requires no special respiratory manoeuvre and is therefore particularly suitable for use in children.[28]

The single-breath method

This method is the most frequently used in clinical practice and has a long history of progressive refinement. There are many variations on the exact method used, which yield broadly similar results,[39] but the multitude of techniques and factors affecting the results have led to attempts to standardize the method between centres.[1,23,40]

The patient is first required to exhale maximally. He then draws in a vital-capacity breath of a gas mixture containing about 0.3% carbon monoxide and about 10% helium. The breath is held for 10 seconds and a gas sample is then taken after the exhalation of the first 0.75 litre, which is sufficient to wash out the patient's dead space. The breath-holding time is sufficient to overcome maldistribution of the inspired gas.

It is assumed that no significant amount of helium has passed into the blood and, therefore, the ratio of the concentration of helium in the inspired gas to the concentration in the end-expiratory gas, multiplied by the volume of gas drawn into the alveoli during the maximal inspiration, will indicate the total alveolar volume during the period of breath holding. The alveolar P_{CO} at the commencement of breath holding is equal to the same ratio multiplied by the P_{CO} of the inspired gas mixture. The end-expiratory P_{CO} is measured directly.

From these data, together with the time of breath holding, it is possible to calculate the carbon monoxide uptake and the mean alveolar P_{CO}. Lung diffusing capacity for carbon monoxide can then be calculated and normalized for lung volume using the alveolar volume measured at the same time with helium. These calculations are now usually performed automatically by computer, which will also provide a 'normal' value based on the patient's gender, height, age and smoking status.

The rebreathing method

Somewhat similar to the single-breath method is the rebreathing method by which a gas mixture containing about 0.3% carbon monoxide and 10% helium is rebreathed rapidly from a rubber bag. The bag and the patient's lungs are considered as a single system, with gas exchange occurring in very much the same way as during breath holding. The calculation proceeds in a similar way to that for the single-breath method.

References

1. American Thoracic Society. Single breath carbon monoxide diffusing capacity (transfer factor). Recommendations for a standard technique – 1995 update. *Am J Respir Crit Care Med* 1995; **152**: 2185–98.
2. Milledge JS. The great oxygen secretion controversy. *Lancet* 1985; **2**: 1408–11.
3. Georg G, Lassen NA, Mellemgaard K, Vinther A. Diffusion in the gas phase of the lungs in normal and emphysematous subjects. *Clin Sci* 1965; **29**: 525–32.
4. Landon MJ, Matson AM, Royston BD, Hewlett AM, White DC, Nunn JF. Components of the inspiratory-arterial isoflurane partial pressure difference. *Br J Anaesth* 1993; **70**: 605–11.
5. Weibel ER, Federspiel WJ, Fryder-Doffey F, Hsia CCW, König M, Stalder-Navarro V, Vock R. Morphometric model for pulmonary diffusing capacity I. Membrane diffusing capacity. *Respir Physiol* 1993; **93**: 125–49.
6. Gil J, Bachofen H, Gehr P, Weibel ER. Alveolar volume–surface area relation in air- and saline-filled lungs fixed by vascular perfusion. *J Appl Physiol* 1979; **47**: 990–1001.
7. Weibel ER. Morphometrische Bestimmung von Zahl, Volumen und Oberfläche der Alveolen und Kapillaren der menschlichen Lunge. *Z Zellforsch Mikrosk Anat* 1962; **57**: 648.
8. Hsia CCW, Chuong CJC, Johnson RL. Critique of conceptual basis of diffusing capacity estimates: a finite element analysis. *J Appl Physiol* 1995; **79**: 1039–47.
9. Sarelius I. Invited editorial on 'Effect of RBC shape and deformability on pulmonary O_2 diffusing capacity and resistance to flow in rabbit lungs'. *J Appl Physiol* 1995; **78**: 763–4.
10. Geiser J, Betticher DC. Gas transfer in isolated lungs perfused with red cell suspension or haemoglobin solution. *Respir Physiol* 1989; **77**: 31–40.
11. Yamaguchi K, Nguyen-Phu D, Scheid P, Piiper J. Kinetics of O_2 uptake and release by human erythrocyte studied by a stopped-flow technique. *J Appl Physiol* 1985; **58**: 1215–24.
12. Betticher DC, Reinhart WH, Geiser J. Effect of RBC shape and deformability on pulmonary O_2 diffusing capacity and resistance to flow in rabbit lungs. *J Appl Physiol* 1995; **78**: 778–83.
13. Staub NC, Bishop JM, Forster RE. Velocity of O_2 uptake by human red blood cells. *J Appl Physiol* 1961; **16**: 511–16.
14. Forster RE. Diffusion of gases across the alveolar membrane. *Handbook of Physiology, Section 3* 1987; **4**: 71–88.
15. Bohr C. Über die spezifische Tätigkeit der Lungen bei der respiratorischen Gasaufnahme. *Skand Arch Physiol* 1909; **22**: 221.
16. Staub NC. Alveolar–arterial oxygen tension gradient due to diffusion. *J Appl Physiol* 1963; **18**: 673–80.
17. Staub NC, Bishop JM, Forster RE. Importance of diffusion and chemical reaction rates in O_2 uptake in the lung. *J Appl Physiol* 1962; **17**: 21–7.

18. Riley RL, Lilienthal JL, Proemmel DD, Franke RE. On the determination of the physiologically effective pressures of oxygen and carbon dioxide in alveolar air. *Am J Physiol* 1946; **147**: 191–8.

19. Asmussen E, Nielsen M. Alveolo-arterial gas exchange at rest and during work at different O_2 tensions. *Acta Physiol Scand* 1960; **50**: 153–66.

20. Wagner PD. Vascular transit times in the lung. *J Appl Physiol* 1995; **79**: 380–1.

21. McHardy GJR. Diffusing capacity and pulmonary gas exchange. *Br J Dis Chest* 1972; **66**: 1–20.

22. Cain SM, Otis AB. Carbon dioxide transport in anaesthetised dogs during inhibition of carbonic anhydrase. *J Appl Physiol* 1961; **16**: 1023–8.

23. Neas LM, Schwartz J. The determinants of pulmonary diffusing capacity in a national sample of US adults. *Am J Respir Crit Care Med* 1996; **153**: 656–64.

24. Weibel ER. Morphometric estimation of pulmonary diffusion capacity. I. Model and method. *Respir Physiol* 1970; **11**: 54–75.

25. Reeves RB, Park HK. CO uptake kinetics of red cells and CO diffusing capacity. *Respir Physiol* 1992; **88**: 1–21.

26. Forster RE. Rate of gas uptake by red cells. *Handbook of Physiology, Section 3* 1964; **1**: 827.

27. Roughton FJW, Forster RE. Relative importance of diffusion and chemical reaction rates in determining rate of exchange of gases in the human lung, with special reference to true diffusing capacity of pulmonary membrane and volume of blood in the lung capillaries. *J Appl Physiol* 1957; **11**: 291–302.

28. Cotes JE. *Lung function. Assessment and application in medicine*, 5th edn. Oxford: Blackwell Scientific Publications, 1993.

29. Stam H, Hrachovina V, Stijnen T, Versprille A. Diffusing capacity dependent on lung volume and age in normal subjects. *J Appl Physiol* 1994; **76**: 2356–63.

30. Gurtner GH, Fowler WS. Interrelationships of factors affecting pulmonary diffusing capacity. *J Appl Physiol* 1971; **30**: 619–24.

31. Cotton DJ, Sparkar GR, Graham BL. Diffusing capacity in the clinical assessment of chronic airflow limitation. *Med Clin North Am* 1996; **80**: 549–64.

32. Kay JM, Edwards FR. Ultra-structure of the alveolar–capillary wall in mitral stenosis. *J Pathol* 1973; **111**: 239–45.

33. Puri S, Baker BL, Dutka DP, Oakley CM, Hughes JMB, Cleland JGF. Reduced alveolar–capillary membrane diffusing capacity in chronic heart failure. *Circulation* 1995; **91**: 2769–74.

34. Sansores RH, Abboud RT, Kennell C, Haynes N. The effect of menstruation on the pulmonary carbon monoxide diffusing capacity. *Am J Respir Crit Care Med* 1995; **152**: 381–4.

35. Effros RM, Mason GR. Measurements of pulmonary epithelial permeability in vivo. *Am Rev Respir Dis* 1983; **127**: S59–65.

36. Jones JG, Royston D, Minty BD. Changes in alveolar–capillary barrier function in animals and humans. *Am Rev Respir Dis* 1983; **127**: S51–9.

37. Staub NA. Alveolar flooding and clearance. *Am Rev Respir Dis* 1983; **127**: S44–51.

38. Gilbert R, Arafat N, Williams L. False-low carbon monoxide diffusing capacity measurement after general anaesthesia. *Chest* 1996; **109**: 592.

39. Beck KC, Offord KP, Scanlon PD. Comparison of four methods for calculating diffusing capacity by the single breath method. *Chest* 1994; **105**: 594–600.

40. British Thoracic Society and Association of Respiratory Technicians and Physiologists. Guidelines for the measurement of respiratory function. *Respir Med* 1994; **88**: 165–94.

Chapter 10

Carbon dioxide

Carbon dioxide is the end-product of aerobic metabolism. It is produced almost entirely in the mitochondria, where the Pco_2 is highest. From its point of origin, there are a series of tension gradients as carbon dioxide passes through the cytoplasm and the extracellular fluid into the blood. In the lungs, the Pco_2 of the blood entering the pulmonary capillaries is normally higher than the alveolar Pco_2, and therefore carbon dioxide diffuses from the blood into the alveolar gas, where a dynamic equilibrium is established. The equilibrium concentration equals the ratio between carbon dioxide output and alveolar ventilation (page 130). Blood leaving the alveoli has, for practical purposes, the same Pco_2 as alveolar gas, and arterial blood Pco_2 is usually very close to 'ideal' alveolar Pco_2.

Abnormal levels for arterial Pco_2 occur in a number of pathological states and have many important physiological effects throughout the body, some as a result of changes in pH, and these are discussed in Chapter 22. Fundamental to all problems relating to Pco_2 is the mechanism by which carbon dioxide is carried in the blood.

Carriage of carbon dioxide in blood

In physical solution

Carbon dioxide belongs to the group of gases with moderate solubility in water. According to Henry's law of solubility:

$$Pco_2 \times \text{solubility coefficient} = CO_2 \text{ concentration in solution} \qquad ...(1)$$

The solubility coefficient of carbon dioxide (α) is expressed in units of $mmol.l^{-1}.kPa^{-1}$ (or $mmol.l^{-1}.mmHg^{-1}$). The value depends on temperature, and examples are listed in Table 10.1. The contribution of dissolved carbon dioxide to the total carriage of the gas in blood is shown in Table 10.2.

As carbonic acid

In solution, carbon dioxide hydrates to form carbonic acid:

$$CO_2 + H_2O \rightleftharpoons H_2CO_3 \qquad ...(2)$$

The equilibrium of this reaction is far to the left under physiological conditions. Published work shows some disagreement on the value of the equilibrium constant, but it seems

Table 10.1 Values for solubility of carbon dioxide in plasma and pK' at different temperatures

Temperature (°C)	Solubility of CO_2 in plasma		pK'		
	$mmol.l^{-1}.kPa^{-1}$	$mmol.l^{-1}.mmHg^{-1}$	at pH 7.6	at pH 7.4	at pH 7.2
40	0.216	0.0288	6.07	6.08	6.09
39	0.221	0.0294	6.07	6.08	6.09
38	0.226	0.0301	6.08	6.09	6.10
37	0.231	0.0308	6.08	6.09	6.10
36	0.236	0.0315	6.09	6.10	6.11
35	0.242	0.0322	6.10	6.11	6.12
25	0.310	0.0413	6.15	6.16	6.17
15	0.416	0.0554	6.20	6.21	6.23

(Data from references 1 and 2)

Table 10.2 Normal values for carbon dioxide carriage in blood

	Arterial blood (Hb sat. 95%)	Mixed venous blood (Hb sat. 95%)	Arterial/venous difference
Whole blood			
pH	7.40	7.367	−0.033
P_{CO_2} (kPa)	5.3	6.1	+0.8
(mmHg)	40.0	46.0	+6.0
Total CO_2 ($mmol.l^{-1}$)	21.5	23.3	+1.8
($ml.dl^{-1}$)	48.0	52.0	+4.0
Plasma ($mmol.l^{-1}$)			
Dissolved CO_2	1.2	1.4	+0.2
Carbonic acid	0.0017	0.0020	+0.0003
Bicarbonate ion	24.4	26.2	+1.8
Carbamino CO_2	Negligible	Negligible	Negligible
Total	25.6	27.6	+2.0
Erythrocyte fraction of 1 litre of blood			
Dissolved CO_2	0.44	0.51	+0.07
Bicarbonate ion	5.88	5.92	+0.04
Carbamino CO_2	1.10	1.70	+0.60
Plasma fraction of 1 litre of blood			
Dissolved CO_2	0.66	0.76	+0.10
Bicarbonate ion	13.42	14.41	+0.99
Total in 1 litre of blood ($mmol.l^{-1}$)	21.50	23.30	+1.80

These data represent the mean values reported in numerous studies.

likely that less than 1 per cent of the molecules of carbon dioxide are in the form of carbonic acid. There is a very misleading medical convention by which both forms of carbon dioxide in equation (2) are sometimes shown as carbonic acid. Thus the term H_2CO_3 may, in some situations, mean the total concentrations of dissolved CO_2 and H_2CO_3; to prevent confusion, it is preferable to use αP_{CO_2} as in equation (7) below. This does not apply to equations (4) and (5) below, where H_2CO_3 has its correct meaning. It would be theoretically more correct to indicate the thermodynamic activities rather than concentrations, the two quantities being related as:

$$\frac{\text{activity}}{\text{concentration}} = \text{activity coefficient}$$

At infinite dilution the activity coefficient is unity, but in physiological concentrations it is significantly less than unity. Activity is therefore less than the concentration. However, in practice it is usual to work in concentrations, and values for the various equilibrium constants are adjusted accordingly, as indicated by a prime after the symbol K thus – K'. This is one of the reasons why these 'constants' are not in fact constant but should be considered as parameters that vary slightly under physiological conditions.

Carbonic anhydrase.[3,4] The reaction of carbon dioxide with water (equation 2) is non-ionic and slow, requiring a period of minutes for equilibrium to be attained. This would be far too slow for the time available for gas exchange in pulmonary and systemic capillaries if the reaction were not speeded up enormously in both directions by the enzyme carbonic anhydrase, which is present in pulmonary capillary endothelium,[5] erythrocytes and many other tissues[4] but not in plasma. In addition to its role in the respiratory transport of carbon dioxide, this enzyme is concerned with the generation of hydrogen and bicarbonate ions in secretory organs, including the kidney, and the transfer of carbon dioxide in both skeletal and cardiac muscle.[4] Carbonic anhydrase, first isolated in 1933,[6] is a zinc-containing enzyme of low molecular weight, now known to have seven isoenzyme forms found in various cytoplasmic, cell membrane and mitochondrial sites.[7] It is inhibited by a large number of unsubstituted sulphonamides (general formula $R—SO_2NH_2$) but not the later antibacterial sulphonamides which are substituted ($R—SO_2NHR'$), and therefore inactive. Active sulphonamides include the thiazide diuretics and various heterocyclic sulphonamides, of which acetazolamide is the most important. This drug produces complete inhibition of carbonic anhydrase in all organs at a dose of $5–20\,mg.kg^{-1}$ and has no other pharmacological effects of importance. Acetazolamide has been much used in the study of carbonic anhydrase and has revealed the surprising fact that it is not essential to life. With total inhibition, P_{CO_2} gradients between tissues and alveolar gas are increased, pulmonary ventilation is increased and alveolar P_{CO_2} is decreased.

As bicarbonate ion

The largest fraction of carbon dioxide in the blood is in the form of bicarbonate ion, which is formed by ionization of carbonic acid:

$$H_2CO_3 \rightleftharpoons \underset{\substack{\text{first}\\\text{dissociation}}}{H^+ + HCO_3^-} \rightleftharpoons \underset{\substack{\text{second}\\\text{dissociation}}}{2H^+ + CO_3^{2-}} \quad\quad \ldots(3)$$

The second dissociation occurs only at high pH (above 9) and is not a factor in the carriage of carbon dioxide by the blood. The first dissociation is, however, of the greatest importance within the physiological range. The pK_1' is about 6.1 and carbonic acid is about 96 per cent dissociated under physiological conditions.

According to the law of mass action:

$$\frac{[H^+] \times [HCO_3^-]}{[H_2CO_3]} = K_1' \quad\quad \ldots(4)$$

where K_1' is the equilibrium constant of the first dissociation. The subscript 1 indicates that it is the first dissociation, and the prime indicates that we are dealing with concentrations rather than the more correct activities.

Rearrangement of equation (4) gives the following:

$$[H^+] = K_1' \frac{[H_2CO_3]}{[HCO_3^-]} \qquad \ldots (5)$$

The left-hand side is the hydrogen ion concentration, and this equation is the non-logarithmic form of the Henderson–Hasselbalch equation.[8] The concentration of carbonic acid cannot be measured and the equation may be modified by replacing this term with the total concentration of dissolved CO_2 and H_2CO_3, most conveniently quantified as αP_{CO_2} as described above. The equation now takes the form:

$$[H^+] = K' \frac{\alpha P_{CO_2}}{[HCO_3^-]} \qquad \ldots (6)$$

The new constant K' is the *apparent* first dissociation constant of carbonic acid, and includes a factor that allows for the substitution of total dissolved carbon dioxide concentration for carbonic acid.

The equation is now in a useful form and permits the direct relation of plasma hydrogen ion concentration, P_{CO_2} and bicarbonate concentration, all quantities that can be measured. The value of K' cannot be derived theoretically and is determined experimentally by simultaneous measurements of the three variables. Under normal physiological conditions, if $[H^+]$ is in $nmol.l^{-1}$, P_{CO_2} in kPa and HCO_3^- in $mmol.l^{-1}$, the value of the combined parameter $(\alpha K')$ is about 180. If P_{CO_2} is in mmHg, the value of the parameter is 24.

Most people prefer to use the pH scale and so follow the approach described by Hasselbalch in 1916 and take logarithms of the reciprocal of each term in equation (6) with the following familiar result:[9]

$$pH = pK' + \log \frac{[HCO_3^-]}{\alpha P_{CO_2}} = pK' + \log \frac{[CO_2] - \alpha P_{CO_2}}{\alpha P_{CO_2}} \qquad \ldots (7)$$

where pK' has an experimentally derived value of the order of 6.1, but varies with temperature and pH (see Table 10.1). '$[CO_2]$' refers to the total concentration of carbon dioxide in all forms (dissolved CO_2, H_2CO_3 and bicarbonate) in plasma and not in whole blood.

Carbamino carriage

Amino groups in the uncharged $R—NH_2$ form have the ability to combine directly with carbon dioxide to form a carbamic acid.[10] At body pH, the carbamic acid then dissociates almost completely to carbamate:

In a protein, the amino groups involved in the peptide linkages between amino acid residues cannot combine with carbon dioxide. The potential for carbamino carriage is therefore restricted to the one terminal amino group in each protein and to the side chain amino groups of lysine and arginine. Because both hydrogen ions and carbon dioxide compete to react with uncharged amino groups, the ability to combine with carbon dioxide is markedly pH dependent. The terminal α-amino groups are the most effective at physiological pH, and one binding site per protein monomer is more than sufficient to account for the quantity of carbon dioxide carried as a carbamino compound.

Carbamino carriage and haemoglobin.[3] Only very small quantities of CO_2 are carried in carbamino compounds with plasma protein. Almost all is carried by haemoglobin, and reduced haemoglobin is about 3.5 times as effective as oxyhaemoglobin (Figure 10.1), this being a major component of the Haldane effect (see below). Carbon dioxide binds to α-amino groups at the ends of both the α- and β-chains of haemoglobin. Earlier studies of CO_2–haemoglobin reactions using free haemoglobin solution overestimated the magnitude of carbamino binding with haemoglobin, as later work showed that 2,3-diphosphoglycerate (2,3-DPG) present *in vivo* antagonizes the binding of CO_2 with haemoglobin. This antagonism results from direct competition between CO_2 and 2,3-DPG for the end-terminal valine of the β-chain of haemoglobin, an effect that is not observed on the α-chains.

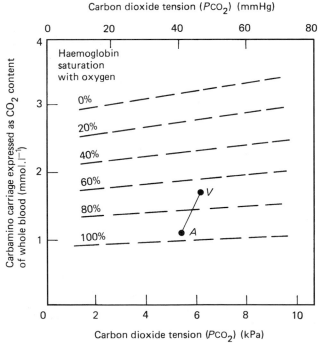

Figure 10.1 The broken lines on the graph indicate the carbamino carriage of carbon dioxide at different levels of oxygen saturation of haemoglobin (15 g Hb per dl blood). It will be seen that this has a far greater influence on carbamino carriage than the actual $P\text{co}_2$ (abscissa). Points *A* and *V* represent the saturation and $P\text{co}_2$ of arterial and venous blood respectively. Note that the arterial/venous difference in carbamino carriage is large in relation to the actual amounts of carbamino carriage.

The Haldane effect is the difference in the quantity of carbon dioxide carried, at constant P_{CO_2}, in oxygenated and deoxygenated blood (Figure 10.2). Although the amount of carbon dioxide carried in the blood in carbamino carriage is small, the *difference* between the amount carried in venous and arterial blood is about a third of the total arterial venous difference (Table 10.2). This therefore accounts for the major part of the Haldane effect, the remainder being due to the increased buffering capacity of reduced haemoglobin, which is discussed below. When the Haldane effect was described by Christiansen, Douglas and Haldane in 1914, they believed that the whole effect was due to altered buffering capacity:[11] carbamino carriage was not demonstrated until much later (1934).[12]

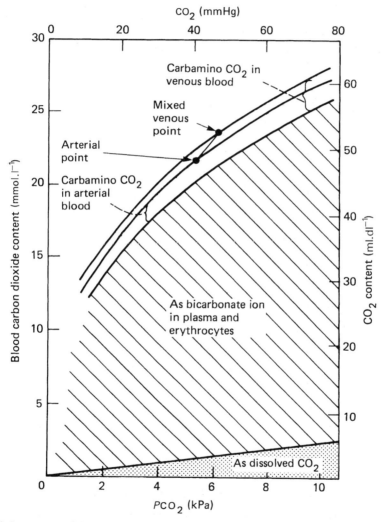

Figure 10.2 Components of the CO_2 dissociation curve for whole blood. Dissolved CO_2 and bicarbonate ion vary with P_{CO_2} but are little affected by the state of oxygenation of the haemoglobin. (Increased basic properties of reduced haemoglobin cause a slight increase in formation of bicarbonate ion.) Carbamino carriage of CO_2 is strongly influenced by the state of oxygenation of haemoglobin but hardly at all by P_{CO_2}.

Formation of carbamino compounds does not require the dissolved carbon dioxide to be hydrated and so is independent of carbonic anhydrase. The reaction is very rapid and would be of particular importance in a patient who had received a carbonic anhydrase inhibitor.

Effect of buffering power of proteins on carbon dioxide carriage

Amino and carboxyl groups concerned in peptide linkages have no buffering power. Neither have most side chain groups (e.g. in lysine and glutamic acid) because their pK values are far removed from the physiological range of pH. In contrast is the imidazole group of the amino acid histidine, which is almost the only amino acid to be an effective buffer in the normal range of pH. Imidazole groups constitute the major part of the considerable buffering power of haemoglobin, each tetramer containing 38 histidine residues. The buffering power of plasma proteins is less and is directly proportional to their histidine content.

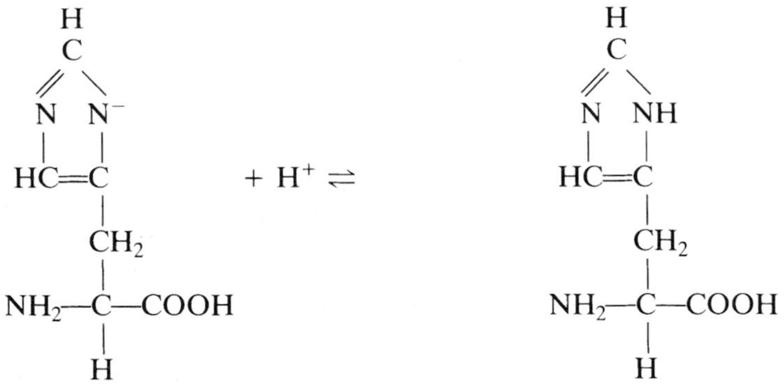

Basic form of histidine   *Acidic form of histidine*

The four haem groups of a molecule of haemoglobin are attached to the corresponding four amino acid chains at one of the histidine residues on each chain (page 263). The following is a section of a β-chain of human haemoglobin:

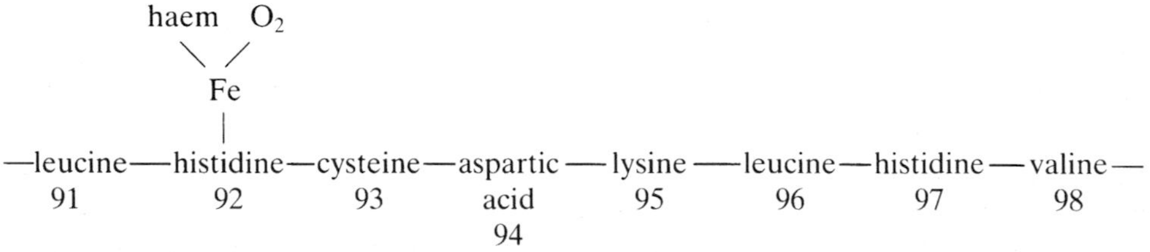

The figures indicate the position of the amino acid residue in the chain. The histidine in position 92 is one to which a haem group is attached, whilst that in position 97 is not. Both have buffering properties but the dissociation constant of the imidazole groups of the four histidine residues to which the haem groups are attached is strongly influenced by the state of oxygenation of the haem. Reduction causes the corresponding imidazole group to become more basic. The converse is also true: in the acidic form of the imidazole group of the histidine, the strength of the oxygen bond is weakened. Each reaction is of great physiological interest and both effects were noticed many decades before their mechanisms were elucidated.

1. *The reduction of haemoglobin causes it to become more basic.* This results in increased carriage of carbon dioxide as bicarbonate, because hydrogen ions are removed, permitting increased dissociation of carbonic acid (first dissociation of equation 3). This accounts for part of the Haldane effect, the other and greater part being due to increased carbamino carriage (see above).
2. *Conversion to the basic form of histidine causes increased affinity of the corresponding haem group for oxygen.* This is, in part, the cause of the Bohr effect (page 267).

Total deoxygenation of the haemoglobin in blood would raise the pH by about 0.03 if the P_{CO_2} were held constant at 5.3 kPa (40 mmHg), and this would correspond roughly to the addition of 3 mmol of base to 1 litre of blood. The normal degree of desaturation in the course of the change from arterial to mixed venous blood is about 25%, corresponding to a pH increase of about 0.007 if P_{CO_2} remains constant. In fact, P_{CO_2} rises by about 0.8 kPa (6 mmHg), which would cause a decrease of pH of 0.040 if the oxygen saturation were to remain the same. The combination of an increase of P_{CO_2} of 0.8 kPa and a decrease of saturation of 25% thus results in a fall of pH of 0.033 (Table 10.2).

Distribution of carbon dioxide in the blood

Table 10.2 shows the forms in which carbon dioxide is carried in normal arterial and mixed venous blood. Although the amount carried in solution is small, most of the carbon dioxide enters and leaves the blood as CO_2 itself (Figure 10.3). Within the plasma there is little chemical combination of carbon dioxide, for three reasons. First, there is no carbonic anhydrase in plasma and therefore carbonic acid is formed only very slowly. Secondly, there is little buffering power in plasma to promote the dissociation of carbonic acid. Thirdly, the formation of carbamino compounds by plasma proteins is not great, and must be almost identical for arterial and venous blood.

Carbon dioxide can, however, diffuse freely into the erythrocyte, where two courses are open. First, increasing intracellular P_{CO_2} will increase carbamino carriage of CO_2 by haemoglobin, an effect greatly enhanced by the fall in oxygen saturation, which is likely to be occurring at the same time (Figure 10.1). The second course is hydration and dissociation of CO_2 to produce hydrogen and bicarbonate ions, facilitated by the presence of carbonic anhydrase in the erythrocyte, which, as a catalyst, speeds up the rate at which the reaction reaches equilibrium by a factor of 13 000.[3] However, accumulation of intracellular hydrogen and bicarbonate ions will quickly tip the equilibrium of the reaction against further dissociation of carbonic acid, a situation that is avoided in the red cell by two mechanisms, as follows:

Haemoglobin buffering. Hydrogen ions produced by carbonic anhydrase are quickly buffered by the imidazole groups on the histidine residues of the haemoglobin, as described above. Once again, the concomitant fall in haemoglobin saturation enhances this effect by increasing the buffering capacity of the haemoglobin.

Hamburger shift. Hydration of CO_2 and buffering of the hydrogen ions results in the formation of considerable quantities of bicarbonate ion within the erythrocyte. These excess bicarbonate ions diffuse out of the cell into the plasma in exchange for chloride ions which diffuse in the opposite direction, to maintain electrical neutrality across the erythrocyte membrane. This ionic exchange was first suggested by Hamburger in 1918,[13] and believed to be a passive process. It is now known to be facilitated by a complex

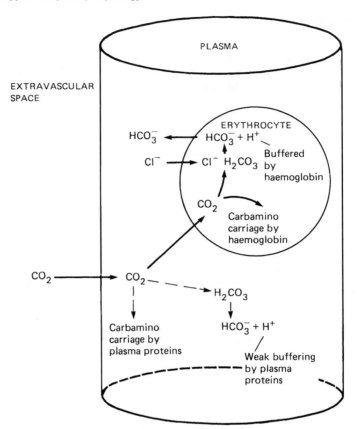

Figure 10.3 How carbon dioxide enters the blood in molecular form. Within the plasma, there is only negligible carbamino carriage by plasma proteins and a slow rate of hydration to carbonic acid due to the absence of carbonic anhydrase. The greater part of CO_2 diffuses into the erythrocyte where conditions for carbamino carriage (by haemoglobin) are more favourable. In addition, formation of carbonic acid is facilitated by carbonic anhydrase, the removal of hydrogen ions by haemoglobin buffering and the transfer of bicarbonate out of the erythrocyte by the Hamburger shift.

membrane-bound protein, which has been extensively studied and named Band 3 after its position on a gel electrophoresis plate.[3,14,15] Band 3 exchanges bicarbonate and chloride ions by a 'ping-pong' mechanism in which one ion first moves out of the cell before the other ion moves inwards, in contrast to most other ion pumps which simultaneously exchange the two ions. Each Band 3 protein is estimated to turn over 50 000 ions per second.[3] Band 3 protein is also intimately related to the proteins ankyrin and spectrin which are involved in the maintenance of cell shape and membrane stability, such that a genetically engineered deficiency of Band 3 in animals results in small, fragile, spherical erythrocytes.[15] Erythrocyte shape and deformability are now known to be important in oxygen transport at a cellular level (page 205), and future developments may reveal involvement of Band 3 in bringing about these shape changes.

In the pulmonary capillary, where P_{CO_2} is low, the series of events described above goes into reverse and the carbon dioxide released from the erythrocyte diffuses into the alveolus and is excreted.

Dissociation curves of carbon dioxide

Figure 10.2 shows the classic form of the dissociation curve of carbon dioxide relating blood content to tension. For 30 years there has been great interest in curves that relate any pair of the following: (1) plasma bicarbonate concentration; (2) P_{CO_2}; (3) pH. These three quantities are related by the Henderson–Hasselbalch equation (equation 7) and therefore

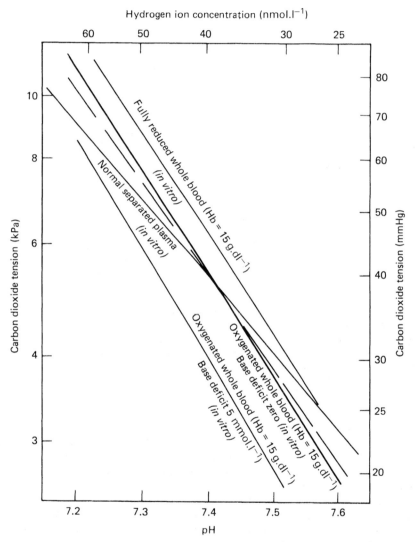

Figure 10.4 A number of CO_2 equilibrium curves plotted on the coordinates pH/log P_{CO_2}.[16] For most biological fluids the plot is linear over the physiological range. pH = 7.40 and P_{CO_2} = 5.3 kPa (40 mmHg) is the accepted normal value through which all the curves for normal oxygenated blood or plasma pass. The steepest curve passing through this point is that of normal oxygenated blood; the flattest is that of plasma, both curves being obtained *in vitro*. The uppermost curve is that of reduced but otherwise normal blood equilibrated *in vitro*. The lowermost curve is that of oxygenated blood with a metabolic acidosis (base deficit) of 5 mmol.l^{-1} equilibrated *in vitro*. The broken curve is the only *in vivo* curve, obtained from a normal anaesthetized patient (Hb 15 g.dl^{-1}) whose P_{CO_2} is acutely changed.[17]

the third variable can always be derived from the other two. The most famous is the Siggaard-Andersen plot which relates log P_{CO_2} to pH (Figure 10.4), though many others have been described (see previous editions of this book). These graphs can be used to explore the effects of changes in respiratory and metabolic acid–base balance, but care must be taken in using these *in vitro* data in intact subjects. For example, if the P_{CO_2} of an entire patient is altered, the pH changes are not the same as those of a blood sample of which the P_{CO_2} is altered *in vitro*. This is because the blood of a patient is in continuity with the extracellular fluid (of very low buffering capacity) and also with intracellular fluid (of high buffering capacity). Bicarbonate ions pass rapidly and freely across the various interfaces, and experimental studies have shown the following changes to occur in the arterial blood of an intact subject when the P_{CO_2} is acutely changed.

1. The arterial pH reaches a steady state within minutes of establishment of the new level of P_{CO_2}.
2. The change in arterial pH is intermediate between the pH changes obtained *in vitro* with plasma and whole blood after the same change in P_{CO_2}. That is to say, the *in vivo* change in pH is greater than the *in vitro* change in the patient's blood when subjected to the same change in P_{CO_2}.

Transfer of carbon dioxide across cell membranes

Membranes made of most plastic materials (e.g. polytetrafluorethylene – PTFE) permit the free diffusion of carbon dioxide but will not permit the passage of hydrogen ions. This is the principle of the CO_2-sensitive electrode (page 242). Somewhat similar selectivity exists across cell membranes in the living body and particularly in the case of the blood–brain barrier, which is impervious to hydrogen and bicarbonate ions but permits the rapid diffusion of CO_2. Therefore, the intracellular hydrogen ion concentration is relatively uninfluenced by changes in extracellular pH, but does respond to changes in P_{CO_2}. Carbon dioxide passes through the membrane and, once inside the cell, is able to hydrate and ionize, thus producing hydrogen ions. This property is unique to CO_2, which is the only substance normally present in the body that is able to diffuse through cell membranes and alter the intracellular pH in this manner.

Factors influencing the carbon dioxide tension in the steady state

In common with other catabolites, the level of carbon dioxide in the body fluids depends upon the balance between production and elimination. There is a continuous gradient of P_{CO_2} from the mitochondria to the expired air and thence to ambient air. The P_{CO_2} in all cells is not identical, but is lowest in tissues with the lowest metabolic activity and the highest perfusion (e.g. skin) and highest in tissues with the highest metabolic activity for their perfusion (e.g. the myocardium). Therefore the P_{CO_2} of venous blood differs from one tissue to another, and the mixed venous P_{CO_2} is the mean for the whole body, integrated with respect to organ perfusion.

In the pulmonary capillaries, carbon dioxide passes into the alveolar gas and this causes the alveolar P_{CO_2} to rise steadily during expiration. During inspiration, the inspired gas dilutes the alveolar gas and the P_{CO_2} falls by about 0.4 kPa, imparting a sawtooth curve to the alveolar P_{CO_2} when it is plotted against time (Figure 10.5).

Blood leaving the pulmonary capillaries has a P_{CO_2} that is very close to that of alveolar gas and, therefore, varies with time in the same manner as the alveolar P_{CO_2}.

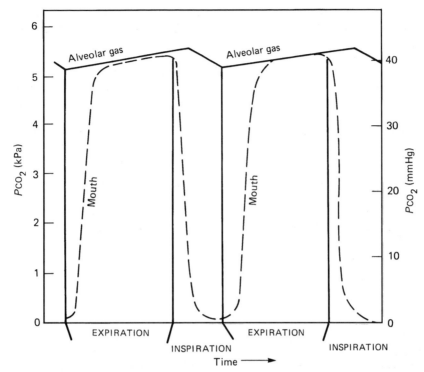

Figure 10.5 Changes in alveolar and mouth P_{CO_2} during the respiratory cycle. The alveolar P_{CO_2} is shown by a continuous curve, and the mouth P_{CO_2} by the broken curve. The mouth P_{CO_2} falls at the commencement of inspiration but does not rise during expiration until the anatomical dead space gas is washed out. The alveolar P_{CO_2} rises during expiration and also during the early part of inspiration until fresh gas penetrates the alveoli after the anatomical dead space is washed out. The alveolar P_{CO_2} then falls until expiration commences. This imparts a sawtooth curve to the alveolar P_{CO_2}.

There is also a regional variation with P_{CO_2} inversely related to the ventilation/perfusion ratio of different parts of the lung (see Figure 8.13). The mixed arterial P_{CO_2} is the integrated mean of blood from different parts of the lung, and a sample drawn over several seconds will average out the cyclical variations.

It is more convenient to consider tension than content, because carbon dioxide always moves in accord with tension gradients even if they are in the opposite direction to concentration gradients. Also, the concept of tension may be applied with equal significance to gas and liquid phases, content having a rather different connotation in the two phases. Furthermore, the effects of carbon dioxide (e.g. upon respiration) are a function of tension rather than content. Finally, it is easier to measure blood P_{CO_2} than carbon dioxide content. Normal values for tension and content are shown in Figure 10.6.

Each factor that influences the P_{CO_2} has already been mentioned in this book and in this chapter they are drawn together, illustrating their relationship to one another. It is convenient first to summarize the factors influencing the alveolar P_{CO_2}, and then to consider the factors that influence the relationship between the alveolar and the arterial P_{CO_2} (Figure 10.7).

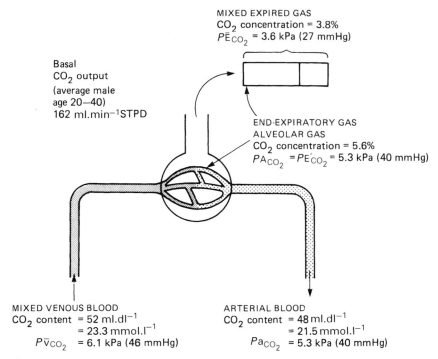

Figure 10.6 Normal values of CO_2 levels. These normal values are rounded off and ignore the small difference in P_{CO_2} between end-expiratory gas, alveolar gas and arterial blood. Actual values of P_{CO_2} depend mainly on alveolar ventilation but the differences depend on maldistribution; the alveolar/end-tidal expiratory P_{CO_2} difference depends on alveolar dead space and the very small arterial/alveolar P_{CO_2} difference on shunt. Scatter of $\dot{V}/\dot{Q}$ ratios makes a small contribution to both alveolar/end-expiratory and arterial/alveolar P_{CO_2} gradients. The arterial/mixed venous CO_2 content difference is directly proportional to CO_2 output and inversely proportional to cardiac output. Secondary symbols: A, alveolar; a, arterial; E, mixed expired; E', end-expiratory; $\bar{v}$, mixed venous.

The alveolar P_{CO_2} ($P_{A_{CO_2}}$)

Carbon dioxide is constantly being added to the alveolar gas from the pulmonary arterial blood, and removed from it by the alveolar ventilation. Therefore, ignoring inspired carbon dioxide, it follows that:

$$\text{alveolar } CO_2 \text{ concentration} = \frac{\text{carbon dioxide output}}{\text{alveolar ventilation}}$$

This axiomatic relationship is the basis for prediction of the alveolar concentration of any gas that enters or leaves the body. With inclusion of the inspired concentration, it may be written as the universal air equation (page 130), for which the version for carbon dioxide is:

$$\begin{array}{l} \text{alveolar} \\ P_{CO_2} \end{array} = \begin{array}{l} \text{dry} \\ \text{barometric} \\ \text{pressure} \end{array} \left(\begin{array}{l} \text{mean} \\ \text{inspired } CO_2 \\ \text{concentration} \end{array} + \frac{CO_2 \text{ output}}{\text{alveolar ventilation}} \right)$$

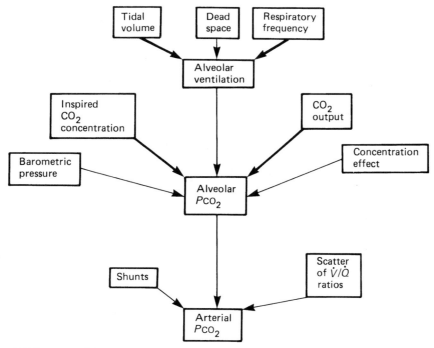

Figure 10.7 Summary of factors that influence P_{CO_2}; the more important ones are indicated with the thicker arrows. In the steady state, the CO_2 output of a resting subject usually lies in the range 150–200 ml.min^{-1} and the alveolar P_{CO_2} is largely governed by the alveolar ventilation, provided that the inspired CO_2 concentration is zero. See text for explanation of the concentration effect.

This equation includes all the more important factors influencing P_{CO_2} (Figure 10.7); examples of the hyperbolic relationship between P_{CO_2} and alveolar ventilation are shown in Figure 10.8. Individual factors will now be considered.

The dry barometric pressure is not a factor of much importance in the determination of alveolar P_{CO_2}, and normal variations of barometric pressure at sea level are unlikely to influence the P_{CO_2} by more than 0.3 kPa (2 mmHg). At high altitude, the hypoxic drive to ventilation lowers the P_{CO_2} (Chapter 16).

The mean inspired CO_2 concentration is a more difficult concept than it seems at first sight;[18] it has been considered in relation to physiological dead space on page 181. Essentially the effect of inspired carbon dioxide on the alveolar P_{CO_2} is additive. If, for example, a patient breathes gas containing 4.2% carbon dioxide (P_{CO_2} = 4.0 kPa or 30 mmHg), the alveolar P_{CO_2} will be raised 4.0 kPa above the level that it would be if there were no carbon dioxide in the inspired gas, *and other factors, including ventilation, remained the same.*

Carbon dioxide output. It is carbon dioxide output and not production that directly influences the alveolar P_{CO_2}. Output equals production in a steady state, but they may be quite different during unsteady states. During acute hypoventilation, much of the carbon dioxide production is diverted into the body stores, so the output may temporarily fall to

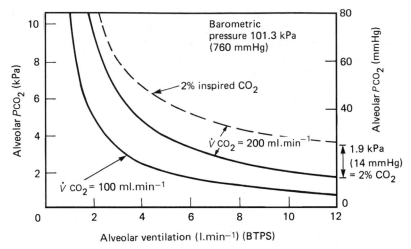

Figure 10.8 The effect of CO_2 output, alveolar ventilation and inspired CO_2 concentration on alveolar PCO_2. The lowest continuous curve shows the relationship between ventilation and alveolar PCO_2 for a CO_2 output of 100 ml.min^{-1} (STPD). The upper continuous curve shows the relationship when the CO_2 output is 200 ml.min^{-1}. The broken curve represents the relationship when the CO_2 output is 200 ml.min^{-1} and there is an inspired CO_2 concentration of 2 per cent. Two per cent CO_2 is equivalent to about 1.9 kPa (14 mmHg) and each point on the broken curve is 1.9 kPa above the upper of the two continuous curves.

very low figures until the alveolar carbon dioxide concentration has risen to its new level. Conversely, acute hyperventilation results in a transient increase in carbon dioxide output. A sudden fall in cardiac output decreases the carbon dioxide output until the carbon dioxide concentration in the mixed venous blood rises. The unsteady state is considered in more detail later in this chapter.

Alveolar ventilation for present purposes means the product of the respiratory frequency and the difference between the tidal volume and the physiological dead space (page 129). It can change over very wide limits and is the most important factor influencing alveolar PCO_2. Factors governing ventilation are considered in Chapter 5, and dead space in Chapter 8.

The concentration effect. Apart from the factors shown in the equation above and in Figure 10.8, the alveolar PCO_2 may be temporarily influenced by net transfer of soluble inert gases across the alveolar/capillary membrane. Rapid uptake of an inert gas increases the concentration (and tension) of carbon dioxide (and oxygen) in the alveolar gas. This occurs, for example, at the beginning of an anaesthetic, when large quantities of nitrous oxide are passing from the alveolar gas into the body stores and a much smaller quantity of nitrogen is passing from the body into the alveolar gas. The converse occurs during elimination of the inert gas and results in transient reduction of alveolar PCO_2 and PO_2.

The end-expiratory PCO_2 (PE'_{CO_2})

In the normal, healthy, conscious subject, the end-expiratory gas consists almost entirely of alveolar gas. If, however, appreciable parts of the lung are ventilated but not perfused, they will contribute a significant quantity of CO_2-free gas from the alveolar dead space to the end-expiratory gas (see Figure 8.10). As a result, the end-expiratory $P\text{CO}_2$ will have a lower $P\text{CO}_2$ than that of the alveoli which are perfused. Gas cannot be sampled selectively from the perfused alveoli. However, because arterial $P\text{CO}_2$ usually approximates closely to $P\text{CO}_2$ of the perfused alveoli (see below), it is possible to compare arterial and end-expiratory $P\text{CO}_2$ to demonstrate the existence of an appreciable proportion of under-perfused alveoli. Studies during anaesthesia have shown, for example, an arterial/end-expiratory $P\text{CO}_2$ gradient between 0.7 and 1.3 kPa (5–10 mmHg).[19,20]

The alveolar/arterial $P\text{CO}_2$ gradient

For reasons that have been discussed in Chapter 9, we may discount the possibility of any significant gradient between the $P\text{CO}_2$ of alveolar gas and that of pulmonary end-capillary blood. Arterial $P\text{CO}_2$ may, however, be slightly greater than the mean alveolar $P\text{CO}_2$ because of shunting or scatter of ventilation/perfusion ratios. Factors governing the magnitude of the gradient were considered in Chapter 8, where it was shown that a shunt of 10 per cent will cause an alveolar/arterial $P\text{CO}_2$ gradient of only about 0.1 kPa (0.7 mmHg) (see Figure 8.11). Because the normal degree of ventilation/perfusion ratio scatter causes a gradient of the same order, neither has much significance for carbon dioxide (in contrast to oxygen), and there is an established convention by which the arterial and 'ideal' alveolar $P\text{CO}_2$ values are taken to be identical. It is only in exceptional patients with, for example, a shunt in excess of 30 per cent that the gradient is likely to exceed 0.3 kPa (2 mmHg).

The arterial $P\text{CO}_2$ (Pa_{CO_2})

Pooled results for the normal arterial $P\text{CO}_2$ reported by various authors show a mean of 5.1 kPa (38.3 mmHg) with 95 per cent limits (2 s.d.) of ±1.0 kPa (7.5 mmHg). Some 5 per cent of normal patients will lie outside these limits and it is therefore preferable to call it the reference range rather than the normal range. There is no evidence that $P\text{CO}_2$ is influenced by age in the healthy subject.

Carbon dioxide stores and the unsteady state

The quantity of carbon dioxide and bicarbonate ion in the body is very large – about 120 litres, which is almost 100 times greater than the volume of oxygen. Therefore, when ventilation is altered out of accord with metabolic activity, carbon dioxide levels change only slowly and new equilibrium levels are attained only after about 20–30 minutes. In contrast, corresponding changes in oxygen levels are very rapid.

Figure 10.9 shows a three-compartment hydraulic model in which depth of water represents $P\text{CO}_2$ and the volume in the various compartments corresponds to volume of carbon dioxide. The metabolic production of carbon dioxide is represented by the variable flow of water from the supply tank. The outflow corresponds to alveolar ventilation, and the controller watching the $P\text{CO}_2$ represents the central chemoreceptors. The rapid compartment represents circulating blood, brain, kidneys and other well-perfused tissues. The medium compartment represents skeletal muscle (resting) and other tissues with a moderate blood flow. The slow compartment includes bone, fat and other tissues with a large capacity for carbon dioxide. Each compartment has its own time constant (see Appendix F), and the long time constants of the medium and slow compartments buffer changes in the rapid compartment.

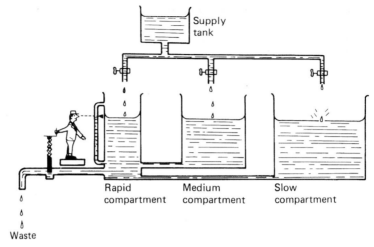

Figure 10.9 A hydrostatic analogy of the elimination of carbon dioxide. See text for full description.

Hyperventilation is represented by a wide opening of the outflow valve with subsequent exponential decline in the levels in all three compartments, the rapid compartment falling most quickly. The rate of decrease of P_{CO_2} is governed primarily by ventilation and the capacity of the stores. Hypoventilation is fundamentally different. The rate of increase of P_{CO_2} is now limited by the metabolic production of carbon dioxide, which is the *only* factor directly increasing the quantity of carbon dioxide in the body compartments. Therefore, the time course of the increase of P_{CO_2} following step decrease of ventilation is not the mirror image of the time course of decrease of P_{CO_2} when ventilation is increased. The rate of rise is much slower than the rate of fall, which is fortunate for patients in asphyxial situations.

When *all* metabolically produced carbon dioxide is retained, the rate of rise of arterial P_{CO_2} is of the order of $0.4-0.8\,\text{kPa.min}^{-1}$ ($3-6\,\text{mmHg.min}^{-1}$). This is the resultant of the rate of production of carbon dioxide and the capacity of the body stores for carbon dioxide. During hypoventilation, the rate of increase in P_{CO_2} will be less than this; Figure 10.10 shows typical curves for P_{CO_2} increase and decrease following step changes in ventilation of anaesthetized patients. The time course of rise of P_{CO_2} after step reduction of ventilation is faster when the previous level of ventilation has been of short duration.[21]

The difference in the rate of change of P_{CO_2} and P_{O_2} after a step change in ventilation (see Figure 11.20) has two important implications for monitoring and measurement. First, changes in P_{O_2} (or the output of a pulse oximeter) will often provide an earlier warning of acute hypoventilation than will the capnogram, provided that the alveolar P_{O_2} is not much above the normal range. However, *in the steady state* P_{CO_2} gives the best indication of the adequacy of ventilation, because oxygenation is so heavily influenced by intrapulmonary shunting and the inspired oxygen concentration. Secondly, step changes in ventilation are followed by temporary changes in the respiratory exchange ratio because, in the unsteady state, carbon dioxide output changes more than oxygen uptake. However, if the ventilation is held constant at its new level, the respiratory exchange ratio must eventually return to the value determined by the metabolic process of the body.

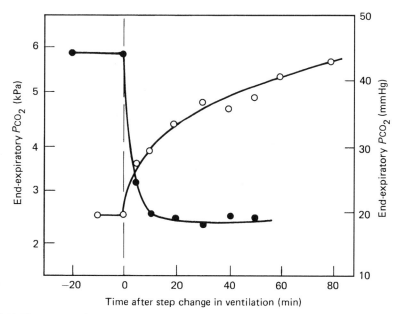

Figure 10.10 Time course of changes in end-expiratory P_{CO_2} following step changes in ventilation. The solid circles indicate the changes in end-expiratory P_{CO_2} that followed a change in ventilation from 3.3 to 14 l.min^{-1}. The open circles show the change following a reduction in ventilation from 14 to 3.3 l.min^{-1} in the same patient. During the fall in P_{CO_2}, half the total change is completed in about 3 minutes; during the rise in P_{CO_2}, half-change takes approximately 16 minutes.

Cardiac output and CO$_2$ transport. In the normal subject, fluctuations in cardiac output have little effect on arterial, alveolar or end-expiratory P_{CO_2} because of the efficiency of the chemical control of breathing. However, with a constant level of artificial ventilation, for example during anaesthesia or cardiopulmonary resuscitation, the situation is quite different. In the extreme circumstance of a total cessation of cardiac output, alveolar and end-expiratory P_{CO_2} will fall dramatically as the delivery of blood containing carbon dioxide to the lung also ceases. In a similar fashion, a sudden reduction in cardiac output during anaesthesia causes an abrupt reduction in end-expiratory P_{CO_2},[22] an observation first made as long ago as 1957.[23] This almost certainly results from increased alveolar dead space caused by an increase in the number of non-perfused but ventilated alveoli (zone 1, page 146). If low cardiac output is sustained for more than a few minutes, arterial P_{CO_2} will rise and the expired P_{CO_2} return towards normal as the blood passing through perfused lung releases more carbon dioxide into the expired gas. Apart from being a useful early warning of cardiovascular catastrophe during anaesthesia, the measurement of expired carbon dioxide has also been advocated during cardiopulmonary resuscitation both as a method of monitoring the efficacy of chest compressions and as an indicator of the return of spontaneous cardiac output.[24]

Apnoea

When a patient becomes apnoeic while breathing air, alveolar gas reaches equilibrium with mixed venous blood within a few minutes. Assuming normal starting conditions and ignoring changes in the composition of the recirculated mixed venous blood, this would entail a rise of alveolar P_{CO_2} from 5.3 to 6.1 kPa (40 to 46 mmHg) and a fall of P_{O_2} from 14 to 5.3 kPa (105 to 40 mmHg). These changes correspond to the uptake of 230 ml of oxygen but the output of only 21 ml of carbon dioxide. Carbon dioxide appears to reach equilibrium within about 10 seconds,[25] while oxygen would take about a minute, being limited by the ability of the cardiac output and the arterial/mixed venous oxygen content difference to remove some two-thirds of the oxygen in the alveolar gas (normally about 450 ml).

These calculations assume that alveolar gas is not replenished from outside the patient. What actually happens to the arterial blood gases in apnoea depends upon the patency of the airway and the composition of the ambient gas if the airway is patent.

With airway occlusion. As described above, there is rapid attainment of equilibrium between alveolar and mixed venous P_{CO_2}. Thereafter, arterial, alveolar and mixed venous P_{CO_2} values remain close, and, with recirculation of the blood, increase together at the rate of about $0.4–0.8\,kPa.min^{-1}$ ($3–6\,mmHg.min^{-1}$), more than 90 per cent of the metabolically produced carbon dioxide passing into the body stores. Alveolar P_{O_2} decreases close to the mixed venous P_{O_2} within about a minute, and then decreases further as recirculation continues. The lung volume falls by the difference between the oxygen uptake and the carbon dioxide output. Initially the rate would be $230 - 21 = 209\,ml.min^{-1}$. The change in alveolar P_{O_2} may be calculated, and gross hypoxia supervenes after about 90 seconds if apnoea with airway occlusion follows air breathing at the functional residual capacity.

With patent airway and air as ambient gas. The initial changes are as described above. However, instead of the lung volume falling by the net gas exchange rate (initially $209\,ml.min^{-1}$), this volume of ambient gas is drawn in by mass movement down the trachea. If the ambient gas is air, the oxygen in it will be removed but the nitrogen will accumulate and rise above its normal concentration until gross hypoxia supervenes after about 2 minutes. This is likely to occur when the accumulated nitrogen has reached 90%, as the alveolar carbon dioxide concentration will then have reached about 8%. Carbon dioxide elimination cannot occur as there is mass movement of air down the trachea, preventing loss of carbon dioxide by either convection or diffusion. Measured at the mouth, there is oxygen uptake but no carbon dioxide output: the respiratory exchange ratio is thus zero.

With patent airway and oxygen as the ambient gas. Oxygen is continuously removed from the alveolar gas as described above, but is replaced by oxygen drawn in by mass movement. No nitrogen is added to the alveolar gas, and the alveolar P_{O_2} falls only as fast as the P_{CO_2} rises (about $0.4–0.8\,kPa.min^{-1}$ or $3–6\,mmHg.min^{-1}$). Therefore the patient will not become seriously hypoxic for several minutes. If the patient has been breathing 100% oxygen prior to the respiratory arrest, the starting alveolar P_{O_2} would be of the order of 88 kPa (660 mmHg) and therefore the patient could theoretically survive about 100 minutes of apnoea *provided that his airway remained clear and he remained connected to a supply of 100% oxygen.* This does, in fact, happen and has been demonstrated in both animals and humans,[26] and is referred to as apnoeic mass-movement oxygenation or diffusion respiration. The phenomenon enjoyed a brief vogue in anaesthetic practice as a means of maintaining oxygenation during apnoea, particularly for bronchoscopy,[27] and remains a useful technique for short periods during airway surgery such as laryngectomy.

However, hypercapnia is an inevitable feature of the technique, and arterial P_{CO_2} values as high as 18.7 kPa (140 mmHg) have been reported.[27]

Carbon dioxide carriage during hypothermia

Understanding the carriage of CO_2 during hypothermia is of importance both to clinicians involved in the care of hypothermic patients and to the comparative physiologist studying differences between warm-blooded (homoeothermic) and cold-blooded (poikilothermic) animals. These two diverse areas of physiology have, over recent years, converged to produce two alternative theories regarding the optimal system for CO_2 carriage at low temperature.

In common with most gases, CO_2 becomes more soluble in water as temperature decreases (Table 10.1) such that, in plasma, maintenance of the same P_{CO_2} under hypothermic conditions will require a greater total CO_2 content. In addition, decreasing temperature reduces the ionization of water into H^+ and OH^- ions, so pH increases by approximately 0.016 per degree Celsius.[28] If CO_2 production and excretion remain constant, hypothermia would therefore be expected to result in alkalotic conditions in both the intra- and extracellular spaces. Different animals are believed to respond to these changes in two ways, as follows.

The pH-stat hypothesis,[29] as the name suggests, involves the animal responding to hypothermia by maintaining the same blood pH regardless of its body temperature. This is achieved by hypoventilation, which increases the P_{CO_2} to maintain pH at close to 7.4, and is seen in hibernating mammals. Indeed it is thought possible that the high P_{CO_2}, and the resulting intracellular acidosis, may contribute to the hypothermic 'sleep' state.

The alpha-stat hypothesis is more complex.[28,30] In this situation, the pH of the animal is allowed to change in keeping with the physical chemistry laws described above. As temperature falls, the blood pH, again measured at the animal's body temperature, increases. Studies of protein function and acid–base disturbances have revealed the importance of the α-imidazole moiety of histidine in buffering changes in pH, and that the state of dissociation of these α-imidazole groups is crucial to protein function. The pK of α-imidazole is unique among amino acids in that it changes with temperature to a similar degree as the dissociation of water.[30] Thus as temperature decreases, blood and tissue pH rise but the dissociative state of α-imidazole, and thus protein function, remains close to normal. Most poikilothermic animals use an alpha-stat system and can function well through a broad range of temperatures. Even hibernators, with their pH-stat regulation, maintain an alpha-stat type control of some vital tissues such as heart and brain.[31]

There is controversy about whether the blood gases of humans undergoing cardiac surgery during hypothermia should be managed by the alpha-stat or pH-stat techniques.[32,29] In the former case, arterial blood drawn from the cold patient is warmed to 37°C before measurement of P_{CO_2}, and the cardiopulmonary bypass adjusted to achieve normal values. For pH-stat control, P_{CO_2} is again measured at 37°C but mathematically corrected to the patient's temperature, and then CO_2 administered to the patient to achieve a pH of 7.4. Increased arterial P_{CO_2} during pH-stat will in theory improve cerebral perfusion, and possibly thereby improve cerebral function.[32] However, there remains little evidence that the two forms of blood gas management result in differences in patient well-being during or after hypothermic surgery except at very low temperatures, when pH-stat may be superior.[33]

Outline of methods of measurement of carbon dioxide

Fractional concentration in gas mixtures

Chemical absorption. This remains the reference method of analysis. In medical circles the most accurate method usually employed is Lloyd's modification of the Haldane apparatus.[34] Chemical methods are markedly influenced by the presence of nitrous oxide in gas samples, and modifications of technique are required.[35]

Infrared analysis. This is the most widely used method for rapid breath-to-breath analysis and is also very convenient for analysis of discrete gas samples. Most diatomic gases absorb infrared radiation, and errors may arise owing to overlap of absorption bands and collision broadening.[36] These effects are best overcome by filtering and calibrating with a known concentration of carbon dioxide in a diluent gas mixture that is similar to the gas sample for analysis. Infrared analysers are available with a response time of less than 300 μs, and will follow the respiratory cycle provided the respiratory frequency is not too high. Breathe-through cells (placed near the patient's airway) have a better frequency response than systems that draw gas from the airway for analysis in a distant machine, as mixing of the inspired and expired gases occurs along the sampling tube. Capnography is described in more detail below (page 243).

Mass spectrometry. This powerful technique is established as an alternative method for the rapid analysis of carbon dioxide. The cost is much greater than for infrared analysis, but response times tend to be shorter and there is usually provision for analysis of up to four gases at the same time. In spite of this, mass spectrometry for measurement of respiratory gases remains essentially a research tool.

Blood CO$_2$ partial pressure

The long and fascinating history of measurement of $P\text{CO}_2$ and acid–base has been recorded by others,[37] and only a brief overview is described here.

Historically, $P\text{CO}_2$ was measured by allowing blood to equilibrate with gas, in which the CO$_2$ concentration was then measured. The first practical method, called bubble tonometry, was described as early as 1866 by Plüger and progressively refined for over 100 years. However, the technique always remained very difficult to master and disappeared from use after 1960. For many years $P\text{CO}_2$ was derived indirectly from the Henderson–Hasselbalch equation given earlier in this chapter. It was a most laborious procedure requiring measurements of both pH and CO$_2$ content, and there was always uncertainty of the value that should be taken for pK'.

The interpolation technique. The death knell of the methods described above was sounded by the development of the interpolation method by Siggaard-Andersen and Astrup in Copenhagen. In their approach, $P\text{CO}_2$ of blood was measured by interpolating the actual pH in a plot of log $P\text{CO}_2$ against pH derived from aliquots of the same blood sample. The plot is linear and the whole operation became a practical proposition following the introduction of the microapparatus described by Siggaard-Andersen et al. in 1960.[38]

The $P\text{CO}_2$-sensitive electrode. All the above methods have given way to the $P\text{CO}_2$-sensitive electrode which, in its automated form, has removed the requirement for technical expertise. Analysis may now be performed satisfactorily by untrained staff on a do-it-yourself basis, with results available within 2 minutes.[39] The technique, first described by

Severinghaus and Bradley in 1958,[40] allows the P_{CO_2} of any gas or liquid to be determined directly. The P_{CO_2} of a film of bicarbonate solution is allowed to come into equilibrium with the P_{CO_2} of a sample on the other side of a membrane permeable to carbon dioxide but not to hydrogen ions, usually PTFE. The pH of the bicarbonate solution is constantly monitored by a glass electrode and the log of the P_{CO_2} is inversely proportional to the recorded pH.

Handling of blood samples.[41] It is important that samples be preserved from contact with air, including bubbles and froth in the syringe, to which they may lose carbon dioxide, and either lose or gain oxygen depending on the relative P_{O_2} of the sample and the air. Dilution with excessive volumes of heparin or 'dead space' fluids from indwelling arterial cannulae should be avoided. Analysis should be undertaken quickly, as the P_{CO_2} of blood *in vitro* rises by about 0.013 kPa (0.1 mmHg) per minute at 37°C, whilst P_{O_2} declines at 0.07–0.3 kPa (0.5–2.3 mmHg) per minute, depending on the P_{O_2}. These changes result from metabolic activity, mainly in the white cells.[42] If rapid analysis is not possible (within 10 minutes), the specimen should be stored on ice, which reduces this carbon dioxide production and oxygen consumption by about 90 per cent. Modern blood gas analysers invariably work at 37°C, so for patients with abnormal body temperatures a correction factor should be applied. Nomograms allow correction for both pre-analytic metabolism and patient temperature;[43] they will be found in Appendix E (Figures E.1 and E.2).

Continuous measurement of arterial P_{CO_2} using indwelling arterial catheters is rapidly becoming a realistic clinical technique.[44,45,46] The method uses a 'photochemical optode', which consists of a small optical fibre (140 μm diameter) along which light of a specific wavelength is passed to impinge on a dye incorporated into the tip of the fibre, which lies within the patient's artery. The dye may either absorb the light or fluoresce (give off light of a different wavelength) in a pH-sensitive fashion, and these changes are transmitted back to the analyser via the same or a second optical fibre. For analysis of Pa_{CO_2}, the pH-sensitive optode is again enclosed in a CO_2-permeable PTFE membrane with a bicarbonate buffer in the same way as for the P_{CO_2} electrode but on a very small scale. The current generation of intra-arterial sensors are reasonably accurate with a precision of 0.4–0.8 kPa (3–6 mmHg).

Capnography[47]

Capnograms consist of plots of CO_2 concentration in airway gas against either time or expired volume. Despite the curves being of similar shape (see Figures 8.17 and 10.11), they contain quite different information; for example, time capnography has both inspiratory and expiratory phases whilst CO_2 volume plots only involve expiration. Plots of CO_2 and expired volume allow calculation of anatomical dead space (see Figure 8.17), physiological dead space and tidal volume, but this form of capnography is not commonly used clinically.

In the past there has been confusion over the nomenclature of a normal time capnogram, but the most widely accepted terms are shown in Figure 10.11a. There is an inspiratory phase (0), and expiration is divided into three phases: I represents CO_2-free gas from the apparatus and anatomical dead space; II a rapidly changing mixture of alveolar and dead space gas; III the alveolar plateau, the peak of which represents end-expiratory P_{CO_2}

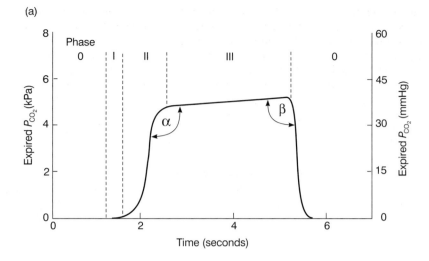

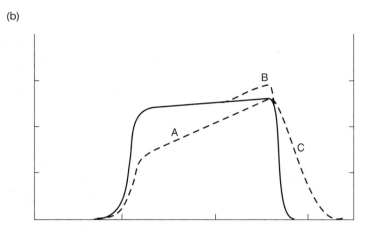

Figure 10.11 Time capnography. (a) Normal trace showing the phases of the respiratory cycle and the angles used to quantify the shape of the capnogram. See text for details. (b) Dashed lines show abnormalities of the trace, which may occur separately or together. A, varying alveolar time constants (page 168) such as asthma; B, phase IV terminal upswing seen in pregnancy and obesity; C, rebreathing of expired gases.

(PE'_{CO_2}). The alpha and beta angles allow quantification of abnormalities of the capnogram. Much information may be obtained from a time capnogram:

1. The inspiratory carbon dioxide concentration.
2. Respiratory rate.
3. The demonstration of the capnogram is a reliable indication of the correct placement of a tracheal tube.
4. PE'_{CO_2} is related to arterial P_{CO_2} (see below).
5. Sudden decrease in PE'_{CO_2} at a fixed level of ventilation is a valuable indication of a sudden reduction in cardiac output (page 239) or a pulmonary embolus (Chapter 28).
6. Cardiac arrest during artificial ventilation will cause PE'_{CO_2} to fall to zero.

There are three principal abnormalities of a capnogram,[47] which may occur separately or together; they are shown in Figure 10.11b. Line A, with an increased alpha angle and phase III slope, results from sequential emptying of fast and slow alveoli. Almost any lung pathology may result in a sloping phase III, and a common clinical cause is acute asthma: line A is typical of a patient with bronchospasm. The gradient of phase III on a capnogram has been proposed as a non-effort-dependent test of the severity of acute asthma.[48] Line B, sometimes referred to as phase IV, is seen in pregnancy and severe obesity. The cause of this appearance is uncertain but may relate to continued evolution of CO_2 from fast alveoli being recorded at the mouth because of the small FRC in which the CO_2 would normally be retained.[47] Line C and an increase in the beta angle occur with rebreathing from either excessive apparatus dead space or a malfunctioning anaesthetic breathing system.

Technical considerations should always be borne in mind when considering abnormalities of a capnogram. The response time of the analyser, excessive lengths of sampling tube and inadequate sampling rates will all tend to 'blunt' the normal capnogram trace. This is a particular problem when the tidal volume is low – for example, in children or tachypnoeic patients.

Arterial to end-expiratory Pco_2 gradient[20] has already been mentioned above (page 237) and occurs to some extent in almost all subjects, but particularly in elderly patients, smokers, those with lung disease or during anaesthesia.[49,50] The magnitude of the difference is greatest in patients with significant alveolar dead space (page 179),[20] who can be identified from the slope of phase III. Attempts to reduce the gradient by forced or prolonged expiration have generally been unsuccessful.[19] Use of $PE'co_2$ as a monitor of absolute arterial Pco_2 is therefore unhelpful, but the assessment remains useful for following changes within a subject.

Other indirect measurements of arterial Pco_2

Measurement of mixed venous Pco_2 may be estimated indirectly with very simple apparatus, using a rebreathing technique described by Campbell and Howell in 1960.[51] There are many problems with the technique, which has been extensively re-evaluated since.[52] Most important is the fact that the rebreathing method measures the Pco_2 of venous blood as it would be if fully oxygenated. The Haldane effect then raises the Pco_2 0.5–1 kPa (3.8–7.5 mmHg) higher than the true mixed venous Pco_2 (see Figure 10.2). Furthermore, the mixed venous/arterial Pco_2 gradient will be increased in hypercapnia (owing to the curvature of the carbon dioxide dissociation curve), as well as with arterial hypoxaemia, reduced cardiac output and anaemia. In general, the observed mixed venous Pco_2 (as measured by the rebreathing technique) is likely to exceed the arterial Pco_2 by 1–2 kPa (7.5–15 mmHg) in the normal resting subject, and this systematic error will be even greater in hypercapnia. Nowadays it is usually simpler to measure arterial Pco_2 directly.

Transcutaneous Pco_2. This technique uses a CO_2-sensitive electrode heated to about 44°C to maximize blood flow to the skin but which is, however, close to the temperature that causes burns. Transcutaneous Pco_2 should be within about 0.5 kPa (3.8 mmHg) of the simultaneous arterial value, but it is necessary to apply a large correction factor for the difference in temperature between body and electrode.[53]

Venous Pco_2. Blood draining skin has a very small arterial/venous Po_2 difference and results are quite acceptable for clinical purposes.[54] However, it is surprisingly difficult to collect a good sample of blood anaerobically from the veins on the back of the hand, and blood from veins draining muscles (e.g. the median cubital vein) has a P_{CO_2} much higher than the arterial level and is useless as an indication of the arterial P_{CO_2}.

Capillary P_{CO_2}. Blood obtained from a skin prick suffers from the same uncertainties that surround cutaneous venous P_{CO_2}. However, the technique is clearly useful in neonates. The likely error (say 0.6 kPa or 4.5 mmHg) is seldom of much consequence in the management of a patient.

References

1. Severinghaus JW, Stupfel M, Bradley AF. Accuracy of blood pH and P_{CO_2} determinations. *J Appl Physiol* 1956; **9**: 189–96.
2. Severinghaus JW, Stupfel M, Bradley AF. Variations in serum carbonic acid pK' with pH and temperature. *J Appl Physiol* 1956; **9**: 197–200.
3. Klocke RA. Carbon dioxide transport. In: Fishman AP, ed. *Handbook of physiology: Section 3: The respiratory system.* Bethesda MD: American Physiological Society, 1987; 173–97.
4. Henry RP. Multiple roles of carbonic anhydrase in cellular transport and metabolism. *Annu Rev Physiol* 1996; **58**: 523–38.
5. Effros RM, Mason G, Silverman P. Asymmetric distribution of carbonic anhydrase in the alveolar–capillary barrier. *J Appl Physiol* 1981; **51**: 190–3.
6. Meldrum NU, Roughton FJW. Carbonic anhydrase: its preparation and properties. *J Physiol* 1933; **80**: 113–42.
7. Sly WS, Hu PY. Human carbonic anhydrases and carbonic anhydrase deficiencies. *Annu Rev Biochem* 1995; **64**: 375–401.
8. Henderson LJ. Das Gleichgewicht zwischen Basen und Säuren im tierischen Organismus. *Ergebn Physiol* 1909; **8**: 254.
9. Hasselbalch KA. Die Berechnung der Wasserstoffzahl des Blutes usw. *Biochem Z* 1916; **78**: 112–44.
10. Klocke RA. Carbon dioxide. In: Crystal RG, West JB, eds. *The lung: scientific foundations.* New York: Raven, 1991; 1233.
11. Christiansen J, Douglas CG, Haldane JS. The adsorption and dissociation of carbon dioxide by human blood. *J Physiol* 1914; **48**: 244–71.
12. Ferguson JKW, Roughton FJW. The direct chemical estimation of carbamino compounds of CO_2 with haemoglobin. *J Physiol* 1934; **83**: 68–86.
13. Hamburger HJ. Anionenwanderungen in serum und Blut unter dem Einfluss von CO_2. Säure und Alkali. *Biochem Z* 1918; **86**: 309.
14. Tanner MJA. Molecular and cellular biology of the erythrocyte anion exchanger (AE1). *Semin Hematol* 1993; **30**: 34–57.
15. Jay DG. Role of band 3 in homeostasis and cell shape. *Cell* 1996; **86**: 853–4.
16. Siggaard-Andersen O. *The acid base status of blood.* Copenhagen: Munksgaard, 1964.
17. Prys-Roberts C, Kelman GR, Nunn JF. Determination of the in vivo carbon dioxide titration curve of anaesthetized man. *Br J Anaesth* 1966; **38**: 500–9.
18. Nunn JF, Newman HC. Inspired gas, rebreathing and apparatus dead space. *Br J Anaesth* 1964; **36**: 5–10.
19. Tavernier B, Rey D, Thevenin D, Triboulet J-P, Scherpereel P. Can prolonged expiration manoeuvres improve the prediction of arterial P_{CO_2} from end-tidal P_{CO_2}? *Br J Anaesth* 1997; **78**: 536–540.
20. Nunn JF, Hill DW. Respiratory dead space and arterial to end tidal CO_2 tension difference in anesthetized man. *J Appl Physiol* 1960; **15**: 383–9.
21. Ivanov SD, Nunn JF. Influence of the duration of hyperventilation on rise time of P_{CO_2} after step reduction of ventilation. *Respir Physiol* 1968; **5**: 243–9.
22. Shibutani K, Muraoka M, Shirasaki S, Kubal K, Sanchala VT, Gupte P. Do changes in end-tidal P_{CO_2} quantitatively reflect changes in cardiac output. *Anesth Analg* 1994; **79**: 829–33.

23. Leigh MD, Jenkins LC, Belton MK, Lewis GB. Continuous alveolar carbon dioxide analysis as a monitor of pulmonary blood flow. *Anesthesiology* 1957; **18**: 878–82.
24. Sanders AB. Capnometry in emergency medicine. *Ann Emerg Med* 1989; **18**: 1287–90.
25. Stock MC, Downs JB, McDonald JS, Silver MJ, McSweeney TD, Fairley DS. The carbon dioxide rate of rise in awake apneic humans. *J Clin Anesth* 1988; **1**: 96–9.
26. Frumin MJ, Epstein RM, Cohen G. Apneic oxygenation in man. *Anesthesiology* 1959; **20**: 789–98.
27. Payne JP. Apnoeic oxygenation in anaesthetised man. *Acta Anaesth Scand* 1962; **6**: 129–42.
28. Nattie EE. The alphastat hypothesis in respiratory control and acid–base balance. *J Appl Physiol* 1990; **69**: 1201–7.
29. Burrows FA. Con: pH-stat management of blood gases is preferable to alpha-stat in patients undergoing brain cooling for cardiac surgery. *J Cardiothorac Vasc Anesth* 1995; **9**: 219–21.
30. Reeves RB. An imidazole alphastat hypothesis for vertebrate acid–base regulation: tissue carbon dioxide content and body temperature in bullfrogs. *Respir Physiol* 1972; **14**:219–36
31. Swain JA, McDonald TJ, Robbins RC, Balaban RS. Relationship of cerebral and myocardial intracellular pH to blood pH during hypothermia. *Am J Physiol* 1991; **260**: H1640–4.
32. Kern FH, Greeley WJ. Pro: pH-stat management of blood gases is not preferable to alpha-stat in patients undergoing brain cooling for cardiac surgery. *J Cardiothorac Vasc Anesth* 1995; **9**: 215–18.
33. Jonas RA, Bellinger PC, Rappaport LA, Wernovsky G, Hickey PR, Farrell DM, Newburger JW. Relation of pH strategy and developmental outcome after hypothermic circulatory arrest. *J Thorac Cardiovasc Surg* 1993; **106**: 362–8.
34. Cormack RS. Eliminating two sources of error in the Lloyd–Haldane apparatus. *Respir Physiol* 1972; **14**: 382–90.
35. Meade F, Owen-Thomas JB. The estimation of carbon dioxide concentration in the presence of nitrous oxide using the Lloyd–Haldane apparatus. *Br J Anaesth* 1975; **47**: 22–4.
36. Cooper EA. Infra-red analysis for the estimation of carbon dioxide in the presence of nitrous oxide. *Br J Anaesth* 1957; **29**: 486–90.
37. Severinghaus JW, Astrup PB. History of blood gas analysis. III. Carbon dioxide tension. *J Clin Monit* 1986; **2**: 60–73.
38. Siggaard-Andersen O, Engel K, Jorgensen K, Astrup P. A micro-method for determination of pH, carbon dioxide tension, base excess and standard bicarbonate in capillary blood. *Scand J Clin Lab Invest* 1960; **12**: 172–6.
39. Minty BD, Barrett AM. Accuracy of automated blood-gas analyser operated by untrained staff. *Br J Anaesth* 1978; **50**: 1031–9.
40. Severinghaus JW, Bradley AF. Electrodes for blood Po_2 and Pco_2 determination. *J Appl Physiol* 1958; **13**: 515–20.
41. Szaflarski NL. Preanalytic error associated with blood gas/pH measurement. *Crit Care Nurse* 1996; **16**: 89–100.
42. Nunn JF, Sturrock JE, Jones AJ, O'Morain C, Segal AW, Coade SB et al. Halothane does not inhibit human neutrophil function in vitro. *Br J Anaesth* 1979; **51**: 1101–5.
43. Kelman GR, Nunn JF. Nomograms for correction of blood Po_2, Pco_2, pH and base excess for time and temperature. *J Appl Physiol* 1966; **21**: 1484–90.
44. Szaflarski NL. Emerging technology in critical care: continuous intra-arterial blood gas monitoring. *Am J Crit Care* 1996; **5**: 55–65.
45. Gravenstein N. Monitoring of blood gases: blood gas measurement, oximetry and capnometry. *Curr Opin Anaesthesiol* 1990; **3**: 881–5.
46. Weiss IK, Fink S, Edmunds S, Harrison R, Donnelly K. Continuous arterial gas monitoring: initial experience with the Paratrend 7 in children. *Intensive Care Med* 1996; **22**: 1414–17.
47. Bhavani-Shankar K, Kumar AY, Moseley HSL, Ahyee-Hallsworth R. Terminology and the current limitations of time capnography: a brief review. *J Clin Monit* 1995; **11**: 175–82.
48. Yaron M, Padyk P, Hutsinpiller M, Cairns CB. Utility of the expiratory capnogram in the assessment of bronchospasm. *Ann Emerg Med* 1996; **28**: 403–7.
49. Wahba RWM, Tessler MJ. Misleading end-tidal CO_2 tensions. *Can J Anaesth* 1996; **43**: 862–6.
50. Fletcher R. Smoking, age and the arterial–end tidal Pco_2 difference during anaesthesia and controlled ventilation. *Acta Anaesthesiol Scand* 1987; **31**: 355–6.

51. Campbell EJM, Howell JBL. Simple rapid methods of estimating arterial and mixed venous P_{CO_2}. *BMJ* 1960; **1**: 458–62.

52. McEvoy JDS, Jones NL, Campbell EJM. Mixed venous and arterial P_{CO_2}. *BMJ* 1974; **4**: 687–90.

53. Severinghaus JW. A combined transcutaneous P_{O_2}–P_{CO_2} electrode with electrochemical HCO_3^- stabilization. *J Appl Physiol* 1981; **51**: 1027–32.

54. Forster HV, Dempsey JA, Thomson J, Vidruk E, doPico GA. Estimation of arterial P_{O_2}, P_{CO_2}, pH and lactate from arterialized venous blood. *J Appl Physiol* 1972; **32**: 134–7.

Chapter 11

Oxygen

The appearance of oxygen in the atmosphere of this planet has played a crucial role in the development of life (see Chapter 1). The whole of the animal kingdom is totally dependent on oxygen, not only for function but also for survival. This is notwithstanding the fact that oxygen is extremely toxic in the absence of elaborate defence mechanisms at a cellular level (see Chapter 25). Before considering the role of oxygen in the cell, it is necessary to bring together many strands from previous chapters and outline the transport of oxygen all the way from the atmosphere to the cell.

The oxygen cascade

The Po_2 of dry air at sea level is 21.2 kPa (159 mmHg). Oxygen moves down a partial pressure gradient from air, through the respiratory tract, the alveolar gas, the arterial blood, the systemic capillaries, the tissues and the cell. It finally reaches its lowest level in the mitochondria, where it is consumed (Figure 11.1). At this point, the Po_2 is probably in the range 0.5–3 kPa (3.8–22.5 mmHg), varying from one tissue to another, from one cell to another, and from one part of a cell to another.

The steps by which the Po_2 decreases from air to the mitochondria are known as the oxygen cascade and are of great practical importance. Any one step in the cascade may be increased under pathological circumstances and this may result in hypoxia. The steps are now considered *seriatim*.

Dilution of inspired oxygen by water vapour

Analysis of oxygen concentration by a chemical method such as the Haldane apparatus indicates the fractional concentration of oxygen in a *dry* gas mixture. If the gas sample is humidified, the added water vapour is ignored and the indicated fractional concentration of oxygen is still that of the dry part of the mixture. Thus the normally quoted value for the concentration of atmospheric oxygen (20.94% or 0.2094 fractional concentration) indicates the concentration of oxygen in dry gas.

As gas is inhaled through the respiratory tract, it becomes humidified at body temperature and the added water vapour dilutes the oxygen, and so reduces the Po_2 below its level in the ambient air. When dry gas at normal barometric pressure becomes fully saturated with water vapour at 37°C, 100 volumes of the dry gas take up about 6 volumes of water vapour, giving a total gas volume of 106 units but containing the same number

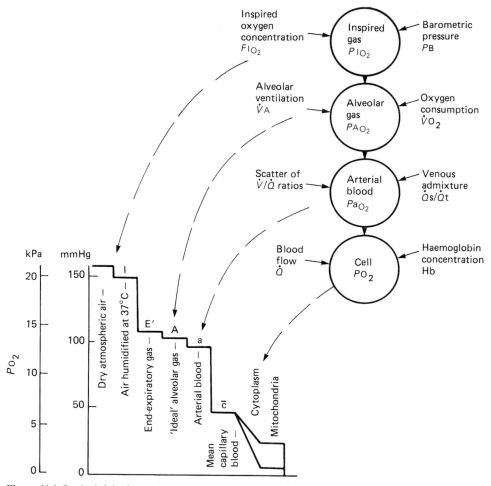

Figure 11.1 On the left is shown the oxygen cascade with Po_2 falling from the level in the ambient air down to the level in mitochondria. On the right is a summary of the factors influencing oxygenation at different levels in the cascade.

of molecules of oxygen. The Po_2 is thus reduced by the fraction 6/106. It follows from Boyle's law that Po_2 after humidification is indicated by the following expression:

$$\text{fractional concentration of oxygen in the dry gas phase (Haldane value)} \times \left(\text{barometric pressure} - \text{saturated water vapour pressure} \right)$$

(the quantity in parentheses is known as the dry barometric pressure)

Therefore the effective Po_2 of inspired air at a body temperature of 37°C is:

$$0.2094 \times (101.3 - 6.3) = 0.2094 \times 95$$
$$= 19.9\,\text{kPa}$$

or, in old units:

$$0.2094 \times (760 - 47) = 0.2094 \times 713$$
$$= 149\,\text{kPa}$$

Primary factors influencing alveolar oxygen tension

The general equation for the calculation of the alveolar tension of a gas has been stated on pages 130 *et seq.* In the case of oxygen:

$$\text{alveolar } Po_2 \doteqdot \begin{pmatrix} \text{dry} \\ \text{barometric} \\ \text{pressure} \end{pmatrix} \left(\begin{matrix} \text{inspired} \\ \text{oxygen} \\ \text{concentration} \end{matrix} - \frac{\text{oxygen uptake}}{\text{alveolar ventilation}} \right) \quad \ldots(1)$$

This equation is only approximate and does not include the second order correction factor due to the small difference in volume between the inspired and the expired gas. Normally this factor is small but, during the exchange of a soluble gas such as nitrous oxide, the difference may be quite large.

Various forms of the alveolar air equation may be used to correct for this difference (pages 192 *et seq.*). The commonest forms assume that the number of molecules of nitrogen inhaled equals the number exhaled. This is not the case when the composition of the inspired gas has been changed, as for example during anaesthesia and intensive care. Therefore, in these circumstances it is necessary to use a special form of the equation introduced by Filley and colleagues in 1954,[1] which makes no assumptions of inert gas equilibrium and is appropriate to most of the varied conditions likely to be encountered in clinical practice:

$$P_{A_{O_2}} = P_{I_{O_2}} - P_{A_{CO_2}} \left(\frac{P_{I_{O_2}} - P_{\bar{E}_{O_2}}}{P_{\bar{E}_{CO_2}}} \right) \quad \ldots(2)$$

In its more accurate forms (e.g. equation 2), the alveolar air equation is used principally for calculation of the 'ideal' alveolar Po_2, a theoretical entity that was introduced on page 173 and explained in greater detail on pages 192 *et seq.* 'Ideal' alveolar gas has the same composition as gas from an imaginary alveolus with the ventilation/perfusion ratio of the lungs as a whole. In practice, it is defined as having a Pco_2 equal to that of arterial blood and a respiratory exchange ratio equal to that of mixed expired gas. Comparison of 'ideal' alveolar Po_2 with arterial Po_2 is the basis of quantification of 'venous admixture' (pages 181 *et seq.*).

In its simplified form (equation 1), the alveolar air equation is particularly useful for consideration of the important quantitative relationships between alveolar Po_2 and the factors that directly influence it, which will now be considered.

Dry barometric pressure. If other factors remain constant, the alveolar Po_2 will be directly proportional to the dry barometric pressure. Thus with increasing altitude, alveolar Po_2 falls progressively to become zero at 19 kilometres where the actual barometric pressure equals the saturated vapour pressure of water at body temperature (see Table 16.1). The effect of increased pressure is complex (see Chapter 17); for example, a pressure of 10 atmospheres (absolute) increases the alveolar Po_2 by a factor of about 15 if other factors remain constant (see Table 17.2).

Inspired oxygen concentration. The alveolar Po_2 will be raised or lowered by an amount equal to the change in the inspired gas Po_2, provided that other factors remain constant. Because the concentration of oxygen in the inspired gas should always be under control, it is a most important therapeutic tool, which may be used to counteract a number of different factors that may impair oxygenation.

Figure 11.2 shows the effect of an increase in the inspired oxygen concentration from 21 to 30% on the relationship between alveolar Po_2 and alveolar ventilation. For any

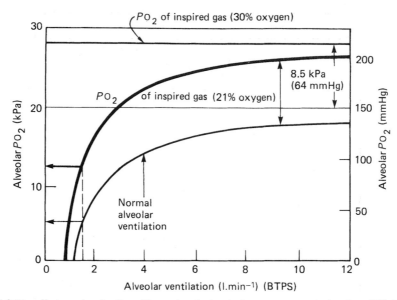

Figure 11.2 The effect on alveolar P_{O_2} of increasing the inspired oxygen concentration from 21% (thin curve) to 30% (heavy curve). In this example, the alveolar P_{O_2} is reduced to a dangerously low level when breathing air at an alveolar minute ventilation of $1.5 \, l.min^{-1}$. In this situation, oxygen enrichment of the inspired gas to 30% is sufficient to raise the alveolar P_{O_2} almost to within the normal range. Oxygen consumption is assumed to be $200 \, ml.min^{-1}$ (STPD).

alveolar ventilation, the improvement of alveolar P_{O_2} will be 8.5 kPa (64 mmHg). This will be of great importance if, for example, hypoventilation while breathing air has reduced the alveolar P_{O_2} to 4 kPa (30 mmHg), a value that is close to the lowest level compatible with life. Oxygen enrichment of inspired gas to 30 per cent will then increase the alveolar P_{O_2} to 12.5 kPa (94 mmHg), which is almost within the normal range. However, at this level of hypoventilation, P_{CO_2} would be about 13 kPa (98 mmHg) and might well have risen further on withdrawal of the hypoxic drive to ventilation. In fact, 30 per cent is the maximum concentration of oxygen in the inspired gas that should be required to correct the alveolar P_{O_2} of a patient breathing air, who has become hypoxaemic purely as a result of hypoventilation. This problem is discussed at some length in Chapter 26 (pages 522 *et seq.*). Figure 6.12 shows ventilation/alveolar P_{O_2} curves for a wide range of inspired oxygen concentrations, indicating the protection against hypoxaemia (due to hypoventilation) that is afforded by different concentrations of oxygen in the inspired gas.

An entirely different problem is hypoxaemia due to venous admixture. This results in an increased alveolar/arterial P_{O_2} difference, which, within limits, can be offset by increasing the alveolar P_{O_2}. Quantitative aspects are quite different from the problem of hypoventilation and are considered later in this chapter.

Oxygen consumption. In the past there has been an unfortunate tendency to consider that all patients consume 250 ml of oxygen per minute under all circumstances. Oxygen consumption must, of course, be raised by exercise but is often well above basal in a patient supposedly 'at rest'. This may be due to restlessness, pain, increased work of breathing or the formation of oxygen-derived free radicals. These factors may well coexist

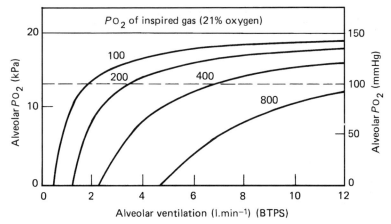

Figure 11.3 The relationship between alveolar ventilation and alveolar P_{O_2} for different values of oxygen consumption for a patient breathing air at normal barometric pressure. The figures on the curves indicate the oxygen consumption in ml.min^{-1} (STPD). A value of 100 ml.min^{-1} is typical of a hypothermic patient at 30°C, 200 ml.min^{-1}, a normal subject at rest or during anaesthesia, and higher values result from exercise or fever. Note that the alveolar ventilation required to maintain any particular alveolar P_{O_2} is directly proportional to the oxygen consumption. (In calculations of this type it is important to make the correction required by the fact that oxygen consumption and alveolar ventilation values are commonly expressed at different temperatures and pressures – see Appendix C.)

with failure of other factors controlling the arterial P_{O_2}. Thus, for example, a patient may be caught by the pincers of a falling ventilatory capacity and a rising ventilatory requirement (see Figure 26.4).

Figure 11.3 shows the effect of different values for oxygen consumption on the relationship between alveolar ventilation and alveolar P_{O_2} for a patient breathing air, and clearly reveals the potential for an increase in oxygen consumption to cause hypoxia. Altered oxygen consumption is very common in patients, being substantially increased with fever, thyrotoxicosis or convulsions, all situations that may lead to difficulties with weaning patients from artificial ventilation. Oxygen consumption is reduced with anaesthesia, hypothyroidism or hypothermia, the last of which causes a marked reduction in oxygen consumption, with values of about 50 per cent of normal at 31°C.

Alveolar ventilation. The alveolar air equation for oxygen in the form given in equation (1) implies a hyperbolic relationship between alveolar P_{O_2} and alveolar ventilation. This relationship, which is considered in Appendix F, has very important clinical relevance. As ventilation is increased, the alveolar P_{O_2} rises asymptotically towards (but never reaches) the P_{O_2} of the inspired gas (Figure 11.2). It will be seen from the shape of the curves that changes in ventilation above normal level have comparatively little effect on alveolar P_{O_2}. In contrast, changes in ventilation below the normal level may have a very marked effect. At very low levels of ventilation, the alveolar ventilation becomes critical and small changes may precipitate gross hypoxia. Note that there is a finite alveolar ventilation at which alveolar P_{O_2} becomes zero.

Secondary factors influencing alveolar oxygen tension

Cardiac output. In the short term, cardiac output can influence the alveolar P_{O_2}. For example, if other factors remain constant, a sudden reduction in cardiac output will temporarily increase the alveolar P_{O_2}, because less blood passes through the lungs to remove oxygen from the alveolar gas. However, the reduced cardiac output also causes increased oxygen extraction in the tissues supplied by the systemic circulation, and before long the mixed venous oxygen level is decreased. When that has happened, the removal of oxygen from the alveolar gas returns to its original level as the reduction in blood flow rate is compensated by the greater amount of oxygen that is taken up per unit volume of blood flowing through the lungs. Thus, in the long term, cardiac output does not directly influence the alveolar P_{O_2}, and therefore it does not appear in equation (1).

The 'concentration', third gas or Fink effect. The diagrams and equations above have ignored a factor that influences alveolar P_{O_2} during exchanges of large quantities of soluble gases such as nitrous oxide. This effect was mentioned briefly in connection with carbon dioxide on page 236 but its effect on oxygen is probably more important. During the early part of the administration of nitrous oxide, large quantities of the more soluble gas replace smaller quantities of the less soluble nitrogen previously dissolved in body fluids. There is thus a net transfer of 'inert' gas from the alveoli into the body, causing a *temporary* increase in the concentration of both oxygen and carbon dioxide, which will thus *temporarily* exert a higher tension than would otherwise be expected. Conversely, during recovery from nitrous oxide anaesthesia, large quantities of nitrous oxide leave the body to be replaced with smaller quantities of nitrogen. There is thus a net outpouring of 'inert' gas from the body into the alveoli, causing dilution of oxygen and carbon dioxide, both of which will *temporarily* exert a lower tension than would otherwise be expected. There may then be *temporary* hypoxia, the direct reduction of alveolar P_{O_2} sometimes being exacerbated by ventilatory depression due to decreased alveolar P_{CO_2}. Fortunately, such effects last only a few minutes and hypoxia can easily be prevented by increasing the inspired oxygen concentration when nitrous oxide administration is stopped.

The alveolar/arterial P_{O_2} difference

The next step in the oxygen cascade is of great clinical relevance. In the healthy young adult breathing air, the alveolar/arterial P_{O_2} difference does not exceed 2 kPa (15 mmHg) but it may rise to above 5 kPa (37.5 mmHg) in aged but healthy subjects. These values may be exceeded in a patient with any lung disease that causes shunting or mismatching of ventilation to perfusion. An increased alveolar/arterial P_{O_2} difference is the commonest cause of arterial hypoxaemia in clinical practice and is therefore a very important step in the oxygen cascade.

Unlike the alveolar P_{O_2}, the alveolar/arterial P_{O_2} difference cannot be predicted from other more easily measured quantities. There is no simple means of knowing the magnitude of the alveolar/arterial P_{O_2} difference in a particular patient other than by measurement of the arterial blood gas tensions and calculation of alveolar P_{O_2}. Therefore, it is particularly important to understand the factors that influence the difference, and the principles of restoration of arterial P_{O_2} by increasing the inspired oxygen concentration when hypoxia is due to an increased alveolar/arterial P_{O_2} difference.

Factors influencing the magnitude of the alveolar/arterial P_{O_2} difference

In Chapter 8 it was explained how the alveolar/arterial P_{O_2} difference results from venous admixture (or physiological shunt), which consists of two components: (1) shunted venous blood that mingles with the oxygenated blood leaving the pulmonary capillaries; (2) a component due to scatter of ventilation/perfusion ratios in different parts of the lungs. Any component due to impaired diffusion across the alveolar/capillary membrane is likely to be very small and in most circumstances can probably be ignored.

Figure 8.11 shows the derivation of the following axiomatic relationship for the first component, shunted venous blood:

$$\frac{\dot{Q}s}{\dot{Q}t} = \frac{Cc'_{O_2} - Ca_{O_2}}{Cc'_{O_2} - C\bar{v}_{O_2}}$$

Two points should be noted.

1. The equation gives a slightly false impression of precision because it assumes that all the shunted blood has the same oxygen content as mixed venous blood. This is not the case, thebesian and bronchial venous blood being obvious exceptions (see Figure 7.1).
2. Oxygen content of pulmonary end-capillary blood (Cc'_{O_2}) is, in practice, calculated on the basis of the end-capillary oxygen tension (Pc'_{O_2}) being equal to the 'ideal' alveolar P_{O_2}, which is derived by means of the alveolar air equation (see page 192).

The equation may be cleared and solved for the pulmonary end-capillary/arterial oxygen content difference as follows:

$$Cc'_{O_2} - Ca_{O_2} = \frac{\dfrac{\dot{Q}s}{\dot{Q}t}(Ca_{O_2} - C\bar{v}_{O_2})}{1 - \dfrac{\dot{Q}s}{\dot{Q}t}} \qquad \ldots(3)$$

(scaling factors are required to correct for the inconsistency of the units that are customarily used for the quantities in this equation).

$Ca_{O_2} - C\bar{v}_{O_2}$ is the arterial/mixed venous oxygen content difference and is a function of the oxygen consumption and the cardiac output thus

$$\dot{Q}t(Ca_{O_2} - C\bar{v}_{O_2}) = \dot{V}_{O_2} \text{ (Fick Equation)} \qquad \ldots(4)$$

Substituting for $Ca_{O_2} - C\bar{v}_{O_2}$ in equation (3), we have:

$$Cc'_{O_2} - Ca_{O_2} = \frac{\dot{V}_{O_2}\dfrac{\dot{Q}s}{\dot{Q}t}}{\dot{Q}t\left(1 - \dfrac{\dot{Q}s}{\dot{Q}t}\right)} \qquad \ldots(5)$$

This equation shows the content difference in terms of oxygen consumption ($\dot{V}_{O_2}$), the venous admixture ($\dot{Q}s/\dot{Q}t$) and the cardiac output ($\dot{Q}t$).

The final stage in the calculation is to convert the end-capillary/arterial oxygen *content* difference to the *tension* difference. The oxygen content of blood is the sum of the oxygen in physical solution and that which is combined with haemoglobin:

$$\text{oxygen content of blood} = \alpha P_{O_2} + (S_{O_2} \times [\text{Hb}] \times 1.31)$$

where: α is the solubility coefficient of oxygen in blood (not plasma); S_{O_2} is the haemoglobin saturation, and varies with P_{O_2} according to the oxygen dissociation curve,

Table 11.1 Oxygen content of human blood (ml.dl^{-1}) as a function of Po_2 and other variables

	Haemoglobin concentration (g.dl^{-1})		
	10	*14*	*18*
Normal			
Po_2 at pH 7.4, 37°C, base excess zero:			
6.7 kPa (50 mmHg)	11.99	16.72	21.45
13.3 kPa (100 mmHg)	13.85	19.27	24.69
26.7 kPa (200 mmHg)	14.41	19.94	25.47
Respiratory acidosis			
Po_2 at pH 7.2, 37°C, base excess zero:			
6.7 kPa (50 mmHg)	10.45	14.57	18.69
13.3 kPa (100 mmHg)	13.62	18.94	24.27
26.7 kPa (200 mmHg)	14.37	19.87	25.38
Hypothermia			
Po_2 at pH 7.4, 34°C, base excess zero:			
6.7 kPa (50 mmHg)	12.81	17.87	22.93
13.3 kPa (100 mmHg)	13.96	19.43	24.89
26.7 kPa (200 mmHg)	14.44	19.98	25.51

The fourth significant figure is not of clinical importance but is useful for interpolation. Data are from reference 2.

which itself is influenced by temperature, pH and base excess (Bohr effect); [Hb] is the haemoglobin concentration (g.dl^{-1}); and 1.31 is the volume of oxygen (ml) that has been found to combine with 1 g of haemoglobin (page 264). Carriage of oxygen in the blood is discussed in detail on pages 261 *et seq.*

Derivation of the oxygen content from the Po_2 is laborious if due account is taken of pH, base excess, temperature and haemoglobin concentration. Derivation of Po_2 from content is even more laborious, as an iterative approach is required. Tables of tension/content relationships are therefore particularly useful; Table 11.1 is an extract from one such table to show the format and general influence of the several variables.[2]

The principal factors influencing the magnitude of the alveolar/arterial Po_2 difference caused by venous admixture may be summarized as follows.

The magnitude of the venous admixture increases the alveolar/arterial Po_2 difference with direct proportionality for small shunts, although this is lost with larger shunts (Figure 11.4). The resultant effect on arterial Po_2 is shown in Figure 8.12. Different forms of venous admixture are considered on pages 181 *et seq.*

$\dot{V}/\dot{Q}$ scatter. It was explained in Chapter 8 that scatter in ventilation/perfusion ratios produces an alveolar/arterial Po_2 difference for the following reasons:

1. More blood flows through the underventilated overperfused alveoli, and the mixed arterial blood is therefore heavily weighted in the direction of the suboxygenated blood from areas of low $\dot{V}/\dot{Q}$ ratio. The smaller amount of blood flowing through areas of high $\dot{V}/\dot{Q}$ ratio cannot compensate for this (see Figure 8.13).
2. Owing to the bend in the dissociation curve around a Po_2 of 8 kPa the fall in saturation in blood from areas of low $\dot{V}/\dot{Q}$ ratio tends to be greater than the rise in saturation in blood from areas of correspondingly high $\dot{V}/\dot{Q}$ (see Figure 8.14).

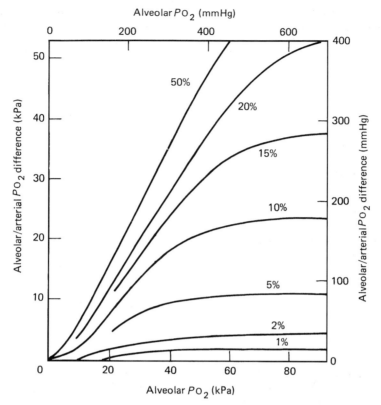

Figure 11.4 Influence of shunt on alveolar/arterial Po_2 difference at different levels of alveolar Po_2. For small shunts, the difference (at constant alveolar Po_2) is roughly proportional to the magnitude of the shunt. For a given shunt, the alveolar/arterial Po_2 difference increases with alveolar Po_2 in a non-linear manner governed by the oxygen dissociation curve. At high alveolar Po_2, a plateau of alveolar/arterial Po_2 difference is reached, but the alveolar Po_2 at which the plateau is reached is higher with larger shunts. Note that, with a 50% shunt, an increase in alveolar Po_2 produces an almost equal increase in alveolar/arterial Po_2 difference. Therefore, the arterial Po_2 is virtually independent of changes in alveolar Po_2, if other factors remain constant. Constants incorporated into the diagram: arterial/venous oxygen content difference, 5ml.dl^{-1}; Hb concentration 14 g.dl^{-1}; temperature of blood, 37°C; pH of blood, 7.40; base excess, zero. Figures in the graph indicate shunt as percentage of total pulmonary blood flow.

These two reasons in combination explain why blood from alveoli with a high $\dot{V}/\dot{Q}$ ratio cannot compensate for blood from alveoli with a low $\dot{V}/\dot{Q}$ ratio.

The actual alveolar Po_2 has a profound but complex and non-linear effect on the alveolar/arterial Po_2 gradient (Figure 11.4). The alveolar/arterial oxygen *content* difference for a given shunt is uninfluenced by the alveolar Po_2 (equation 5), and the effect on the *tension* difference arises entirely in conversion from content to tension: it is thus a function of the slope of the dissociation curve at the Po_2 of the alveolar gas. For example, a loss of 1 ml per 100 ml of oxygen from blood with a Po_2 of 93 kPa (700 mmHg) causes a fall of Po_2 of about 43 kPa (325 mmHg), most of the oxygen being lost from physical solution. However, if the initial Po_2 were 13 kPa (100 mmHg), a loss of 1 ml per 100 ml would cause a fall of Po_2 of only 4.6 kPa (35 mmHg), most of the oxygen being lost from combination with haemoglobin. If the initial P_{O_2} is only 6.7 kPa (50 mmHg), a loss of 1 ml per 100 ml would cause a very small change in P_{O_2} of the order of 0.7 kPa (5 mmHg), drawn almost entirely from combination with haemoglobin at a point where the dissociation curve is steep.

The quantitative considerations outlined in the previous paragraph have most important clinical implications. Figure 11.4 clearly shows that, for the same degree of shunt, the alveolar/arterial P_{O_2} difference will be greatest when the alveolar P_{O_2} is highest. If the alveolar P_{O_2} is reduced (e.g. by underventilation), the alveolar/arterial P_{O_2} gradient will also be diminished if other factors remain the same. The arterial P_{O_2} thus falls less than the alveolar P_{O_2}. This is fortunate and may be considered as one of the many benefits deriving from the shape of the oxygen dissociation curve. With a 50 per cent venous admixture, changes in the alveolar P_{O_2} are almost exactly equal to the resultant changes in the alveolar/arterial P_{O_2} difference (Figure 11.4). Therefore, the arterial P_{O_2} is almost independent of changes in alveolar P_{O_2}, and administration of oxygen will do little to relieve cyanosis (see Figure 8.12).

Cardiac output changes have extremely complex effects on the alveolar/arterial P_{O_2} difference. The Fick relationship (equation 4, page 255) tells us that a reduced cardiac output *per se* must increase the arterial/mixed venous oxygen content difference if the oxygen consumption remains the same. This means that the shunted blood will be more desaturated, and will therefore cause a greater decrease in the arterial oxygen level than would less desaturated blood flowing through a shunt of the same magnitude. Equation (5) shows an inverse relationship between the cardiac output and the alveolar/arterial oxygen content difference if the venous admixture is constant (Figure 11.5b). However, when the content difference is converted to tension difference, the relationship to cardiac output is no longer truly inverse, but assumes a complex non-linear form in consequence of the shape of the oxygen dissociation curve. An example of the relationship between cardiac output and alveolar/arterial P_{O_2} difference is shown in Figure 11.5a but this applies only to the conditions specified, with an alveolar P_{O_2} of 24 kPa (180 mmHg).

Unfortunately, the influence of cardiac output is even more complicated because it has been observed that a reduction in cardiac output is almost always associated with a reduction in the shunt fraction. Conversely, an increase in cardiac output usually results in an increased shunt fraction. This approximately counteracts the effect on mixed venous desaturation, so arterial P_{O_2} tends to be relatively little influenced by changes in cardiac output (see Chapter 8, page 185). Nevertheless, it must be remembered that, even if the arterial P_{O_2} is unchanged, the oxygen delivery (flux) will be reduced in proportion to the change in cardiac output.

Temperature, pH and base excess of the patient's blood influence the dissociation curve (page 266). In addition, temperature affects the solubility coefficient of oxygen in blood. Thus all three factors influence the relationship between tension and content (see Table 11.1), and therefore the effect of venous admixture on the alveolar/arterial P_{O_2} difference, although the effect is not usually important except in extreme deviations from normal.

Haemoglobin concentration influences the partition of oxygen between physical solution and chemical combination. Although the haemoglobin concentration does not influence the pulmonary end-capillary/arterial oxygen *content* difference (equation 5), it does alter the *tension* difference. An increased haemoglobin concentration causes a small decrease in the alveolar/arterial P_{O_2} difference. Table 11.2 shows an example with a cardiac output of 5 l.min^{-1}, oxygen consumption of 200 ml.min^{-1} and a venous admixture of 20 per cent.

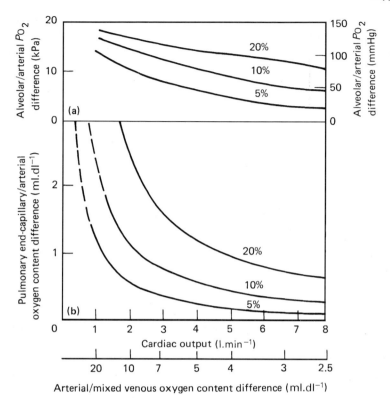

Figure 11.5 Influence of cardiac output on the alveolar/arterial Po_2 difference in the presence of shunts (values indicated for each curve). In this example it is assumed that the patient has an oxygen consumption of 200 ml.min^{-1} and an alveolar Pco_2 of 24 kPa (180 mmHg). Changes in cardiac output produce an inverse change in the pulmonary end-capillary/arterial oxygen content difference (graph b). When converted to tension differences, the inverse relationship is distorted by the effect of the oxygen dissociation curve in a manner which is applicable only to the particular alveolar Po_2 of the patient (graph a). (Alveolar Po_2 is assumed to equal pulmonary end-capillary Po_2.)

Table 11.2 Effect of different haemoglobin concentrations on the arterial Po_2 under venous admixture conditions defined in the text

Haemoglobin concentration (g.dl^{-1})	Alveolar/arterial Po_2 difference		Arterial Po_2	
	kPa	mmHg	kPa	mmHg
8	15.0	113	9.0	67
10	14.5	109	9.5	71
12	14.0	105	10.0	75
14	13.5	101	10.5	79
16	13.0	98	11.0	82

This would result in a pulmonary end-capillary/arterial oxygen content difference of 0.5 ml per 100 ml. Assuming an alveolar Po_2 of 24 kPa (180 mmHg), the alveolar/arterial Po_2 difference is influenced by haemoglobin concentration as shown in Table 11.2. (Different figures would be obtained by selection of a different value for alveolar Po_2.)

Alveolar ventilation. The overall effect of changes in alveolar ventilation on the arterial Po_2 presents an interesting problem and serves to illustrate the integration of the separate aspects of the factors discussed above. An increase in the alveolar ventilation may be expected to have the following results.

1. *The alveolar Po_2 must be raised provided the barometric pressure, inspired oxygen concentration and oxygen consumption remain the same (equation 1 on page 251 and Figure 11.2).*
2. *The alveolar/arterial Po_2 difference is increased for the following reasons:*
    a. the increase in the alveolar Po_2 will increase the alveolar/arterial Po_2 difference by the same proportion if other factors remain the same (see Figure 11.4);
    b. under many conditions it has been demonstrated that a fall of Pco_2 (resulting from an increase in alveolar ventilation) reduces the cardiac output, with the consequent changes that have been outlined above;
    c. the change in arterial pH resulting from the reduction in Pco_2 causes a small, unimportant increase in alveolar/arterial Po_2 difference.

Thus an increase in alveolar ventilation may be expected to increase both the alveolar Po_2 and the alveolar/arterial Po_2 difference. The resultant change in arterial Po_2 will depend on the relative magnitude of the two changes. Figure 11.6 shows the changes in arterial Po_2 caused by variations of alveolar ventilation at an inspired oxygen concentration of 30% in the presence of varying degrees of venous admixture, assuming that cardiac output is influenced by Pco_2 as described in the legend. Up to an alveolar ventilation of $1.5\,l.min^{-1}$, an increase in ventilation will always raise the arterial Po_2. Beyond that, in the example cited, further increases in alveolar ventilation will increase the arterial Po_2 only if the venous admixture is less than 3 per cent. For larger values of venous admixture, the increase in the alveolar/arterial Po_2 difference exceeds the increase in the alveolar Po_2 and the arterial Po_2 is thus decreased.

Compensation for increased alveolar/arterial Po_2 difference by raising the inspired oxygen concentration

Many patients with severe respiratory dysfunction are hypoxaemic while breathing air. The main objective of treatment is clearly to remove the cause of the hypoxaemia but, when this is not immediately possible, it is often possible to relieve the hypoxaemia by increasing the inspired oxygen concentration. The principles for doing so depend on the cause of the hypoxaemia. As a broad classification, hypoxaemia may be due to hypoventilation or to venous admixture or to a combination of the two. When hypoxaemia is primarily due to hypoventilation, and when it is not appropriate or possible to restore the normal ventilation, the arterial Po_2 can usually be restored by elevation of the inspired oxygen within the range 21–30% as explained above (page 251 and Figure 11.2) and also in Chapter 26.

Quantitatively, the situation is entirely different when hypoxaemia is primarily due to venous admixture. It is then possible to restore the arterial Po_2 by oxygen enrichment of the inspired gas only when the venous admixture does not exceed the equivalent of a shunt

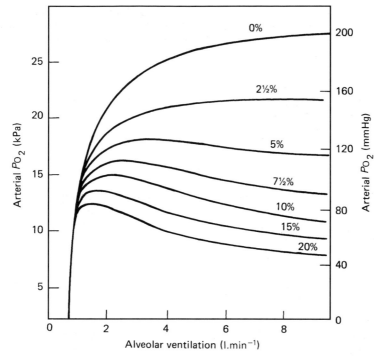

Figure 11.6 The effect of alveolar ventilation on arterial Po_2 is the algebraic sum of the effect on the alveolar Po_2 (Figure 11.2) and the consequent change in alveolar/arterial Po_2 difference (Figure 11.4). When the increase in the latter exceeds the increase in the former, the arterial Po_2 will be diminished. The figures in the diagram indicate the percentage venous admixture. The curve corresponding to 0% venous admixture will indicate alveolar Po_2. Constants incorporated in the design of this figure: inspired O_2 concentration, 30%; O_2 consumption, 200 ml.min^{-1}; respiratory exchange ratio, 0.8. It has been assumed that the cardiac output is influenced by the Pco_2 according to the equation $\dot{Q} = 0.039 \times Pco_2 + 2.23$ (mmHg). (Reproduced from reference 3 by permission of the Editor of *British Journal of Anaesthesia*.)

of 30% of the cardiac output, and at this level may require up to 100% inspired oxygen (page 186). The quantitative aspects of the relationship are best considered in relation to the iso-shunt diagram (see Figure 8.12).

The carriage of oxygen in the blood

The preceding section considered at some length the factors that influence the Po_2 of the arterial blood. It is now necessary to consider how oxygen is carried in the blood and, in particular, the relationship between the Po_2 and the quantity of oxygen that is carried. The latter is crucially important to the delivery of oxygen and is no less important than the partial pressure at which it becomes available to the tissue.

Oxygen is carried in the blood in two forms. Much the greater part is in reversible chemical combination with haemoglobin, while a smaller part is in physical solution in plasma and intracellular fluid. The ability to carry large quantities of oxygen in the blood is of great importance to the organism. Without haemoglobin the amount carried would be so small that the cardiac output would need to be increased by a factor of about 20 to give an adequate delivery of oxygen. Under such a handicap, animals could not have developed to their present extent. The biological significance of the haemoglobin-like compounds is thus immense. It is interesting that the tetrapyrrole ring, which contains iron in haemoglobin, is also a constituent of chlorophyll (which has magnesium in place of iron) and the cytochromes responsible for cellular oxygen metabolism. This chemical structure is thus concerned with production, transport and utilization of oxygen.

Physical solution of oxygen in blood

Oxygen is carried in physical solution in both erythrocytes and plasma. There does not seem to have been any recent determination of the solubility coefficient, and we tend to rely on earlier studies indicating that the amount carried in normal blood in solution at 37°C is about $0.0225 \, ml.dl^{-1}.kPa^{-1}$ or $0.003 \, ml.dl^{-1}.mmHg^{-1}$. At normal arterial Po_2, the oxygen in physical solution is thus about $0.25-0.3 \, ml.dl^{-1}$ or rather more than 1% of the total oxygen carried in all forms. However, when breathing 100% oxygen, the level rises to about $2 \, ml.dl^{-1}$. Breathing 100% oxygen at 3 atmospheres pressure absolute (303 kPa), the amount of oxygen in physical solution rises to about $6 \, ml.dl^{-1}$, which is sufficient for the normal resting arteriovenous extraction. The amount of oxygen in physical solution rises with decreasing temperature for the same Po_2.

Haemoglobin[4]

Haemoglobin was the subject of many years of detailed X-ray crystallographic analysis by the team led by Perutz in Cambridge. Its structure is now well understood and this provides the molecular basis for its remarkable properties.[5]

The haemoglobin molecule consists of four protein chains, each of which carries a haem group (Figure 11.7a), the total molecular weight being 64 458. The amino acids comprising the chains have been identified and it is known that, in the commonest type of adult human haemoglobin (HbA), there are two types of chain, two of each occurring in each molecule. The two α-chains each have 141 amino acid residues, with the haem attached to a histidine residue occupying position 87. The two β-chains each have 146 amino acid residues, with the haem attached to a histidine residue occupying position 92. Figure 11.7b shows details of the point of attachment of the haem in the α-chain.

The four chains of the haemoglobin molecule lie in a ball like a crumpled necklace. However, the form is not random and the actual shape (the quaternary structure) is of critical importance and governs the reaction with oxygen. The shape is maintained by loose bonds between certain amino acids on different chains and also between some amino acids on the same chain. One consequence of these bonds is that the haem groups lie in crevices formed by weak bonds between the haem groups and histidine residues, other than those to which they are attached by normal valency linkages. For example, Figure 11.7c shows a section of an α-chain with the haem group attached to the iron atom that is bound to the histidine residue in position 87. However, the haem group is also attached by a loose bond to the histidine residue in position 58 and also by non-polar bonds to many other amino acids. This forms a loop and places the haem group in a crevice that limits and controls the ease of access for oxygen molecules.

Structural basis of the Bohr effect (page 267). The precise shape of the haemoglobin molecule is altered by factors that influence the strength of the loose bonds; such factors include temperature, pH, ionic strength and carbon dioxide binding to the *N*-terminal amino acid residues as carbamate.[5,6] This alters the accessibility of the haem groups to

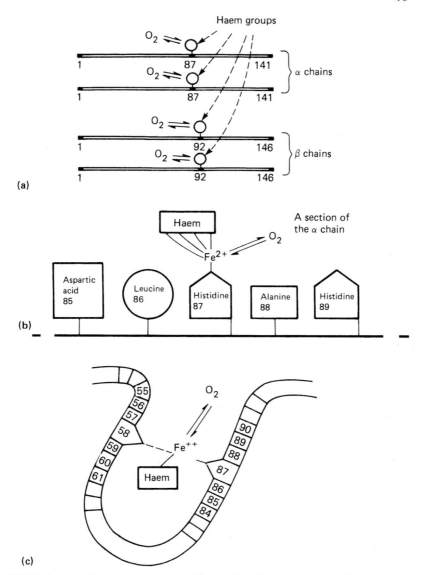

Figure 11.7 The haemoglobin molecule consists of four amino acid chains, each carrying a haem group. (a) There are two pairs of identical chains: α-chains each with 141 amino acid residues and β-chains each with 146 amino acid residues. (b) The attachment of the haem group to the α-chain. (c) The crevice that contains the haem group.

oxygen and is believed to be the basis of the mechanism by which the affinity of haemoglobin for oxygen is altered by these factors, an effect that is generally considered in terms of its influence on the dissociation curve (see Figure 11.10, below). The molecular basis of the Bohr effect has interested biochemists for many years. Crystallographic studies have shown that in deoxyhaemoglobin the histidine in position 146 of the β-chain is loosely bonded to the aspartine residue at position 94, and that oxygenation of the molecule moves the histidine 10 Å further away from the aspartine, which is sufficient distance to change its pK value.[5,7] Proton nuclear magnetic resonance techniques, which allow the precise measurement of hydrogen ion positions in large proteins, do not require the protein to be crystallized before analysis and so allow a more physiological assessment of these conformational changes.[7] These studies have shown that many different areas of the haemoglobin structure contribute to the Bohr effect, depending on the physiological circumstances.

Structural basis of the Haldane effect (page 227). The quaternary structure of the haemoglobin molecule is also altered by the uptake of oxygen to form oxyhaemoglobin. It is believed that this increases the ionization of certain —NH2 or =NH groups and so reduces their ability to undertake carbamino carriage of carbon dioxide (see Figure 10.1).

Oxygen-combining capacity of haemoglobin. There is still confusion over the oxygen-combining capacity of haemoglobin. Until 1963 the value was taken to be 1.34 ml.g^{-1}. Following the precise determination of the molecular weight of haemoglobin, the theoretical value of 1.39 ml.g^{-1} was derived and passed into general use. However, it gradually became clear that this value was not obtained when direct measurements of haemoglobin concentration and oxygen capacity were compared. After an exhaustive study of the subject, Gregory in 1974 proposed the values of 1.306 ml.g^{-1} for human adult blood and 1.312 ml.g^{-1} for fetal blood,[8] and these values are now generally accepted for clinical use.[9] Haemoglobin concentrations are ultimately compared with the International Cyan-methaemoglobin Standard, which is based on iron content and not on oxygen-combining capacity. Because some of the iron is likely to be in the form of haemochromogens, it is not surprising that the observed oxygen-combining capacity is less than the theoretical value of 1.39.

Kinetics of the reaction of oxygen with haemoglobin

Over 70 years ago Adair first proposed that the oxidation of haemoglobin proceeds in four separate stages:[10]

$$\text{Hb} + 4\text{O}_2 \underset{}{\overset{K_1}{\rightleftharpoons}} \text{HbO}_2 + 3\text{O}_2 \underset{}{\overset{K_2}{\rightleftharpoons}} \text{Hb(O}_2)_2 + 2\text{O}_2 \underset{}{\overset{K_3}{\rightleftharpoons}} \text{Hb(O}_2)_3 + \text{O}_2 \underset{}{\overset{K_4}{\rightleftharpoons}} \text{Hb(O}_2)_4$$

For each of the four reactions there are two velocity constants with small k indicating the reverse reaction (towards deoxyHb) and small k prime (k') indicating the forward reaction. Large K is used to represent the ratio of the forward and reverse reactions, thus for example $K_1 = k'_1/k_1$. In this way, the dissociation between deoxy- and oxyhaemoglobin may be represented by the four velocity constants K_1–K_4.

The Adair equation described assumes that the α- and β-chains of haemoglobin behave identically in their chemical reactions with oxygen, which is unlikely *in vivo*. When α- and β-chains are taken into account, there are many different reaction routes that may be followed between deoxy- and oxyhaemoglobin, in theory giving rise to 16 different reversible reactions (Figure 11.8).[11] However, the multiple separate forward and reverse reactions can again be combined to give a single value for K that does not differ significantly from that obtained using the simpler Adair equation.

In both cases, the separate velocity constants have been measured[11] and values for K_1–K_4 are shown in Figure 11.8. It can be seen that the last reaction has a forward velocity that is many times higher than that of the other reactions. During the saturation of the last

Hb   HbO₂   Hb(O₂)₂   Hb(O₂)₃   Hb(O₂)₄

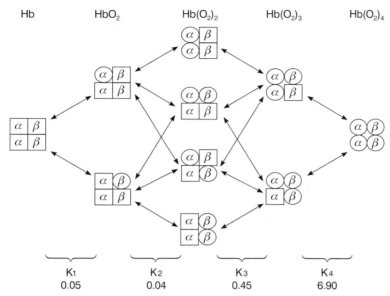

	K₁	K₂	K₃	K₄
	0.05	0.04	0.45	6.90

Figure 11.8 Oxygenation of tetrameric haemoglobin. If chemical interactions with oxygen differ between α- and β-chains, the transition from deoxyHb to fully oxygenated Hb can take a variety of routes as shown. Arrows indicate the 16 possible separate dissociation equilibria, which must be combined to derive the four Adair constants $K_1–K_4$, the values of which are indicated. It can be clearly seen that the final stage of oxygenation is considerably faster than the previous three.[11]

75% of reduced haemoglobin, the last reaction will predominate and the high velocity constant counteracts the effect of the ever-diminishing number of oxygen receptors, which would otherwise slow the reaction rate by the law of mass action.[12] The magnitude of the forward reaction for K_4 also explains why the dissociation of oxyhaemoglobin is somewhat slower than its formation.

    The velocity constant of the combination of carbon monoxide with haemoglobin is of the same order, but the rate of dissociation of carboxyhaemoglobin is extremely slow by comparison.

The oxyhaemoglobin dissociation curve

As a result of the complex kinetics of the chemical reaction between oxygen and haemoglobin, the relationship between Po_2 and percentage saturation of haemoglobin is non-linear, and the precise form of the non-linearity is of fundamental biological importance. It is shown, under standard conditions, in graphical form for adult and fetal haemoglobin and also for myoglobin and carboxyhaemoglobin in Figure 11.9.

Equations to represent the dissociation curve. In 1925, Adair[10] was the first to develop an equation that would reproduce the observed oxygen dissociation curve, using four coefficients as described in the previous section. Forty years later, this was modified by Kelman,[13] who used seven coefficients, each determined to eight significant figures. His equation generates a curve indistinguishable from the true curve above a Po_2 of about 1 kPa (7.5 mm Hg) and this has remained the standard. Calculation of Po_2 from saturation requires an iterative approach, but saturation may be conveniently determined from Po_2

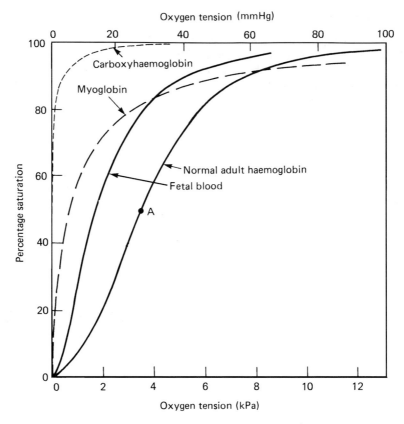

Figure 11.9 Dissociation curves of normal adult haemoglobin compared with fetal blood. Curves for myoglobin and carboxyhaemoglobin are shown for comparison. Point A is the P_{50} for this curve, and shows the oxygen tension at which the Hb saturation is 50%. Note: (1) Fetal blood is adapted to operate at a lower Po_2 than adult blood. (2) Myoglobin approaches full saturation at Po_2 levels normally found in voluntary muscle (2–4 kPa, 15–30 mmHg); the bulk of its oxygen can be released only at very low Po_2 during exercise. (3) Carboxyhaemoglobin can be dissociated only by the maintenance of very low levels of Pco.

by computer, a calculation that is automatically carried out by most blood gas analysers in clinical use, very few of which actually measure saturation. The following simplified version of the Kelman equation is convenient to use and yields similar results at Po_2 values above 4 kPa (30 mmHg):[14]

$$So_2 = \frac{100(Po_2^3 + 2.667 \times Po_2)}{Po_2^3 + 2.667 \times Po_2 + 55.47}$$

(Po_2 values here are in kilopascals; So_2 is percentage).

This equation takes no account of the position of the dissociation curve as described in the next section, so must be used with caution in clinical situations.

Factors causing displacement of the dissociation curve

Several physiological and pathological changes to blood chemistry cause the normal dissociation curve to be displaced in either direction along its X axis. A convenient approach to quantifying a shift of the dissociation curve is to indicate the Po_2 required for 50% saturation and, under the standard conditions shown in Figure 11.9, this is 3.5 kPa (26.3 mmHg). Referred to as the P_{50}, this is the usual method of reporting shift of the dissociation curve.

The Bohr effect, as a result of changes in blood pH, is shown in Figure 11.10. Shifts may be defined as the ratio of the Po_2 that produces a particular saturation under standard conditions, to the Po_2 that produces the same saturation with a particular shift of the curve. Standard conditions include pH 7.4, temperature 37°C and zero base excess. In Figure 11.10, a saturation of 80% is produced by Po_2 6 kPa (45 mmHg) at pH 7.4 (standard). At pH 7.0 the Po_2 required for 80% saturation is 9.4 kPa (70.5 mmHg). The ratio is 0.64 and this applies to all saturations at pH 7.0.

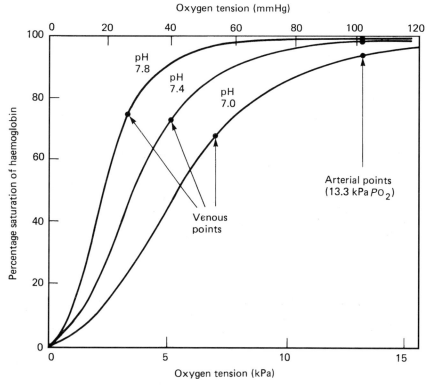

Figure 11.10 The Bohr effect and its effect on oxygen tension. The centre curve is the normal curve under standard conditions; the other two curves show the displacement caused by differing blood pH as indicated, other factors remaining constant. The venous points have been determined on the basis of a fixed arterial/mixed venous oxygen saturation difference of 25%. They are thus 25% saturation less than the corresponding arterial saturation, which is equivalent to a Po_2 of 13.3 kPa (100 mmHg) in each case. Under the conditions shown, alkalosis lowers venous Po_2 and acidosis raises venous Po_2. Tissue Po_2 is related to venous Po_2. Temperature 37°C; base excess, zero.

Temperature has a large influence on the dissociation curve with a left shift in hypothermia and *vice versa*.

Base excess is a parameter derived from blood pH and P_{CO_2} to quantify the metabolic (as opposed to respiratory) component of an observed change in blood pH. Compared with pH itself, alterations in base excess have only a small effect on the position of the dissociation curve but must be taken into account for accurate results.

Quantifying displacement of the haemoglobin dissociation curve. Estimation of haemoglobin saturation from P_{O_2} using the modified Kelman equation has been shown above.

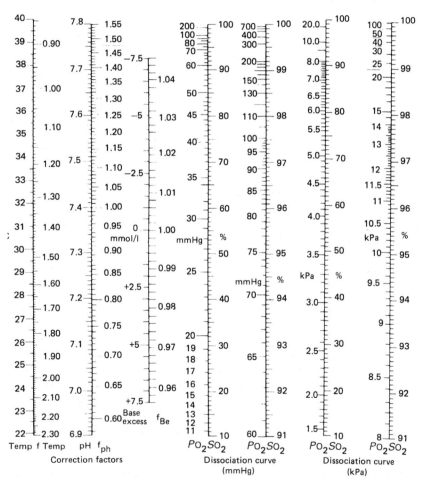

Figure 11.11 Numerical representation of the standard oxyhaemoglobin dissociation curve and the factors that displace it. The two pairs of right-hand line charts give corresponding values of P_{O_2} and saturation for standard conditions with all other factors being normal. The remaining lines indicate the factors by which the actual measured P_{O_2} should be multiplied before entering into the standard curve to determine the saturation. Where more than one factor is required, they should be multiplied together before being applied to the P_{O_2}. (Reproduced from reference 97 by permission of the Editor of the *Journal of Applied Physiology*, modified in accord with the data of reference 15.)

However, this equation assumes a normal P_{50}, so will yield erroneous results in all but the most 'normal' physiological circumstances. Correction may be done manually by reference to Figure 11.11, which shows the factor to be applied for alterations in either pH, temperature or base excess. With multiple abnormalities, the usual practice is to derive a factor for the influence of each and then to multiply them together. This combined factor is then multiplied by the observed P_{O_2} to give the apparent P_{O_2}, which may be entered into the standard dissociation curve to indicate the saturation (as shown on the right of Figure 11.11 or graphically in Figure 11.9).

In clinical practice, the type of patient who requires blood gas measurement invariably also has abnormalities of pH, temperature and base excess. Automated calculation of saturation from P_{O_2} by blood gas machines therefore routinely takes these factors into account, using a variety of equations to correct for dissociation curve displacement, of which one example[16,17] is:

$$\text{Corrected } P_{O_2} = P_{O_2} \times 10^{[0.48\,(pH-7.4)-0.024\,(T-37)-0.0013\times BE]}$$

where P_{O_2} is in kPa and temperature (T) in °C. The corrected P_{O_2} may then be entered into any version of the haemoglobin dissociation curve equation as shown above (page 266).[17]

Clinical significance of displacement of the haemoglobin dissociation curve. The important effect is on tissue P_{O_2}, and the consequences of a shift in the dissociation curve are not intuitively obvious. It is essential to think quantitatively. For example, a shift to the right (caused by low pH or high temperature) impairs oxygenation in the lungs but aids release of oxygen in the tissues. Do these effects in combination increase or decrease tissue P_{O_2}? An illustrative example is set out in Figure 11.10. The arterial P_{O_2} is assumed to be 13.3 kPa (100 mmHg) and there is a decrease in arterial saturation with a reduction of pH. At normal arterial P_{O_2} the effect on arterial saturation is relatively small, but at the venous point the position is quite different, and the examples in Figure 11.10 show the venous oxygen tensions to be very markedly affected. Assuming that the arterial/venous oxygen saturation difference is constant at 25%, it will be seen that at low pH the venous P_{O_2} is raised to 6.9 kPa (52 mmHg) whereas at high pH the venous P_{O_2} is reduced to 3.5 kPa (26 mmHg). This is important, as the tissue P_{O_2} equates more closely to the venous P_{O_2} than to the arterial P_{O_2}. Thus, in the example shown, the shift to the right is beneficial for tissue oxygenation.

It is a general rule that a shift to the right (increased P_{50}) will benefit venous P_{O_2}, provided that the arterial P_{O_2} is not critically reduced. Below an arterial P_{O_2} of about 5 kPa (38 mmHg), the arterial point is on the steep part of the dissociation curve, and the deficiency in oxygenation of the arterial blood would outweigh the improved off-loading of oxygen in the tissues. Thus, with severe arterial hypoxaemia, the venous P_{O_2} would tend to be reduced by a shift to the right and a *leftward* shift would then be advantageous. It is therefore of great interest that a spontaneous leftward shift occurs at extreme altitude when arterial P_{O_2} is critically reduced (see below).

2,3-Diphosphoglycerate (DPG). In 1967 it was found that the presence of certain organic phosphates in the erythrocyte has a pronounced effect on the P_{50}.[18,19] The most important of these compounds is DPG,[20] one molecule of which becomes clamped between the β-chains of one tetramer of deoxyhaemoglobin,[5] resulting in a conformational change that reduces oxygen affinity, and so displaces the dissociation curve to the right. The percentage of haemoglobin molecules containing a DPG molecule governs the overall P_{50} of a blood sample within the range 2–4.5 kPa (15–34 mmHg).

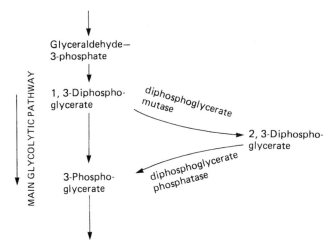

Figure 11.12 Rapoport–Luebering shunt for synthesis of 2,3-diphosphoglycerate.

DPG is formed in the Rapoport–Luebering shunt off the glycolytic pathway, and its level is determined by the balance between synthesis and degradation (Figure 11.12). Activity of DPG mutase is enhanced and DPG phosphatase diminished at high pH, which thus increases the level of DPG.

The relationship between DPG levels and P_{50} suggested that DPG levels would have a most important bearing on clinical practice. Throughout the early 1970s much research effort was devoted to investigating the conditions that might result in substantial changes in DPG levels and possible therapeutic avenues involving manipulation of DPG levels.[21] In general, it may be said that this research failed to substantiate the theoretical importance of DPG for oxygen delivery. In fact, the likely effects of changes in P_{50} mediated by DPG seem to be of marginal significance in comparison with changes in arterial Po_2, acid–base balance and tissue perfusion.

Blood storage and transfusion remains the only area where red cell DPG levels may have significant effects in clinical practice. Storage of blood for transfusion at below 6°C reduces glycolysis to less than 5 per cent of normal rates, and so reduces DPG production by a similar amount. Thus, after one to two weeks of storage, red cell DPG levels are effectively zero. Blood-preservation solutions have evolved through the years to include the addition of dextrose to encourage glycolytic activity, citrate to buffer the resulting lactic acid and adenine or phosphate to maintain ATP levels. Thus storage of blood with citrate–phosphate–dextrose (CPD) reduces the rate of DPG depletion when compared with older preservation solutions,[22] but levels still become negligible within two weeks.

Once transfused, the red blood cells are quickly warmed and provided with all required metabolites, and the limiting factor for return to normal DPG levels will be reactivation of DPG mutase (Figure 11.12). *In vivo* studies in healthy volunteers indicate that red cell DPG levels in transfused red cells are about 50 per cent of normal 7 hours after transfusion, and pretransfusion levels not achieved until 48 hours (Figure 11.13).[23] This ingenious study involved the administration of 35-day-old CPD–adenine preserved type O blood to type A volunteers, and then in repeated venous samples red cells were separated according to their blood group before measuring DPG levels. In this way, DPG

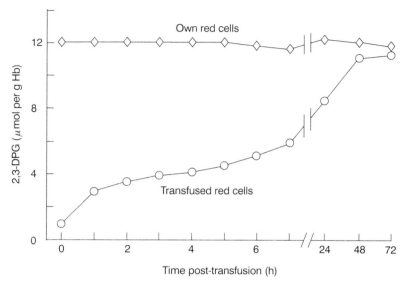

Figure 11.13 Restoration of red cell 2,3-diphosphoglycerate (2,3-DPG) levels following blood transfusion. The type O transfused red cells were stored for 35 days in CPD-A preservative solution before being given to type A volunteers. Red cells could subsequently be separated into the transfused cells and the volunteers' own cells before analysis. The clinical implications of this slow return to normal DPG levels are unclear, see text for details. (Redrawn from reference 23 by permission of the authors and the publishers of *British Journal of Haematology.*)

levels of both the recipient's own cells and the transfused cells could be monitored separately (Figure 11.13).

The clinical significance of the slow return to normal DPG levels is uncertain, and in most cases likely to be minimal, as the proportion of the patient's haemoglobin that consists of transfused blood will usually be small. However, rapid transfusion of large volumes of DPG-depleted blood does result in a reduced P_{50} in both rats and humans,[24,25] which will in theory impair tissue oxygenation (page 269). However, in humans, little evidence has been found of tissue hypoxia in these circumstances, with no changes in cardiac output or oxygen consumption after transfusion with DPG-depleted blood.[26,27] Changes in the P_{50} of a patient do not usually exceed 0.5 kPa (3.8 mmHg), and it is possible that changes in the haemoglobin dissociation curve are compensated for by changes in blood flow at a capillary level.[28]

Other causes of altered DPG levels. Anaemia results in a raised DPG level, with P_{50} of the order of 0.5 kPa (3.8 mmHg) higher than control levels.[29] The problem of oxygen delivery in anaemia is considered in Chapter 24.

Altitude causes an increased red cell concentration of DPG. However, there is a progressive respiratory alkalosis with increasing altitude, which has an opposite and much more pronounced effect on displacement of the dissociation curve. There is now a firm consensus that there is a *leftward* displacement of the haemoglobin dissociation curve at high altitude (see Chapter 16).

Abnormal forms of haemoglobin

There are a great number of alternative amino acid sequences in the haemoglobin molecule. Most animal species have their own peculiar haemoglobins while, in humans, γ- and δ-chains occur in addition to the α- and β-monomers already mentioned. γ- and δ-chains occur normally in combination with α-chains. The combination of two γ-chains with two α-chains constitutes fetal haemoglobin (HbF), which has a dissociation curve well to the left of adult haemoglobin (Figure 11.9). The combination of two δ-chains with two α-chains constitutes A_2 haemoglobin (HbA_2), which forms 2 per cent of the total haemoglobin in normal adults. Other variations in the amino acid chains can be considered abnormal, and, although over 600 have been reported and named, only one-third of these have any clinical effects.[30] Some abnormal haemoglobins (such as San Diego and Chesapeake) have a high P_{50} but it is more common for the P_{50} to be lower than normal (such as Sickle and Kansas). In the long term, a reduced P_{50} results in excessive production of red blood cells (erythrocytosis), presumed to result from cellular hypoxia in the kidney leading to erythropoietin production.[31] However, many abnormal haemoglobins also have a deranged quaternary protein structure and so are unstable, a situation that leads to haemoglobin chains becoming free within the red cell cytoplasm and membrane, causing cell lysis.[31] These patients therefore have a higher than normal rate of red cell production but are generally anaemic because of even greater degrees of red cell destruction. This combination of abnormalities results in severe problems with body iron metabolism.

Sickle cell anaemia is caused by the presence of HbS in which valine replaces glutamic acid in position 6 on the β-chains. This apparently trivial substitution is sufficient to cause critical loss of solubility of reduced haemoglobin, causing red cells to take on the characteristic 'sickle' shape. It is a hereditary condition and in the homozygous state is a grave abnormality, sickling occurring at a Pao_2 of less than 5.5 kPa (40 mmHg), which is close to the normal venous Po_2. Thus any condition that increases the arterial/venous oxygen difference, such as infection, risks precipitating a sickle 'crisis'. Heterozygous carriers of the disease sickle only below a Pao_2 of 2.7 kPa (20 mmHg) and so are usually asymptomatic.

Thalassaemia is another hereditary disorder of haemoglobin. It consists of a suppression of formation of HbA with a compensatory production of fetal haemoglobin (HbF), which persists throughout life instead of falling to low levels after birth. The functional disorder thus includes a shift of the dissociation curve to the left (Figure 11.9).

Methaemoglobin[32] consists of haemoglobin in which the iron has been oxidized and assumes the trivalent ferric form. One way in which methaemoglobin forms is when oxyhaemoglobin acts as a nitric oxide (NO) scavenger (see below), a process that occurs physiologically to limit the biological activity of endogenous NO, or pharmacologically during treatment with inhaled NO. Other drugs may cause methaemoglobinaemia, most notably some local anaesthetics (prilocaine, benzocaine) but also nitrites and dapsone.[33] Methaemoglobin is unable to combine with oxygen but is slowly reconverted to haemoglobin in the normal subject by the action of four different systems:

1. NADH-methaemoglobin reductase system of enzymes, which is present in erythrocytes and uses NADH generated by glycolysis (Figure 11.14) to reduce methaemoglobin. This system is by far the most important in normal subjects, accounting for over two-thirds of methaemoglobin-reducing activity, and is deficient in familial methaemoglobinaemia.

2. Ascorbic acid may also bring about the reduction of methaemoglobin by a direct chemical effect, though the rate of this reaction is slow and normally accounts for only 16 per cent of total red cell methaemoglobin reduction.[32]

3. Glutathione-based reductive enzymes have a small amount of methaemoglobin reductase activity.

4. NADPH-dehydrogenase enzyme in erythrocytes can reduce methaemoglobin using NADPH generated from the pentose phosphate pathway. Under physiological conditions, this system has almost no effect and is regarded as the 'reserve' methaemoglobin reductase.

Elevated methaemoglobin levels of whatever cause may be treated by the administration of either ascorbic acid (to encourage natural erythrocyte conversion) or methylene blue $(1-2\,mg.kg^{-1})$.[32,33] The latter is extremely effective and brings about methaemoglobin reduction by activation of NADPH-dehydrogenase.

Abnormal ligands

The iron in haemoglobin is able to combine with other inorganic molecules apart from oxygen. Compounds so formed are, in general, more stable than oxyhaemoglobin and therefore block the combination of haemoglobin with oxygen. The most important of these abnormal compounds is carboxyhaemoglobin but ligands may also be formed with nitric oxide, cyanide, sulphur, ammonia and a number of other substances. In addition to the loss of oxygen-carrying power, there is also often a shift of the dissociation curve to the left.

Carboxyhaemoglobin. Carbon monoxide is well known to displace oxygen from combination with haemoglobin, the affinity being approximately 300 times greater than the affinity for oxygen. Thus in subjects with 20 per cent of their haemoglobin bound to carbon monoxide, blood oxygen content will be reduced by a similar amount (the small contribution from dissolved oxygen will be unchanged). However, the presence of carboxyhaemoglobin also causes a leftward shift of the dissociation curve of the remaining oxyhaemoglobin, partly mediated by a reduction in DPG levels. Tissue oxygenation is therefore impaired to an even greater extent than simply reducing the amount of haemoglobin available for oxygen carriage. This situation contrasts with that of anaemia, where P_{50} is increased so the reduced oxygen-carrying capacity is partially alleviated by an improved unloading of oxygen in the tissues (page 483). Atmospheric exposure to carbon monoxide is considered in Chapter 20.

Nitric oxide and haemoglobin. The enormous interest over recent years in both endogenous and exogenous NO has inevitably led to research into its interaction with haemoglobin. It has been known for some time that NO binds to haemoglobin very rapidly,[34] and this observation is fundamental to its therapeutic use when inhaled NO exerts its effects in the pulmonary vasculature but is inactivated by binding to haemoglobin before it reaches the systemic circulation (page 584). There are two quite separate chemical reactions between NO and the haemoglobin molecule:[35]

1. NO binds to the haem moiety of each haemoglobin chain, but the resulting reaction differs with the state of oxygenation. For deoxyhaemoglobin a fairly stable HbNO complex is rapidly formed which has little vasodilator activity, whilst for oxyhaemo-

globin the oxygen is displaced by NO and in doing so the iron atom is oxidized to methaemoglobin and a nitrate ion produced:

$$Hb[Fe^{2+}] + NO \rightarrow Hb[Fe^{2+}]NO$$

or

$$Hb[Fe^{2+}]O_2 + NO \rightarrow Hb[Fe^{3+}] + NO_3^-$$

These reactions are so rapid that there is doubt that endogenous NO itself can exert any effects within blood (e.g. on platelets) before being bound by haemoglobin, and must therefore act via an intermediate substance.

2. Nitric oxide is also known to form stable compounds with sulphydryl groups termed S-nitrosothiols with the general formula R—S—NO, where the R group may be glutathione or sulphur containing amino acid residues within proteins. Nitrosothiols retain biological activity as vasodilators[36] and can survive for longer than free NO within the blood vessels. NO forms a nitrosothiol group with the cysteine residue at position 93 on the β-chains, producing S-nitrosohaemoglobin (SNO-Hb). As a result of conformational changes in haemoglobin the reaction is faster with oxyhaemoglobin and under alkaline conditions.[35]

Thus *in vivo*, NO in arterial blood is predominantly in the form of SNO-Hb whilst in venous blood haem-bound HbNO predominates.[35] The biological implications of this are yet to be determined. It would seem that, as haemoglobin passes through the pulmonary capillary, changes in oxygenation and hydrogen ion concentration favour the intra-molecular transfer of NO from the haem to cysteine-bound positions. In the peripheral capillaries, both deoxygenation of SNO-Hb and scavenging of free NO by its haem centre will encourage release of the RSNO group either directly across the red cell membrane or via glutathione transport. The released RSNO groups act as local vasodilators, and this may represent one mechanism by which capillary blood flow is regulated,[36,37] effectively improving flow to vessels with the greatest demand for oxygen. The mechanism of action of NO in peripheral capillaries is the same as in pulmonary capillaries; it is described on page 149.

Blood substitutes[38]

There are obvious advantages in the provision of an artificial oxygen-carrying solution that would avoid the infectious and antigenic complications seen with transfusion of another individual's red cells. The search for a blood substitute has followed two quite different parallel paths.

Perfluorocarbons.[39] Oxygen is highly soluble in these hydrophobic compounds, which, with an 8- to 10-carbon chain, are above the critical molecular size to act as anaesthetics. Fluosol DA20 is a 20% emulsion, which will carry about 7 ml of oxygen per 100 ml on equilibration with 100% oxygen at normal atmospheric pressure. Because oxygen is in physical solution in fluorocarbons, its 'dissociation curve' is a straight line, the quantity of dissolved oxygen being directly proportional to Po_2. Thus in a patient with their entire blood volume replaced with Fluosol DA20, and the maximum achievable arterial Po_2 of about 75 kPa (560 mmHg), oxygen carriage will still only be 5 ml.dl^{-1}. This will just provide sufficient oxygen in physical solution to satisfy the normal mean arteriovenous extraction of 5 ml.dl^{-1}, assuming that the tissues are able to extract all the oxygen. When fluorocarbons function alongside the recipient's remaining blood, the overall relationship between tension and content would depend upon their relative proportions. Clinical experience with Fluosol DA20 at the maximal permitted dose (currently only 40 ml.kg^{-1})

in grossly anaemic patients who were unwilling to receive transfusion has been unsatisfactory, with poor or absent improvements in oxygen delivery.

Droplet size in the emulsion is of the order of 0.1 μm, compared with the 5 μm diameter of an erythrocyte. The flow resistance is considerably less than that of blood and, as it is virtually unaffected by shear rate, the rheological properties are particularly favourable at low flow rates. Fluorocarbons may therefore be useful in partial obstruction of the circulation; for example, in myocardial infarction and during percutaneous transluminal coronary angioplasty, the latter of which remains the only use for which the products are licensed.[40]

Second generation perfluorocarbons such as perflubron has four to five times the oxygen-carrying capacity of Fluosol DA20 and may therefore be more effective.[39,41]

Perfluorocarbons are cleared from the circulation into the reticuloendothelial system, where they reside for varying lengths of time before being excreted unchanged from the lungs. Because of the requirement to maintain adequate blood constituents apart from red cells (e.g. platelets, clotting factors, blood chemistry and oncotic pressure), it is unlikely that perfluorocarbons will ever become established for use in the circulation. However, successful use of perflubron in the lungs for liquid or partial liquid ventilation has been reported in animals, premature babies (page 327), children and adults.[42]

Modified haemoglobin solutions.[43,44] Early attempts at using erythrocyte haemolysates resulted in acute renal failure due to the stroma from the erythrocyte rather than the free haemoglobin. Development of stroma-free haemoglobin solutions failed to solve the problem because, although relatively stable *in vitro*, the haemoglobin tetramer dissociates in the body into dimers, which are excreted in the urine. This results in a half-life of only 2–4 hours.[41] Other problems include the absence of DPG resulting in a low P_{50}, and a high colloid oncotic pressure limiting their use to a maximum concentration of 7 g.dl^{-1}.[38] The short half-life and high oncotic pressure can be improved by either polymerization of haemoglobin molecules or encapsulation within liposomes, and several products are now undergoing extensive trials. In addition, the haemoglobin molecules used for production may include recombinant human haemoglobin prepared by expression in genetically modified *Escherichia coli* such that both the α- and β-chains are produced to form tetramers with a full complement of haem groups.[45] Clearly, this approach opens up possibilities for producing large quantities of blood without using donors, and also modifying the properties of the haemoglobin. An example of this is the deliberate production of a specific variant of human haemoglobin (Presbyterian Hb) that has a naturally higher P_{50}.[46] Bovine haemoglobin has attracted interest because of its unique property of not needing DPG to lower oxygen affinity, having a P_{50} of 3.7 kPa (28 mmHg) in conditions found in the human circulation.[38]

Clinical trials in humans of various modified haemoglobin solutions are advanced, and side effects seem to be mostly trivial.[38] Some solutions have been found to produce pulmonary and systemic vasoconstriction, which is believed to result from the free haemoglobin acting as a NO scavenger, but the precise mechanism of this observation is not yet elucidated.[40,44]

Bubbles.[47,48] The intriguing possibility of transporting oxygen in the form of micro-bubbles has been proposed, but has not yet been explored *in vivo*. Bubbles that are permeable to gases and less than 5 μm in diameter would in theory be able to transport oxygen through the circulation in sufficient quantities to sustain life. Such bubbles can be produced using small amounts of intravenous lipid, in effect forming a gaseous emulsion.

Intravenous bubbles can exist for up to 30 minutes and are currently under investigation as a radiological contrast medium for use in ultrasound investigations.

Effect of age on blood oxygen carriage

In contrast to the arterial Pco_2, the arterial Po_2 shows a progressive decrease with age. Using the pooled results from 12 studies of healthy subjects, one review[49] suggested the following relationship in subjects breathing air:

$$\text{mean arterial } Po_2 = 13.6 - 0.044 \times \text{age in years (kPa)}$$

or
$$102 - 0.33 \times \text{age in years (mmHg)}$$

About this regression line there are 95% confidence limits (2 s.d.) of ± 1.33 kPa (10 mmHg) (Table 11.3). Some 5 per cent of normal patients will lie outside these limits, so it is preferable to refer to this as the reference range rather than the normal range.

It seems likely that some of the scatter of values for Po_2 is due to transient changes in ventilation, perhaps associated with arterial puncture. Because of the meagre body oxygen stores, such changes have a greater effect on Po_2 than on Pco_2.

Table 11.3 Normal values for arterial Po_2

Age (years)	Mean and 95% confidence intervals	
	kPa	mmHg
20–29	12.5 (11.2–13.9)	94 (84–104)
30–39	12.1 (10.8–13.5)	91 (81–101)
40–49	11.7 (10.4–13.1)	88 (78–98)
50–59	11.2 (9.9–12.5)	84 (74–94)
60–69	10.8 (9.5–12.1)	81 (71–91)

(Figures derived from reference 49)

When breathing oxygen the scatter of normal values for arterial Po_2 is even greater, usually because of technical problems with delivering an accurate concentration of oxygen (see below). To attain an F_{IO_2} of 1.0 great care must be taken to prevent dilution with air, and very high values of arterial Po_2 may be obtained in the healthy subject. Breathing oxygen alone, mean values for arterial Po_2 range from 80 to 86.7 kPa (600 to 650 mmHg), but individual values range from 73.3 kPa (550 mmHg) to values that are (no doubt erroneously) in excess of the alveolar Po_2. Prediction of a 'normal' value against which to compare a measured arterial Po_2 is therefore difficult for different inspired oxygen concentrations, and 'abnormalities' of oxygenation must be interpreted against the high degree of scatter in normal subjects under normal conditions.

The role of oxygen in the cell

Dissolved molecular oxygen (dioxygen) enters into many metabolic processes in the mammalian body. Quantitatively much the most important is the cytochrome c oxidase system, which is responsible for about 90 per cent of the total oxygen consumption of the body. However, cytochrome c oxidase is but one of more than 200 oxidases, which may be classified as follows.

Electron transfer oxidases. As a group, these oxidases involve the reduction of oxygen to superoxide anion, hydrogen peroxide or water, the last being the fully reduced state (see Chapter 25, Figure 25.2). The most familiar of this group of enzymes is cytochrome c oxidase. It is located in the mitochondria and is concerned in the production of the high energy phosphate bond in adenosine triphosphate (ATP), which is the main source of biological energy. This process is described in greater detail below under the heading 'Oxidative phosphorylation'. Another member of this group of oxidases is NADPH oxidase, which is concerned in the generation of superoxide anion in phagocytes. Whilst the superoxide anion and its derivatives are potentially toxic, they play a major role in bacterial killing (see Chapter 25).

Oxygen transferases (dioxygenases). This group of oxygenases incorporates oxygen into substrates without the formation of any reduced oxygen product. Familiar examples are cyclooxygenase and lipoxygenase, which are concerned in the first stage of conversion of arachidonic acid into prostaglandins and leukotrienes (see Chapter 12).

Mixed function oxidases. These oxidases result in oxidation of both a substrate and a co-substrate, which is most commonly NADPH. Well known examples are the cytochrome P-450 hydroxylases, which play an important role in detoxification. Mixed function oxidases are also concerned in the conversion of phenylalanine to tyrosine and of dopamine to noradrenaline, the co-substrate being NADPH for the former and ascorbate for the latter.

Energy production

Most of the energy deployed in the mammalian body is derived from the oxidation of food fuels, of which the most important is glucose:

$$C_6H_{12}O_6 + 6O_2 \rightarrow 6CO_2 + 6H_2O + energy$$

The equation accurately describes the combustion of glucose *in vitro*, but is only a crude, overall representation of the oxidation of glucose in the body. The direct reaction would not produce energy in a form in which it could be used by the body. The biological oxidation proceeds by a large number of stages, with phased production of energy. This energy is not released immediately but is stored mainly by means of the reaction of adenosine diphosphate (ADP) with inorganic phosphate ion to form adenosine triphosphate (ATP):

$$ADP + inorganic\ phosphate\ ion + energy = ATP$$

The third phosphate group in ATP is held by a high energy bond that releases its energy when ATP is split back into ADP and inorganic phosphate ion during any of the myriad biological reactions requiring energy input. ADP is thus recycled indefinitely, ATP acting as a short-term store of energy available in a form that may be used directly for work such as muscle contraction, ion pumping, protein synthesis and secretion. ATP is commonly transported short distances between the sites of synthesis and utilization. For example, in voluntary muscles, it is formed in the mitochondria and used in the myofibrils.

There is no large store of ATP in the body and it must be synthesized continuously as it is being used. The ATP/ADP ratio is an indication of the level of energy that is currently carried in the ADP/ATP system, and the ratio is normally related to the state of oxidation of the cell. The ADP/ATP system is not the only short-term energy store in the body but it is the most important.

The uses of ATP in the body lie outside the scope of this book, but its production from ADP is highly relevant to this chapter because the most efficient methods of production of ATP require the consumption of oxygen. Complete oxidation of glucose requires a three-stage process, the first of which, glycolysis, is independent of oxygen supply.

Glycolysis and anaerobic energy production

Figure 11.14 shows details of the glycolytic pathway for the conversion of glucose to lactic acid. The whole comprises the Embden–Meyerhof pathway for the anaerobic metabolism of glucose, and occurs entirely within the cytoplasm. This pathway is completed either when the Po_2 falls below its critical level or, in the case of erythrocytes, when there is an absence of the respiratory enzymes located in the mitochondria. Figure 11.14 shows that, over all, four molecules of ATP are produced, but two of these are consumed in the priming stages prior to the formation of fructose-1,6-diphosphate, 6-phosphofructokinase being the rate-limiting enzyme. The conversion of glyceraldehyde-3-phosphate to 3-phosphoglyceric acid produces a hydrogen ion, which becomes bound to extramitochondrial nicotinamide adenine dinucleotide (NAD). This hydrogen cannot enter the mitochondria for further oxidative metabolism, so is taken up lower down the pathway by the reduction of pyruvic acid to lactic acid.

This series of changes is therefore associated with the net formation of only two molecules of ATP from one of glucose:

$$\text{Glucose} + 2Pi + 2ADP \rightarrow 2\text{Lactic acid} + 2ATP + 2H_2O$$

(Pi = inorganic phosphate).

However, considerable chemical energy remains in the lactic acid, which, in the presence of oxygen, can be reconverted to pyruvic acid and then oxidized in the citric acid cycle (see below), producing a further 36 molecules of ATP. Alternatively, lactic acid may be converted into liver glycogen to await more favourable conditions for oxidation. Conversion of glucose to ethyl alcohol (fermentation) provides energy without the consumption of oxygen in certain organisms but not in animals. This pathway also yields two molecules of ATP for one of glucose.

In spite of their inefficiency for ATP production, anaerobic metabolism is of great biological importance and was universal before the atmospheric Po_2 was sufficiently high for aerobic pathways (Chapter 1). Anaerobic metabolism is still the rule in anaerobic bacteria and also in the mammalian body when energy requirements outstrip oxygen supply as, for example, during severe exercise and in hypoxia.

Aerobic energy production

The aerobic pathway permits the release of far greater quantities of energy from the same amount of substrate and is therefore used whenever possible. Under aerobic conditions, most reactions of the glycolytic pathway remain unchanged, with two very important exceptions. The conversion of glyceraldehyde-3-phosphate to 3-phosphoglyceric acid occurs in the mitochondrion, when the two NADH molecules formed may enter oxidative phosphorylation (see below) rather than producing lactic acid. Similarly, pyruvate does

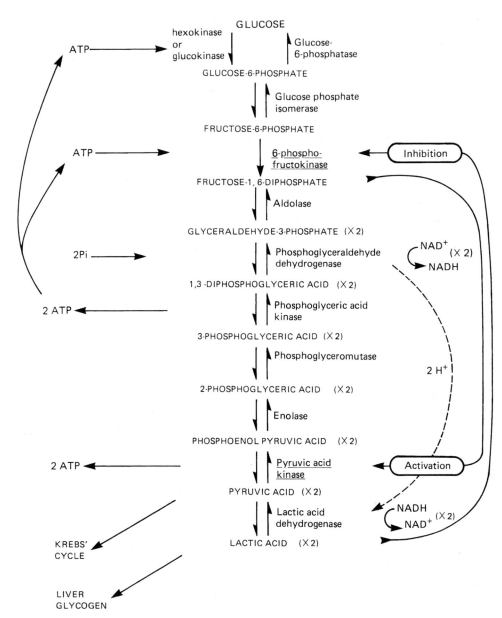

Figure 11.14 The glycolytic (Embden–Meyerhof) pathway for anaerobic metabolism of glucose. From glyceraldehyde-3-phosphate downwards, two molecules of each intermediate are formed from one of glucose. Note the consumption of two molecules of ATP in the first three steps. These must be set against the total production of four molecules of ATP, leaving a net gain of only two molecules of ATP from each molecule of glucose. All the acids are largely ionized at tissue pH.

not continue along the pathway to lactic acid but diffuses into the mitochondria and enters the next stage of oxidative metabolism.

The citric acid (Krebs') cycle occurs in the mitochondria, as shown in Figure 11.15. It consists of a series of reactions to reduce the length of the carbon chain of the molecules before adding a new 2-carbon chain (acetyl CoA) derived from glycolysis. During these reactions, six molecules of carbon dioxide are produced (for each molecule of glucose) along with a further eight molecules of NADH and one molecule of $FADH_2$. Therefore in total, each glucose molecule yields 12 hydrogen ions bound to either NAD or FAD carrier molecules.

The scheme shown in Figure 11.15 also accounts for the consumption of oxygen in the metabolism of fat. After hydrolysis, glycerol is converted into pyruvic acid while the fatty acids shed a series of 2-carbon molecules in the form of acetyl CoA. Pyruvic acid and acetyl CoA enter the citric acid cycle and are then degraded in the same manner as though they had been derived from glucose. Amino acids are dealt with in similar manner after deamination.

Oxidative phosphorylation is the final stage of energy production and again occurs in the mitochondria. The hydrogen ions from $NADH_2$ or $FADH_2$ are passed along a chain of

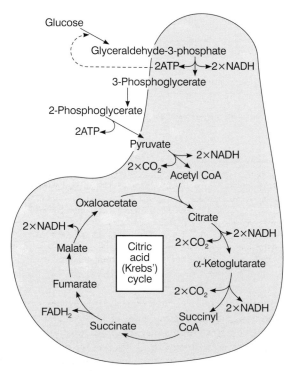

Figure 11.15 Oxidative metabolic pathway of glucose by the citric acid cycle. The shaded area represents the mitochondria and indicates the reactions that can take place only within them. The names of substances that straddle the shaded area show those that are capable of diffusion across the mitochondrial membrane. Many stages of the glycolytic pathway (Figure 11.14) have been omitted for clarity. Note that one molecule of glucose will produce two molecules of all the other intermediate substances. Only 2 molecules of ATP are produced, along with 12 molecules of $NADH_2$, each of which enters oxidative phosphorylation within the mitochondria producing 3 molecules of ATP (Figure 11.16).

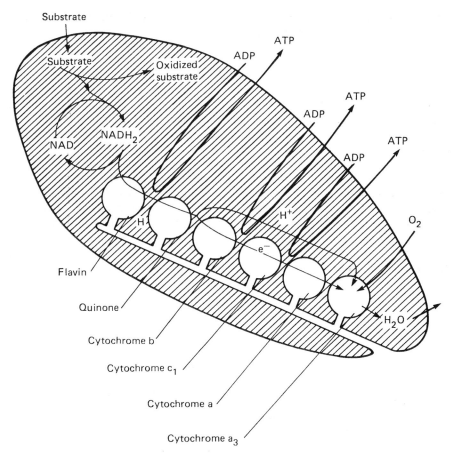

Figure 11.16 Diagrammatic representation of oxidative phosphorylation within the mitochondrion. Intramitochondrial $NADH_2$ produced from glycolysis and the citric acid cycle provides hydrogen to the first of a chain of hydrogen carriers which are attached to the cristae of the mitochondria. When the hydrogen reaches the cytochromes, ionization occurs; the proton passes into the lumen of the mitochondrion while the electron is passed along the cytochromes where it converts ferric iron to the ferrous form. The final stage is at cytochrome a_3 where the proton and the electron combine with oxygen to form water. Three molecules of ADP are converted to ATP at the stages shown in the diagram. ADP and ATP can cross the mitochondrial membrane freely while there are separate pools of intra- and extramitochondrial NAD that cannot interchange.

hydrogen carriers to combine with oxygen at cytochrome a_3, which is the end of the chain. Figure 11.16 shows the transport of hydrogen along the chain, which consists of structural entities just visible under the electron microscope and arranged in rows along the cristae of the mitochondria. Three molecules of ATP are formed at various stages of the chain during the transfer of each hydrogen ion. The process is not associated directly with the production of carbon dioxide, which is formed only in the citric acid cycle. Oxidative phosphorylation can take place only when the P_{O_2} within the mitochondrion is above a critical level, thought to be of the order of 0.1 kPa.

Cytochromes have a structure similar to that of haemoglobin, with an iron-containing haem complex bound within a large protein. Their activity is controlled by the availability of oxygen and hydrogen molecules, and different cytochromes have different values for

P_{50} and so may act as oxygen sensors in several areas of the body. Recent studies have shown an important interaction between NO and several cytochromes, NO forming nitrosyl complexes in a similar fashion to its reaction with haemoglobin.[37] It is postulated that NO, or NO-derived nitrosyl compounds, may play an important role in controlling oxygen consumption at a mitochondrial level. High levels of endogenous NO, for example during sepsis, may produce sufficient inhibition of cytochrome activity and therefore oxygen consumption to contribute to the impaired tissue function seen in vital organs such as the heart.[37] The reduction of oxygen to water by cytochrome a_3 is inhibited by cyanide, whilst a similar but less dramatic effect is seen with barbiturates that reduce oxygen consumption significantly by an effect on the electron transport chain.

Significance of aerobic metabolism. Glycolysis under aerobic conditions and the citric acid cycle yields a total of 12 hydrogen molecules for each glucose molecule used. In turn, each hydrogen molecule enters oxidative phosphorylation to yield three ATP molecules. These, along with the two produced during glycolysis (Figure 11.14), result in a total production of 38 ATP molecules.

In simplified form, the contrasting pathways can be shown as follows:

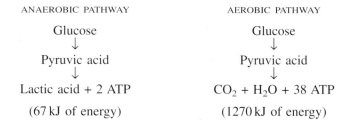

ANAEROBIC PATHWAY	AEROBIC PATHWAY
Glucose	Glucose
↓	↓
Pyruvic acid	Pyruvic acid
↓	↓
Lactic acid + 2 ATP	CO_2 + H_2O + 38 ATP
(67 kJ of energy)	(1270 kJ of energy)

In vitro combustion of glucose liberates $2820\,kJ.mol^{-1}$ as heat. Thus, under conditions of oxidative metabolism, 45 per cent of the total energy is made available for biological work, which compares favourably with most machines.

Use of anaerobic pathways must therefore either consume very much larger quantities of glucose or, alternatively, yield less ATP. In high energy consuming organs such as brain, kidney and liver it is not possible to transfer the increased quantities of glucose, and therefore these organs suffer ATP depletion under hypoxic conditions. In contrast, voluntary muscle is able to function satisfactorily on anaerobic metabolism during short periods of time and this is normal in the diving mammals.

The critical oxygen tension for aerobic metabolism. When the mitochondrial Po_2 is reduced, oxidative phosphorylation continues normally down to a level of about 0.3 kPa (2 mmHg). Below this level, oxygen consumption falls and the various members of the electron transport chain tend to revert to the reduced state. NADH/NAD$^+$ and lactate/ pyruvate ratios rise and the ATP/ADP ratio falls. The critical Po_2 varies between different organs and different species but, as an approximation, a mitochondrial Po_2 of about 0.13 kPa (1 mmHg) may be taken as the level below which there is serious impairment of oxidative phosphorylation and a switch to anaerobic metabolism. This level is, of course, far below the critical arterial Po_2, because there normally exists a large gradient of Po_2 between arterial blood and the site of utilization of oxygen in the mitochondria, as part of the oxygen cascade (see Figure 11.1). Tissue hypoxia is discussed further on page 476. The critical Po_2 for oxidative phosphorylation, also known as the Pasteur point, has applications beyond the pathophysiology of hypoxia in humans. In particular, it has a powerful bearing on putrefaction, many forms of which are anaerobic metabolism resulting from a fall of Po_2 below the Pasteur point in, for example, polluted rivers.

Tissue Po_2

It is almost impossible to quantify tissue Po_2. It is evident that there are differences between different organs, with the tissue Po_2 influenced not only by arterial Po_2 but also by the ratio of tissue oxygen consumption to perfusion. However, even greater difficulties arise from the regional variations in tissue Po_2 in different parts of the same organ, which are again presumably caused by regional variations in tissue perfusion and oxygen consumption. Nor is this the whole story. An advancing Po_2-sensitive microelectrode detects variations in Po_2 that can be interpreted in relation to the proximity of the electrode to small vessels (see Figure 9.5). Very large variations have been demonstrated with exploring electrodes in the brain.[50] As described on page 216, movement of oxygen from capillaries into the tissue is by simple diffusion.[51] For a single cell, the capillary Po_2 will be that of the nearest section of capillary and so anywhere between the local arterial and venous values, and the final tissue Po_2 will also depend on the distance between the capillary and the cell, which may be up to 200 μm. These factors explain why the largest drop in Po_2 of the oxygen cascade is the final stage between capillary and mitochondrial Po_2 (see Figure 11.1). In spite of this sometimes long diffusion path, and low value for mitochondrial Po_2, oxygen supply is extremely efficient, and it is believed to be the supply of metabolic substrates (fatty acids and glucose) that normally limit cellular energy production.[51] Tissue Po_2 is thus an unsatisfactory quantitative index of the state of oxygenation of an organ, and indirect assessments must be made (page 297).

Transport of oxygen from the lungs to the cell

The concept of oxygen delivery

The most important function of the respiratory and circulatory systems is the supply of oxygen to the cells of the body in adequate quantity and at a satisfactory partial pressure. The quantity of oxygen made available to the body in one minute is known as oxygen delivery ($\dot{D}o_2$) or oxygen flux, and is equal to cardiac output × arterial oxygen content.

At rest, the numerical values are approximately:

$$5000 \text{ ml blood per min} \times 20 \text{ ml } O_2 \text{ per dl blood} = 1000 \text{ ml } O_2 \text{ per min}$$
$$\text{(cardiac output)} \qquad \text{(arterial oxygen content)} \qquad \text{(oxygen delivery)}$$

Of this 1000 ml.min^{-1}, approximately 250 ml.min^{-1} are used by the conscious resting subject. The circulating blood thus loses 25 per cent of its oxygen and the mixed venous blood is approximately 70% saturated (i.e. 95−25). The 70 per cent of unextracted oxygen forms an important reserve that may be drawn on under the stress of such conditions as exercise, to which additional extraction forms one of the integrated adaptations (see Figure 14.3).

Oxygen consumption must clearly depend on delivery but the relationship is non-linear. Modest reduction of oxygen delivery is well tolerated by the body, which is, within limits, able to draw on the reserve of unextracted venous oxygen without reduction of oxygen consumption. However, below a critical value for delivery, consumption is decreased and the subject shows signs of hypoxia. The important quantitative aspects of the relationship between oxygen consumption and delivery are considered below.

Quantification of oxygen delivery

The arterial oxygen content consists predominantly of oxygen in combination with haemoglobin, and this fraction is given by the following expression:

$$Ca_{O_2} = Sa_{O_2} \times [Hb] \times 1.31$$

where Ca_{O_2} is the arterial oxygen content, Sa_{O_2} is the arterial oxygen saturation (as a fraction) and [Hb] is the haemoglobin concentration of the blood; 1.31 is the volume of oxygen (ml) that has been found to combine with 1 g of haemoglobin (see above, page 264).

To the combined oxygen must be added the oxygen in physical solution, which will be of the order of 0.3 ml.dl^{-1}, and the expression for total arterial oxygen concentration may now be expanded thus:

$$
\begin{array}{cccccc}
Ca_{O_2} & = & (Sa_{O_2} & \times [Hb] & \times 1.31) & + & 0.3 \qquad \ldots(6)\\
\text{ml.dl}^{-1} & & \%/100 & \text{g.dl--1} & \text{ml.g}^{-1} & & \text{ml.dl}^{-1}
\end{array}
$$

e.g.
$$19 = (0.97 \times 14.7 \times 1.31) + 0.3$$

Because oxygen delivery is the product of cardiac output and arterial oxygen content:

$$
\begin{array}{ccccc}
\dot{D}o_2 & = & \dot{Q} & \times & Ca_{O_2} \qquad \ldots(7)\\
\text{ml.min}^{-1} & & \text{l.min}^{-1} & & \text{ml.dl}^{-1}
\end{array}
$$

e.g.
$$1000 = 5.25 \times 19$$

$\dot{Q}$ is cardiac output. (The right-hand side is multiplied by a scaling factor of 10).

By combining equations (6) and (7) the full expression for oxygen delivery is as follows:

$$
\begin{array}{ccccccc}
\dot{D}o_2 & = & \dot{Q} & \times \{(Sa_{O_2} & \times [Hb] & \times 1.31) & + & 0.3\} \qquad \ldots(8)\\
\text{ml.min}^{-1} & & \text{l.min}^{-1} & \%/100 & \text{g.dl}^{-1} & \text{ml.g}^{-1} & & \text{ml.dl}^{-1}
\end{array}
$$

e.g.
$$1000 = 5.25 \times \{(0.97 \times 14.7 \times 1.31) + 0.3\}$$

(RH side is multiplied by a scaling factor of 10).

For comparison between subjects, values for oxygen delivery must be related to body size, which is done by relating the value to body surface area. Oxygen delivery divided by surface area is known as oxygen delivery index and has units of ml.min^{-1}.m^{-2}.

Interaction of the variable factors governing oxygen delivery. Equation (8) contains, on the right-hand side, three variable factors that govern oxygen delivery.

1. Cardiac output (or, for a particular organ, the regional blood flow). Failure of this factor has been termed 'stagnant anoxia'.
2. Arterial oxygen saturation. Failure of this (for whatever reason) has been termed 'anoxic anoxia'.
3. Haemoglobin concentration. Reduction as a cause of tissue hypoxia has been termed 'anaemic anoxia'.

The classification of 'anoxia' into stagnant, anoxic and anaemic was proposed by Barcroft in 1920[52] and has stood the test of time. The three types of 'anoxia' may be conveniently displayed on a Venn diagram (Figure 11.17), which shows the possibility of combinations

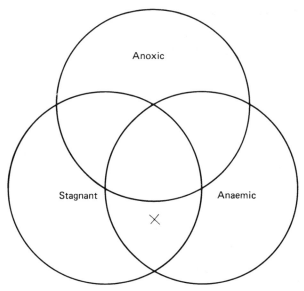

Figure 11.17 Barcroft's classification of causes of hypoxia displayed on a Venn diagram to illustrate the possibility of combinations of more than one type of hypoxia. The lowest overlap, marked with a cross, shows coexistent anaemia and low cardiac output. The central area illustrates a combination of all three types of hypoxia (e.g. a patient with sepsis resulting in anaemia, circulatory failure and lung injury).

of any two types of anoxia or all three together. For example, the combination of anaemia and low cardiac output, which occurs in untreated haemorrhage, would be indicated by the overlapping area of the stagnant and anaemic circles (indicated by X). If the patient also suffered from lung injury, he might then move into the central area, indicating the addition of anoxic anoxia. On a more cheerful note, compensations are more usual. Patients with anaemia normally have a high cardiac output; subjects resident at altitude have polycythaemia, and so on. Such considerations provide a classic example of the importance of viewing a patient as a whole. Clinical implications of oxygen delivery are considered in Chapter 23.

It is important to note that oxygen delivery equals the product of three variables and one constant. If one variable is halved, delivery is halved; but if all three variables are simultaneously halved, delivery is reduced to one-eighth of the original value. One-eighth of 1000 is $125\,\text{ml.min}^{-1}$ – a value that, if maintained for any length of time, is incompatible with life, although the reduction of each individual variable is not in itself lethal.

The relationship between oxygen delivery and consumption

The relationship between oxygen delivery ($\dot{D}o_2$) and consumption ($\dot{V}o_2$) is best illustrated on the coordinates shown in Figure 11.18. The abscissa shows oxygen delivery as defined above, while consumption is shown on the ordinate. The fan of lines originating from the zero point indicate different values for oxygen extraction ($\dot{D}o_2/\dot{V}o_2$) expressed as a percentage. Because the mixed venous oxygen saturation is the arterial saturation less the extraction, it is a simple matter to indicate the mixed venous saturation, which corresponds to a particular value for extraction. The black dot indicates a typical normal resting point,

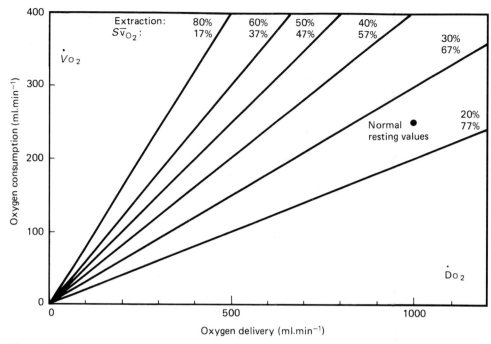

Figure 11.18 Grid relating oxygen delivery and consumption to extraction and mixed venous oxygen saturation, on the assumption of 97% saturation for arterial blood. The spot marks the normal resting values.

with delivery of $1000 \, \text{ml.min}^{-1}$, consumption of $250 \, \text{ml.min}^{-1}$ and extraction 25 per cent. With an arterial saturation of 95%, the mixed venous saturation will therefore be about 70%.

When oxygen delivery is moderately reduced, for whatever reason, oxygen consumption tends to be maintained at its normal value by increasing oxygen extraction and therefore decreasing mixed venous saturation. There should be no evidence of additional anaerobic metabolism, such as increased lactate production. This is termed 'supply-independent oxygenation', a condition that applies provided that delivery remains above a critical value. This is shown by the horizontal line in Figure 11.19. Below the critical level of oxygen delivery, oxygen consumption decreases as a linear function of delivery. This is termed 'supply-dependent oxygenation' and is usually accompanied by evidence of hypoxia, such as increased lactate in peripheral blood and organ failure.

Pathological supply dependency of oxygen consumption has been the source of great controversy for many years.[53] In critically ill patients, the transition between supply-dependent and supply-independent oxygen consumption shown in Figure 11.19 is believed to move to the right, such that increasing oxygen delivery continues to increase oxygen consumption even at 'supranormal' levels, greater than those seen in normal healthy subjects.[54,55] Early work in these critically ill patients revealed an association between high oxygen consumption and the likelihood of survival,[53,56] and aggressive manipulation of oxygen delivery, and therefore consumption, was widely adopted by intensive care units. Subsequent, much larger, randomized studies have failed to confirm the benefits of aggressive management of oxygen delivery.[57,58] A study of 10 726 patients

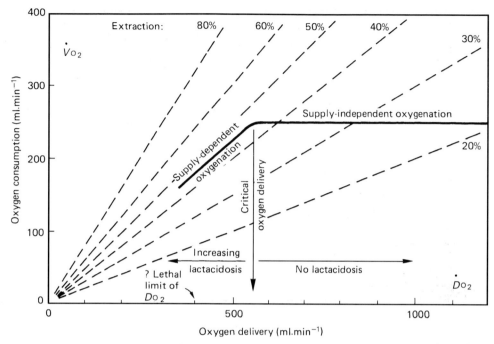

Figure 11.19 This diagram is based on the grid shown in Figure 11.18. For an otherwise healthy subject, the thick horizontal line shows the extent to which oxygen delivery can be reduced without reducing oxygen consumption and causing signs of cellular hypoxia (supply-independent oxygenation). Below the postulated critical delivery, oxygen consumption becomes supply-dependent and there are signs of hypoxia. There is uncertainty of the exact values for critical delivery in otherwise healthy subjects.

found no difference in mortality or morbidity between three different methods of manipulating oxygen delivery and consumption.[57]

A value for the critical oxygen delivery in ill patients has remained elusive.[59] There are many obvious difficulties in assessing the relationship between oxygen consumption and delivery in pathological situations, including the following.

1. To reproduce the line shown in Figure 11.19 in a single patient requires measurement of $\dot{D}o_2$ and $\dot{V}o_2$ at several different values for $\dot{D}o_2$. This is fraught with practical and ethical difficulties, particularly at lower values for oxygen delivery.
2. Measurement of $\dot{D}o_2$ using the product of cardiac output and arterial oxygen content (page 301) and $\dot{V}o_2$ by the reverse Fick technique (page 300) involves sharing two of the three variables used (cardiac output and arterial oxygen content). It is possible that this mathematical coupling explains much of the correlation seen between $\dot{D}o_2$ and $\dot{V}o_2$ measured in this way.[55,59,60]
3. Measurement of $\dot{V}o_2$ by direct means such as indirect calorimetry (page 298) yields different results from those obtained with the reverse Fick technique, mainly because the latter method excludes oxygen consumption by the lung (page 300),[9] which may be significant in patients with extensive lung disease (page 574). Pathological supply-dependency of $\dot{V}o_2$ has never been demonstrated when direct methods are used to measure $\dot{V}o_2$.[55,61,62]

4. Achieving a supranormal $\dot{D}o_2$ requires an increase in cardiac output, which may in itself be responsible for extra oxygen consumption as a result of increased cardiac work. Similarly, administration of adrenoreceptor agonists as cardiac inotropes may increase metabolic requirements elsewhere in the body.

It is therefore possible that pathological oxygen supply-dependency may not exist at all, much of the earlier data resulting from methodological problems and mathematical coupling of the variables being measured. This complex problem, with a potentially large impact on clinical practice, continues to generate controversy,[53] particularly with respect to deliberately increasing $\dot{D}o_2$. However, benefits to patients do now seem to be minimal or non-existent,[57,58] and current advice is to concentrate more closely on achieving normal values for cardiac output, haemoglobin and blood volume,[53] rather than pursuing supranormal targets.

Oxygen stores and the steady state

In spite of its great biological importance, oxygen is a very difficult gas to store in a biological system. There is no satisfactory method of physical storage in the body. Haemoglobin is the most efficient chemical carrier, but more than 0.5 kg is required to carry 1 g of oxygen. The concentration of haemoglobin in blood far exceeds the concentration of any other protein in any body fluid. Even so, the quantity of oxygen in the blood is barely sufficient for three minutes' metabolism in the resting state. It is a fact of great clinical importance that the body oxygen stores are so small and that, if replenishment ceases, they are normally insufficient to sustain life for more than a few minutes. The principal stores are shown in Table 11.4.

While breathing air, not only are the total oxygen stores very small but also, to make matters worse, only part of the stores can be released without an unacceptable reduction in Po_2. Half of the oxygen in blood is still retained when the Po_2 is reduced to 3.5 kPa (26 mmHg). Myoglobin is even more reluctant to part with its oxygen, and very little can be released above a Po_2 of 2.7 kPa (20 mmHg).

Breathing oxygen causes a substantial increase in total oxygen stores. Most of the additional oxygen is accommodated in the alveolar gas from which 80 per cent may be withdrawn without causing the Po_2 to fall below the normal value. With 2400 ml of easily available oxygen after breathing oxygen, there is no difficulty in breath holding for several minutes without becoming hypoxic.

The small size of the oxygen stores means that changes in factors affecting the alveolar or arterial Po_2 will produce their full effects very quickly after the change. This is in

Table 11.4 Principal stores of body oxygen

	While breathing air	While breathing 100% oxygen
In the lungs (FRC)	450 ml	3000 ml
In the blood	850 ml	950 ml
Dissolved in tissue fluids	50 ml	? 100 ml
Combined with myoglobin	? 200 ml	? 200 ml
Total	1550 ml	4250 ml

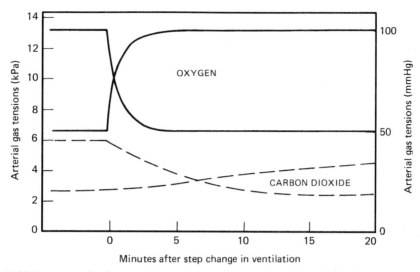

Figure 11.20 The upper pair of curves indicate the rate of change of arterial P_{O_2} following step changes in ventilation. Half of the total change occurs in about 30 seconds. The rising curve could be produced by an increase of alveolar ventilation from 2 to 4 l.min^{-1} while breathing air (see Figure 11.2). The falling curve could result from the corresponding reduction of alveolar ventilation from 4 to 2 l.min^{-1}. The lower pair of broken curves indicate the time course of changes in P_{CO_2}, which are much slower than for oxygen. These changes are shown in greater detail in Figure 10.10.

contrast to carbon dioxide where the size of the stores buffers the body against rapid changes (page 237). Figure 11.20 compares the time course of changes in P_{O_2} and P_{CO_2} produced by the same changes in ventilation. Figure 10.10 showed how the time course of changes of P_{CO_2} is different for falling and rising P_{CO_2}.

Factors that reduce the P_{O_2} always act rapidly, but two examples of changes that produce anoxia illustrate different degrees of 'rapid'.

Circulatory arrest. When the circulation is arrested, hypoxia supervenes as soon as the oxygen in the tissues and stagnant capillaries has been exhausted. In the case of the brain, with its high rate of oxygen consumption, there is only about 10 seconds before consciousness is lost. If the eyeball is gently compressed with a finger to occlude its vessels, vision commences to be lost at the periphery within about 6 seconds. Circulatory arrest also differs from other forms of hypoxia in the failure of clearance of products of anaerobic metabolism (e.g. lactic acid) which, with the exception of the brain, should not occur in arterial hypoxaemia.

Apnoea. The rate of onset of anoxia depends on the initial alveolar P_{O_2}, the lung volume and the rate of oxygen consumption. It is, for example, more rapid while swimming underwater than while breath holding at rest in the laboratory. Generally speaking, after breathing air, 90 seconds of apnoea results in a substantial fall of P_{O_2} to a level that threatens loss of consciousness. If a patient has previously inhaled a few breaths of oxygen, the arterial P_{O_2} should remain above 13.3 kPa (100 mmHg) for at least 3 minutes of apnoea, and this is the basis of the usual method of protection against hypoxia during any deliberate interference with ventilation, as for example during tracheal intubation. If a patient breathes 100% oxygen for a few minutes and is then connected to a supply of oxygen while apnoeic, the arterial Po_2 is well maintained for a long time by the process of apnoeic mass-movement oxygenation (page 240).

In view of the rapid changes shown in Figure 11.20, it follows that, for a patient breathing air, a pulse oximeter will probably give an earlier indication of underventilation than will a carbon dioxide analyser. However, if the patient is protected from hypoxia by the inhalation of a gas mixture enriched with oxygen, the carbon dioxide will give the earlier indication of hypoventilation. It should be remembered that oxygen levels change quickly and are potentially much more dangerous. Carbon dioxide levels change only slowly (in response to a change in ventilation) and are usually less dangerous.

Because a steady state for oxygen is attained very rapidly, it follows that oxygen uptake is seldom appreciably different from consumption in the tissues. Therefore, measurement of oxygen uptake usually gives a satisfactory estimate of the oxygen consumption. In contrast, measured values of carbon dioxide output may be very different from the simultaneous level of metabolic production of carbon dioxide production when the ventilation has just changed. Thus the respiratory exchange ratio may be very low during acute under-ventilation, and well above unity during a brief period of hyperventilation (page 238).

Control of the inspired oxygen concentration

Much of this chapter has been concerned with the theoretical basis for selection of the optimal inspired oxygen concentration for a particular pathophysiological state. It now remains to be considered how this should be put into effect.

Gas mixing

The most satisfactory technique for delivery of a designated inspired oxygen concentration is to mix the required proportions of air and oxygen. Gas mixtures may be conveniently obtained from air and oxygen pipeline installations using a pair of rotameters and appropriate humidification. Mixing devices are available, such as the Quantiflex with separate controls for total flow rate and oxygen concentration. It is a valuable safety feature if such devices have a visible indication of oxygen flow.[63] Air/oxygen mixtures can be delivered to ventilators, passed over a T-piece for patients breathing spontaneously with a cuffed tracheal tube or delivered to the patient by means of a non-rebreathing gas delivery system. Nowadays, most ventilators incorporate their own electronically controlled gas inlet valves on high pressure oxygen and air supplies, allowing the required inspired oxygen concentration to simply be entered into the ventilator settings.

Fixed performance systems

These allow the delivery of a known concentration of oxygen, independent of the patient's respiratory system – that is, the oxygen concentration delivered is unaffected by respiratory rate, tidal volume and inspiratory flow rate. Methods may be divided into low flow (closed) or high flow (open) delivery systems.

Closed delivery systems. A crucial factor in oxygen therapy is the nature of the seal between the patient's airway and the external breathing apparatus. Airtight seals may be obtained with cuffed tracheal or tracheostomy tubes or at low airway pressures with a laryngeal mask airway. These devices should give complete control over the composition of the inspired gas. An anaesthetic facemask will usually provide an airtight seal with the face, but it must be held by a trained person and is at best a temporary measure. Various patterns of masks intended for use by non-trained personnel such as aircrew can give an excellent seal, but there is no mask generally available for clinical use that can be guaranteed to provide an airtight fit to a patient's face.

Any closed delivery system requires the use of a breathing system that provides suitable separation of inspired and expired gases to prevent rebreathing, and does not present significant resistance to breathing.

Open delivery systems. Most disposable oxygen masks do not attempt to provide an airtight fit. An alternative solution to the problem of the airtight seal is to provide a high flow of gas that can vent to atmosphere between the mask and the face, thus preventing the inflow of air. The required flow of air/oxygen mixture needs to be in excess of the peak inspiratory flow rate. For normal resting ventilation this is approximately $30\,l.min^{-1}$ but in patients with respiratory distress may be considerably greater.

Oxygen may be passed through the jet of a Venturi to entrain air. Venturi-based devices are a convenient and highly economical method of preparing high flows of oxygen mixtures in the range 25–40% concentration. For example, $1\,l.min^{-1}$ of oxygen passed through the jet of a Venturi with an entrainment ratio of 8:1 will deliver $9\,l.min^{-1}$ of 30% oxygen. Higher oxygen concentrations require a lower entrainment ratio and therefore a higher oxygen flow in order to maintain an adequate total delivered flow rate. Commercially available Venturi masks now have a variety of colour coded Venturi attachments that indicate the required oxygen flow rate, the inspired oxygen concentration achieved and the total gas flow rate.

With an adequate flow rate of the air/oxygen mixture, the Venturi mask need not fit the face with an airtight junction. The high flow rate escapes round the cheeks as well as through the holes in the mask, and room air is effectively excluded. Numerous studies have indicated that the Venturi mask gives excellent control over the inspired oxygen concentration with an accuracy of ± 1% unaffected by variations in the ventilation of the patient.[64] There is no doubt that this is the most satisfactory method of controlling the inspired oxygen concentration of a patient who is breathing spontaneously without tracheal intubation.

Control of the patient's gaseous environment. The popularity of oxygen tents declined because of their large volume and high rate of leakage, which made it difficult to attain and maintain a high oxygen concentration unless the volume was reduced and a high gas flow rate used. In addition, the fire hazard cannot be ignored. These problems are minimized when the patient is an infant, and oxygen control in an incubator is a satisfactory way to administer a precise oxygen concentration.

Hyperbaric oxygenation. Two systems are in use. One-person chambers are filled with 100% oxygen and the patient is entirely exposed to 100% oxygen at high pressure, no mask being required. Larger chambers are pressurized with air that is breathed by staff: 100% oxygen is made available to the patient by means of a tight-fitting facemask. The quality of the airtight fit is obviously crucial and has caused considerable difficulties in the past.

Variable performance devices

Simple disposable oxygen masks and nasal catheters aim to blow oxygen at or into the air passages. The oxygen is mixed with inspired air to give an inspired oxygen concentration that is a complex function of the geometry of the device, the oxygen flow rate, the patient's ventilation and whether the patient is breathing through his mouth or nose. The effective inspired oxygen concentration is impossible to predict and may vary within very wide limits.[64] These devices cannot be used for oxygen therapy when the exact inspired oxygen concentration is critical (e.g. ventilatory failure), but may be useful in less critical situations such as recovery from routine anaesthesia. Nasal prongs are the preferred method for delivering sleeping oxygen.[65] With simple oxygen masks a small inspiratory reservoir will store fresh gas during expiration for use during inspiration, which will tend to increase the inspired oxygen concentration but, again, in a somewhat unpredictable fashion.

With a device such as a nasal catheter or prongs, the lower the ventilation, the greater will be the fractional contribution of the fixed flow of oxygen to the inspired gas mixture. There is thus an approximate compensation for hypoventilation, with greater oxygen concentrations being delivered at lower levels of ventilation. Arterial P_{O_2} may then be maintained in spite of a progressively falling ventilation. However, this will do nothing to prevent the rise in P_{CO_2}, which may reach a dangerous level without the appearance of cyanosis to warn that all is not well.[66]

Monitoring oxygen concentrations

When the inspired gas has a fixed composition (e.g. in oxygen tents and with Venturi masks), there is no problem in sampling inspired gas and measuring the oxygen concentration (see below). With variable performance devices it is extremely difficult to determine the inspired oxygen, which may not be constant throughout the duration of inspiration. Furthermore, the measured oxygen concentration may be highly dependent on the point from which the sample is taken and whether the patient is breathing through his nose or his mouth. In the face of these difficulties, it may be preferable to measure the end-expiratory oxygen concentration or even the arterial blood P_{O_2}. However, if such measures are necessary, it would be wiser to use a device with a fixed performance.

Cyanosis

Cyanosis describes a blue discoloration of a subject's skin and mucous membranes, and is almost universally caused by arterial hypoxaemia. Though now regarded as a sign of rather advanced hypoxia, there must have been countless occasions in which the appearance of cyanosis has given warning of hypoventilation, pulmonary shunting, stagnant circulation or decreased oxygen concentration of inspired gas. Indeed, it is interesting to speculate on the additional hazards to life if gross arterial hypoxaemia could occur without overt changes in the colour of the blood.

Central and peripheral cyanosis

If shed arterial blood looks purple, this is a reliable indication of arterial desaturation. However, when skin or mucous membrane is inspected, most of the blood that colours the tissue is lying in veins (i.e. sub-papillary venous plexuses) and its oxygen content is related to the arterial oxygen content as follows:

$$\begin{array}{c}\text{venous oxygen} \\ \text{content}\end{array} = \begin{array}{c}\text{arterial oxygen} \\ \text{content}\end{array} - \begin{array}{c}\text{arterial/venous oxygen} \\ \text{content difference}\end{array}$$

The last term may be expanded in terms of the tissue metabolism and perfusion:

$$\frac{\text{venous oxygen}}{\text{content}} = \frac{\text{arterial oxygen}}{\text{content}} - \frac{\text{tissue oxygen consumption}}{\text{tissue blood flow}}$$

In normal circumstances, the oxygen consumption by the skin is usually low in relation to its circulation, so the second term on the right-hand side of the second equation is generally small. Therefore, the cutaneous venous oxygen content is close to that of the arterial blood and inspection of the skin usually gives a reasonable indication of arterial oxygen content. However, when circulation is reduced in relation to skin oxygen consumption, cyanosis may occur in the presence of normal arterial oxygen levels. This occurs typically in patients with low cardiac output or in cold weather. Vigorous coughing, particularly when lying flat, or placing a patient in the Trendelenburg position causes the skin capillaries of the upper body to become engorged with venous blood, once again causing the appearance of cyanosis with normal arterial oxygen content.

The influence of anaemia

In 1923 Lundsgaard and Van Slyke stressed the importance of anaemia in appearance of cyanosis.[67] Much credence is attached to their statement that cyanosis is apparent when there are 5 g of reduced haemoglobin per 100 ml of *capillary* blood. They defined capillary blood as having a desaturation equal to the mean of the levels in arterial and venous blood. If, for example, the arterial blood contained 3 g.dl^{-1} of reduced haemoglobin (80% saturation at normal haemoglobin concentration) and the arterial/venous difference for the skin were 2 ml of oxygen per 100 ml blood (corresponding to the reduction of a further 1.5 g.dl^{-1} of haemoglobin), the 'capillary' blood would contain only 3.75 g.dl^{-1} of reduced haemoglobin, well below the threshold at which cyanosis should be evident. This seems improbable for an arterial saturation of 80%. In cases of severe anaemia, it might be impossible for the reduced haemoglobin concentration of the capillary blood to attain the level of 5 g.dl^{-1}, which is said to be required for the appearance of cyanosis and, clearly, cyanosis could never occur if the haemoglobin concentration were only 5 g.dl^{-1}.

There seems little doubt that Lundsgaard and Van Slyke were right to stress the importance of the total haemoglobin concentration, although there has been little confirmation of 5 g of reduced haemoglobin being the critical value for detection. It is generally found that cyanosis can be detected when *arterial* blood contains greater than 1.5 g.dl^{-1} of reduced haemoglobin,[68] or at an arterial oxygen saturation of 85–90%, although there is much variation. Such levels would probably correspond to a 'capillary' reduced haemoglobin concentration of about 3 g.dl^{-1}.

Sensitivity of cyanosis as an indication of hypoxaemia

The importance of the source of illumination.[69] Different types of fluorescent lighting used in hospitals affect the perceived colour of a patient's skin. Some lamps tend to make the patient look pinker and others impart a bluer tinge to the patient. The former gives false negatives (no cyanosis in the presence of hypoxaemia), while the latter gives false positives (cyanosis in the absence of hypoxaemia). However, the total number of false results is approximately the same with all tubes. Provided all areas of the same hospital are illuminated with the same type of tube this effect is unlikely to adversely affect the assessment of a patient's colour.

Thus the appearance of cyanosis is considerably influenced by the circulation, patient position, haemoglobin concentration and lighting conditions. Even when all these are optimal, cyanosis is by no means a precise indication of the arterial oxygen level and it should be regarded as a warning sign rather than a measurement. Cyanosis is detected in about half of patients who have an arterial saturation of 93%, and about 95 per cent of patients with a saturation of 89%.[69] In other words, cyanosis is not seen in 5 per cent of patients at or below a saturation of 89% (arterial $P_{O_2} \approx 7.5\,kPa$ or 56 mmHg). It is quite clear that absence of cyanosis does not necessarily mean normal arterial oxygen levels.

Non-hypoxic cyanosis has several causes, all of which are rare but worth considering in a patient who seems cyanosed yet displays no other evidence of hypoxia. Sulph-haemoglobin and, more importantly, methaemoglobin (at concentrations of $1.5\,g.dl^{-1}$) cause a blue–grey appearance,[32] and chronic use of drugs or remedies that include gold or silver have been reported to cause 'pseudo-cyanosis'.[71,77]

Principles of measurement of oxygen levels

Oxygen concentration in gas samples

Chemical methods based on Lloyd's modification of the Haldane apparatus was for many years the standard method of measurement of oxygen concentrations in physiological gas samples. However, analysers working on three different physical principles mostly replaced chemical techniques over 30 years ago.[72]

Paramagnetic analysers rely on the fact that oxygen will influence an electrically generated magnetic field in direct proportion to its concentration in a mixture of gases.[72] A particularly attractive feature of the method for physiological use is the complete lack of interference by other gases likely to be present, as significant paramagnetic properties are unique to oxygen. Early paramagnetic analysers were cumbersome and delicate and had slow response times, but technological progress has led to the availability of inexpensive, accurate and robust analysers that are now found in a whole range of anaesthetic and intensive care equipment.

Measurement of breath-to-breath changes in oxygen concentrations of respired gases requires an instrument with a response time of less than about 300 ms. Formerly the only suitable technique for oxygen measurement was the mass spectrometer, but modern paramagnetic analysers have much faster response times, so are easily capable of tracking breath-by-breath oxygen concentration.

Fuel cells have similarities to the polarographic electrode described below. An oxygen-permeable membrane covers a cell, made up of a gold cathode and a lead anode separated by potassium hydroxide, which generates a current in proportion to the oxygen concentration. The response time is many seconds, so these analysers are not suitable for measuring inspired and expired oxygen concentrations. No electrical input is needed, the fuel cell acting like a battery generating its own power from the absorption of oxygen. However, the cell therefore also has a limited lifespan, depending on the total amount of oxygen to which it is exposed over time, but, in normal clinical use, fuel cells last several months.

Polarographic monitors will measure oxygen concentrations in gas samples but are used almost exclusively in medicine for analysis of blood samples (see below).

Blood P_{O_2}

Previous chemical-based analyses have now been completely replaced by a single method.

Polarography. This method, first described by Clark in 1956,[73] is based on a cell formed by a silver anode and a platinum cathode, both in contact with an electrolyte in dilute solution. If a potential difference of about 700 mV is applied to the cell, a current is passed that is directly proportional to the P_{O_2} of the electrolyte in the region of the cathode. In use, the electrolyte is separated from the sample by a thin membrane that is permeable to oxygen. The electrolyte rapidly attains the same P_{O_2} as the sample, and the current passed by the cell is proportional to the P_{O_2} of the sample, which may be gas, blood or other liquids. It has been of immense value in anaesthesia, because it is uninfluenced by the presence of anaesthetic agents. Gas mixtures are normally used for calibration, and an important source of error is the difference in reading between blood and gas of the same P_{O_2}. Estimates of the ratio vary between 1.0 and 1.17 but it may change unexpectedly owing to changes in the position of the membrane. This source of error has been greatly reduced in modern microelectrodes, which consume much less oxygen at the cathode. The error may be detected and prevented by calibration with tonometer-equilibrated blood, which is simple to perform. It is possible to calibrate with a solution of 30% glycerol in water, which gives the same reading as blood of the same P_{O_2}. Frequent measurement of P_{O_2} in blood samples leads to protein deposition on the membrane, which over time forms a diffusion barrier between the sample and the electrolyte. Regular cleaning with a proteolytic solution is therefore required.

Polarographic electrodes may now be made small enough to facilitate intra-arterial monitoring of P_{O_2}. Along with pH, P_{CO_2} and temperature sensors (page 243), the intra-arterial catheter remains less than 0.5 mm in diameter.[74]

Derivation from saturation. If the dissociation curve is known, including its position (P_{50}), the P_{O_2} may be derived from the saturation (see above). This method is quite accurate on the steep part of the dissociation curve, but is of limited value when the P_{O_2} is greater than about 10 kPa (75 mmHg).

Blood oxygen content. The reliability and simplicity of measurements of P_{O_2} and saturation have decreased the demand for measurement of oxygen content, which is now often derived from saturation and haemoglobin concentration. Techniques for direct measurement of oxygen content were based on the chemical liberation of oxygen from haemoglobin followed by measurement of P_{O_2} either in the solution or an equilibrated gas phase. Details may be found in previous editions of this book.

Errors in measuring oxygen levels. Errors arising from the handling of samples for blood gas analysis are considered on page 243. Temperature has a marked effect on P_{O_2} measurement. If blood P_{O_2} is measured at a lower temperature than the patient's, the measured P_{O_2} will be less than the P_{O_2} of the blood while it was in the patient. It is usual to maintain the measuring apparatus at 37°C, and, if the patient's body temperature differs from this by more than 1°C, a significant error will result. Correction is possible but the factor is variable, depending upon the saturation.[75] Automated blood gas machines will perform this correction, provided the patient's temperature is entered; alternatively, a nomogram may be used and is included in Appendix E as Figure E.2.

Transcutaneous P_{O_2}.[76] Cutaneous venous or capillary blood P_{O_2} may, under ideal conditions, be close to the arterial P_{O_2}, but a modest reduction in skin perfusion will cause a substantial fall in P_{O_2}, because the oxygen is consumed at the flat part of the dissociation curve, where small changes in content correspond to large changes in P_{O_2}. As for transcutaneous P_{CO_2} (page 245), heating of skin to 44°C minimizes differences between arterial and capillary/skin P_{O_2}, which can be measured by a directly applied polarographic electrode. Measurement of P_{O_2} at this high temperature requires correction for changes in oxygen solubility.

Oxygen saturation

The classic method of measurement of saturation is as the ratio of content to capacity (with dissolved oxygen subtracted from each):

$$\text{saturation} = \frac{\text{HbO}_2}{\text{Hb} + \text{HbO}_2}$$

$$= \frac{\text{oxygen content} - \text{dissolved oxygen}}{\text{oxygen capacity} - \text{dissolved oxygen}}$$

Blood oxygen saturation. Oxygen capacity is determined as the content after saturation of the blood by exposure to 100% oxygen at room temperature. Both content and capacity were measured by the chemical methods mentioned above.

Nowadays, it is more usual to measure saturation photometrically. Methods are based on the fact that the absorption of monochromatic light of certain wavelengths (e.g. 805 nm) is the same (isobestic) for reduced and oxygenated haemoglobin. At other wavelengths (particularly 650 nm) there is a marked difference between the absorption of transmitted or reflected light by the two forms of haemoglobin. Many devices are marketed that depend on the simultaneous absorption of light at two wavelengths and so indicate the saturation directly. Use of other different wavelengths also allows the detection and quantification of other commonly present haemoglobins such as carboxy-haemoglobin and methaemoglobin.

Saturation may be derived from P_{O_2}, a process that is performed automatically by modern blood gas analysers (page 266). This is reasonably accurate above a P_{O_2} of about 7.3 kPa (55 mmHg) but is inaccurate at lower tensions because, on the steep part of the curve, the saturation changes by 3% for a P_{O_2} change of only 0.13 kPa (1 mmHg).

Pulse oximetry.[77] Saturation may be measured photometrically *in vivo* as well as *in vitro*. Light at the appropriate wavelengths is either transmitted through a finger or an ear lobe or else is reflected from the skin, usually on the forehead. With the original techniques, most of the blood that was visualized was venous or capillary rather than arterial, and the result therefore depended on there being a brisk cutaneous blood flow to minimize the arterial/venous oxygen difference. The older techniques have now been completely replaced by pulse oximeters, which relate the optical densities (at different wavelengths) to the pulse wave detected by the same sensor. The signal between the pulse waves is subtracted from the signal at the height of the pulse wave, the difference being due to the inflowing arterial blood and so reflecting the saturation of the arterial blood.

Instruments currently available continue to function down to levels of severe arterial hypotension, although there is usually a delayed indication of changes in saturation.[78]

Anaemia tends to exaggerate desaturation readings. At a haemoglobin concentration 8 g.dl^{-1}, normal saturations were correctly recorded, but there was a mean bias of -15% at a true saturation of 53.6%.[79] The problem was only clinically important below a saturation of about 75%. Pulse oximeters cannot distinguish between carboxy- and oxyhaemoglobin.[77] Methaemoglobin is read as though it were half oxyhaemoglobin and half reduced haemoglobin up to about 20% methaemoglobin. At higher levels of methaemoglobin, pulse oximeter readings tend to become fixed at about 85%.

Calibration of cutaneous oximeters presents a problem. Optical filters may be used for routine calibration, but the gold standard is calibration against arterial blood Po_2 or saturation, which is seldom undertaken. When oxygenation is critical, there is no substitute for direct measurement of arterial Po_2.

Tissue Po_2

Clearly the tissue Po_2 is of greater significance than the Po_2 at various intermediate stages higher in the oxygen cascade. It would therefore seem logical to attempt the measurement of Po_2 in the tissues, but this has proved difficult both in technique and in interpretation. As described above, for experimental procedures needle electrodes may be inserted directly into tissue, and Po_2 measured on the tip of a needle. Difficulties of interpretation arise from the fact that Po_2 varies immensely in the tissue, and even in a single cell. Thus direct measurement of tissue Po_2 has no place in clinical monitoring.

Tissue surface electrodes. A miniaturized polarographic electrode may be placed on or attached to the surface of an organ to indicate the Po_2. Interpretation of the reading is subject to many of the same limitations as with the needle electrode described previously. Nevertheless, tissue surface Po_2 may provide the surgeon with useful information regarding perfusion and viability in cases of organ ischaemia. Changes in Po_2 may also provide useful information on the efficacy of surgical techniques to improve circulation.[80]

Near infra-red spectroscopy.[81] The biochemical state of tissue oxidation may be determined by the use of transmission spectroscopy in the near infrared (700–1000 nm), where tissues are relatively translucent. The state of relative oxidation of haemoglobin and cytochrome a$_3$ may be determined within this wave band. At present it is feasible to study *transmission* spectroscopy over a path length up to about 9 cm, which is sufficient to permit monitoring the brain of newborn infants. Use in adults requires *reflectance* spectroscopy and does allow assessment of oxygenation in, for example, an area of a few cubic centimetres of brain tissue. This is particularly useful during surgery on the carotid arteries, when changes in oxygenation in the area supplied by the artery concerned can be followed. However, the technique has failed to gain widespread acceptance because of interference from extracranial tissue, particularly scalp blood flow, and difficulties with calibrating the readings and defining any 'normal' values.

Indirect assessment of tissue oxygenation.[82] Such are the difficulties of measurements of tissue Po_2 that in clinical practice it is more usual simply to seek evidence of anaerobic tissue metabolism. In the absence of this, tissue perfusion and oxygenation can be assumed to be acceptable. Indirect methods that assess global (i.e. whole body) tissue perfusion include mixed venous oxygen saturation measured either by sampling pulmonary arterial blood or using a fibreoptic catheter to measure oxygen saturation continuously in the pulmonary artery. Blood lactate levels also provide a global indication of tissue perfusion.

However, acceptable global tissue oxygenation provides no reassurance about function either of regions in an individual organ or an entire organ. Methods of assessing oxygenation in a specific tissue have focused on the gut because of ease of access and the observation that gut blood flow is often the first to be reduced when oxygen delivery is inadequate. Gastric intramucosal pH measurement allows an assessment to be made of cellular pH in the stomach mucosa, which has been shown to correlate with other assessments of tissue oxygenation and patient well-being during critical illness.

Measurement of oxygen consumption and delivery

Oxygen consumption

There are four main methods for the measurement of oxygen consumption:

1. Oxygen loss from (or replacement into) a closed breathing system.
2. Subtraction of the expired from the inspired volume of oxygen.
3. The ventilated hood.
4. Multiplication of cardiac output by arterial/mixed venous oxygen content difference.

Oxygen loss from (or replacement into) a closed breathing system. Probably the simplest method of measuring oxygen consumption is by observing the loss of volume from a closed-circuit spirometer, with expired carbon dioxide absorbed by soda lime. Alternatively, a known flow rate of oxygen may be added to maintain the volume of the spirometer and its oxygen concentration constant: under these conditions, the oxygen

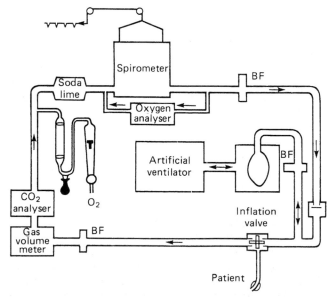

Figure 11.21 A closed-circuit spirometer system for measurement of oxygen consumption of a patient ventilated artificially by means of a box/bag system. When the system is in equilibrium, oxygen consumption is indicated by the oxygen added to the system, and carbon dioxide output is measured as the product of expired minute volume and mean carbon dioxide concentration in the expired gas. BF, bacterial filter. (Reproduced from reference 85 by permission of the Editor and publishers of *Critical Care Medicine.*)

inflow rate must equal the oxygen consumption. It is essential that the spirometer initially contains an oxygen-enriched mixture so that the inspired oxygen concentration does not fall to a level that is dangerous for the subject or patient. The subject's nitrogen stores will exchange with the spirometer gas if the partial pressures are different, and this may introduce a small error when the subject is first connected to the spirometer. The technique may be adapted to the conditions of artificial ventilation (Figure 11.21), but the technique, although accurate, is cumbersome.[83]

Subtraction of expired from inspired volume of oxygen (Indirect calorimetry). The essence of the technique is subtraction of the volume of oxygen breathed out (expired minute volume × mixed expired oxygen concentration) from the volume of oxygen breathed in (inspired minute volume × inspired oxygen concentration). The difference between the inspired and expired minute volumes is a very important factor in achieving accuracy with the method, particularly when a high concentration of oxygen is inhaled. Inspired and expired minute volumes differ as a result of the respiratory exchange ratio, and also any exchange of inert gas (e.g. nitrogen) that might occur. On the assumption that the patient is in equilibrium for nitrogen, and the mass of nitrogen inspired is the same as that expired, it follows that the ratio of inspired/expired minute volumes is inversely proportional to the respective ratios of nitrogen concentrations. Therefore:

$$\text{insp. minute volume} = \text{exp. minute volume} \times \frac{\text{exp. nitrogen concentration}}{\text{insp. nitrogen concentration}}$$

The ratio of the nitrogen concentrations is known as the Haldane transformation factor, which is used to calculate the inspired minute volume from the expired minute volume that is normally measured. Use of Haldane factors is valid only if the subject is in equilibrium with regard to nitrogen.

This is the basis of the classic Douglas bag technique, in which expired gas is measured for volume, and analysed for oxygen and carbon dioxide concentrations. The expired nitrogen concentration is determined by subtraction and the inspired minute volume derived. The approach has been automated by several manufacturers, and their systems can be used satisfactorily during artificial ventilation.[85] The essential feature is the measurement of gas composition of inspired and expired gas by the same analysers under the same conditions of humidity, temperature and pressure, with a very high level of accuracy. The potential for error is theoretically increased when the inspired oxygen concentration and minute volume are increased, but the manufacturers have had considerable success in overcoming the formidable practical problems.

The ventilated hood. In this approach, the subject's head is covered by a hood, through which is drawn a known high flow rate of air, sufficient to capture all the expired air. The gas drawn into the hood is expired air mixed with entrained air, and is treated in the calculations as though it were expired air. The surplus entrained air is like a very large dead space, but it does not alter the essential calculations. Clearly, the product of the air flow rate and the concentration of carbon dioxide in the gas drawn through the hood must equal the carbon dioxide output of the subject. Similarly, it is possible to derive oxygen consumption and respiratory exchange ratio. The system is virtually non-invasive and potentially very accurate. However, it can be used only when the subject is breathing air.

Multiplication of cardiac output by arterial/mixed venous oxygen content difference This approach is the reverse of using the Fick principle for measurement of cardiac output (see page 157) and is commonly known as the reversed Fick technique.

$$\dot{V}_{O_2} = \dot{Q}(Ca_{O_2} - C\bar{v}_{O_2})$$

where $\dot{V}_{O_2}$ is the oxygen consumption, $\dot{Q}$ is the cardiac output, Ca_{O_2} is the arterial oxygen content and $C\bar{v}_{O_2}$ is the mixed venous oxygen content.

The technique is essentially invasive because the cardiac output must be measured by an independent method (usually thermodilution), and it is also necessary to sample arterial and mixed venous blood, the latter preferably from the pulmonary artery. Nevertheless, it is convenient in the intensive care situation where the necessary vascular lines are commonly in place.

The method has a larger random error than the gasometric techniques described above,[84] but also has a systematic error because it excludes the oxygen consumption of the lungs (Figure 11.22).[9] In animal studies, the difference is negligible in the case of healthy lungs but is substantial when the lungs are infected.[86] Studies comparing the two methods in humans are presented in Table 11.5, showing the wide variations obtained by different groups. The necessity for invasive monitoring prevents the study of normal awake subjects, but results from patients in intensive care (with presumed lung pathology) do not seem to differ from patients with normal lungs undergoing cardiac surgery. Lung oxygen consumption measured as the difference between oxygen consumption by direct and

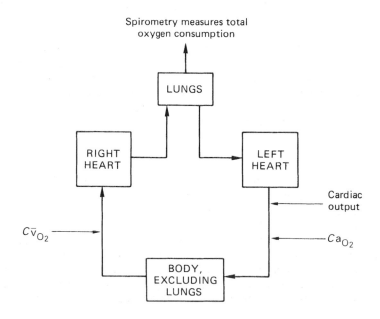

Oxygen delivery = cardiac output × Ca_{O_2}
Oxygen consumption (by reversed Fick technique)
= cardiac output $(Ca_{O_2} - C\bar{v}_{O_2})$

Figure 11.22 Schematic representation of the essential differences in measurement of oxygen consumption by spirometry and by the reversed Fick technique, which measures the oxygen consumption of the body *excluding* the lungs.

Table 11.5 Comparisons of oxygen consumption measured simultaneously by direct (spirometry or indirect calorimetry) or calculated (reverse Fick) methods

Patients studied	Direct measurement	Indirect measurement (reverse Fick)	Difference
Intensive care[87]	319	298	21
Intensive care[88]	320	253	67
Intensive care[84]	286	249	37
Intensive care[89]	262	262	0
Intensive care[62]	262	246	6
Anaesthetized, normal lungs[90]	216	190	26
Anaesthetized, normal lungs[91]	190	131	59
Intensive care[92]	218	173	45
Fulminant hepatic failure[93]	–	–	70

The difference is presumed to be due to the oxygen uptake of the lung. All values are mean results expressed as $ml.min^{-1}$. Where appropriate, body surface area is assumed to be 1.70 m^2.

reversed Fick techniques (Table 11.5) is similar to results obtained by measurement of lung oxygen consumption during cardiopulmonary bypass when the lungs are isolated from the rest of the circulation. The contribution of the lungs to total oxygen consumption therefore remains to be fully elucidated. Table 11.5 would seem to indicate that the pulmonary contribution may be very variable, depending on many physiological and pathological factors.

Validation of methods of measurement of oxygen consumption. Meticulous attention to detail is required if oxygen consumption is to be measured with a satisfactory degree of accuracy. Various metabolic simulators have been described for the validation of techniques under different circumstances of use. These include the combustion of known flow rates of an inflammable gas[83,94] and the preparation of a mock 'expired gas' by nitrogen dilution and addition of carbon dioxide.[88,95]

Oxygen delivery

Oxygen delivery is measured as the product of cardiac output and arterial oxygen content. This excludes oxygen delivered for consumption in the lung. In the intensive care situation, cardiac output is now commonly measured by thermal dilution and simultaneously an arterial sample is drawn for measurement of oxygen content by any of the methods described above. If oxygen delivery is determined at the same time that oxygen consumption is measured by the reversed Fick technique, it should be remembered that two of the variables (cardiac output and arterial oxygen content) are common to both measurements. This linking of data is a potential source of error in inferring the consequences of changes in one product on the other (see page 287).[60,96]

References

1. Filley GF, Mackintosh DJ, Wright GW. Carbon monoxide uptake and pulmonary diffusing capacity in normal subjects at rest and during exercise. *J Clin Invest* 1954; **33**: 530–9.
2. Kelman GR, Nunn JF. *Computer produced physiological tables*. London and Boston MA: Butterworth, 1968.

3. Kelman GR, Nunn JF, Prys-Roberts C, Greenbaum R. The influence of cardiac output on arterial oxygenation. *Br J Anaesth* 1967; **39**: 450–8.

4. Hsia CCW. Respiratory function of hemoglobin. *N Engl J Med* 1998; **338**: 239–47.

5. Perutz MF. Stereochemistry of cooperative effects in haemoglobin. *Nature* 1970; **228**: 726–39.

6. Kilmartin JV, Rossi-Bernardi L. Interaction of haemoglobin with hydrogen ions, carbon dioxide, and inorganic phosphates. *Physiol Rev* 1973; **53**: 836–90.

7. Ho C, Perussi JR. Proton nuclear magnetic resonance studies of haemoglobin. *Methods Enzymol* 1994; **232**: 97–139.

8. Gregory IC. The oxygen and carbon monoxide capacities of foetal and adult blood. *J Physiol* 1974; **236**: 625–34.

9. Nunn JF. Pulmonary oxygen consumption. *Intensive Care Med* 1996; **22**: 275–6.

10. Adair GS. The hemoglobin system. VI. The oxygen dissociation curve of hemoglobin. *J Biol Chem* 1925; **63**: 529–45.

11. Imai, K. Adair fitting to oxygen equilibration curves of hemoglobin. *Methods Enzymol* 1994; **232**: 559–76.

12. Staub NC, Bishop JM, Forster RE. Velocity of O_2 uptake by human red blood cells. *J Appl Physiol* 1961; **16**: 511–16.

13. Kelman GR. Digital computer subroutine for the conversion of oxygen tension into saturation. *J Appl Physiol* 1966; **21**: 1375–6.

14. Severinghaus JW, Stafford M, Thunstrom AM. Estimation of skin metabolism and blood flow with tcPO₂ and tcPCO₂ electrodes by cuff occlusion of the circulation. *Acta Anaesthiol Scand Supp* 1978; **68**: 9–15.

15. Roughton FJW, Severinghaus JW. Accurate determination of O_2 dissociation curve of human blood above 98.7% saturation with data on O_2 solubility in unmodified human blood from 0°C to 37°C. *J Appl Physiol* 1973; **35**: 861–9.

16. Severinghaus JW. Blood gas calculator. *J Appl Physiol* 1966; **21**: 1108–16.

17. Thomas LJ. Algorithms for selected blood acid–base and blood gas calculations. *J Appl Physiol* 1972; **33**: 154–8.

18. Chanutin A, Curnish R. Effect of organic and inorganic phosphates on the oxygen equilibrium of human erythrocytes. *Arch Biochem Biophys* 1967; **121**: 96–9.

19. Benesch R, Benesch RE. The effects of organic phosphate from human erythrocyte on the allosteric properties of hemoglobin. *Biochem Biophys Res Commun* 1967; **26**: 162–7.

20. MacDonald R. Red cell 2,3-diphosphoglycerate and oxygen affinity. *Anaesthesia* 1977; **32**: 544–53.

21. Shappell SD, Lenfant CJM. Adaptive, genetic and iatrogenic alterations of the oxyhaemoglobin-dissociation curve. *Anesthesiology* 1972; **37**: 127–39.

22. Shafer AW, Tague LL, Welch MH, Guenter CA. 2,3-Diphosphoglycerate in red cells stored in acid–citrate–dextrose and citrate–phosphate–dextrose: implications regarding delivery of oxygen. *J Lab Clin Med* 1971; **77**: 430–7.

23. Heaton A, Keegan T, Holme S. *In vivo* regeneration of red cell 2,3-diphosphoglycerate following transfusion of DPG-depleted AS-1, AS-3 and CPDA-1 red cells. *Br J Haematol* 1989; **71**: 131–6.

24. Valeri CR. Blood components in the treatment of acute blood loss: use of freeze-preserved red cells, platelets and plasma proteins. *Anesth Analg* 1975; **54**: 1–14.

25. Guy JT, Brombert PA, Metz EN, Ringle R, Balcerzak SP. Oxygen delivery following transfusion of stored blood. I. Normal rats. *J Appl Physiol* 1974; **37**: 60–3.

26. Valeri CR, Collins FB. Physiologic effects of 2,3-DPG-depleted red cells with high affinity for oxygen. *J Appl Physiol* 1971; **31**: 823–7.

27. Sheldon GF. Diphosphoglycerate in massive transfusion and erythrophoresis. *Crit Care Med* 1979; **7**: 407–11.

28. Bowen JC, Fleming WH. Increased oxyhaemoglobin affinity after transfusion of stored blood: evidence for circulatory compensation. *Ann Surg* 1974; **180**: 760–4.

29. Torrance J, Jacobs P, Restrepo A, Eschbach J, Lenfant C, Finch CA. Intraerythrocytic adaptation to anemia. *N Engl J Med* 1970; **283**: 165–9.

30. Huisman TH. The structure and function of normal and abnormal haemoglobins. *Baillière's Clin Haematol* 1993; **6**: 1–30.

31. Wajcman H, Galacteros F. Abnormal haemoglobins with high oxygen affinity and erythrocytosis. *Hematol Cell Ther* 1996; **38**: 305–12.

32. Jaffé ER. Methaemoglobinaemia. *Clin Haematol* 1981; **10**: 99–122.

33. Coleman MD, Coleman NA. Drug-induced methaemoglobinaemia. Treatment issues. *Drug Saf* 1996; **14**: 394–405

34. Toothill C. The chemistry of the in vivo reaction between haemoglobin and various oxides of nitrogen. *Br J Anaesth* 1967; **39**: 405–12.

35. Jia L, Bonaventura C, Bonaventura J, Stamler JS. *S*-Nitrosohaemoglobin: a dynamic activity of blood involved in vascular control. *Nature* 1996; **380**: 221–6.

36. Stamler JS, Simon DL, Osborne JA, Mullins ME, Jaraki O, Michel T et al. *S*-Nitrosylation of proteins with nitric oxide: synthesis and characterisation of biologically active compounds. *Proc Natl Acad Sci USA* 1992; **89**: 444–8.

37. Shen W, Hintze TH, Wolin MS. Nitric oxide: an important signaling mechanism between vascular endothelium and parenchymal cells in the regulation of oxygen consumption. *Circulation* 1995; **92**: 3505–12.

38. Mallick A, Bodenham AR. Modified haemoglobins as oxygen transporting blood substitutes. *Br J Hosp Med* 1996; **55**: 443–8.

39. Spiess BD. Perfluorocarbon emulsions: one approach to intravenous artificial respiratory gas transport. *Int Anesthesiol Clin* 1995; **33**: 103–13.

40. Tobias MD, Longnecker DE. Recombinant haemoglobin and other blood substitutes. *Baillière's Clin Anaesth* 1995; **9**: 165–79.

41. Urbaniak SJ. Artificial blood. *BMJ* 1991; **303**: 1348–50.

42. Hirschl RB, Pranikoff T, Gauger P, Schreiner RJ, Dechert R, Bartlett RH. Liquid ventilation in adults, children, and full-term neonates. *Lancet* 1995; **346**: 1201–2.

43. Ogden JE, Parry ES. The development of hemoglobin solutions as red cell substitutes. *Int Anesthesiol Clin* 1995; **33**: 115–29.

44. Tremper KK. Hemoglobin-based oxygen carriers: problems and promise. *J Cardiothorac Vasc Anesth* 1997; **11**: 1–2.

45. Hoffman SJ, Looker DL, Roehrich JM, Cozart PE, Durfee SL, Tedesco JL, Stetler GL. Expression of fully functional tetrameric human haemoglobin in *Escherichia coli. Proc Natl Acad Sci USA* 1990; **87**: 8521–5.

46. Looker D, Abbott-Brown D, Kozart P, Durfee S, Hoffman S, Mathews AJ, et al. A human recombinant hemoglobin designed for use as a blood substitute. *Nature* 1992; **356**: 258–60.

47. Burkard ME, Van Liew HD. Oxygen transport to tissues by persistent bubbles: theory and simulations. *J Appl Physiol* 1994; **77**: 2874–8.

48. D'Arrigo JS, Ho S-Y, Simon RH. Detection of experimental rat liver tumors by contrast-assisted ultrasonography. *Invest Radiol* 1993; **28**: 218–22.

49. Marshall BE, Whyche MQ. Hypoxemia during and after anesthesia. *Anesthesiology* 1972; **37**: 178–209.

50. Lübbers DW, Baumgärtl H. Heterogeneities and profiles of oxygen pressure in brain and kidney as examples of the pO_2 distribution in living tissue. *Kidney Int* 1997; **51**: 372–80.

51. Weibel ER, Taylor CR, Weber J-M, Vock R, Roberts TJ, Hoppeler H. Design of the oxygen substrate pathways. VII. Different structural limits for oxygen and substrate supply to muscle mitochondria. *J Exp Biol* 1996; **199**: 1699–709.

52. Barcroft J. Physiological effects of insufficient oxygen supply. *Nature* 1920; **106**: 125–9.

53. Hinds C, Watson D. Manipulating hemodynamics and oxygen transport in critically ill patients. *N Engl J Med* 1995; **333**: 1074–5.

54. Soni N, Fawcett WJ, Halliday FC. Beyond the lung: oxygen delivery and tissue oxygenation. *Anaesthesia* 1993; **48**: 704–11.

55. Pinsky MR. Beyond global oxygen supply–demand relations: in search of measures of dysoxia. *Intensive Care Med* 1994; **20**: 1–3.

56. Shoemaker WC, Bland RD, Apel PL. Therapy of critically ill postoperative patients based on outcome prediction and prospective clinical trials. *Surg Clin North Am* 1985; **65**: 811–33.

57. Gattinoni L, Brazzi L, Pelosi P, Latini R, Tognoni G, Pesenti A, Fumagalli R. A trial of goal-oriented hemodynamic therapy in critically ill patients. *N Engl J Med* 1995; **333**: 1025–32.

58. Hayes MA, Timmins AC, Yau EHS, Palazzo M, Hinds CJ, Watson D. Elevation of systemic oxygen delivery in the treatment of critically ill patients. *N Engl J Med* 1994; **330**: 1717–22.

59. Steltzer H, Hiesmayr M, Mayer N, Krafft P, Hammerle AF. The relationship between oxygen delivery and

uptake in the critically ill: is there a critical or optimal therapeutic value? A meta-analysis. *Anaesthesia* 1994; **49**: 229–36.

60. Walsh TS, Lee A. Mathematical coupling in medical research: lessons from studies of oxygen kinetics. *Br J Anaesth* 1998; **81**: 118–20.

61. Russell JA, Phang PT. The oxygen delivery/consumption controversy. *Am J Respir Crit Care Med* 1994; **149**: 533–7.

62. Hanique G, Dugernier T, Laterre PF, Dougnac A, Roesler J, Reynaert MS. Significance of pathologic oxygen supply dependency in critically ill patients: comparison between measured and calculated methods. *Intensive Care Med* 1994; **20**: 12–18.

63. Richardson FJ, Chinn S, Nunn JF. Performance and application of the quantiflex air/oxygen mixer. *Br J Anaesth* 1976; **48**: 1057–64.

64. Leigh JM. Variation in performance of oxygen therapy devices. *Ann R Coll Surg Engl* 1973; **52**: 234–53.

65. Flenley DC. Disordered breathing during sleep: discussion paper. *J R Soc Med* 1985; **78**: 1031–3.

66. Davies RJO, Hopkin JM. Nasal oxygen in exacerbations of ventilatory failure: an underappreciated risk. *BMJ* 1989; **299**: 43–4.

67. Lundsgaard C, Van Slyke DD. *Cyanosis*. Baltimore: Williams & Wilkins, 1923.

68. Goss GA, Hayes JA, Burdon JGW. Deoxyhaemoglobin in the detection of central cyanosis. *Thorax* 1988; **43**: 212–13.

69. Kelman GR, Nunn JF. Clinical recognition of hypoxaemia under fluorescent lamps. *Lancet* 1966; **1**: 1400–3.

70. Familton MJG, Armstrong RF. Pseudo-cyanosis: time to reclassify cyanosis. *Anaesthesia* 1989; **44**; 257.

71. Timmins AC, Morgan GAR. Argyria or cyanosis. *Anaesthesia* 1988; **43**: 755–6.

72. Ellis FR, Nunn JF. The measurement of gaseous oxygen tension utilising paramagnetism: an evaluation of the Servomex OA 150 analyser. *Br J Anaesth* 1968; **40**: 569–78.

73. Clark LC. Monitor and control of tissue oxygen tensions. *Trans Am Soc Artif Intern Organs* 1956; **2**: 41–8.

74. Weiss IK, Fink S, Edmunds S, Harrison R, Donnelly K. Continuous arterial gas monitoring: initial experience with the Paratrend 7 in children. *Intensive Care Med* 1996; **22**: 1414–17.

75. Nunn JF, Bergman NA, Bunatyan A, Coleman AJ. Temperature coefficients for Pco_2 and Po_2 of blood in vitro. *J Appl Physiol* 1965; **20**: 23–6.

76. Severinghaus JW. A combined transcutaneous Po_2–Pco_2 electrode with electrochemical HCO_3^- stabilization. *J Appl Physiol* 1981; **51**: 1027–32.

77. Severinghaus JW, Kelleher JF. Recent developments in pulse oximetry. *Anesthesiology* 1992; **76**: 1018–38.

78. Severinghaus JW, Spellman MJ. Pulse oximeter failure thresholds in hypotension and vasoconstriction. *Anesthesiology* 1990; **73**: 532–7.

79. Severinghaus JW, Koh SO. Effect of anemia on pulse oximeter accuracy at low saturation. *J Clin Monit* 1990; **6**: 85–8.

80. Kram HB, Shoemaker WC. Method for intraoperative assessment of organ perfusion and viability using a miniature oxygen sensor. *Am J Surg* 1984; **148**: 404–7.

81. Harris DNF. Near infra-red spectroscopy. *Anaesthesia* 1995; **50**: 1015–16.

82. Vincent JL. Monitoring tissue perfusion. *Can J Anaesth* 1996; **43**: R55–7.

83. Nunn JF, Makita K, Royston B. Validation of oxygen consumption measurements during artificial ventilation. *J Appl Physiol* 1989; **67**: 2129–34.

84. Smithies MN, Royston B, Makita K, Konieczko K, Nunn JF. Comparison of oxygen consumption measurements: indirect calorimetry versus the reversed Fick method. *Crit Care Med* 1991; **19**:1401–6.

85. Makita K, Nunn JF, Royston B. Evaluation of metabolic measuring instruments for use in critically ill patients. *Crit Care Med* 1990; **18**: 638–44.

86. Light RB. Intrapulmonary oxygen consumption in experimental pneumococcal pneumonia. *J Appl Physiol* 1988; **64**: 2490–5.

87. Behrendt W, Weiland C, Kalff J, Giani G. Continuous measurement of oxygen uptake. Evaluation of the Engstrom metabolic computer and clinical experiences. *Acta Anaesthesiol Scand* 1987; **31**:10–14.

88. Takala J, Keinanen O, Vaisanen P, Kari A. Measurement of gas exchange in intensive care: laboratory and clinical validation of a new device. *Crit Care Med* 1989; **17**:1041–7.

89. Hanique G, Dugernier T, Laterre PF, Roeseler J, Dougnac A, Reynaert MS. Evaluation of oxygen uptake and delivery in critically ill patients: a statistical reappraisal. *Intensive Care Med* 1994; **20**: 19–26.

90. Bizouarn P, Blanloeil Y, Pinaud M. Comparison between oxygen consumption calculated by Fick's principle using continuous thermodilution technique and measured by indirect calorimetry. *Br J Anaesth* 1995; **75**: 719–23.

91. Oudemans-van Straaten HM, Scheffer GJ, Eysman L, Wildevuur ChRH. Oxygen consumption after cardiopulmonary bypass – implications of different measuring methods. *Intensive Care Med* 1993; **19**: 105–10.

92. Jolliet P, Thorens JB, Nicod L, Pichard C, Kyle U, Chevrolet JC. Relationship between pulmonary oxygen consumption, lung inflammation, and calculated venous admixture in patients with acute lung injury. *Intensive Care Med* 1996; **22**: 277–85.

93. Walsh TS, Hopton P, Lee A. Comparison between reverse Fick and indirect calorimeter measurements of oxygen consumption in patients with fulminant hepatic failure. *Br J Anaesth* 1997; **79**: 131P–2P.

94. Svensson KL, Sonander HG, Stenqvist O. Validation of a system for measurement of metabolic gas exchange during anaesthesia with controlled ventilation in an oxygen consuming lung model. *Br J Anaesth* 1990; **64**: 311–19.

95. Braun U, Zundel J, Freiboth K, Weyland W, Turner E, Heidelmeyer CF, Hellige G. Evaluation of methods for indirect calorimetry with a ventilated lung model. *Intensive Care Med* 1989; **15**: 196–202.

96. Archie JP. Mathematical coupling of data. A common source of error. *Ann Surg* 1981; **193**: 296–303.

97. Kelman GR, Nunn JF. Nomograms for correction of blood P_{O_2}, P_{CO_2}, pH and base excess for time and temperature. *J Appl Physiol* 1996; **21**: 1484.

Chapter 12

Non-respiratory functions of the lung

The lungs are primarily adapted to subserve the purpose of gas exchange, and to achieve this with such efficiency almost the entire blood volume passes through the lungs during a single circulation. This characteristic makes the lungs ideally suited to undertake many other important functions. The location of the lungs in the circulatory system is ideal for its role as a filter to protect the systemic circulation, not only from particulate matter but also from a wide range of chemical substances that undergo removal or biotransformation in the pulmonary circulation. The pulmonary arterial tree is well adapted for the reception of emboli without resultant infarction, and the very large area of endothelium gives the lung a metabolic role out of proportion to its total mass. This large interface between the external atmosphere and the circulation is not without its own hazards, and the lung must protect the circulation from many potentially harmful inhaled substances.

Filtration

Sitting astride the whole output of the right ventricle, the lung is ideally situated to filter out particulate matter from the systemic venous return. Without such a filter, there would be a constant risk of particulate matter entering the arterial system, where the coronary and cerebral circulations are particularly vulnerable to damaging emboli. Desirable though this function seems at first sight, it cannot be essential to life, as it is partially bypassed in patients with a right-to-left intracardiac shunt.

Pulmonary capillaries have a diameter of about 7 μm, but this does not seem to be the effective pore size of the pulmonary circulation when considered as a filter. There is no clear agreement on the maximal diameter of particles that can traverse the pulmonary circulation. Animal studies have demonstrated the passage through perfused lungs of glass beads up to 500 μm.[1] It is well known that small quantities of gas and fat emboli may gain access to the systemic circulation in patients without intracardiac shunting. More extensive invasion of the systemic arteries may occur in the presence of an overt right-to-left intracardiac shunt, which is potentially quite common. Post mortem studies show that over 25 per cent of the population have a 'probe-patent' foramen ovale, which is normally kept closed by the left atrial pressure being slightly greater than the right. In more than 10 per cent of normal subjects, a simple Valsalva manoeuvre or cough results in easily demonstrable blood flow between the right and left atria.[2] Paradoxical embolism may therefore result from a relative increase in right atrial pressure caused by physiological events (page 553). Furthermore, emboli may bypass the alveoli as a result of the opening of 'sperr' arteries (page 139).

So far as the survival of the lung is concerned, the geometry of the pulmonary microcirculation is particularly well adapted to maintaining alveolar perfusion in the face of quite large degrees of embolization. However, a significant degree of embolization inevitably blocks the circulation to parts of the lung, disturbing the balance between ventilation and perfusion. This situation is considered in Chapter 28. Pulmonary microembolism with small clumps of fibrin and/or platelets will not have a direct effect on gas exchange until it is very extensive. Plugging of pulmonary capillaries by microemboli does, however, initiate neutrophil activation in the area that leads to an increase in endothelial permeability and alveolar oedema,[3] and has been implicated in the aetiology of acute lung injury (Chapter 30).

Thrombi are cleared more rapidly from the lungs than from other organs. The lung possesses well-developed proteolytic systems not confined to the removal of fibrin. Pulmonary endothelium is known to be rich in plasmin activator, which converts plasminogen into plasmin which in turn converts fibrin into fibrin degradation products. However, the lung is also rich in thromboplastin, which converts prothrombin to thrombin. To complicate the position further, the lung is a particularly rich source of heparin, and bovine lung is used in its commercial preparation. The lung can thus produce high concentrations of substances necessary to promote or delay blood clotting and also for fibrinolysis. Apart from the lung's ability to clear itself of thromboemboli, it may play a role in controlling the overall coagulability of the blood.

Defence against inhaled substances

The skin, gastrointestinal tract and lungs form the major interfaces between the outside world and the carefully controlled internal body systems. Efficient gas exchange in the lung requires a physically very thin interface between air and blood, which leaves the lung vulnerable to invasion by many airborne hazards, both chemical and biological.

Biological hazards

Inhaled bacteria, viruses, fungi and spores are effectively dealt with by the respiratory mucosa, as described on page 26. Most pathogens are large enough (over 5 μm) to be impacted on the mucous layer in the airways, which allows them to be removed intact. Some will penetrate deeper in the bronchial tree, particularly when the infective load is high during respiratory infections, and must be dealt with by neutrophils, macrophages and other phagocytes.

Protease transport system. Activation of neutrophils in the lung leads to the release of dangerous proteases, particularly elastase and trypsin. These enzymes are highly effective at destroying pathogens, but if left unchecked may also damage lung tissues. There are at least two mechanisms to protect against this eventuality. First, the proteases are mostly confined to the mucous layer, which is continually swept towards the larynx by the flow of mucus. Secondly, they are conjugated by α_1-antitrypsin, present in plasma. Conjugated proteases are then removed in the pulmonary circulation and lymph, and transferred to conjugation with α_2-macroglobulin, which is finally destroyed in the liver.

In 1963 a group of patients were described whose plasma proteins were deficient in α_1-antitrypsin and who had developed emphysema.[4] The enzyme deficiency is inherited as an autosomal recessive gene and the incidence of homozygous patients is about 1:3000 of the population, though many of these are believed to succumb to pulmonary and liver disease before the α_1-antitrypsin deficiency is ever found.[5] Homozygotes do form a higher proportion of patients with emphysema and estimates range from 3 to 26 per cent. These patients tend to have basal emphysema, onset at a younger age and a severe form of the disease.[6] It thus seems that α_1-antitrypsin deficiency is an aetiological factor in a small proportion of patients with emphysema (page 532). Smoking, which increases neutrophil protease production (page 412) and inactivates α_1-antitrypsin, is associated with more severe lung disease in patients with a deficiency of α_1-antitrypsin.[5]

Phagocytosis of pathogens. Neutrophils are common in the mucous of the bronchial tree, and it is well established that, with more widespread infection, neutrophils, macrophages and certain other cells can marginate on the pulmonary capillary endothelium. Following immunological activation, these phagocytic cells throughout the lung are responsible for killing pathogens, and do so by the formation of oxygen-derived free radicals. Very substantial quantities of oxygen are consumed in the formation of free radicals and related species derived from molecular oxygen. The mechanism is described elsewhere (page 499) in relation to oxygen toxicity. Though not yet conclusively proven, it is possible that pulmonary oxygen consumption is higher in infected lungs (see Table 11.5), and this is likely to result, at least in part, from oxygen consumed in killing pathogens.[7]

Chemical hazards

Many factors will influence the fate of inhaled chemicals.[8]

Particle size, as with biological particles, will affect where in the lung deposition occurs: above 5 μm deposit in the nose and large airways; less than 1 μm enter the alveoli; whilst the remainder are spread between the two.

Water solubility. Once incorporated into the lung tissue, water solubility affects the rate at which chemicals are cleared from the lung, water-soluble substances taking longer than lipid soluble ones to be absorbed into the blood for disposal elsewhere.

Concentration of inhaled chemicals is important, as metabolic activity within the lung is easily saturated.

Metabolism of inhaled chemicals is poorly understood in the human lung, and, though it has been extensively investigated in animals, there are known to be large species differences.[8] Metabolic activity is found in all cell types of the respiratory mucosa, but in animals is particularly well developed in Clara cells and type II alveolar cells (page 31).[8,9] As in the liver, metabolism of toxic chemicals involves two stages:

1. Phase I metabolism in which the toxic molecule is converted to a different compound, usually by oxidative reactions. This is achieved in the lung by the cytochrome P-450 monoxygenase and, to a much lesser extent, flavin-based monoxygenase systems. The lung is one of the major extrahepatic sites of mixed function oxidation by the cytochrome P-450 systems but, gram for gram, remains considerably less active than the liver.
2. Phase II metabolism involves conjugation of the resulting compounds to 'carrier' molecules, which render them less biologically active, more water soluble and

therefore easier to excrete. In the lung, phase II metabolism is normally by conjugation with glucuronide or glutathione.[8]

Metabolic changes to inhaled chemicals may not be beneficial, especially with many synthetic organic compounds and several chemicals in cigarette smoke (page 407). Bioactivation by phase I metabolism converts some quite innocuous compounds into potent carcinogens, whilst slightly different metabolic conversions may do the reverse.[8,10] The balance between activating and inactivating pathways varies between species. What little data are available on human lungs indicate that we are fortunate in having a very favourable ratio, the inactivation of potential carcinogens being 100-fold greater than in rodents.[8] Presumably, without this evolutionary advantage, the history of cigarette smoking would have been considerably different.

Processing of endogenous compounds by the pulmonary vasculature[11,12]

As long ago as 1925, Starling and Verney observed that passage of blood through the lungs was essential for maintenance of adequate circulation through an isolated perfused kidney.[13] It was later found that the 'detoxification of a serum vasoconstrictor substance' in the blood was due to removal of 5-hydroxytryptamine (serotonin) in the pulmonary circulation. Much recent research has now shown that certain hormones pass through the lung unchanged, others may be almost entirely removed from the blood during a single pass, and some may be activated during transit (Table 12.1).

Of the many types of cell in the lungs, it is the endothelium that is most active metabolically. The most important location is the pulmonary capillary but it must be stressed that endothelium from a very wide range of vessels has been shown to possess a very similar repertoire of metabolic processes.[14] This is fortunate because it is not possible to harvest pulmonary capillary endothelium, so cultures must be prepared from vascular endothelial cells harvested from other sites (e.g. human umbilical vein). However, there are some important differences in activity between endothelium from different vessels.

Table 12.1 Summary of metabolic changes to hormones on passing through the pulmonary circulation

Group	Effect of passing through pulmonary circulation		
	Activated	*No change*	*Inactivated*
Amines		Dopamine Adrenaline Histamine	5-Hydroxytryptamine Noradrenaline
Peptides	Angiotensin I	Angiotensin II Oxytocin Vasopressin	Bradykinin Atrial natriuretic peptide Endothelins
Arachidonic acid derivatives	Arachidonic acid	PGI_2 (prostacyclin) PGA_2	PGD_2 PGE_2 $PGF_{2\alpha}$ Leukotrienes
Purine derivatives			Adenosine ATP, ADP, AMP

For example, endothelium grown from various non-pulmonary vessels will not inactivate PGE_2, although this is well known to occur in the pulmonary circulation. The extensive metabolic activity of the pulmonary endothelium takes place in spite of the paucity of organelles, which are normally associated with metabolic activity, in particular mitochondria and smooth endoplasmic reticulum or microsomes (see Figure 2.8). Nevertheless, the caveolae result in a major increase in the already extensive surface area of these cells (about $126\,m^2$),[15] which is particularly advantageous for membrane-bound enzymes.

Catecholamines and acetylcholine

Noradrenaline (norepinephrine). There is a striking difference in the handling of noradrenaline and adrenaline. Although each catecholamine has a half-life of about 20 seconds in blood, some 30 per cent of noradrenaline is removed in a single pass through the lungs,[16] while adrenaline (and isoprenaline and dopamine) are unaffected. Monoamine oxidase and catechol-*O*-methyl transferase in the endothelial cells will metabolize all amine derivatives with equal efficiency. The specificity of pulmonary endothelium for noradrenaline therefore lies with the cell membrane, which selectively takes up only noradrenaline and 5-hydroxytryptamine.[17] Extraneuronal uptake of noradrenaline is not confined to the endothelium of the lungs, but uptake by the pulmonary circulation differs from extraneuronal uptake (uptake 2) in other tissues, which is less specific for noradrenaline.[18]

5-Hydroxytryptamine (5-HT, serotonin) is removed very effectively by the lungs, up to 98 per cent being removed in a single pass.[19] There are considerable similarities to the processing of noradrenaline. 5-HT is taken up by the endothelium, mainly in the capillaries,[18] and is then rapidly metabolized by monoamine oxidase. The half-life of 5-HT in blood is about 1–2 minutes, and pulmonary clearance plays the main role in preventing its recirculation. If the uptake of 5-HT is inhibited (e.g. by cocaine or tricyclic antidepressant drugs), its pulmonary clearance is greatly reduced.[20]

Histamine, dopamine and adrenaline are not removed from blood on passage through the pulmonary circulation, in spite of the high concentrations of monoamine oxidase in lung tissue. Their removal from the circulation is limited by the lack of a transport mechanism across the blood/endothelium barrier.

Acetylcholine is rapidly hydrolysed in blood where it has a half-life of less than 2 seconds. This tends to overshadow any changes attributable to the lung, which nevertheless does contain acetylcholinesterases and pseudocholinesterases.

Peptides

Angiotensin. It has long been known that angiotensin I, a decapeptide formed by the action of renin on a plasma α_2-globulin (angiotensinogen), was converted into the vasoactive octapeptide angiotensin II by incubation with plasma (Figure 12.1). In 1967, Ng and Vane[21] found greatly increased conversion in the pulmonary circulation, some 80 per cent being converted in a single pass. Enhanced conversion of angiotensin is not peculiar to the pulmonary circulation but the lung is certainly a major site for angiotensin conversion. Angiotensin-converting enzyme (ACE) is free in the plasma but is also bound to the surface of endothelium. This seems to be a general property of endothelium but ACE is

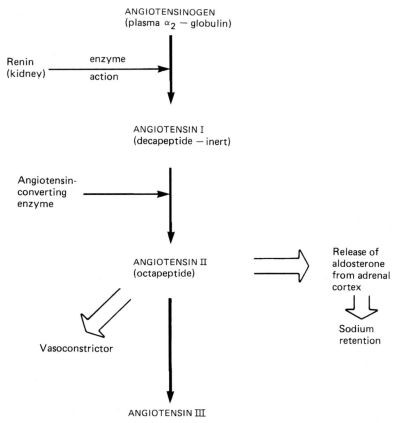

ANGIOTENSINOGEN
(plasma α_2 − globulin)

Renin
(kidney)

enzyme

action

ANGIOTENSIN I
(decapeptide − inert)

Angiotensin-
converting
enzyme

ANGIOTENSIN II
(octapeptide)

Release of
aldosterone
from adrenal
cortex

Sodium
retention

Vasoconstrictor

ANGIOTENSIN III

Figure 12.1 Renin–angiotensin–aldosterone axis. Angiotensin-converting enzyme is found in plasma and on systemic vascular endothelium, but is present in much larger quantities on the endothelium of pulmonary vessels.

present in abundance on the vascular surface of pulmonary endothelial cells, also lining the inside of the caveolae and extending onto the projections into the lumen.[14]

Bradykinin, a vasoactive nonapeptide, is also very effectively removed during passage through the lung and other vascular beds. The half-life in blood is about 17 seconds but less than 4 seconds in various vascular beds. Like angiotensin I, ACE is the enzyme responsible for metabolism of bradykinin.

   ACE is inhibited by many substances, many of which now have an enormous clinical role in the treatment of cardiovascular disease. However, this also decreases the degradation of bradykinin by ACE, although other enzymes are capable of handling bradykinin. Even with total inhibition of ACE, there is thought to be an adequate reserve for bradykinin metabolism.[22] Angiotensin II itself passes through the lung unchanged, as do vasopressin and oxytocin.

Atrial natriuretic peptide (ANP) is largely removed by the rabbit lung in a single pass but can then be released from what seems to be binding to a 'silent' receptor – that is, a receptor that specifically binds ANP but in so doing does not initiate any other cellular action.[23]

Endothelins, a group of 21 amino acid peptides with diverse biological activity (page 153), have a plasma half-life of just a few minutes, being cleared by the kidney, liver and lungs. The pulmonary enzymes responsible are not clearly defined, but there are believed to be several different types in humans.[24]

Arachidonic acid derivatives

The lung is a major site of synthesis, metabolism, uptake and release of arachidonic acid metabolites.[25] The group as a whole are 20-carbon carboxylic acids, generically known as eicosanoids. The initial stages of metabolism of arachidonic acid are oxygenations with two main pathways for which the enzymes are respectively cyclo-oxygenase and lipoxygenase. The cyclo-oxygenase pathway (Figure 12.2) commences with oxygenation and cyclization to form the prostaglandin PGG_2, the enzyme being microsomal and found in most cells (the subscript 2 indicates two double bonds in the

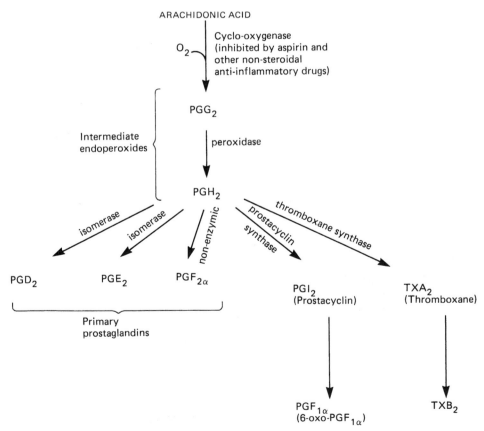

Figure 12.2 The cyclo-oxygenase pathway of metabolism of arachidonic acid to form the prostaglandins and thromboxanes. See text for metabolism taking place in the lungs.

carbon chain). A non-specific peroxidase then converts PGG_2 to PGH_2, which is the parent compound for synthesis of many important derivatives shown in Figure 12.2.

$PGF_{2\alpha}$, PGD_2, PGG_2, PGH_2 and thromboxane TXA_2 are bronchial and tracheal constrictors, $PGF_{2\alpha}$ and PGD_2 being much more potent in asthmatics than in normal subjects. PGE_1 and PGE_2 are bronchodilators, particularly when administered by aerosol. Prostacyclin (PGI_2) has different effects in different species. In humans, it has no effect on airway calibre in doses that have profound cardiovascular effects.[26] PGI_2 and PGE_1 are pulmonary vasodilators. PGH_2 and $PGF_{2\alpha}$ are pulmonary vasoconstrictors.

Eicosanoids are not stored preformed, but are synthesized as required by many cell types in the lung, including endothelium, airway smooth muscle, mast cells, epithelial cells and vascular muscle. Activation of the complement system is a potent stimulus to the metabolism of arachidonic acid. Synthesis from endogenous arachidonic acid in the lung seems to be limited by the rate of formation of arachidonic acid from parent lipids. Steroids decrease the availability of endogenous arachidonic acid. Infusion of exogenous arachidonic acid bypasses this stage and results in both bronchoconstriction and vasoconstriction, mediated by its metabolites and depending on the dose. This effect can

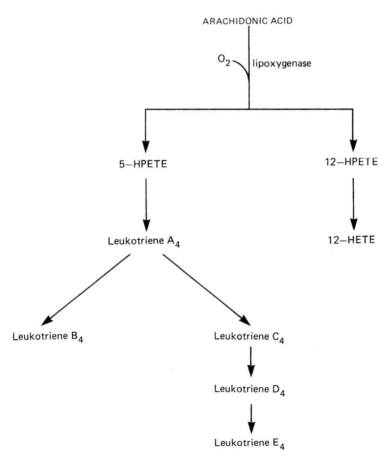

Figure 12.3 The lipoxygenase pathway of metabolism of arachidonic acid to form the leukotrienes. See text for metabolism taking place in the lungs.

be blocked by high-dose aspirin and some other non-steroidal anti-inflammatory drugs that inhibit cyclo-oxygenase. Release of eicosanoids, particularly TXA_2, occurs in anaphylactic reactions in response to complement activation. However, release of cyclo-oxygenase products does not seem to be a major factor in allergic asthma, which is not significantly relieved by inhibition of cyclo-oxygenase. This may well be explained by increased availability of arachidonic acid for the lipoxygenase pathway (see below).

Various specific enzymes in the lung are responsible for extensive metabolism of PGE_2, PGE_1 and $PGF_{2\alpha}$. However, PGA_2 and PGI_2 pass through the lung unchanged but are metabolized on passing through the portal circulation.[25] As for catecholamine metabolism, specificity for pulmonary prostaglandin metabolism is in the uptake pathways rather than with the intracellular enzymes.[12]

Leukotrienes are also eicosanoids derived from arachidonic acid but by the lipoxygenase pathway (Figure 12.3). The leukotrienes LTC_4 and LTD_4 are mainly responsible for the bronchoconstrictor effects of what was formerly known as slow-reacting substance A or SRS-A.[27] SRS-A also contains LTB_4, which is a less powerful bronchoconstrictor but increases vascular permeability. These compounds, which are synthesized by the mast cell, have an important role in asthma; the mechanism of their release is discussed in Chapter 27.

Purine derivatives

Specific enzymes exist on the surface of pulmonary endothelial cells for the degradation of AMP, ADP and ATP to adenosine. Adenosine itself has potent effects on the circulation, but is also inactivated in the lungs by a rapid uptake mechanism into the endothelial cells, where it is either phosphorylated into AMP or deaminated to produce inosine and ultimately uric acid for excretion.

Processing of drugs by the lung

The wide range of mechanisms present in the lung for the processing of endogenous and inhaled substances makes an effect on drug disposition almost inevitable.

Inhaled drugs will be subjected to the same metabolic activity in the airway and alveolar cells as other toxic chemicals described above. Mixed function oxidase and cytochrome P-450 systems are active in the lung and so are presumed to metabolize drugs in the same way as in hepatocytes. Unlike the liver, there is little evidence that these enzymes can be induced to increase their availability when required. Steroids are known to be metabolized in lung airway tissue, as is isoprenaline.[12] Inhalational anaesthetics, in particular those that undergo significant metabolism elsewhere in the body such as methoxyflurane and halothane, undergo biotransformation in the airways by similar pathways producing fluoride ions.[28]

Pulmonary circulation.[12,29] Many drugs are removed from the circulation on passing through the lungs. However, in most cases this occurs by binding of the drug to lung tissue rather than actual metabolism. There are two likely reasons for this. First, access to the metabolic enzymes in endothelial cells is closely controlled by highly specific uptake mechanisms that are vital to allow the highly selective metabolism of endogenous compounds. Secondly, it is possible that the oxidative systems responsible for drug metabolism elsewhere in the body are located mostly in the airways, thus preventing bloodborne drugs gaining access to them. Drugs that are basic and lipophilic tend to be taken up in the pulmonary circulation whereas acidic drugs preferentially bind to plasma proteins.[12] Drug binding in the pulmonary circulation may act as a reservoir for the drug, and give rise to rapid changes in plasma drug levels either when the binding sites become saturated or when one drug is displaced by a different drug with greater affinity for the binding site.

Pulmonary toxicity of drugs. Accumulation of some drugs and other toxic substances in the lung may cause dangerous local toxicity.[30] Paraquat is an outstanding example: it is slowly taken up into alveolar epithelial cells where it promotes the production of reactive oxygen species (page 502), with resulting lung damage. Some drugs cause pulmonary toxicity by a similar mechanism, including nitrofurantoin and bleomycin, toxicity from the latter being strongly associated with exposure to high concentrations of oxygen. Amiodarone, a highly effective and commonly used antiarrhythmic agent, is also associated with pulmonary toxicity which occurs in 6 per cent of patients given the drug.[31] When toxicity occurs, it may be severe and is fatal in up to 10 per cent of cases. The cause is unknown, but formation of reactive oxygen species, immunological activation and direct cellular toxicity are all believed to contribute.[31]

The endocrine lung

To qualify as a true endocrine organ, the lung must secrete a substance into the blood, which brings about a useful physiological response in a distant tissue. In spite of its wide-ranging metabolic activities already described, the endocrine functions of the lung remain ill-defined. Contenders include the following.

Inflammatory mediators. Histamine, endothelin and arachidonic acid derivatives are released from the lung following immunological activation by inhaled allergens (Chapter 27). These mediators are undoubtedly responsible for cardiovascular and other physiological changes in the rest of the body, such as a rash, peripheral vasodilatation and a reduction in blood pressure. However, it is doubtful if this can really be regarded as a desirable physiological effect.

Hypoxic endocrine responses.[32] Animal studies have demonstrated the presence of clusters of peptide- and amine-secreting cells in lung tissue. These cells degranulate in the presence of acute hypoxia, but the substances secreted and their effects are not known. The cells belong to the 'diffuse endocrine system' and are present in humans, but their role is extremely unclear.

Nitric oxide plays an important role in the regulation of airway smooth muscle (page 71) and pulmonary vascular resistance (page 149), and is well known for its effects on platelet function and the systemic vasculature elsewhere in the body. There is no evidence that pulmonary endothelium secretes nitric oxide into the blood in order to exert an effect elsewhere, mainly because of the rapid uptake of nitric oxide by haemoglobin (page 273). This does not rule out an indirect effect of pulmonary production of nitric oxide in influencing peripheral blood flow, which may be controlled by the balance between different forms of nitric oxide–haemoglobin complexes (page 274).

References

1. Niden AH, Aviado DM. Effects of pulmonary embolism on the pulmonary circulation with special reference to arteriovenous shunts in the lung. *Circ Res* 1956; **4**: 67–73.
2. Fisher DC, Fisher EA, Budd JH, Rosen SE, Goldman ME. The incidence of patent foramen ovale in 1000 consecutive patients. *Chest* 1995; **107**: 1504–9.
3. Malik AB. Pulmonary microembolism and lung vascular injury. *Eur Respir J Suppl* 1990; **11**: 499s–506s.
4. Laurell CB, Eriksson S. The electrophoretic α_1-globulin pattern of serum in α_1-antitrypsin deficiency. *Scand J Clin Lab Invest* 1963; **15**: 132–6.
5. Norman MR, Mowat AP, Hutchinson DCS. Molecular basis, clinical consequences and diagnosis of alpha-1 antitrypsin deficiency. *Ann Clin Biochem* 1997; **34**: 230–46.
6. Hutchinson DCS, Cook PJL, Barter CE, Harris H, Hugh-Jones P. Pulmonary emphysema and α_1-antitrypsin deficiency. *BMJ* 1971; **1**: 689–94.
7. Nunn JF. Pulmonary oxygen consumption. *Intensive Care Med* 1996; **22**: 275–6.
8. Bond JA. Metabolism and elimination of inhaled drugs and airborne chemicals from the lungs. *Pharmacol Toxicol* 1993; **72** (Supp 3): 36–47.
9. Dahl AR, Gerde P. Uptake and metabolism of toxicants in the respiratory tract. *Environ Health Perspect* 1994; **102** (Supp 11): 67–70.
10. Kikkawa Y. Diverse role of pulmonary cytochrome P-450 monooxygenase. *Lab Invest* 1992; **67**: 535–9.
11. Davidson JM. Biochemistry and turnover of lung interstitium. *Eur Respir J* 1990; **3**: 1048–68.
12. Bahkle YS. Pharmacokinetic and metabolic properties of the lung. *Br J Anaesth* 1990; **65**: 79–93.
13. Starling EH, Verney EB. The secretion of urine as studied in the isolated kidney. *Proc R Soc* 1925; **97**: 321–63.
14. Ryan US. Structural basis for metabolic activity. *Annu Rev Physiol* 1982; **44**: 223–39.
15. Weibel ER. How does lung structure affect gas exchange? *Chest* 1983; **83**: 657–65.
16. Sole MJ, Dobrac M, Schwartz L, Hussain MN, Vaughan-Neil EF. The extraction of circulating catecholamines by the lungs in normal man and in patients with pulmonary hypertension. *Circulation* 1979; **60**: 160–3.
17. Gillis CN, Pitt BR. The fate of circulating amines within the pulmonary circulation. *Annu Rev Physiol* 1982; **44**: 269–81.
18. Junod AF. 5-Hydroxytryptamine and other amines in the lung. *Handbook of Physiology, Section 3* 1985; **1**: 337–49.
19. Thomas DP, Vane JR. 5-Hydroxytryptamine in the circulation of the dog. *Nature* 1967; **216**: 335–8.
20. Said SI. Metabolic functions of the pulmonary circulation. *Circ Res* 1982; **50**: 325–33.
21. Ng KKF, Vane JR. Conversion of angiotensin I to angiotensin II. *Nature* 1967; **216**: 762–6.
22. Bakhle YS. Pulmonary angiotensin-converting enzyme and its inhibition. In: *Metabolic activities of the lung*, Ciba Foundation symposium 78. Amsterdam: Excerpta Medica, 1980.
23. Needleman P, Blaine EH, Greenwald JE, Michener ML, Saper CB, Stockmann PT, Tolunay HE. The biochemical pharmacology of atrial peptides. *Annu Rev Pharmacol Toxicol* 1989; **29**: 23–54.
24. Michael JR, Markewitz BA. Endothelins and the lung. *Am J Respir Crit Care Med* 1996; **154**: 555–81.
25. Bakhle YS, Ferreira SH. Lung metabolism of eicosanoids: prostaglandins, prostacyclin, thromboxane and leukotrienes. *Handbook of Physiology, Section 3* 1985; **1**: 365–86.
26. Hardy C, Robinson C, Lewis RA, Tattersfield AE, Holgate ST. Airway and cardiovascular responses to inhaled prostacyclin in normal and asthmatic subjects. *Am Rev Respir Dis* 1985; **131**: 18–21.
27. Piper PJ, Samhoun MN, Tippins JR, Williams TJ, Palmer MA, Peck MJ. Pharmacological studies on pure SRS-A and synthetic leukotrienes C_4 and D_4. In: Piper PJ, ed. *SRS-A and leukotrienes*. New York: Wiley, 1981.
28. Blitt CD, Brown BR, Wright BJ, Gandolfi AJ, Sipes G. Pulmonary biotransformation of methoxyflurane: an *in vitro* study in the rabbit. *Anesthesiology* 1979; **51**: 528–31.
29. Bend JR, Serabjit-Singh CJ, Philpot RM. The pulmonary uptake, accumulation and metabolism of xenobiotics. *Annu Rev Pharmacol Toxicol* 1985; **25**: 97–125.
30. Foth H. Role of the lung in accumulation and metabolism of xenobiotic compounds – implications for chemically induced toxicity. *Crit Rev Toxicol* 1995; **25**: 165–205.
31. Reasor MJ, Kacew S. An evaluation of possible mechanisms underlying amiodarone-induced pulmonary toxicity. *Proc Soc Exp Biol Med* 1996; **212**: 297–305.
32. Gosney JR. The endocrine lung and its response to hypoxia. *Thorax* 1994; **49**: S25–6.

Part 2

Applied Physiology

Chapter 13

Pregnancy, neonates and children

Respiratory function in pregnancy[1]

Several physiological changes occur during pregnancy that affect respiratory function. Fluid retention caused by increasing oestrogen levels causes oedema throughout the airway mucosa, and increases blood volume, substantially increasing oxygen delivery. Progesterone levels rise sixfold through pregnancy, and have significant effects on the control of respiration and therefore arterial blood gases. Finally, in the last trimester of pregnancy, the enlarging uterus has a direct impact on respiratory mechanics. A summary of the changes for common respiratory measurements is given in Table 13.1.

Lung volumes. During the last third of pregnancy the diaphragm becomes displaced cephalad by the expansion of the uterus into the abdomen. This reduces both the residual volume (by about 20 per cent) and expiratory reserve volume, such that functional residual capacity is greatly reduced (Table 13.1). This is particularly true in the supine position,

Table 13.1 Respiratory function throughout pregnancy

Variable	Non-pregnant	Pregnant		
		1st trimester	*2nd trimester*	*3rd trimester*
Tidal volume (l)	0.52	0.60	0.65	0.72
Respiratory rate (breaths per min)	18	18	18	18
Minute volume (l.min^{-1})	9.3	11.0	11.8	13.1
Residual volume (l)	1.37	1.27	1.26	1.01
Functional residual capacity (l)	2.69	2.52	2.48	1.95
Vital capacity (l)	3.50	3.45	3.58	3.0
Oxygen consumption (ml.min^{-1})	194	211	242	258
Arterial P_{O_2} (kPa)	12.6	14.2	13.7	13.6
(mmHg)	95	106	103	102
Arterial P_{CO_2} (kPa)	4.70	3.92	3.93	4.05
(mmHg)	35	29	29	31
CO_2 response slope (l.min^{-1}.kPa^{-1})	11.6	15.0	17.3	19.8
Oxygen saturation response slope (l.min^{-1}.%$^{-1}$)	0.64	1.04	1.13	1.33

Figures refer to normal subjects with an average non-pregnant body weight of 60 kg at the end of each trimester of pregnancy. (Derived from references 2 and 3.)

and effectively removes one of the largest stores of oxygen available to the body, making pregnant women very susceptible to hypoxia during anaesthesia or with respiratory disease.

Vital capacity, forced expiratory volume in one second and maximal breathing capacity are normally unchanged during pregnancy.[1,4] In the supine position when the diaphragm is high in the chest, inspiratory capacity and maximal breathing capacity may actually exceed non-pregnant values.

Oxygen consumption. Oxygen consumption increases throughout pregnancy, peaking at between 15 and 30 per cent above normal at full term.[2,5] The increase is mainly attributable to the demands of the fetus, uterus and placenta, such that when oxygen consumption is expressed per kilogram of body weight there is little change.

Ventilation. Respiratory rate remains unchanged whilst tidal volume, and therefore minute volume of ventilation, increase by up to 40 per cent above normal at full term.[1] The increase in ventilation is beyond the requirements of the enhanced oxygen uptake or carbon dioxide production, so alveolar and arterial P_{CO_2} are reduced to about 4 kPa (30 mmHg).[3] This must facilitate clearance of carbon dioxide by the fetus. There is also an increase in alveolar and arterial P_{O_2} of about 1 kPa (7.5 mmHg).[3] Posture has little effect on oxygenation, and in one study mean values for oxygen saturation (by pulse oximetry) in the last four weeks of pregnancy were 97.3% sitting and 96.9% supine.[4]

The hyperventilation is attributable to progesterone levels, and the mechanism is assumed to be a sensitization of the central chemoreceptors. Pregnancy gives rise to a threefold increase in the slope of a P_{CO_2}/ventilation response curve.[2] The hypoxic ventilatory response is increased twofold, most of the change occurring before the mid-point of gestation, at which time oxygen consumption has hardly begun to increase.[6]

Dyspnoea occurs in more than half of pregnant women, beginning early in pregnancy, long before the mass effect of the uterus becomes apparent. Dyspnoeic pregnant women, compared with non-dyspnoeic controls, show a greater degree of hyperventilation in spite of having similar plasma progesterone levels.[2] Dyspnoea therefore seems to arise from an increased sensitivity of the chemoreceptors to the increase in progesterone levels.

The lungs before birth[7]

Embryologically, the lungs develop as an outgrowth from the foregut and first appear at about day 24 of gestation. The lungs begin to contain surfactant and are first capable of function by about 24–26 weeks, this being a major factor in the viability of premature infants. In humans at full term all major elements of the lungs are fully formed, but the number of alveoli present is only 15 per cent of the adult lung. Division of saccules into alveoli continues following birth and is believed to be complete by 2 years of age.[7] This postnatal maturation of lung structure is seen only in altricial mammals (humans, mouse, rabbit), who have the luxury of being able to remain 'helpless' following birth. Precocial species such as range animals are born with a structurally mature lung, ready for immediate activity.[8]

Control of lung development.[9] Fetal lungs contain 'lung liquid' (LL), which is secreted by the pulmonary epithelial cells and flows out through the developing airway into the amniotic fluid or gastrointestinal tract. The main functions of LL seem to be flushing debris out of the lung and preventing the developing lung tissues from collapsing. It is thought that LL maintains the lung at a slight positive pressure, relative to the amniotic fluid, and that this expansion is responsible for stimulating cell division and lung growth. The respiratory tract in late pregnancy contains some 40 ml of LL, but its turnover is rapid, believed to be of the order of 500 ml per day.[10] Its volume corresponds approximately with the functional residual capacity (FRC) after breathing is established.[9]

Fetal breathing movements also contribute to lung development. In humans they begin in the middle trimester of pregnancy, and are present for over 20 minutes per hour in the last trimester,[11] normally during periods of general fetal activity. During episodes of breathing, the frequency is about 45 breaths per minute and the diaphragm seems to be the main muscle concerned, producing an estimated fluid shift of about 2 ml at each 'breath'.[12]

Maintenance of a positive pressure in the developing lung requires the upper airway to offer some resistance to the outflow of LL.[9] During apnoea, both elastic recoil of the lung tissue and continuous production of LL are opposed by intrinsic laryngeal resistance and a collapsed pharynx. Fetal inspiratory activity, as in the adult, includes dilatation of the upper airway. With quiet breathing this would allow increased efflux of LL from the airway, but simultaneous diaphragmatic contraction opposes this. During vigorous breathing movements with the mouth open, pharyngeal fluid may be 'sucked' into the airway, so contributing to the expansion of the lungs. Thus fetal breathing movements are believed to contribute to maintaining lung expansion, and their abolition is known to impair lung development.[9]

The fetal circulation

The fetal circulation differs radically from the postnatal circulation (Figure 13.1). Blood from the right heart is deflected away from the lungs, partly through the foramen ovale and partly through the ductus arteriosus. Less than 10 per cent of the output of the right ventricle reaches the lungs, the remainder passing to the systemic circulation and the placenta. Right atrial pressure exceeds left atrial pressure, and this maintains the patency of the foramen ovale. Furthermore, because the vascular resistance of the pulmonary circulation exceeds that of the systemic circulation before birth, pressure in the right ventricle exceeds that in the left ventricle and these factors control the direction of flow through the ductus arteriosus. The direction may be reversed in abnormal circumstances if the pressure gradient between the ventricles is reversed.

The umbilical veins drain via the ductus venosus into the inferior vena cava, which therefore contains better oxygenated blood than the superior vena cava. The anatomy of the atria and the foramen ovale is such that the better oxygenated blood from the inferior vena cava passes preferentially into the left atrium and thence to the left ventricle, and so to the brain. (This is not shown in Figure 13.1.) Overall gas tensions in the fetus are of the order of 6.4 kPa (48 mmHg) for P_{CO_2} and 4 kPa (30 mmHg) for P_{O_2}. The fact that the fetus remains apnoeic for much of the time *in utero* with these blood-gas levels is probably in part attributable to central hypoxic ventilatory depression[13] (page 102).

Events at birth

Oxygen stores in the fetus are small and it is therefore essential that air breathing and oxygen uptake be established within a few minutes of birth. This requires radical changes in the function of both lungs and circulation.

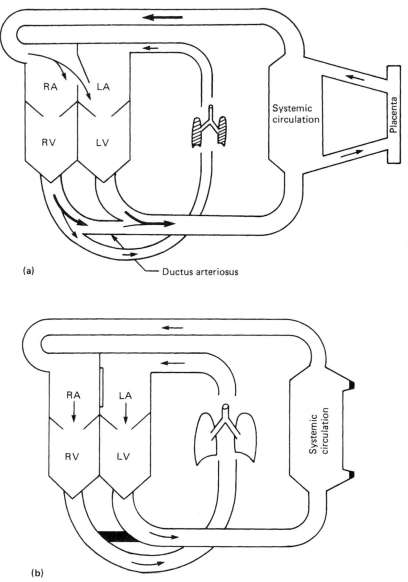

Figure 13.1 Fetal circulation (a) compared with adult circulation (b). The foramen ovale is between right atrium (RA) and left atrium (LA). RV and LV, right and left ventricles.

Factors in the initiation of breathing

Most normal infants take their first breath within 20 seconds of delivery, and rhythmic respiration is usually established within 90 seconds. Thoracic compression during vaginal delivery followed by recoil of the ribcage causes air to be drawn passively into the lungs. However, the major stimuli to breathing are probably the cooling of the skin and mechanical stimulation acting via the respiratory centre. Without this, babies born via caesarean section would suffer greatly from immediate respiratory difficulties, which is not the case in practice. Hypoxaemia, resulting from apnoea or clamping of the cord, is unlikely to be a reliable respiratory stimulus at this time, because of central hypoxic ventilatory depression (see above).

Fate of the fetal lung fluid. The volume of intraluminal fluid decreases just before and during labour. Some of the residual fluid may be expressed during a vaginal delivery but this is not thought to be a major factor.[10] After the first breath, most of the fluid passes into distensible perivascular spaces around blood vessels and bronchi, forming cuffs as in pulmonary oedema (page 542). These spaces are then cleared in the first few hours after delivery.

Changes in the circulation

The geometry of the circulation changes radically and quickly at birth. The establishment of spontaneous breathing causes a massive decrease in the vascular resistance of the pulmonary circulation, due partly to mechanical factors and partly to changes in blood gases. Simultaneously there is an increase in the resistance of the systemic circulation, due partly to vasoconstriction and partly to cessation of the placental circulation. As a result, the right atrial pressure falls below the left atrial pressure, to give the relationship that is then maintained throughout life. This normally results in closure of the foramen ovale (Figure 13.1), which is followed by closure of the ductus arteriosus as a result of active vasoconstriction of its smooth muscle layer in response to increased Po_2. The circulation is thus converted from the fetal mode, in which the lungs and the systemic circulation are essentially in parallel, to the adult mode, in which they are in series.

Mechanism of reduced pulmonary vascular resistance at birth. Pulmonary vascular resistance declines due to a combination of ventilation of the lung and changes in blood gases, particularly increasing Po_2. Clearly this is a difficult area to study in humans, and most work has been performed in other mammals,[9,14,15] but there is no reason to expect humans to differ significantly.

Removal of LL from the lung establishes an air/liquid interface that is responsible for a rapid increase in lung recoil pressure,[9,14] which, possibly along with changes in chest wall compliance, results in a negative intrapleural pressure as in adult lungs. This creates the transmural pressure gradient between the alveoli and pleura, which physically dilates the pulmonary capillaries (page 146). These mechanical forces leading to a reduction in pulmonary vascular resistance are believed to account for over half of the observed changes at birth.[15]

Further reductions in pulmonary vascular resistance, as a result of increased Po_2 and decreased Pco_2, are believed to be endothelium dependent.[16] Though many mediators may be involved, prostaglandins, endothelin and nitric oxide are the most widely studied. The first two groups have conflicting effects on the neonatal pulmonary circulation, with *in vitro* studies showing both vasodilating and vasoconstricting effects of different individual mediators. Prostacyclin seems to be involved in the *in vivo* vasodilatation of pulmonary blood vessels at birth, but the effect is minor. In animals, inhibition of nitric oxide synthase prior to birth attenuates the reduction in pulmonary vascular resistance on delivery. Nitric oxide is believed to mediate the component of pulmonary vasodilatation that occurs in response to oxygen.[17]

Persistent pulmonary hypertension of the newborn (PPHN)[17,18] occurs in over 1 in 1000 births. Pulmonary vascular resistance remains elevated, so right heart pressures remain high and a significant right-to-left shunt continues, with resulting hypoxaemia. Although PPHN may occur with other parenchymal lung problems such as meconium aspiration or respiratory distress syndrome, it also occurs in isolation. Mechanical changes at birth leading to pulmonary vasodilatation, as described above, will still occur and are probably responsible for bringing about sufficient pulmonary blood flow for immediate survival. However, structural abnormalities of pulmonary vessels are common in PPHN, and may limit the vasodilatation obtained by mechanical factors. There is undoubtedly an element of abnormal pulmonary vasoconstriction, or at least a failure of oxygen-stimulated vasodilatation, in babies with PPHN, and abnormalities of both endothelin and nitric oxide activity are implicated.

Treatment is aimed at the correction of any concurrent lung disease, and artificial ventilation to try to improve oxygenation. Extracorporeal membrane oxygenation (Chapter 32) is often required. Inhaled nitric oxide has also had some success in improving hypoxaemia but not all babies respond and its place in the treatment of PPHN is not yet clear.

The Apgar score

The scoring system devised many years ago by Virginia Apgar is still widely accepted as an assessment of the overall condition of the neonate. This is based on scoring of a scale from 0 to 2 for five attributes, two of which are related to respiration (Table 13.2).[19] The total score is the sum of each of the five constituent scores, and is best undertaken one and five minutes after delivery. Scores of 8–10 are regarded as normal.

Table 13.2 The Apgar scoring system

Score	0	1	2
Heart rate	Absent	Less than 100 per min	More than 100 per min
Respiratory effort	Absent	Slow, irregular	Good, crying
Colour	Blue, pale	Body pink, extremities blue	Completely pink
Reflex irritability	Absent	Grimace	Cough, sneeze
Muscle tone	Limp	Some flexion of extremities	Active motion

Add together scores for each section (maximum possible 10). Score at 1 and 5 minutes after delivery. (After reference 19.)

Neonatal lung function

Mechanics of breathing. Functional residual capacity is about $30\,ml.kg^{-1}$ and total respiratory compliance $50\,ml.kPa^{-1}$ ($5\,ml.cmH_2O^{-1}$). Most of the impedance to expansion is due to the lung and depends primarily on the presence of surfactant in the alveoli. The chest wall of the neonate is highly compliant. This contrasts with the adult, in whom compliance of lung and chest wall are approximately equal. Total respiratory resistance is of the order of $7\,kPa.l^{-1}.s$ ($70\,cmH_2O\;kPa.l^{-1}.s$), most of which is in the bronchial tree. Compliance is about one-twentieth that of an adult and resistance about 15 times greater.

At the first breath the infant is capable of generating a subatmospheric intrathoracic pressure of the order of 7 kPa (70 cmH$_2$O).

Ventilation and gas exchange.[20] For a 3 kg neonate, the minute volume is about 0.6 litre, with a high respiratory frequency of 25–40 breaths per minute. Dead space is close to a half of tidal volume, giving a mean alveolar ventilation of about 0.3 l.min^{-1} for a neonate of average size. There is a shunt of about 10% immediately after birth. However, distribution of gas is better than in the adult and there is, of course, a negligible hydrostatic pressure gradient in the vertical axis of the tiny lungs of an infant.

Oxygen consumption is of the order of 20–30 ml.min^{-1}, depending on weight in the range 2–4 kg. Arterial Pco$_2$ is close to 4.5 kPa (34 mmHg) and Po$_2$ 9 kPa (68 mmHg). Because of the shunt of 10%, there is an alveolar/arterial Po$_2$ gradient of about 3.3 kPa (25 mmHg) compared with less than half of this in a young adult. Arterial pH is within the normal adult range.

Control of breathing.[21,22] Animal studies have shown that, in the fetus, carotid chemoreceptors are active but at a much lower Po$_2$ than in adults; the ventilatory response curve is thus displaced far to the left compared with adults. Prolonged periods of apnoea seen *in utero* in spite of this carotid sinus activity occur because of brainstem inhibition of the respiratory centre. In contrast to this, cardiovascular responses to hypoxia are well developed in the fetus, bradycardia and vasoconstriction being well-recognized responses to hypoxia in neonates as shown by the Apgar score. After birth, there is a very rapid transition towards the adult pattern of respiratory control. Brainstem hypoxic ventilatory depression ceases, and the carotid chemoreceptors quickly 'reset' to adult values. Thus hypoxic respiratory stimulation develops, and, soon after birth, ventilation is depressed by the inhalation of 100% oxygen, indicating a tonic drive from the peripheral chemo-receptors. Ventilatory response to carbon dioxide seems to be similar to that in the adult if allowance is made for body size, although the response is depressed in REM sleep.[23]

At birth, changes in respiratory pattern must, by necessity, be substantial because the long periods of apnoea seen *in utero* are incompatible with life in the outside world. Although most changes occur shortly after birth, complete transition to 'adult' respiration may take some weeks to complete, particularly in premature and small babies, and those with other respiratory problems that cause repeated periods of hypoxia. In the meantime, newborn infants have a variety of breathing patterns. For example, 'periodic breathing' consists of slowly oscillating changes in respiratory rate and tidal volume size; 'periodic apnoea' consists of a series of respiratory pauses of over 4 seconds' duration with a few normal breaths in between. In normal babies under 2 months of age, there may be in excess of 200 apnoeic episodes and 50 minutes of periodic breathing per day,[24] and these may be associated with short-lived reductions in saturation.[25] The proportion of time spent with regular breathing increases with age, such that, beyond 3 months old, periodic breathing and apnoeas are significantly less.[24] Moderate reductions in inspired oxygen (15%), similar to that seen during flying or at altitude (Chapter 16), cause a dramatic increase in the amount of time 3-month-old infants spend with periodic apnoea, indicating that adult hypoxic ventilatory responses are not fully developed.[26]

Haemoglobin. Children are normally born polycythaemic with a mean haemoglobin of about 18 g.dl^{-1} and a haematocrit (packed cell volume) of 53%.[27] Some 70 per cent of the haemoglobin is HbF and the resultant P$_{50}$ is well below the normal adult value (see Figure 11.9). Arterial oxygen content is close to the normal adult value in spite of the low arterial Po$_2$. The haemoglobin concentration decreases rapidly, to become less than the normal adult value by 3 weeks of life. HbF gradually disappears from the circulation, to reach negligible values by 6 months, by which time the P_{50} has already attained the normal adult value.

Respiratory distress syndrome (RDS)[28]

The syndrome comprises respiratory distress within a few hours of birth and occurs in 2 per cent of all live births, but with a greatly increased incidence in premature infants. The essential lesion is a deficiency of surfactant, which is first detectable in the fetal lung at 20–24 weeks of gestation but the concentration increases rapidly after week 30. Therefore, prematurity is a major factor in the aetiology of RDS, though male babies, caesarean delivery, perinatal stress or birth asphyxia and maternal diabetes are all additional risk factors for its development.

The disease presents with difficulty in inspiration against the decreased compliance due to the high surface tension of the alveolar lining fluid deficient in surfactant. This progresses to ventilatory failure, alveolar collapse, hyaline membrane deposit, pulmonary oedema leading to denaturing of surfactant and, ultimately, interference with gas exchange resulting in severe hypoxaemia. Increased pulmonary vascular resistance may raise right atrial pressure and reopen the foramen ovale, so increasing the shunt.

Physiological principles of treatment of RDS

The physiological basis of therapy is to supplement surfactant activity and employ artificial ventilation as a temporary expedient to spare the infant the excessive work of breathing against stiff lungs. Results have improved over the years and most infants with a birth weight greater than 1 kg should survive.[29] Overall treatment is very complex and outside the scope of this book, but aspects of treatment with physiological interest are as follows.

Prevention. Amniocentesis allows the measurement of lecithin (derived from pulmonary surfactant) to sphingomyelin ratio, which is highly predictive of lung maturity.[28] If this ratio is less than 2, measures may be taken to prolong pregnancy by administration of tocolytic drugs, and steroids may be given to accelerate the rate at which the fetal lungs mature. This, combined with careful obstetric management to prevent perinatal stress, should significantly reduce the incidence and severity of subsequent RDS.

Artificial ventilation. Artificial ventilation is considered in Chapter 22. For neonates, the usual choice is a time-cycled square-wave pressure generator (page 590), but operating at much higher respiratory frequencies than for the adult. Inspiratory and expiratory durations may be as little as 0.3 second, but inflation pressures are of the same order as those used in adults and do not usually exceed 3 kPa (30 cmH$_2$O). Both the compressible volume of the ventilator circuit and the apparatus dead space tend to be large in relation to the size of very small children. It is for this reason that pressure generators are preferable to volume generators. Furthermore, there is considerable practical difficulty in measuring the very small imposed tidal volumes or expired $P\text{CO}_2$. For this reason, close monitoring of arterial $P\text{O}_2$ and $P\text{CO}_2$ is essential. Positive end-expiratory pressure (PEEP) is widely used, and spontaneous respiration is often undertaken with continuous positive airway pressure (CPAP). Bronchopulmonary dysplasia, a relatively common complication of RDS, seems to be a form of pulmonary barotrauma (page 615) in the ventilated infant.

Normal humidification and monitoring of airway pressure are important. Improved predelivery care and surfactant replacement therapy have reduced the necessity to ventilate infants with RDS.

Surfactant replacement therapy[30] has now been used for about 20 years.[31] Endogenous surfactant is complex, consisting of multiple components divided into phospholipids and proteins (page 40). Currently available synthetic surfactants consist mostly of phospholipids. Alternatively, natural surfactant preparations are obtained from mammalian lungs or human amniotic fluid and contain both phospholipid and some of the surfactant apoproteins, though not necessarily of the same type and proportion as in humans. Surfactant proteins are important to facilitate spreading of the surfactant around the lung after administration by intratracheal instillation, and there is now evidence that natural surfactants are more effective as therapeutic agents.[30] Exogenous surfactant seems to be taken up in type II alveolar cells and recycled, and its clearance is fortunately very slow.[29] Surfactant replacement therapy has now been conclusively shown to improve survival and reduce complication rates in many trials both in the USA[30] and Europe.[32] In addition, the importance of surfactant deficiency is now recognized in many other causes of neonatal respiratory failure such as meconium aspiration and pneumonia, and surfactant replacement seems to be beneficial.[33]

Extracorporeal membrane oxygenation (ECMO) is described in Chapter 32. In contrast to its use in adults, ECMO is of proven benefit in infants (page 629). A recent multicentre study showed ECMO to be effective in reducing mortality and long-term disability in severe neonatal respiratory failure from a variety of causes,[34] including RDS. Unfortunately, most cases of RDS cannot be treated with ECMO because of technical problems in babies of less than 2 kg weight or 35 weeks' gestation.

Partial liquid ventilation with perflubron, a synthetic oxygen carrier (page 274), has been used successfully in neonates with severe RDS. A volume of perflubron approximately equal to the infant's FRC is instilled into the lungs, and positive pressure ventilation by conventional methods continued. The liquid improves lung function by replacing the alveolar air/liquid interface, by physically preventing alveolar collapse and by increasing lung compliance, allowing more effective ventilation. Chest radiographs show the extent to which partial liquid ventilation replaces normal gas-filled lung, and also that clearance of perflubron by evaporation from the lung takes some time (Figure 13.2). Partial liquid ventilation improved oxygenation and caused few side effects.[35] Trials are awaited to confirm improvements in clinical outcome from this technique.

Sudden infant death syndrome (SIDS)[36]

This is defined simply as the sudden death of an infant that is unexplained after review of the clinical history, examination of the circumstances of the death and post-mortem examination. The peak incidence is at 2–3 months of age and there remains a multitude of theories regarding the aetiology, though the respiratory system is implicated in most. Some more common theories include the following.

Apnoea hypothesis remains popular, mainly because of the frequent periods of apnoea and desaturation observed in almost all babies under 3 months old (see above). The peak incidence of SIDS corresponds to the period of development when the fetal and adult

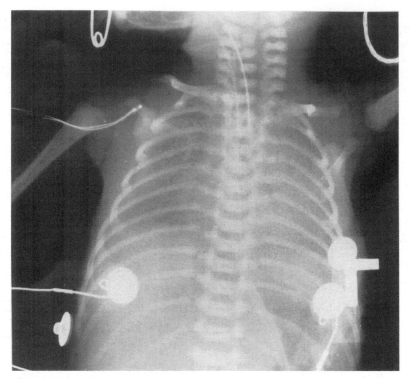

Figure 13.2 Chest radiographs of an infant receiving partial liquid ventilation for severe respiratory distress syndrome. (a) Conventional ventilation for respiratory distress syndrome.

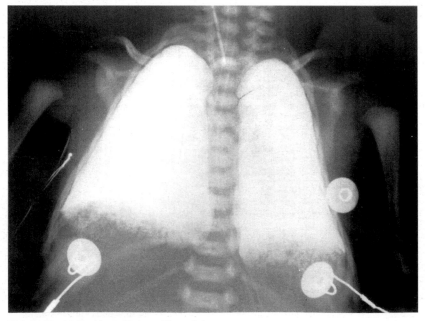

Figure 13.2 (b) Partial liquid ventilation with perflubron.

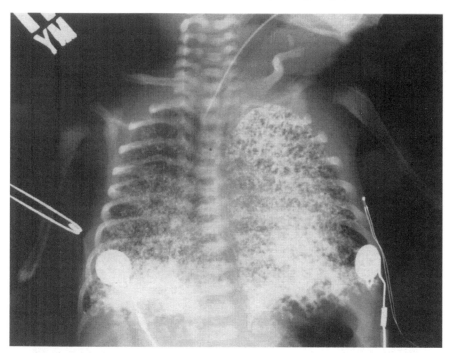

Figure 13.2 (c) Forty eight hours after termination of liquid ventilation.

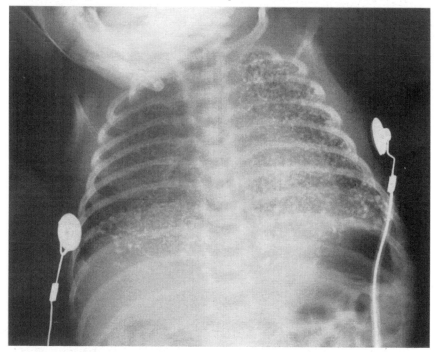

Figure 13.2 (d) Three weeks later. (After reference 35 by permission of the authors and the publishers of *New England Journal of Medicine*.)

Table 13.3 Recent changes in the incidence of sudden infant death syndrome in various countries as a result of health education campaigns

Country	Incidence of SIDS	
	Before health advice	After health advice
United Kingdom	1.9	0.7
New Zealand	3.5	1.4
United States of America	1.3	0.8
Australia (Tasmania)	3.8	1.5
Netherlands	1.0	0.4
Norway	2.0	1.1

All figures are the number of SIDS cases per 1000 live births. Almost all countries advised the *avoidance* of the prone sleeping position, parental smoking, and the use of excessive clothing and bedding at night. (Figures derived from references 36, 39, 40 and 41.)

systems for ventilatory control are swapping over, and it is believed that this may make the infant susceptible to respiratory disturbances.[36] Evidence that these episodes of periodic breathing or apnoeas contribute to SIDS is, however, lacking. Nevertheless, this hypothesis led to the widespread use of 'apnoea alarms' for babies, though again, evidence that this reduces SIDS has so far not been found.[37]

Temperature regulation may be abnormal in SIDS babies, and metabolic rate as a function of body size is particularly high at 3 months of age, leading to the hypothesis that 'heat stress' is responsible.[38]

Infection with common viruses has been implicated in SIDS, though it is believed that SIDS is more likely to occur during the prodromal phase of an infection before symptoms develop.[36]

Smoking by parents is associated with SIDS, particularly if the infant shares the parent's bed. The mechanism is not clear.

Sleeping position. There is a substantial body of agreement that the prone sleeping position is more common in infants dying of SIDS, though the mechanism remains uncertain.[36]

That SIDS is caused by multiple factors is now undisputed. However, its prevention has progressed greatly despite the absence of understanding regarding the aetiology. In the late 1980s many countries introduced national health educational policies to encourage the avoidance of prone sleeping position, parental smoking and overheating in babies. These measures have been spectacularly effective in reducing the incidence of SIDS (Table 13.3).

Development of lung function during childhood

The lungs continue to develop during childhood. Chest wall compliance, which is very high at birth, decreases rapidly for the first two years of life, when it becomes

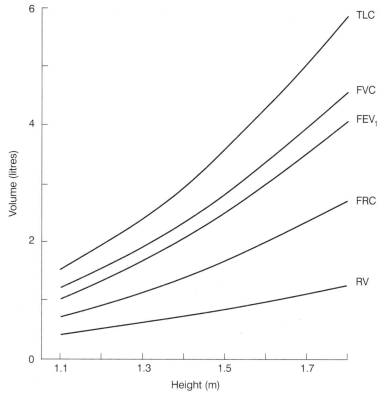

Figure 13.3 Changes in lung volumes as a function of stature. When considering reference values for children, height in metres is used in preference to age to allow for large differences in growth rate. Each graph represents the mean for both boys and girls, though boys generally have greater values at equivalent heights.

approximately equal to lung compliance as in the adult.[42] Between birth and adult life, there is an approximately tenfold increase in the number of airways. Below the age of 8 years, measurement of lung volumes is difficult,[20] but many studies of normal lung function beyond this age are available. Because of the large variations in the rate at which children grow, reference values are usually related to height rather than age or weight. Equations relating lung volumes to height are available,[20] and some are shown in graphical form in Figure 13.3.

Various indices of respiratory function are independent of age and body size so that adult values can be used. These include forced expiratory volume in 1 second (FEV_1) as a fraction of vital capacity, functional residual capacity and peak expiratory flow rate as a fraction of total lung capacity, *specific* airway conductance and *specific* compliance (page 47) and probably dead space/tidal volume ratio.[20]

Blood gases and the control of breathing. Arterial P_{CO_2} and alveolar P_{O_2} do not change appreciably during childhood but arterial P_{O_2} increases from the neonatal value to reach a maximum of about 13 kPa (98 mmHg) at young adulthood. Much of this increase occurs during the first year of life.[43] There are obvious difficulties in determining the normal arterial P_{O_2} in children. Ventilatory responses to both hypercapnia and hypoxia are at their highest in early childhood and decrease progressively into adulthood.[44] The changes are small for hypoxic responses but quite marked for hypercapnia, and are believed to relate to the higher metabolic rate in children.

References

1. Elkus R, Popovich J. Respiratory physiology in pregnancy. *Clin Chest Med* 1992; **13**: 555–65.
2. Garcia-Rio F, Pino JM, Gomez L, Alvarez-Sala R, Villasnate C, Villamor J. Regulation of breathing and perception of dyspnoea in healthy pregnant women. *Chest* 1996; **110**: 446–53.
3. Templeton A, Kelman GR. Maternal blood-gases, ($P_{A_{O_2}}$–$P_{a_{O_2}}$), physiological shunt and V_D/V_T in normal pregnancy. *Br J Anaesth* 1976; **48**: 1001–4.
4. Nørregaard O, Schultz P, Østergaard A, Dahl R. Lung function and postural changes during pregnancy. *Respir Med* 1989; **83**: 467–74.
5. Pernol ML, Metcalfe J, Schlenker TL, Welch JE, Matsumoto JA. Oxygen consumption at rest and during exercise in pregnancy. *Respir Physiol* 1975; **25**: 285–92.
6. Moore LG, McCullough RE, Weil JV. Increased HVR in pregnancy: relationship to hormonal and metabolic changes. *J Appl Physiol* 1987; **62**: 158–63.
7. Merkus PJFM, ten Have-Opbroek AAW, Quanjer PH. Human lung growth: a review. *Ped Pulmonol* 1996; **21**: 383–97.
8. Massaro GD, Massaro D. Formation of pulmonary alveoli and gas-exchange surface area: quantitation and regulation. *Annu Rev Physiol* 1996; **58**: 73–92.
9. Harding R, Hooper SB. Regulation of lung expansion and lung growth before birth. *J Appl Physiol* 1996; **81**: 209–24.
10. Bland RD. Fetal lung liquid and its removal near birth. In: Crystal RG, West JB, eds. *The lung: scientific foundations.* New York: Raven, 1991; 1677.
11. Patrick J, Campbell K, Carmichael L, Natale R, Richardson B. Patterns of human fetal breathing during the last 10 weeks of pregnancy. *Obstet Gynecol* 1980; **56**: 24–30.
12. Harding R. Fetal breathing movements. In: Crystal RG, West JB, eds. *The lung: scientific foundations.* New York: Raven, 1991; 1655.
13. Edelman NH, Neubauer JA. Hypoxic depression of breathing. In: Crystal RG, West JB, eds. *The lung: scientific foundations.* New York: Raven, 1991; 1341.
14. Avery ME, Cook CD. Volume pressure relationships of lungs and thorax in fetal, newborn and adult goats. *J Appl Physiol* 1961; **16**: 1034–8.
15. Teitel DF, Iwamotot HS, Rudolph AM. Changes in the pulmonary circulation during birth-related events. *Pediatr Res* 1990; **27**: 372–8.
16. Ziegler JW, Ivy DD, Kinsella JP, Abman SH. The role of nitric oxide, endothelin, and prostaglandins in the transition of the pulmonary circulation. *Clin Perinatol* 1995; **22**: 387–403.
17. Morin FC, Stenmark KR. Persistent pulmonary hypertension of the newborn. *Am J Respir Crit Care Med* 1995; **151**: 2010–32.
18. Steinhorn RH, Millard SL, Morin FC. Persistent pulmonary hypertension of the newborn. *Clin Perinatol* 1995; **22**: 405–28.
19. McIntosh N. The newborn. In: Campbell AGM, McIntosh N, eds. *Forfar and Arneil's textbook of pediatrics.* Edinburgh: Churchill Livingstone, 1998; 1221–6.
20. Cotes JE. *Lung function: assessment and application in medicine.* Oxford: Blackwell Scientific Publications, 1993; 445–64.
21. Lagercrantz H, Milerad J, Walker D. Control of ventilation in the neonate. In: Crystal RG, West JB, eds. *The lung: scientific foundations.* New York: Raven, 1991; 1711.
22. Hanson M, Kumar P. Chemoreceptor function in the fetus and neonate. *Adv Exp Med Biol* 1994; **360**: 99–108.
23. Cohen G, Xu C, Henderson-Smart D. Ventilatory response of the sleeping newborn to CO_2 during normoxic rebreathing. *J Appl Physiol* 1991; **71**: 168–74.

24. Richards JM, Alexander JR, Shinebourne EA, de Swiet M, Wilson AJ, Southall DP. Sequential 22-hour profiles of breathing patterns and heart rate in 110 full-term infants during their first 6 months of life. *Pediatrics* 1984; **74**: 763–77.

25. Stebbens VA, Poets CF, Alexander JR, Arrowsmith WA, Southall DP. Oxygen saturation and breathing patterns in infancy. 1. Full term infants in the second month of life. *Arch Dis Child* 1991; **66**: 569–73.

26. Parkins KJ, Poets CF, O'Brien LM, Stebbens VA, Southall DP. Effect of exposure to 15% oxygen on breathing patterns and oxygen saturation in infants: interventional study. *BMJ* 1998; **316**: 887–94.

27. Delivoria-Papadopoulos M, Roncevic NP, Oski FA. Postnatal changes in oxygen transport of term, premature, and sick infants. *Pediat Res* 1971; **5**: 235–6.

28. Verma R. Respiratory distress syndrome of the newborn infant. *Obstet Gynecol Survey* 1995; **50**: 542–55.

29. Jobe A, Ikegami M. Surfactant for the treatment of respiratory distress syndrome. *Am Rev Respir Dis* 1987; **136**: 1256–75.

30. Soll RF. Surfactant therapy in the USA: trials and current routines. *Biol Neonate* 1997; **71** (Supp 1): 1–7.

31. Enhoring G. From bubbles to babies: the evolution of surfactant replacement therapy. *Biol Neonate* 1997; **71** (Supp 1): 28–31.

32. Halliday HL. Clinical trials of surfactant replacement in Europe. *Biol Neonate* 1997; **71** (Supp 1): 8–12.

33. Barrington KJ, Finer NN. Care of near term infants with respiratory failure. *BMJ* 1997; **315**: 1215–18.

34. UK Collaborative ECMO Trial Group. UK collaborative trial of neonatal extracorporeal membrane oxygenation. *Lancet* 1996; **348**: 75–82.

35. Leach CL, Greenspan JS, Rubenstein SD, Shaffer TH, Wolfson MR, Jackson JC et al. Partial liquid ventilation with perflubron in premature infants with severe respiratory distress syndrome. The LiquiVent study group. *N Engl J Med* 1996; **335**: 761–7.

36. Sibert J, Fleming PJ. Poisoning, accidents and sudden infant death syndrome. In: Campbell AGM, McIntosh N, eds. *Forfar and Arneil's textbook of pediatrics*. Edinburgh: Churchill Livingstone, 1998; 1719–23.

37. Keens TG, Ward SL. Apnea spells, sudden deaths and the role of the apnea monitor. *Pediat Clin N Am* 1993; **40**: 897–911.

38. Fleming PJ, Levine MR, Azaz Y, Wigfield R. The development of thermoregulation and interactions with the control of respiration in infants: possible relationship to sudden infant death. *Acta Paed Scand* 1993; **389** (Supp): 57–9.

39. de Jonge GA, Burgmeijer RJF, Engelberts AC, Hoogenboezem J, Kostense PJ, Sprij AJ. Sleeping position for infants and cot death in the Netherlands 1985–91. *Arch Dis Child* 1993; **69**: 660–3.

40. Irgens LM, Markestad T, Baste V, Schreuder P, Skjaerven R, Øyen N. Sleeping position and sudden infant death syndrome in Norway 1967–91. *Arch Dis Child* 1995; **72**: 478–82.

41. Dwyer T, Ponsonby AL, Blizzard L, Newman NM, Cochrane JA. The contribution of changes in the prevalence of prone sleeping position to the decline in sudden infant death syndrome in Tasmania. *JAMA* 1995; **273**: 783–9.

42. Papastamelos C, Panitch HB, England SE, Allen JL. Developmental changes in chest wall compliance in infancy and early childhood. *J Appl Physiol* 1995; **78**: 179–84.

43. Mansell A, Bryan AC, Levison H. Airway closure in children. *J Appl Physiol* 1972; **33**: 711–15.

44. Marcus CL, Glomb WB, Basinski DJ, Davidson SL, Keens TG. Developmental pattern of hypercapnic and hypoxic ventilatory responses from childhood to adulthood. *J Appl Physiol* 1994; **76**: 314–20.

Chapter 14

Exercise

The respiratory response to exercise depends on the level of exercise performed, which can be conveniently divided into three grades:[1]

1. *Moderate exercise* is below the subject's anaerobic threshold (see below) and the arterial blood lactate is not raised. He is able to transport all the oxygen required and remain in a steady state. This would correspond to work (more correctly 'power') levels up to about 100 watts (612 kg.m.min^{-1}).
2. *Heavy exercise* is above the anaerobic threshold. The arterial blood lactate is elevated but remains constant. This too may be regarded as a steady state.
3. *Severe exercise* is well above the anaerobic threshold and the arterial blood lactate continues to rise. This is an unsteady state and the level of work cannot long be continued.

Oxygen consumption during exercise

There is a close relationship between the external power that is produced and the oxygen consumption of the subject (Figure 14.1). The oxygen consumption at rest (the basal metabolic rate) is of the order of 200–250 ml.min^{-1}. As work is done, the oxygen consumption increases by approximately 12 ml.min^{-1} per watt. A consumption of about 1 l.min^{-1} is required for walking briskly on the level. About 3 l.min^{-1} is needed to run at 12 km.h^{-1} (7.5 miles per hour).

Time course of the increase in oxygen consumption[4]

Oxygen consumption rises rapidly at the onset of a period of exercise, with an accompanying increase in carbon dioxide production and a small increase in blood lactate. With light or moderate exercise (Figure 14.2a) a plateau is quickly reached and the lactate level remains well below the normal maximum resting level (<3.5 mmol.l^{-1}). With heavy exercise, $\dot{V}_{O_2}$, $\dot{V}_{CO_2}$ and lactate all increase more quickly, again reaching constant levels within a few minutes, the magnitude of which relates to the power generated and the fitness of the subject (Figure 14.2b). If the level of exercise exceeds about 60 per cent of the subject's maximal exercise ability (see below), there is usually a secondary 'slow component' to the increase in oxygen consumption, associated with a continuing increase

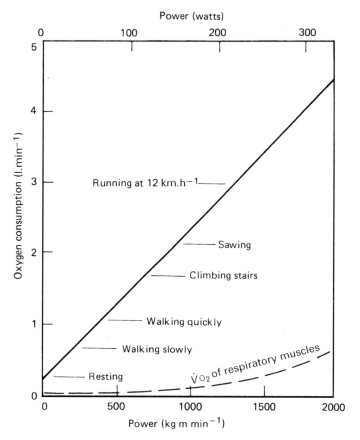

Figure 14.1 Steady state oxygen consumption with varying degrees of exercise. The continuous straight line denotes whole body oxygen consumption as a function of the level of power developed. The broken curve is an estimate of the oxygen cost of breathing for the increasing hyperventilation of exercise.[2,3]

in blood lactate level, which ultimately prevents the exercise from continuing (Figure 14.2c). Many explanations have been proposed for this slow component of $\dot{V}o_2$, including increased temperature, the oxygen cost of breathing,[5] lactacidosis[4] and changes in muscle metabolism secondary to the use of differing fibre types with prolonged exercise.[6] No consensus has been reached.

Maximal oxygen uptake

Maximal oxygen uptake ($\dot{V}o_{2max}$) refers to the oxygen consumption of a subject when exercising as hard as possible for that subject. A fit and healthy young adult of 70 kg should be able to maintain a $\dot{V}o_{2max}$ of about $3\,l.min^{-1}$, but this decreases with age to about $2\,l.min^{-1}$ at the age of 70. A sedentary existence without exercise can reduce $\dot{V}o_{2max}$ to 50 per cent of the expected value. Conversely, $\dot{V}o_{2max}$ can be increased by regular exercise, and athletes commonly achieve values of $5\,l.min^{-1}$. The highest levels (over $6\,l.min^{-1}$) are attained in rowers, who use a greater muscle mass than other athletes. One study reported an elite group of oarsmen who, for a brief period, attained a mean oxygen

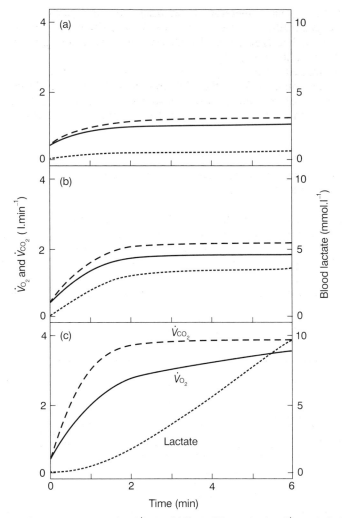

Figure 14.2 Changes in oxygen consumption ($\dot{V}o_2$, solid line), CO_2 production ($\dot{V}co_2$, dashed line) and blood lactate (dotted line) with the onset of varying levels of exercise. (a) Light to moderate exercise with little or no increase in lactate; (b) heavy exercise with an increase in lactate to an increased, but steady, level; (c) severe exercise, above the lactate threshold when levels continue to rise as exercise proceeds. Note that with severe exercise (c) the increase in oxygen consumption is biphasic with a second 'slow' component.

consumption of 6.6l.min^{-1} on the treadmill.[7] This required a minute volume of 200l.min^{-1} (tidal volume 3.29 litres at a frequency of 62 breaths per minute).

$\dot{V}o_{2\text{max}}$ is commonly used in exercise physiology as a measure of cardiorespiratory fitness. Subjects undertake a period of graduated exercise while $\dot{V}o_2$ is measured continuously by a spirometric method (page 298). In all but severe exercise, within a few minutes $\dot{V}o_2$ reaches a plateau (Figure 14.2), which is the subject's $\dot{V}o_{2\text{max}}$. At higher levels of exercise, as seen in athletes, defining when maximal oxygen uptake is reached may be difficult because of the slow component of oxygen consumption. Many varying definitions of $\dot{V}_{O_{2}max}$ have therefore been used over the years,[8] none of which is universally accepted. Elite athletes rarely reach a satisfactory plateau in $\dot{V}_{O_{2}}$, and secondary criteria such as high plasma lactate levels or a raised respiratory exchange ratio need to be used to define $\dot{V}_{O_{2}max}$.[8]

At $\dot{V}_{O_{2}max}$ in trained athletes, approximately 80 per cent of the oxygen consumed is used by locomotor muscles. With the high minute volumes seen during exercise, the oxygen consumption of respiratory muscles also becomes significant, being around 5 per cent of total $\dot{V}_{O_{2}}$ with moderate exercise and 10 per cent at $\dot{V}_{O_{2}max}$ (Figure 14.1).[3,9]

Response of the oxygen delivery system

A 10- or 20-fold increase in oxygen consumption requires a complex adaptation of both circulatory and respiratory systems.

Oxygen delivery or flux is the product of cardiac output and arterial oxygen content (page 283). The latter cannot be significantly increased, so an increase in cardiac output is essential. However, the cardiac output does not, and indeed could not, increase in proportion to the oxygen consumption. For example, an oxygen consumption of 4 l.min^{-1} is a 16-fold increase compared with the resting state. A typical cardiac output at this level of exercise would be only 25 l.min^{-1} (Figure 14.3), which is only five times the resting

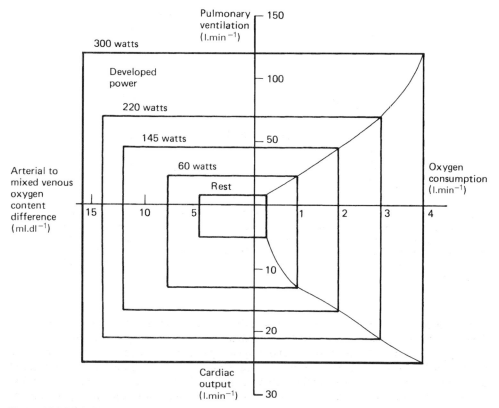

Figure 14.3 Changes in ventilation, oxygen consumption, cardiac output and oxygen extraction at different levels of power developed.

value. Therefore, there must also be increased extraction of oxygen from the blood. Figure 14.3 shows that the largest relative increase in cardiac output occurs at mild levels of exercise. At an oxygen consumption of $1 \, l.min^{-1}$, cardiac output is already close to 50 per cent of its maximal value.

Oxygen extraction. In the resting state, blood returns to the right heart with haemoglobin 70% saturated. This provides a substantial reserve of available oxygen, and the arterial/mixed venous oxygen content difference increases progressively as oxygen consumption is increased, particularly during heavy exercise when the mixed venous saturation may be as low as 20% (Figure 14.3). This decrease in mixed venous saturation covers the steep part of the oxygen dissociation curve (see Figure 11.9) and therefore the decrease in P_{O_2} is relatively less (5 to 2 kPa, or 37.5 to 15 mmHg). High levels of blood lactate seen during heavy exercise (Figure 14.2) may contribute to the increase in oxygen extraction by shifting the dissociation curve to the right at a capillary level.[4]

The additionally desaturated blood returning to the lungs and the greater volume of blood require that the respiratory system transport a larger quantity of oxygen to the alveoli. If there were no increased oxygen transport to the alveoli, the reserve oxygen in the mixed venous blood would be exhausted in one or two circulation times. Fortunately, the respiratory system normally responds rapidly to this requirement.

Anaerobic metabolism

During heavy exercise, the total work exceeds the capacity for aerobic work, which is limited by oxygen transport (see below). The difference is made up by anaerobic metabolism, of which the principal product is lactic acid (see Figure 11.14), which is almost entirely ionized to lactate and hydrogen ions. An increase in blood lactate level is therefore taken as an indication of a significant anaerobic contribution to metabolism. This defines the anaerobic threshold, which depends not only on the power produced but also on many other factors, including altitude, environmental temperature and the degree of training undertaken by the subject. An additional factor is the muscle groups that are used to accomplish the work, as different skeletal muscle fibres, and therefore muscle groups, have different metabolic products.[4] Lactacidosis probably provides part of the stimulus for the excess ventilation required for work in excess of the anaerobic threshold (see below).

During severe exercise the lactate level continues to rise (Figure 14.2c) and begins to cause distress at levels above about $11 \, mmol.l^{-1}$, ten times the normal resting level. Lactate accumulation seems to be the limiting factor for sustained heavy work, and the progressive increase in blood lactate results in the level of work being inversely related to the time for which it can be maintained. Thus there is a reciprocal relationship between the record time for various distances and the speed at which they are run.[10]

Oxygen debt

The difference between the total work and the aerobic work is achieved by anaerobic metabolism of carbohydrates to lactate, which is ultimately converted to citrate, enters the citric acid cycle and is then fully oxidized. Like glucose, lactate has a respiratory quotient of 1.0. Although this process continues during heavy exercise, lactate accumulates and the excess is oxidized in the early stages of recovery. Oxygen consumption remains above the resting level during recovery for this purpose. This constitutes the 'repayment of the oxygen debt' and is related to the lactate level attained by the end of exercise.

There is considerable evidence that some of the early part of the repayment of the oxygen debt is not only concerned with clearing lactate. Apart from oxidation of other products of anaerobic metabolism, there is the restoration of both oxygen stores and levels of high energy phosphate compounds to their normal resting levels.[10]

Repayment of the oxygen debt is especially well developed in the diving mammals such as seals and whales. During a dive, their circulation is largely diverted to heart and brain, and the metabolism of the skeletal muscles is almost entirely anaerobic (page 381). On regaining the surface, very large quantities of lactate are suddenly released into the circulation and are rapidly metabolized while the animal is on the surface between dives.

Excess post-exercise oxygen consumption.[11] Sustained heavy exercise results in an increased $\dot{V}_{O_2}$ even when the subject's blood lactate remains only mildly elevated. Excess oxygen consumption may occur for several hours, and is related to both the intensity and the duration of exercise undertaken. Previous hypotheses put forward to explain the excess $\dot{V}_{O_2}$ included an increase in body temperature and increased fat metabolism, though proof of these is lacking. Exercise at around 75 per cent of $\dot{V}_{O_2max}$ raises levels of catabolic hormones such as cortisol and catecholamines, which may explain the excess $\dot{V}_{O_2}$.[12]

The ventilatory response to exercise

Time course.[13] We have seen in the previous section that exercise without a rapid ventilatory response would be dangerous if not fatal. In fact, the respiratory system does respond with great rapidity (Figure 14.4). There is an instant increase in ventilation at, if

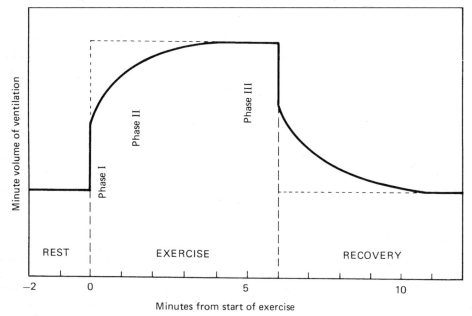

Figure 14.4 The time course of changes in ventilation in relation to a short period of moderate exercise. Note the instant increase in ventilation at the start of exercise before the metabolic consequences of exercise have had time to develop.

not slightly before, the start of exercise (phase I). During moderate exercise, there is then a further increase (phase II) to reach an equilibrium level of ventilation (phase III) within about 3 minutes.[14] With heavy exercise there is a secondary increase in ventilation, which may reach a plateau, but ventilation continues to rise in severe work. At the end of exercise, the minute volume falls to resting levels within a few minutes. After heavy and severe exercise, return to the resting level of ventilation takes longer, as the oxygen debt is repaid and lactate levels return to normal (see above).

The ventilation equivalent for oxygen. The respiratory minute volume is normally very well matched to the increased oxygen consumption, and the relationship between minute volume and oxygen consumption is approximately linear up to an oxygen consumption of about $2 \, l.min^{-1}$ in the untrained subject and more following training (Figure 14.5). The slope of the linear part is the ventilation equivalent for oxygen and is in the range $20-30 \, l.min^{-1}$ ventilation per $l.min^{-1}$ of oxygen consumption.[15,16] The slope does not appear to change with training.

    In heavy exercise, above a critical level of oxygen consumption (Owles point), the ventilation increases above the level predicted by an extrapolation of the linear part of the ventilation/oxygen consumption relationship (Figure 14.5). This is surplus to the

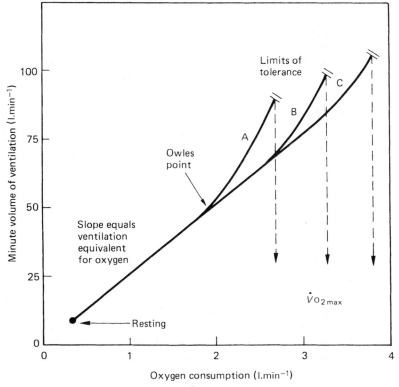

Figure 14.5 Changes in minute volume of ventilation in relation to the increased oxygen consumption of exercise. The break from linearity (Owles point) occurs at higher levels of oxygen consumption in trained athletes, who can also tolerate higher minute volumes. A to C shows progressive levels of training. Both mechanisms combine to enable the trained athlete to increase his maximum oxygen consumption.

requirement for gas exchange and is accompanied by hypocapnia, arterial P_{CO_2} decreasing by levels of the order of 1 kPa (7.5 mmHg). The excess ventilation is probably driven by lactacidosis. In the trained athlete, the break from linearity occurs at higher levels of oxygen consumption. This, together with improved tolerance of high minute volumes, allows the trained athlete to increase his $\dot{V}_{O_{2}max}$ as shown in Figure 14.5.

Minute volume and dyspnoea. It is generally believed that the ventilatory system does not limit exercise in normal subjects, although the evidence for this view is elusive.[17] One study[18] found that 50–60 per cent of maximal breathing capacity (MBC) was required for work at 80 per cent of aerobic capacity. However, the breaking point of exercise is usually determined by breathlessness, which occurs when the exercise ventilation uses a high proportion of the maximal breathing capacity. There is a close correlation between MBC and $\dot{V}_{O_{2}max}$.[16]

Minute volumes as great as 200 l.min^{-1} have been recorded during exercise, although the normal subject cannot maintain a minute volume approaching MBC for more than a very short period. Tidal volume during maximal exercise is about half vital capacity,[16] and 70–80 per cent of MBC can normally be maintained, with difficulty, for 15 minutes by fit young subjects.[18] Ventilation approximates to 60 per cent of MBC at maximal oxygen consumption.[14] The usable fraction of the maximal breathing capacity can, however, be increased by training.

Diffusing capacity. Diffusion across the alveolar/capillary membrane does not normally limit the increased oxygen consumption at sea level but this is a limiting factor at altitude (see Chapters 9 and 16). Exercise-induced hypoxia, which is seen fairly commonly in elite endurance athletes, is believed to be caused, at least in part, by diffusion limitation.[19]

Control of ventilation

Elucidation of the mechanisms that underlie the remarkably efficient adaptation of ventilation to the demands of exercise has been a challenge to generations of physiologists, and a complete explanation remains elusive.[1,13,14,15]

Neural factors

It has long been evident that neural factors play an important role, particularly as ventilation normally increases at or even before the start of exercise (phase I), when no other physiological variable has changed except cardiac output (Figure 14.4). In 1963, Kao and his colleagues[20] reported that in dogs virtually all of the hyperventilation of exercise can be explained by afferents arising from the exercising muscles. This was convincingly shown in crossed-circulation studies. The essential observation was that an anaesthetized dog in neurological continuity with electrically stimulated limb muscles hyperventilated, while another dog receiving the venous drainage from the exercising muscles did not. There is evidence in humans that the phase I ventilatory response may be in part a 'learned' response to the onset of exercise.[21]

Arterial blood gas tensions and the chemoreceptors

There is a large body of evidence that, during exercise at sea level with oxygen consumption up to about 3 l.min^{-1}, there is no significant change in either P_{CO_2} or P_{O_2} of arterial blood. In one study, even at the point of exhaustion (oxygen consumption $3.5\,l.min^{-1}$), the arterial Po_2 was the same as the resting value and Pco_2 was reduced. Blood gas tensions do not therefore seem at first sight to be the main factor governing the increased minute volume. Two caveats must be mentioned.

Inhalation of 100% oxygen during exercise reduces minute volume for a particular oxygen consumption.[22] The Po_2/ventilation response curve is known to be steeper during exercise (see Figure 5.9), so ventilation will respond to small fluctuations in normal arterial Po_2 under these circumstances. Carotid body resection[23] or administration of dopamine to inhibit carotid body activity[24] reduces the ventilatory response to exercise, particularly phase II (Figure 14.4). Thus it seems likely that the peripheral chemoreceptors do contribute, in a small way, to exercise-induced hyperpnoea, particularly during the non-steady state.[13,25]

The second caveat is that during exercise there is an increased respiratory phasic variation in arterial Pco_2, which is known to stimulate the carotid body (page 97).

In spite of these caveats, it is difficult to avoid the conclusion that arterial blood gas tensions acting on the chemoreceptors cannot be the main factor in the increase of ventilation during exercise. This contrasts sharply with their dominant role in the control of resting ventilation.

Humoral mechanisms

Humoral factors play a comparatively minor role in moderate exercise but are more important in heavy and severe exercise, when lactacidosis is an important factor.

Metabolic acidosis causes excess ventilation during heavy and severe exercise (Figure 14.5), causing a slight reduction in arterial Pco_2. However, study of arterial pH may be misleading because the very short transit time from lungs to carotid body during exercise (of the order of 4–6 seconds) is insufficient for the change in Pco_2 in the lungs to result in an equilibrium change in plasma pH by the time the blood reaches the chemoreceptors. The limiting step is the dehydration of carbonic acid (equation 2 in Chapter 10), which takes an appreciable time even in the presence of carbonic anhydrase. However, there is ample time for equilibration to occur in arterial blood sampled for analysis. Therefore the peripheral chemoreceptors see a different pH from that indicated by the pH meter, and blood perfusing the carotid bodies may be 0.02–0.03 pH units more acid, and the Pco_2 slightly higher than indicated by analysis of an arterial blood sample by conventional methods.[26] Slight additional respiratory drive may result from hyperthermia.

It has not escaped notice that the hyperventilation of exercise accords with the blood gas changes of the mixed venous blood. However, there is no evidence of any chemoreceptor in the great veins, the right heart or the input side of the lungs. There is some evidence that there may be metabolic chemoreceptors in the muscles,[1] but their exact role is unclear.

Fitness and training

The definitions of moderate, heavy and severe exercise at the beginning of this chapter are not transferable between individuals. A given amount of energy expenditure that constitutes severe exercise to a sedentary unfit subject is likely to represent less than moderate exercise to a trained athlete. The linear relationship between power generated and $\dot{V}o_2$ (Figure 14.1) is remarkably consistent irrespective of fitness and training, but the distance a subject may progress along this line (i.e. their $\dot{V}o_{2max}$) is extremely variable.

In healthy untrained subjects, rapidly increasing lactate levels normally limit exercise tolerance. Intracellular lactic acidosis in muscles gives rise to weakness and cramp, the respiratory stimulation rapidly takes the subject towards an intolerable minute ventilation, and exhaustion occurs. Training changes many aspects of exercise physiology. For example, improved cardiovascular fitness results in improved oxygen delivery, such that the Vo_2 at which lactate rises is greatly increased. Muscle in trained athletes releases less lactate than in untrained subjects (see below), and animal studies indicate that training may improve the ability of the liver to remove circulating lactate.[4] Finally, trained athletes can tolerate much higher blood lactate levels, up to 20 mmol.l^{-1}, or twice that of untrained subjects. There are two respiratory aspects of training that merit further consideration.

Minute volume of ventilation. Maximal expiratory flow rate is limited by flow-dependent airway closure (page 68), and is relatively unaffected by training.[18] However, within the limits of maximal breathing capacity, it is possible to increase the strength and endurance of the respiratory muscles. It is therefore possible to improve the *fraction* of the maximal breathing capacity that can be sustained during exercise. Highly trained athletes may be able to maintain ventilation by as much as 90 per cent of their maximal breathing capacity.

Ventilation equivalent for oxygen. There is no evidence that training can alter the slope of the plot of ventilation against oxygen consumption (Figure 14.5). However, the upward inflection of the curve (Owles point) is further to the right in the trained subject. This permits the attainment of a higher oxygen consumption for the same minute volume. Prolongation of the straight part of the curve is achieved by improving metabolic processes in skeletal muscle to minimize the stimulant effect of lactacidosis. There is ample evidence that training can improve the aerobic performance of muscles by many adaptations, including, for example, the increased density of the capillary network in the muscles. The consequent reduction in lactacidosis and therefore the excess ventilation, together with an increase in the tolerable minute volume, combine to increase the Vo_{2max} as shown in Figure 14.5. It would seem that the major factor in increasing the Vo_{2max} is improved performance of skeletal muscle and the cardiovascular system, rather than any specific change in respiratory function.

Cardiorespiratory disease[4,6,27]

Patients with cardiovascular or respiratory disease have poor exercise tolerance for three main reasons. First, the ventilatory response to exercise is more rapid, so a greater minute volume is required to achieve a given Vo_2. Secondly, the proportion of MBC that a patient can tolerate is reduced, and when combined with the previous observation this results in an extreme limitation of exercise tolerance before shortness of breath intervenes. Thirdly, a limited increase in cardiac output in response to exercise quickly gives rise to anaerobic metabolism, extra ventilatory requirements and exhaustion.

References

1. Whipp BJ. The control of exercise hyperpnea. In: Hornbein TF, ed. *Regulation of breathing.* New York: Marcel Dekker, 1981.
2. Otis AB. The work of breathing. *Handbook of Physiology, Section 3* 1964; **1**: 463.
3. Aaron EA, Seow KC, Johnson BD, Dempsey JA. Oxygen cost of exercise hyperpnea: implications for performance. *J Appl Physiol* 1992; **72**: 1818–25.

4. Wasserman K. Coupling of external to cellular respiration during exercise: the wisdom of the body revisited. *Am J Physiol* 1994; **266**: E519–39.

5. Hagberg JM, Mullin JP, Nagle FJ. Oxygen consumption during constant-load exercise. *J Appl Physiol* 1978; **45**: 381–4.

6. Poole DC, Barstow TJ, Gaesser GA, Willis WT, Whipp BJ. $\dot{V}o_2$ slow component: physiological and functional significance. *Med Sci Sports Exerc* 1994; **26**: 1354–8.

7. Clark JM, Hagerman FC, Gelfand R. Breathing patterns during submaximal and maximal exercise in elite oarsmen. *J Appl Physiol* 1983; **55**: 440–6.

8. Howley ET, Bassett DR, Welch HG. Criteria for maximal oxygen uptake: review and commentary. *Med Sci Sports Exerc* 1995; **27**: 1292–301.

9. Dempsey JA, Harms CA, Ainsworth DM. Respiratory muscle perfusion and energetics during exercise. *Med Sci Sports Exerc* 1996; **28**: 1123–9.

10. Asmussen E. Muscular exercise. *Handbook of Physiology, Section 3* 1965; **2**: 939.

11. Gaesser GA, Brooks GA. Metabolic basis of excess postexercise oxygen consumption. *Med Sci Sports Exerc* 1984; **16**: 29–43.

12. Quinn TJ, Vroman NB, Kertzer R. Postexercise oxygen consumption in trained females: effect of exercise duration. *Med Sci Sports Exerc* 1994; **26**: 908–13.

13. Whipp BJ. Peripheral chemoreceptor control of exercise hyperpnea in humans. *Med Sci Sports Exerc* 1994; **26**: 337–47.

14. Wasserman K. Breathing during exercise. *N Engl J Med* 1978; **298**: 780–5.

15. Forster HV, Pan LG. Exercise hyperpnea. In: Crystal RG, West JB, eds. *The lung: scientific foundations*. New York: Raven, 1991; 1553.

16. Åstrand P-O, Rodahl K. *Textbook of work physiology*, 3rd edn. New York: McGraw-Hill, 1986.

17. Bye PTP, Farkas GA, Roussos C. Respiratory factors limiting exercise. *Annu Rev Physiol* 1983; **45**: 439–51.

18. Shephard RJ. The maximum sustained voluntary ventilation in exercise. *Clin Sci* 1967; **32**: 167–76.

19. Powers SK, Martin D, Dodd S. Exercise-induced hypoxaemia in elite endurance athletes. *Sports Med* 1993; **16**: 14–22.

20. Kao FF. An experimental study of the pathways involved in exercise hyperpnoea employing cross-circulation techniques. In: Cunningham DJC, Lloyd BB, eds. *The regulation of human respiration*. Oxford: Blackwell Scientific, 1963.

21. Helbling D, Boutellier U, Spengler CM. Modulation of the ventilatory increase at the onset of exercise in humans. *Respir Physiol* 1997; **109**: 219–29.

22. Ward SA, Blesovsky L, Russak S, Ashjian A, Whipp BJ. Chemoreflex modulation of ventilatory dynamics during exercise in humans. *J Appl Physiol* 1988; **63**: 2001–7.

23. Wasserman K, Whipp BJ, Koyal SN, Cleary MG. Effect of carotid body resection on ventilatory and acid–base control during exercise. *J Appl Physiol* 1975; **39**: 354–8.

24. Boetger CL, Ward DS. Effect of dopamine on transient ventilatory response to exercise. *J Appl Physiol* 1986; **61**: 2102–7.

25. Forster HV, Pan LG. The role of carotid chemoreceptors in the control of breathing during exercise. *Med Sci Sports Exerc* 1994; **26**: 328–36.

26. Crandall ED, Bidani A, Forster RE. Postcapillary changes in blood pH in vivo during carbonic anhydrase inhibition. *J Appl Physiol* 1977; **43**: 582–90.

27. Piña IL, Fitzpatrick JT. Exercise and heart failure. *Chest* 1996; **110**: 1317–27.

Chapter 15

Sleep

Since about 1980, there has been a surge of interest in the respiratory physiology of sleep. This has resulted from the recognition that sleep-related breathing disorders are extremely common, and their effects present a major public health challenge.[1] This chapter provides a general review of the effects of sleep on respiration in normal and pathological states.

Normal sleep

Sleep is classified on the basis of the electroencephalogram (EEG) and electro-oculogram (EOG) into non-REM (stages 1–4) and rapid eye movement (REM) sleep.

Stage 1 is dozing from which arousal easily takes place. The EEG is low voltage and the frequency is mixed but predominantly fast. This progresses to stage 2 in which the background EEG is similar to stage 1 but with episodic sleep spindles (frequency 12–14 Hz) and K complexes (large biphasic waves of characteristic appearance). Slow, large amplitude (delta) waves start to appear in stage 2 but become more dominant in stage 3 in which spindles are less conspicuous and K complexes become difficult to distinguish. In stage 4, which is often referred to as deep sleep, the EEG is mainly high voltage (more than 75 μV) and more than 50 per cent slow (delta) frequency.

REM sleep has quite different characteristics. The EEG pattern is the same as in stage 1 but the EOG shows frequent rapid eye movements that are easily distinguished from the rolling eye movements of non-REM sleep. Other forms of activity are manifest in REM sleep and dreaming occurs.

The stage of sleep changes frequently during the night, and the pattern varies between different individuals and on different nights for the same individual (Figure 15.1). Sleep is entered in stage 1 and usually progresses through 2 to 3 and sometimes into 4. Episodes of REM sleep alternate with non-REM sleep throughout the night. On average there are four or five episodes of REM sleep per night, with a tendency for the duration of the episodes to increase towards morning. Conversely, stages 3 and 4 predominate in the early part of the night. The sleeper can pass from any stage to any other stage but it is unusual to pass from stage 1 or REM into either 3 or 4 or from stage 3 or 4 into REM. However, it is not uncommon for the sleeper to pass from any stage into stage 1 or full consciousness.

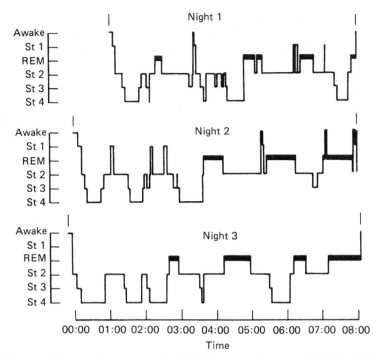

Figure 15.1 Patterns of sleep on three consecutive nights in a young fit man aged 20. The thick horizontal bars indicate rapid eye movement (REM) sleep. (Record kindly supplied by Dr C Thornton.)

Respiratory changes

Ventilation. Tidal volume decreases with deepening levels of non-REM sleep and is minimal in REM sleep, when it is about 25 per cent less than in the awake state.[2] Respiratory frequency increases slightly in all stages of sleep but the minute volume is progressively reduced in parallel with the tidal volume.

Arterial $P\text{co}_2$ is usually slightly elevated by about 0.4 kPa (3 mmHg). In the young healthy adult, arterial $P\text{o}_2$ decreases by about the same amount as the $P\text{co}_2$ is increased, and therefore the oxygen saturation remains reasonably normal. Mean value for ribcage contribution to breathing (page 120) has been found to be 54 per cent in stages 1–2, decreasing slightly in stages 3–4.[3] However, in REM sleep, the value was reduced to 29 per cent, which is close to the normal awake value in the supine position.

Pharyngeal airway resistance. The nasal airway is normally used during sleep, and upper airway resistance is consistently increased, especially during inspiration and in REM sleep. The main sites of increase are across the soft palate and in the hypopharynx.[4] Changes in pharyngeal muscle activity with sleep are complex. Muscles with predominantly tonic activity, such as tensor palati, show a progressive decrease in activity with deepening non-REM sleep,[5] reaching only 20–30 per cent of awake activity in stage 4 sleep. This loss of tonic activity correlates very well with increased upper airway resistance.[5] Unlike in the awake state, the tensor palati also fails to respond to an inspiratory resistive load. The activity of muscles with predominantly phasic inspiratory activity (e.g. geniohyoid and genioglossus) are influenced little by non-REM sleep.[6,7] In spite of maintained phasic activity during sleep, tonic activity of the geniohyoid is reduced whilst that of the genioglossus is well preserved, and responds appropriately to resistive loading.[8,9,10] It thus seems that the major effect is on the tonic activity of nasopharyngeal muscles and the increase in hypopharyngeal resistance seems to be due to secondary downstream collapse. This was clearly shown during application of external resistive loads in normal subjects during non-REM sleep.[11] In one study, pharyngeal collapse occurred at a mean value of 1.3 kPa (13 cmH$_2$O) below atmospheric in normal sleeping subjects.[12] Upper airway dilator muscles are affected more markedly in REM sleep.[13]

Chemosensitivity. In humans, the slope of the hypercapnic and hypoxic ventilatory responses are markedly reduced during sleep.[14,15] In both cases, the slope is reduced by approximately one-third during non-REM sleep, and even further reduced during REM sleep, but fortunately the responses are never abolished completely.

The ventilatory response to increased airway resistance is important in normal sleep because of the increased pharyngeal resistance, and is generally well preserved. There are substantial and rapid increases in both diaphragmatic and genioglossal inspiratory activity following nasal occlusion in normal sleeping adults.[16]

Effect of age. Compared with young subjects, the elderly have more variable ventilatory patterns when awake, which seems to result in more episodes of periodic breathing and apnoea when asleep.[17] Elderly subjects also have significant oscillations in upper airway resistance during sleep,[18] which may contribute to the observed variations in ventilation.[17] Thus as age advances, episodes of transient hypoxaemia occur in subjects who are otherwise healthy, with saturations commonly falling as low as 75% during sleep. Such changes must be regarded as a normal part of the ageing process.

Snoring

Snoring may occur at any age, but the incidence is bimodal, peaking in the first and the fifth to sixth decades of life. It is more common in males than in females, and obesity is an additional factor. It may occur in any stage of sleep, becoming more pronounced as non-REM sleep deepens, though usually attenuated in REM sleep.[19] It has been suggested that about 25 per cent of the population are habitual snorers, but these vary from the occasional snorer (e.g. after alcohol or with an upper respiratory tract infection) to the habitual persistent and heavy snorer.

Snoring originates in the oropharynx and in its mildest form is due to vibration of the soft palate and posterior pillars of the fauces. However, in its more severe forms, during inspiration the walls of the oropharynx collapse and the tongue is drawn back as a result of the subatmospheric pressure generated during inspiration against more upstream airway obstruction.[20] This may be at the level of the palate as described above or may be the result of nasal polyps, nasal infection or enlarged adenoids which are the commonest cause of snoring in children. As obstruction develops, the inspiratory muscles greatly augment their action and intrathoracic pressure may fall as low as –7 kPa (–70 cmH$_2$O).

Rather surprisingly, formal investigation has not shown posture to be a major factor in the production of snoring.[21] Nevertheless, it is widely believed that snoring is worse in the supine position.

Apart from the annoyance to conjugal partners and others, there are strong associations between snoring and a wide range of pathological conditions, including hypertension, heart and chest disease, rheumatism, diabetes and depression.[22] 'Normal' snoring is not associated with either frequent arousal from sleep or apnoea, but is believed to precede the development of more serious sleep-related breathing disorders.

Sleep-related breathing disorders

This term is used to describe a continuum of respiratory abnormalities seen during sleep, which range from simple snoring to life-threatening obstructive sleep apnoea.[1,23,24] All are characterized by airway narrowing or obstruction that leads to repeated episodes of arterial hypoxia and arousal as a result of increased respiratory effort. Repeated arousals throughout the night give rise to excessive daytime sleepiness. Three syndromes are described, but there is considerable overlap between them.

Upper airway resistance syndrome[24,25] in which tidal volume and arterial oxygen saturation (Sa_{O_2}) remain normal, but at the expense of extensive respiratory effort, which causes over 15 arousals per hour.

Obstructive sleep hypopnoea involving frequent (>15 per hour) episodes of airway obstruction of sufficient severity to reduce tidal volume to less than 50 per cent of normal for over 10 seconds. There may be small decreases in Sa_{O_2}.

Obstructive sleep apnoea characterized by more than five episodes per hour of obstructive apnoea lasting over 10 seconds and associated with severe decreases in Sa_{O_2}. In fact, duration of apnoea may be as long as 90 seconds and the frequency of the episodes as high as 160 per hour. In severe cases, 50 per cent of sleep time may be spent without tidal exchange.

The last two syndromes are commonly grouped together as sleep apnoea/hypopnoea syndrome (SAHS). Severity is normally quantified by recording the apnoea/hypopnoea index (AHI), which is simply the number of occurrences per hour of apnoeas or hypopnoeas lasting longer than 10 seconds. Milder forms of sleep-disordered breathing tend to progress to more severe forms as patients grow older and fatter. The prevalence of SAHS, defined as an AHI of over 5, is between 3.5 and 24 per cent in men and between 1.5 and 9 per cent in women, depending on the population studied.[26,27]

Apnoea or hypopnoea may be central (absence of all respiratory movements, as in Figure 15.2b) or obstructive. Differentiation between central and obstructive apnoea is conveniently made by continuous recording of ribcage and abdominal movements. Inductance plethysmography permits calculation of the tidal volume attributable to each compartment (page 120). If, as a result of upper airway obstruction, abdominal and ribcage movements become uncoordinated (Figure 15.2c), hypopnoea results. When these movements are equal but opposite in phase, there is total obstructive apnoea (Figure 15.2d). Obstructive apnoea may occur in REM or non-REM sleep but the longest periods of apnoea tend to occur in REM sleep. Central apnoeas are more common in elderly patients.

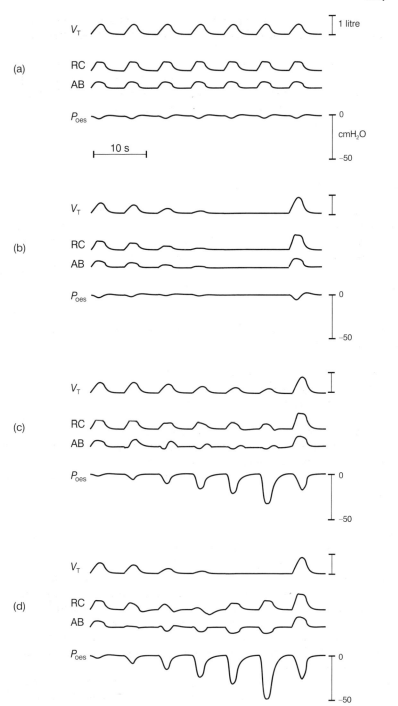

Figure 15.2 Continuous records of breathing during differing types of apnoea and hypopnoea showing tidal volume (*V*T), ribcage (RC) and abdominal (AB) contributions to breathing, and oesophageal pressure (*P*oes). (a) normal; (b) central apnoea; (c) obstructive hypopnoea; (d) obstructive apnoea. See text for details.

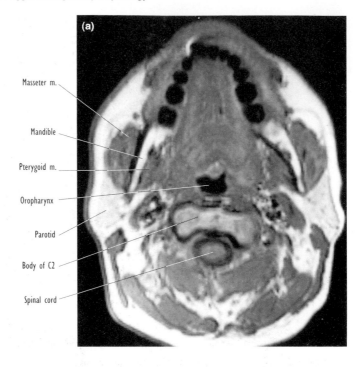

Masseter m.

Mandible

Pterygoid m.

Oropharynx

Parotid

Body of C2

Spinal cord

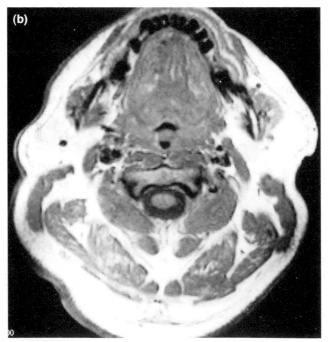

Figure 15.3 Magnetic resonance imaging scan of the neck at level of the oropharynx. In this type of scan, fat tissue appears white. (a) Normal, non-obese subject. (b) Obese patient with obstructive sleep apnoea, showing deposits of adipose tissue throughout the neck (the uvula is seen in the pharynx).

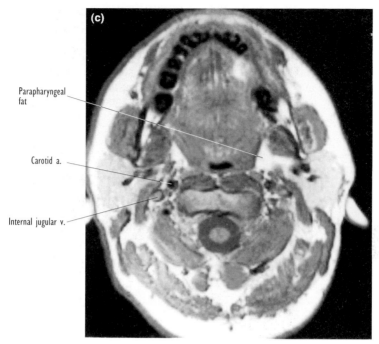

Parapharyngeal
fat

Carotid a.

Internal jugular v.

Figure 15.3 (c) Non-obese patient with sleep apnoea, showing fat deposits lateral to the pharynx with normal amounts of adipose tissue elsewhere. (I am indebted to Dr I Mortimore for providing the scans. Parts (a) and (c) reproduced by permission of the publishers of *American Journal of Respiratory and Critical Care Medicine*.)

The mechanism of airway obstruction[7,28]

Anatomical factors. There is now widespread agreement that, on average, patients with SAHS have anatomically narrower airways than have controls, though there is considerable overlap. Anatomical airway narrowing is believed to relate to two main factors.

First, obesity influences pharyngeal airway size. A central pattern of obesity, commonly seen in males, includes extensive fat deposition in the neck tissues. This accounts for the strong association between SAHS and neck circumference.[29] Adipose tissue is best visualized using magnetic resonance imaging (MRI), and in patients with SAHS, collections of fat are invariably seen lateral to the pharynx, between the pterygoid muscles and the carotid artery (Figure 15.3).[30,31] Pharyngeal fat is increased above normal levels even in non-obese patients with SAHS (Figure 15.3).[32] In addition, the quantity of adipose tissue seen correlates with the AHI, and weight loss predictably reduces both.

Secondly, facial structure may be different in some patients with SAHS, including micrognathia (small mandible) or retrognathia (posterior positioned mandible),[33] both of which will tend to displace the tongue backwards, requiring extra genioglossus activity to maintain a normal sized airway. This hypothesis raises the interesting possibility that SAHS may begin in early childhood, when enlarged adenoids and tonsils can influence facial bone development, and may also go some way to explaining familial 'aggregations' of SAHS and snoring.[23]

Pharyngeal dilator muscles are more active in awake subjects with SAHS when compared with controls, presumably as a physiological response to the anatomically smaller airway. The activity is believed to originate from the usual reflex stimulated by a negative pharyngeal pressure (page 113), which may be present to a greater extent in SAHS subjects even when awake. This requirement for increased pharyngeal muscle activity to maintain airway size may become impossible to maintain during sleep. Coupled with the normal loss of tonic activity of pharyngeal muscles (see above), sleep quickly results in airway obstruction.

Airway collapse occurs only in obstructive sleep apnoea, and normally results from increased upstream resistance behind the soft palate[34] leading to secondary downstream collapse. This is a function of the compliance (collapsibility) of the hypopharyngeal walls opposed by the action of the pharyngeal dilator muscles. Collapse is more likely to occur when pharyngeal compliance is high and particularly when there is increased submucosal fat.[31] Severe collapse of the hypopharynx occurs with the combination of enhanced diaphragmatic contraction, depressed pharyngeal dilator muscle activity and upstream obstruction.[34] Animal studies showed that alcohol induced a significant reduction in hypoglossal and recurrent laryngeal nerve activities in doses that had little or no effect on phrenic nerve activity.[35] This seems relevant to the well-known effect of alcohol on both snoring and SAHS.

Arousal

Apnoea or hypopnoea are terminated when the patient is aroused from sleep, though this arousal is normally subcortical – that is, the patient does not return to full consciousness. Arousal is followed by clearance of the pharyngeal airway, and this is crucially important for survival. In spite of the depressed ventilatory response curves, hypoxia and hypercapnia do contribute to arousal, probably alongside afferent input from pressure-sensitive pharyngeal receptors. Current opinion supports the view that a combination of all these factors results in increased respiratory drive, which brings about arousal.[7] Whatever the mechanism, arousal is accompanied by massive sympathetic discharge.

Medical effects of SAHS[36]

The effects of the SAHS are not trivial and, over a period of years, mortality in patients with SAHS is considerably higher than in controls. However, proving that this excess mortality relates to the SAHS itself has been difficult, as most studies have not adequately controlled for the associated risk factors of smoking, obesity and alcohol consumption.[1,36] There are two main causes of medical problems, as follows.

Arousal. A night's sleep that is disturbed hundreds of times, even subconsciously, leaves the individual with severe daytime somnolence, with decrement of performance in many fields. The ability to drive is impaired, such that patients with SAHS have two to three times as many accidents than other drivers and may endanger themselves and other road users.

   Each arousal is associated with significant secretion of catecholamines, leading to raised systemic blood pressure and tachycardia. These may exacerbate hypertension and ischaemic heart disease or even precipitate cardiac arrhythmias or cerebrovascular accidents.

Hypoxia. Repeated hypoxic episodes may be responsible for the development of pulmonary hypertension and right-sided heart failure, along with some degree of intellectual deterioration. These effects are considerably worse in patients with other, unrelated, pulmonary diseases.

Postoperative sleep apnoea/hypopnoea

Continuous monitoring has shown that transient apnoea occurs very frequently during sleep in the postoperative period.[38] Both central and obstructive apnoea occur but hypoxaemia is more pronounced in the obstructive type (see Figure 15.2). Stage 3 and 4 and REM sleep were not observed in the first 24 hours after operation and apnoea was therefore restricted to stages 1 and 2. Patients tend to catch up on REM sleep on the second and third postoperative nights, and obstructive episodes are often more common at that time. Avoidance of opiates greatly reduced the incidence of episodes of hypoxia, which were seldom seen in patients whose postoperative pain was controlled only with regional analgesia.

Treatment of sleep apnoea/hypopnoea syndrome (SAHS)[39,40]

Weight loss is effective at reducing the AHI in obese patients with SAHS, and is believed to act by reducing peripharyngeal fat, thus increasing airway diameter.[30] Bariatric surgery has been used to produce a dramatic and sustained weight loss in SAHS, but is associated with increased mortality in these patients compared with obese patients with normal respiration. There is some evidence that small amounts of weight loss (10 per cent) are associated with large reductions in AHI (50 per cent).

Nasal continuous positive airway pressure (nCPAP)[41] aims to prevent the development of a subatmospheric pharyngeal pressure sufficient to cause downstream pharyngeal collapse. It requires a well-fitting nasal mask or soft plastic tubes that fit inside the external nares. Compressed air must then be provided at the requisite gas flow, preferably with humidification. nCPAP serves no useful purpose during expiration, and systems have been developed to return airway pressure to atmospheric during expiration. In effect, this provides a modest level of intermittent positive pressure ventilation. Compliance with nCPAP may be poor, but it has proved to be highly effective in the relief of obstructive sleep apnoea, particularly the daytime somnolence that has such a major effect on the patient's life.[37]

Surgical relief of obstruction. For snoring alone, the first approach is the removal of any pathological obstruction such as nasal polyps that cause downstream collapse, though this may not improve patients with SAHS. A more radical approach is uvulo-palato-pharyngoplasty, which reduces the size of the soft palate and so dampens palatal oscillations and reduces pharyngeal collapse at this level. This is usually very effective in the relief of snoring,[42] but its value in SAHS is less impressive, symptoms improving in under 50 per cent of patients. Patients who do improve with surgery are those in whom the site of obstruction is high in the pharynx, and development of the technique is now aimed at better selection of patients who will benefit. Non-obese patients with SAHS who have facial bone abnormalities may benefit from maxillofacial corrective surgery, usually involving advancement of the anterior mandible and/or maxilla. Tracheotomy (opened only at night) has been used in some cases as a last resort.

Drug treatment of SAHS has had limited success. Many antidepressant drugs cause a considerable reduction in REM sleep, so may be beneficial in patients who have episodes of apnoea mostly during REM sleep. Serotonin antagonists such as fluoxetine have also been shown to improve the AHI, and are believed to act as ventilatory stimulants.

Oral appliances are available that can be maintained in the mouth at night to move either the tongue or the mandible forward, thus increasing the size of the airway. They are effective treatments for moderate SAHS and surprisingly well tolerated by patients.[43]

Oxygen has the advantage of increasing the inspired oxygen concentration as minute volume decreases. In fact, oxygen does not decrease the AHI, nor does it delay arousal from obstruction or result in hypercapnia. It will, however, reduce the desaturation that results, so may have a place in preventing the sequelae of the recurrent bouts of hypoxaemia. Current advice on treatment is aimed at reducing the AHI, and therefore the need for oxygen as well.

References

1. Fleetham JA. A wake up call for sleep disordered breathing. *BMJ* 1997; **314**; 839–40.
2. Douglas NJ, White DP, Pickett CK, Weil JV, Zwillich CW. Respiration during sleep in normal man. *Thorax* 1982; **37**: 840–4.
3. Millman RP, Knight H, Kline LR, Shore ET, Chung DC, Pack AI. Changes in compartmental ventilation in association with eye movements during REM sleep. *J Appl Physiol* 1988; **65**: 1196–202.
4. Hudgel DW, Hendricks C. Palate and hypopharynx – sites of inspiratory narrowing of the upper airway during sleep. *Am Rev Respir Dis* 1988; **138**: 1542–7.
5. Tangel DJ, Mezzanotte WS, White DP. Influence of sleep on tensor palatini EMG and upper airway resistance in normal men. *J Appl Physiol* 1991; **70**: 2574–81.
6. Wiegand DA, Zwillich CW, Latz B, Wiegand L. The influence of sleep on geniohyoid muscle activity and supraglottic airway resistance. *Am Rev Respir Dis* 1989; **139**: A447
7. White DP. Pathophysiology of obstructive sleep apnoea. *Thorax* 1995; **50**: 797–804.
8. Tangel DJ, Mezzanotte WS, Sandberg EJ, White DP. The influence of sleep on the activity of tonic postural versus inspiratory phasic muscles in normal men. *J Appl Physiol* 1992; **73**: 1058–66.
9. Wiegand DA, Latz B, Zwillich CW, Wiegand L. Geniohyoid muscle activity in normal man during wakefulness and sleep. *J Appl Physiol* 1990; **69**: 1262–9.
10. Henke KG. Upper airway muscle activity and upper airway resistance in young adults during sleep. *J Appl Physiol* 1998; **84**: 486–91.
11. Wiegand DA, Zwillich CW, White DP. Collapsibility of the human upper airway during normal sleep. *J Appl Physiol* 1989; **66**: 1800–8.
12. Schwartz AR, Smith PL, Wise RA, Gold AR, Permutt S. Induction of upper airway occlusion in sleeping individuals with subatmospheric nasal pressure. *J Appl Physiol* 1988; **64**: 535–42.
13. Dempsey JA, Skatrud JB, Badr S, Henke KG. Effects of sleep on the regulation of breathing and respiratory muscle function. In: Crystal RG, West JB, eds. *The lung: scientific foundations*. New York: Raven, 1991; 1615.

14. Douglas NJ, White DP, Weil JV, Pickett CK, Zwillich CW. Hypercapnic ventilatory response in sleeping adults. *Am Rev Respir Dis* 1982; **126**: 758–62.
15. Douglas NJ, White DP, Weil JV, Pickett CK, Martin RJ, Hudgel DW, Zwillich CW. Hypoxic ventilatory response decreases during sleep in normal men. *Am Rev Respir Dis* 1982; **125**: 286–9.
16. Kuna ST, Smickley J. Response of genioglossus muscle activity to nasal airway occlusion in normal sleeping adults. *J Appl Physiol* 1988; **64**: 347–53.
17. Shore ET, Millman RP, Silage DA, Chung DCC, Pack AI. Ventilatory and arousal patterns during sleep in normal young and elderly subjects. *J Appl Physiol* 1985; **59**: 1607–15.
18. Hudgel DW, Devadatta P, Hamilton H. Pattern of breathing and upper airway mechanics during wakefulness and sleep in healthy elderly humans. *J Appl Physiol* 1993; **74**: 2198–204.
19. Lugaresi E, Cirignotta F, Coccagna G, Montagna P. Clinical significance of snoring. In: Saunders NA, Sullivan CE, eds. *Sleep and breathing.* New York: Marcel Dekker, 1984.
20. Jennett S. Snoring and its treatment. *BMJ* 1984; **289**: 335–6.
21. Sullivan CE, Berthon-Jones M, Issa FG. Remission of severe obesity hypoventilation syndrome following short-term treatment during sleep with nasal continuous positive airway pressure. *Am Rev Respir Dis* 1983; **128**: 177–87.
22. Norton PG, Dunn EV. Snoring as a risk factor for disease: an epidemiological survey. *BMJ* 1985; **291**: 630–2.
23. Stradling JR. Obstructive sleep apnoea: definitions, epidemiology, and natural history. *Thorax* 1995; **50**: 683–9.
24. Strollo PJ, Rogers RM. Obstructive sleep apnea. *N Engl J Med* 1996; **334**: 99–104.
25. Guilleminault C, Stoohs R, Duncan S. Snoring: daytime sleepiness in regular heavy snorers. *Chest* 1991; **99**: 40–48.
26. Strohl KP, Redline S. Recognition of obstructive sleep apnea. *Am J Respir Crit Care Med* 1996; **154**: 279–89.
27. Ohayon MM, Guilleminault C, Priest RG, Caulet M. Snoring and breathing pauses during sleep: telephone interview survey of United Kingdom population sample. *BMJ* 1997; **314**: 860–3.
28. Douglas NJ. Pathogenesis of obstructive sleep apnoea/hypopnoea syndrome. *Lancet* 1994; **344**: 653–5.
29. Davies RJO, Stradling JR. The relationship between neck circumference, radiographic pharyngeal anatomy, and the obstructive sleep apnoea syndrome. *Eur Respir J* 1990; **3**: 509–14.
30. Shelton KE, Woodson H, Gay S, Suratt PM. Pharyngeal fat in obstructive sleep apnoea. *Am Rev Respir Dis* 1993; **148**: 462–6.
31. Horner RL, Mohiaddin RH, Lowell DG, Shea SA, Burman ED, Longmore DB, Guz A. Sites and sizes of fat deposits around the pharynx in obese patients with obstructive sleep apnoea and weight matched controls. *Eur Respir J* 1989; **2**: 613–22.
32. Mortimore IL, Marshall I, Wraith PK, Sellar RJ, Douglas NJ. Neck and total body fat deposition in nonobese and obese patients with sleep apnea compared with that in control subjects. *Am J Respir Crit Care Med* 1998; **157**: 280–3.
33. Jamieson A, Guilleminault C, Partinen M, Quera-Salva MA. Obstructive sleep apneic patients have craniomandibular abnormalities. *Sleep* 1986; **9**: 469–78.
34. Horner RL, Shea SA, McIvor J, Guz A. Pharyngeal size and shape during wakefulness and sleep in patients with obstructive sleep apnoea. *QJM* 1989; **72**: 719–35.
35. Bonora M, Shields GI, Knuth SL, Bartlett D, St John WM. Selective depression by ethanol of upper airway respiratory motor activity in cats. *Am Rev Respir Dis* 1984; **130**: 156–61.
36. Ferguson KA, Fleetham JA. Consequences of sleep disordered breathing. *Thorax* 1995; **50**: 998–1004.
37. Wright J, Johns R, Watt I, Melville A, Sheldon T. Health effects of obstructive sleep apnoea and the effectiveness of continuous positive airway pressure: a systematic review of the research evidence. *BMJ* 1997; **314**: 851–60.
38. Catley DM, Thornton C, Jordan C, Lehane JR, Royston D, Jones JG. Pronounced, episodic oxygen desaturation in the postoperative period: its association with ventilatory pattern and analgesic regimen. *Anesthesiology* 1985; **63**: 20–8.
39. Hudgel DW. Treatment of obstructive sleep apnoea. *Chest* 1996; **109**: 1346–58.
40. Aboussouan LS, Golish JA, Dinner DS, Strome M, Mendelson WB. Limitations and promise in the diagnosis and treatment of obstructive sleep apnoea. *Respir Med* 1997; **91**: 181–91.

41. Grunstein RR. Nasal continuous positive airway pressure treatment for obstructive sleep apnoea. *Thorax* 1995; **50**: 1106–13.
42. Sharp JF, Jalaludin M, Murray JAM, Maran AGD. The uvulopalatopharyngoplasty operation: the Edinburgh experience. *J R Soc Med* 1990; **83**: 569–70.
43. Ferguson KA, Ono T, Lowe AA, Keenan SP, Fleetham JA. A randomised crossover study of an oral appliance vs nasal continuous positive airway pressure in the treatment of mild–moderate obstructive sleep apnoea. *Chest* 1996; **109**: 1269–75.

Chapter 16

High altitude and flying

With increasing altitude, the barometric pressure falls, but the fractional concentration of oxygen in the air (0.21) and the saturated vapour pressure of water at body temperature (6.3 kPa or 47 mmHg) remain constant. The Po_2 of the inspired air is related to the barometric pressure as follows:

$$\text{Inspired gas } Po_2 = 0.21 \text{ (Barometric pressure} - 6.3) \text{ kPa}$$

or $\quad\quad$ Inspired gas $Po_2 = 0.21$ (Barometric pressure $-$ 47) mmHg

The influence of the saturated vapour pressure of water becomes relatively more important until, at an altitude of about 19 000 m or 63 000 ft, the barometric pressure equals the water vapour pressure, and alveolar Po_2 and Pco_2 become zero.

Table 16.1 is based on the standard table relating altitude and barometric pressure. However, there are important deviations from the predicted barometric pressure under certain circumstances, particularly at low latitudes. At the summit of Everest, the barometric pressure was found to be 2.4 kPa (18 mmHg) greater than predicted, and this was crucial to reaching the summit without oxygen. The uppermost curve in Figure 16.1 shows the expected Po_2 of air as a function of altitude, while the crosses indicate observed values that have been consistently higher than expected in the Himalayas.

Equivalent oxygen concentration

The acute effect of altitude on inspired Po_2 may be simulated by reduction of the oxygen concentration of gas inspired at sea level (Table 16.1). This provides the basis for much experimental work. Conversely, up to 10 000 m (33 000 ft), it is possible to restore the inspired Po_2 to the sea level value by an appropriate increase in the oxygen concentration of the inspired gas (also shown in Table 16.1). Lower inspired Po_2 values may be obtained between 10 000 and 19 000 m, above which body fluids boil.

Respiratory system responses to altitude

Ascent to altitude presents three main challenges to the respiratory system, resulting from progressively reduced inspired Po_2, low relative humidity and, in outdoor environments, extreme cold. Hypoxia is by far the most important of these, and requires significant

Table 16.1 Barometric pressure relative to altitude

Altitude		Barometric pressure		Inspired gas P_{O_2}		Equivalent oxygen % at sea level	Percentage oxygen required to give sea level value of inspired gas P_{O_2}
feet	metres	kPa	mmHg	kPa	mmHg		
0	0	101	760	19.9	149	20.9	20.9
2 000	610	94.3	707	18.4	138	19.4	22.6
4 000	1 220	87.8	659	16.9	127	17.8	24.5
6 000	1 830	81.2	609	15.7	118	16.6	26.5
8 000	2 440	75.2	564	14.4	108	15.1	28.8
10 000	3 050	69.7	523	13.3	100	14.0	31.3
12 000	3 660	64.4	483	12.1	91	12.8	34.2
14 000	4 270	59.5	446	11.1	83	11.6	37.3
16 000	4 880	54.9	412	10.1	76	10.7	40.8
18 000	5 490	50.5	379	9.2	69	9.7	44.8
20 000	6 100	46.5	349	8.4	63	8.8	49.3
22 000	6 710	42.8	321	7.6	57	8.0	54.3
24 000	7 320	39.2	294	6.9	52	7.3	60.3
26 000	7 930	36.0	270	6.3	47	6.6	66.8
28 000	8 540	32.9	247	5.6	42	5.9	74.5
30 000	9 150	30.1	226	4.9	37	5.2	83.2
35 000	10 700	23.7	178	3.7	27	3.8	–
40 000	12 200	18.8	141	2.7	20	2.8	–
45 000	13 700	14.8	111	1.8	13	1.9	–
50 000	15 300	11.6	87	1.1	8	1.1	–
63 000	19 200	6.3	47	0	0	0	–

100% oxygen restores sea level inspired P_{O_2} at 10 000 m (33 000 ft).

physiological changes to allow continuation of normal activities at altitude. The efficiency of these changes depends on many factors such as the normal altitude at which the subject lives, the rate of ascent, the altitude attained and the health of the subject.

Acute exposure to altitude

Transport technology now permits altitude to be attained quickly and without the exertion of climbing. Rail, air, cable car or motor transport may take a passenger within a few hours from near sea level to as high as 4000 m (13 100 ft), or 5000 m (16 400 ft) in certain exceptional locations. Aircraft, helicopters and balloons can take the traveller very much higher and faster, but passengers in unpressurized commercial aircraft are not normally exposed to altitudes exceeding 3700 m (12 000 ft).

Ventilatory changes. At high altitude the decrease in inspired gas P_{O_2} reduces alveolar and therefore arterial P_{O_2}. The actual decrease in alveolar P_{O_2} is mitigated by hyperventilation caused by the hypoxic drive to ventilation. However, on acute exposure to altitude, the ventilatory response to hypoxia is very short lived, owing to a combination of the resultant hypocapnia and hypoxic ventilatory decline (page 101 and Figure 5.8). During the first

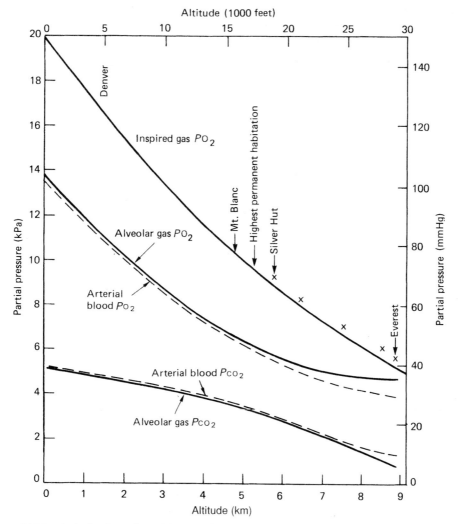

Figure 16.1 Inspired, alveolar and arterial gas tensions at rest, as a function of altitude. The curve for inspired Po_2 is taken from standard data in Table 16.1, but the crosses show actual measurements in the Himalayas. The alveolar gas data are from reference 1, and agree remarkably well with the arterial blood data from the simulated ascent of Everest.[2]

few days at altitude, this disadvantageous negative feedback is reversed by acclimatization (see below).

Signs and symptoms. Impairment of night vision is the earliest sign of hypoxia, and may be detected as low as 1200 m (4000 ft). However, the most serious aspect of acute exposure to altitude is impairment of mental performance, culminating in loss of consciousness, which usually occurs on acute exposure to altitudes in excess of 6000 m (about 20 000 ft). The time to loss of consciousness varies with altitude and is of great practical importance to pilots in the event of loss of pressurization (Figure 16.2). The shortest possible time to loss of consciousness (about 15 s) is governed by lung-to-brain

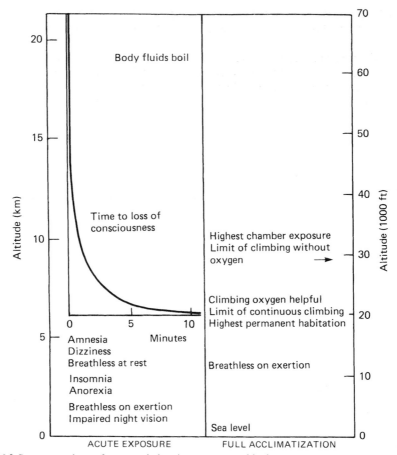

Figure 16.2 Symptomatology of acute and chronic exposure to altitude.

circulation time and the capacity of high energy phosphate stores in the brain (page 472). This applies above about 16 000 m (52 000 ft).

Acclimatization to altitude

Acclimatization refers to the processes by which tolerance and performance are improved over a period of hours to weeks after an individual who normally lives at relatively low altitude ascends to a much higher area. Everest has been climbed without oxygen by well-acclimatized lowlanders, although the barometric pressure on the summit would cause rapid loss of consciousness without acclimatization (Figure 16.2). Adaptation to altitude (described below) refers to physiological differences in permanent residents at high altitude and is quite different from acclimatization.

Earlier studies of acclimatization took place in the attractive, though somewhat hostile, environment of high altitude expeditions in many mountain ranges. Technical limitations in these conditions led, in 1985, to Operation Everest II in which eight volunteers spent over 32 days in a decompression chamber in which an ascent to the summit of Everest was simulated.[3] These conditions permitted extensive physiological research to be undertaken, including arterial and Swan–Ganz catheterization at rest and during exercise.

Ventilatory control. Prolonged hypoxia results in several complex changes in ventilation and arterial blood gases which are shown in Figure 16.3.[4,5] The initial hypoxic drive to ventilation on acute exposure is short lived, and after about 30 minutes ventilation returns to only slightly above normoxic levels with Pco_2 just below control levels (Figure 16.3).

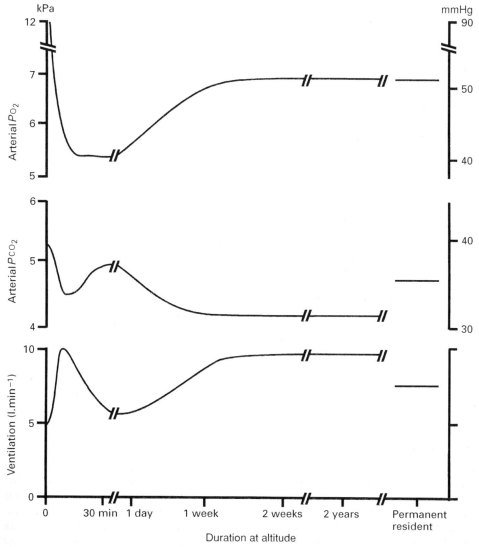

Figure 16.3 Effects of prolonged hypoxia (equivalent to 4300 m) on ventilation and blood gases. The first section of the graph shows the acute hypoxic response and hypoxic ventilatory decline described in Chapter 5. Acclimatization then takes place, partially restoring Po_2 by means of long-term hyperventilation and hypocapnia, a situation that is maintained indefinitely while remaining at altitude. Individuals who reside throughout life at this altitude maintain similar Po_2 values with lesser degrees of hyperventilation, but still have a minute ventilation greater than sea level normal. (Redrawn from reference 4.)

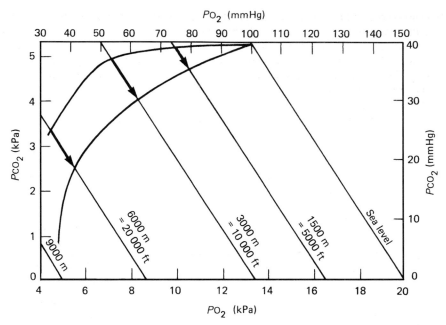

Figure 16.4 Magnitude of Po_2 changes with acclimatization. Straight lines representing the respiratory exchange ratio (R) have been drawn for various altitudes through inspired gas points at the bottom of the graph. Intersections between the R lines and the upper curve indicate alveolar gas tensions on acute exposure to altitude. Hyperventilation from early acclimatization results in the alveolar points moving down the R lines (as shown by the arrows) until they lie on the lower curve, thus decreasing Pco_2 and improving Po_2. (Data from references 1 and 6.)

This poor ventilatory response causes significant arterial hypoxaemia and results in many of the symptoms seen during the first few hours and days at altitude. Over the next few days, ventilation slowly increases with an accompanying reduction of Pco_2 and increase in arterial Po_2. This increase in Po_2 is of relatively small magnitude and can never correct Po_2 to normal (sea level) values (Figure 16.4), but it does seem to be enough to ameliorate most of the symptoms of exposure to acute altitude.

There are significant differences between species in the rate at which acclimatization takes place, being just a few hours in most animals, and several days or weeks in humans.[4] Both the rate of ascent and the altitude attained influence the speed at which ventilatory acclimatization occurs,[7] but in humans, most subjects are fully acclimatized within one week.

There are many possible mechanisms to explain ventilatory changes with acclimatization.[4] In spite of the low blood Pco_2, stimulation of the central chemoreceptors almost certainly plays a part in the hyperventilation that occurs with acclimatization. It was first suggested, in 1963, that the restoration of cerebrospinal fluid (CSF) pH, by means of bicarbonate transport, might explain this acclimatization of ventilation to altitude.[8,9] Shortly afterwards Severinghaus and his colleagues measured their own CSF pH during acclimatization to altitude and showed that it did indeed tend to return towards its initial value of 7.2.[10] (The mechanism of the shift in CSF bicarbonate is considered on page 94.) Subsequent work showed that the time course of changes in CSF pH do not match changes in ventilation,[4] and, as acclimatization becomes complete, CSF pH does not return to normal (non-hypoxic) levels. Changes in CSF pH therefore seem unlikely to represent the only mechanism of acclimatization.[11] Other studies, mainly in animals, have provided other explanations involving stimulation of the central chemoreceptors, which include the development of either interstitial or intracellular lactic acidosis in response to hypoxia.[12] In spite of the use of elaborate magnetic resonance techniques, these findings have not been confirmed in humans.[13]

In addition to changes affecting the central chemoreceptors, there is evidence that peripheral chemoreceptor influence is increased during prolonged hypoxia, so contributing to the progressive hyperventilation seen with acclimatization. In humans, the acute hypoxic ventilatory response is increased during the first few days at altitude and for several days after return to sea level. The mechanism of this increased sensitivity to hypoxia is not known, but is independent of changes in $P\text{CO}_2$,[14] and may reside either with increased sensitivity of the carotid bodies themselves or increased sensitivity of the central nervous system to normal carotid body afferent input.[4]

Respiratory alkalosis at altitude is counteracted, over the course of a few days, by renal excretion of bicarbonate, resulting in a degree of metabolic acidosis that will tend to increase respiratory drive (see Figure 5.6). This was formerly thought to be the main factor in the ventilatory adaptation to altitude but it now appears to be of minor importance compared with the changes in the central and peripheral chemoreceptors.

Blood gas tensions. Figure 16.3 shows the time course of blood gas changes during acclimatization and Figure 16.1 shows changes in alveolar gas tensions with altitude in fully acclimatized mountaineers at rest. Alveolar $P\text{O}_2$ was found to be unexpectedly well preserved at extreme altitude, and above 8000 m (26 000 ft) tended to remain close to 4.8 kPa (36 mmHg).[1] Operation Everest II found a mean arterial $P\text{O}_2$ of 4 kPa (30 mmHg) at a pressure equivalent to the summit of Everest (32 kPa or 240 mmHg) (Table 16.2), with an alveolar/arterial $P\text{O}_2$ difference of less than 0.3 kPa (2 mmHg) at rest.[15] Operation Everest II fully confirmed West's observation[1] of extreme hypocapnia both at rest and exercise at the equivalent altitude of the summit of Everest (Table 16.2).

Haemoglobin concentration and oxygen affinity. An increase in haemoglobin concentration was the earliest adaptation to altitude to be demonstrated. Operation Everest II reported an increase from 13.5 to 17 g.dl^{-1} which, at the resting value of 58% saturation, maintained an arterial oxygen content of 12 ml.dl^{-1}.[2] Plasma erythropoietin levels begin to increase within a few hours at altitude, reaching a maximum at 24–48 hours and then declining.[18] Haemoglobin concentrations may also be influenced by changes in plasma volume. Increases in haemoglobin concentration above about 18 g.dl^{-1} are probably detrimental because of the increased viscosity of the blood.

The haemoglobin dissociation curve at altitude is affected by changes in both pH and 2,3-diphosphoglycerate (DPG) concentration (page 269). 2,3-DPG concentrations increased from 1.7 to 3.8 mmol.l^{-1} on Operation Everest II.[2] However, it has been estimated that the overall effect is a leftward shift at extreme altitude, where oxygen loading in the lung takes priority over maintaining $P\text{O}_2$ at the point of release.[18,19]

Adaptation to altitude[20]

Adaptation refers to physiological and genetic changes that occur over a period of years to generations by those who have taken up permanent residence at high altitude. There are qualitative as well as quantitative differences between acclimatization and adaptation but each is remarkably effective. High altitude residents, Sherpas in particular, have a

Table 16.2 Cardiorespiratory data obtained at rest and exercise at extreme reduction of ambient pressure during the simulated ascent of Everest in a low pressure chamber

	Sea level equivalent		Extreme altitude equivalent	
Ambient pressure (kPa)	101		33.7	
(mmHg)	760		253	
Haemoglobin concentration (g.dl^{-1})	13.5		17.0	
$\dot{V}_{O_2max}$ (ml.min^{-1}, STPD)	3980		1170	
State	Rest	Exercise	Rest	Exercise
Exercise intensity (watts)	0	281	0	90
Ventilation (l.min^{-1}, BTPS)	11	107	42.3	157.5
$\dot{V}_{O_2}$ (ml.min^{-1}, STPD)	350	3380	386	1002
Ventilation equivalent	31	32	110	157
Arterial P_{O_2} (kPa)	13.2	12.0	4.0	3.7
(mmHg)	33.9	90.0	11.2	27.7
Arterial P_{CO_2} (kPa)	4.5	4.7	1.5	1.3
(mmHg)	33.9	35.0	11.2	10.1
(a/v) O_2 content difference (ml.dl^{-1})	5.7	15.0	4.6	6.7
Mixed venous P_{O_2} (kPa)	4.7	2.6	2.9	1.9
(mmHg)	35.1	19.7	22.1	14.3
Cardiac output (l.min^{-1})	6.7	27.2	8.4	15.7
Pulm. arterial pressure (mean, mmHg)	15	33	33	48

(Data from references 2, 16 and 17)

Notes
1. Actual ambient pressure at simulated high altitude was 32 kPa (240 mmHg) but leakage of oxygen from masks worn by investigators had caused the oxygen concentration in the chamber to rise to 22%, the equivalent of 33.7 kPa at 21%, which is equivalent to the summit of Everest.
2. Study 16 reported cardiovascular data for a mean exercise intensity of 90 watts at the highest altitude. Data from other studies have been interpolated to give values corresponding to the same exercise intensity in order to achieve compatibility.

remarkable ability to exercise under grossly hypoxic conditions, but their adaptations show many striking differences from those in acclimatized lowlanders.

Long-term residence at altitude leads to a reduced ventilatory response to hypoxia, the magnitude of which relates to the product of altitude level and years of residence there.[4] This results in a reduction of ventilation compared with an acclimatized lowlander and a rise in P_{CO_2}, though neither of these returns to sea level values (Figure 16.3). High altitude residents maintain similar arterial P_{O_2} values as acclimatized lowlanders in spite of the reduced ventilation and therefore lower alveolar P_{O_2}. Pulmonary diffusing capacity must therefore be increased, and depends on anatomical pulmonary adaptations increasing the area available for diffusion by the generation of greater numbers of alveoli and associated capillaries. This adaptation seems not to be inherited, but occurs in children and infants who spend their formative years at altitude. An adult moving permanently to high altitude will therefore never achieve the same degree of adaptation as a native of the area, thus explaining the ability of Sherpas to exercise to a much greater degree than their non-resident visitors.

Hypoxic pulmonary vasoconstriction is preserved at altitude, leading to chronic pulmonary hypertension and right ventricular hypertrophy.[21] This does not seem beneficial and has been lost by the yak. Polycythaemia is normal and the highest levels (haemoglobin concentrations of 22.9 g.dl^{-1}) occur in Andean miners living at 5300 m (17 500 ft). Lower haemoglobin concentrations have been found more recently in residents of the Himalayas and Tibetan plateau.[18]

Another major adaptation to altitude by long-term residents seems to be increased vascularity of heart and striated muscles, a change that is also important for the trained athlete. For the high altitude resident, increased perfusion seems to compensate very effectively for the reduced oxygen content of the arterial blood.

Limits for residence and work.[22] The upper limit for sustained work seems to be 5950 m (19 500 ft) at the Aucanquilcha sulphur mine in the Andes. The upper limit for elective permanent habitation is lower, and the Andean miners declined to live in accommodation built for them near the mine, preferring to live at 5330 m (17 500 ft) and climb every day to their work. Increased commercial pressure for mining has led to an increase in high altitude activity, and West has suggested the use of oxygen enrichment of sleeping quarters to reduce altitude-induced illness (see below), each 1 per cent increase in oxygen concentration being equivalent to 300 m (1000 ft) of descent.[23]

Monge's disease. A small minority of people who dwell permanently at very high altitude in certain locations develop a characteristic condition known as Monge's disease or chronic mountain sickness. The condition is well recognized in miners living above 4000 m in the Andes. It is characterized by an exceptionally poor ventilatory response to hypoxia, resulting in low arterial Po_2 and high Pco_2. There is cyanosis, high haematocrit (packed cell volume), finger clubbing, pulmonary hypertension, right heart failure, dyspnoea and lethargy.

Exercise at high altitude

The summit of Everest was attained without the use of oxygen in 1978 by Messner and Habeler, and by many other climbers since that date. Studies of exercise have been made at various altitudes up to and including the summit, and on the simulated ascent in Operation Everest II. Of necessity, these observations are largely confined to very fit subjects.

Capacity for work performed. There is a progressive decline in the external work that can be performed as altitude increases. On Operation Everest II, 300–360 watts was attained at sea level, 240–270 watts at 440 mmHg pressure (equivalent to 4300 m, 14 000 ft) and 120 watts at 280 mmHg (Everest summit), very close to the results obtained on Everest.[24] $\dot{V}o_{2max}$ declined in accord with altitude to 1177 ml.min^{-1} at 240 mmHg pressure.[17] Resting cardiac output is unchanged at moderate altitude and only slightly increased at extreme altitude. For a given power expenditure, cardiac output at altitude is the same as at sea level.[2] Surprisingly, exercise at altitude (up to 70 per cent of $\dot{V}o_{2max}$) results in no higher blood lactate levels than at sea level,[2] possibly owing to inhibition of phosphofructokinase.[19]

Ventilation equivalent of oxygen consumption. Figure 14.1 shows that ventilation as a function of $\dot{V}o_2$ is comparatively constant. The length of the line increases with training but the slope of the linear portion remains the same. With increasing altitude, the slope and intercept are both dramatically increased up to four times the sea level value[2,17] with maximal ventilation approaching 200 l.min^{-1} (Figure 16.5). This is because ventilation is

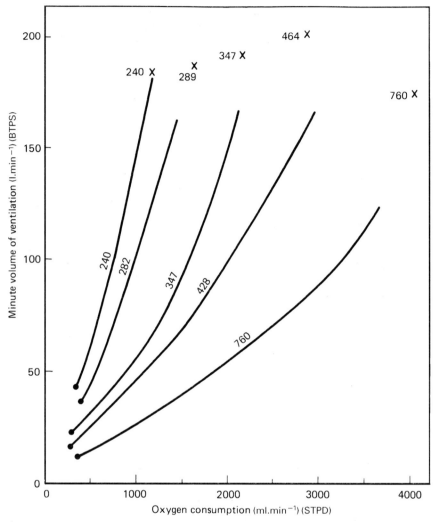

Figure 16.5 The relationship between minute volume of ventilation and oxygen consumption at rest and during exercise at altitude. The relationship is radically changed at altitude primarily because ventilation is reported at body temperature and pressure (saturated), whereas oxygen consumption is reported at standard temperature and pressure (dry). Numbers in the Figure indicate barometric pressure. ●, resting points; ×, values at $\dot{V}_{O_{2}max}$ from reference 17. (Curves are derived from reference 2)

reported at body temperature and pressure saturated (BTPS) and oxygen consumption at standard temperature and pressure dry (STPD) – see Appendix C. Fortunately, the density of air is reduced in proportion to the barometric pressure at altitude. Resistance to turbulent flow is decreased and therefore the work of breathing at a particular minute volume of respiration is less.

$P_{CO_{2}}$ *and* $P_{O_{2}}$. During exercise at altitude, alveolar $P_{CO_{2}}$ falls and $P_{O_{2}}$ rises (Figure 16.6).[2,25] Arterial $P_{CO_{2}}$ falls with alveolar $P_{CO_{2}}$ but oxygenation of the pulmonary end-capillary blood is diffusion-limited during exercise at high altitude. The alveolar/arterial

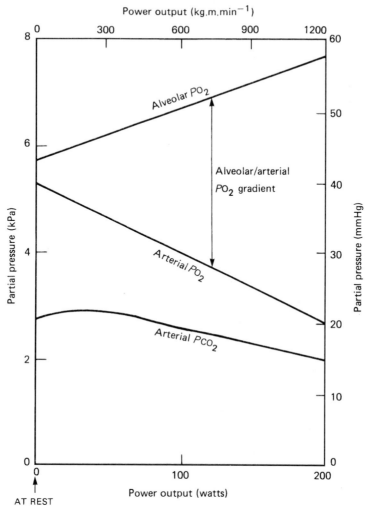

Figure 16.6 Po_2 and Pco_2 changes during exercise in a single subject (Dr John West) at 5800 m (19 000 ft). (Data from reference 25.)

Po_2 difference increases more than the alveolar Po_2 rises[25] and there is a consistent decrease in arterial Po_2 during exercise at altitude, leading to very low values for Po_2 (Figure 16.6).

Altitude illness[26]

Acute mountain sickness

Acute mountain sickness (AMS) is characterized by headache, nausea, fatigue, anorexia, dyspnoea and difficulty in sleeping (see below), and climbing performance may be impaired (Figure 16.2). Symptoms normally begin to occur at above 2000 m (6600 ft). At

5000 m (16 000 ft), there are feelings of unreality (often enhanced by the environment!), amnesia and dizziness. The unacclimatized person has extreme dyspnoea on exertion at this level and has dyspnoea at rest. Severity varies greatly from a mild inconvenient headache to a severe life-threatening illness involving cerebral and pulmonary oedema.

The likelihood of developing AMS relates to altitude (particularly sleeping altitude), the rate of ascent and the degree of exertion. The mountaineer is therefore affected by altitude in a manner that differs from that of the aviator because his physical exertion is much greater and the time course of exposure is different. Rate of ascent seldom exceeds 2000 m (6500 ft) per day from sea level, decreasing to only 300 m (1000 ft) per day at very high altitude. Over half of mountaineers develop AMS above 4000 m (13 000 ft),[26] whilst one-quarter of tourists travelling to resorts between 2000–3000 m (6300–9700 ft) high develop it.[27]

High altitude pulmonary oedema (HAPE)

About 1 per cent of climbers develop HAPE[26] following acute exposure to altitudes in excess of about 3000 m (10 000 ft), usually following rapid ascent and strenuous exercise. It is most commonly seen in the unacclimatized and overambitious climber. It also occurs in high altitude residents following their return from low altitude travel. Clinical features include cough, dyspnoea and hypoxia with clinical and radiological signs of pulmonary oedema. Untreated, HAPE has a mortality rate of almost 50 per cent, but with appropriate treatment this is normally less than 3 per cent.

The aetiology of HAPE is complex.[28,29,30] There is general agreement that subjects with HAPE have significant pulmonary hypertension secondary to hypoxia and low pulmonary capillary wedge pressures indicating normal left ventricular function. The site of increased pulmonary resistance is believed to be at the precapillary arterioles. A recent study performed at high altitude showed that inhaled nitric oxide produced a greater amount of pulmonary vasodilatation in subjects susceptible to HAPE compared with those who were not.[31] It is therefore possible that these subjects have an excessive hypoxic pulmonary vasoconstriction response to hypoxia. Pulmonary shadows on chest radiographs of people with HAPE are typically patchy, indicating that pulmonary vasoconstriction is non-uniform, such that some areas of lung have little blood flow whilst others have greatly increased blood flow. High capillary flow in some areas is postulated to lead to 'stress failure' of capillaries. Animal studies have shown disruption of endothelial cell tight junctions with increased capillary pressure,[32] which could occur in the high flow areas of lung in HAPE. Disruption of endothelial cell architecture will lead to pulmonary oedema either directly or via activation of inflammatory mediators. This mechanism would explain the association between exercise and HAPE, with increased cardiac output causing huge blood flows through vasodilated sections of lung.

Other respiratory problems at altitude

Cerebral oedema is also potentially lethal and is manifest in the early stages by ataxia, irritability and irrational behaviour, and may progress to hallucinations, drowsiness and coma. Post-mortem studies have shown that cerebral oedema may be accompanied by intracranial thrombosis and haemorrhage.[18] Both pulmonary and cerebral forms of severe acute mountain sickness may be present in the same patient, but a common aetiology has not been elucidated.[30] Mild, or localized, cerebral oedema probably contributes to the symptoms of AMS.

Following return to low altitude, cerebral disturbance may persist. Investigations up to 30 days after expeditions to very high altitudes have found a variety of impairments, including visual long-term memory.[33] Changes were more marked in people with a vigorous hypoxic ventilatory response, perhaps because of hypocapnic decrease in cerebral blood flow. Some defects persisted for years after high altitude expeditions.[19]

Cough.[34] Almost half of trekkers in Nepal complain of a cough, which may be severe. Coughing normally develops after a few days at altitude, and airway sensitivity to irritants is increased as a result of hyperventilation of low humidity cold air. Development of a cough may, however, be the first manifestation of impending HAPE.

Sleep disturbance. Periodic breathing occurs in most individuals during the first few nights above about 4000 m (13 000 ft). Breathing patterns are very similar to those of the sleep apnoea/hypopnoea syndrome (page 348). There are cyclical changes in tidal volume, often associated with central (rather than obstructive) apnoeas with or without arousal from sleep (see Figure 15.2). Apnoeas may result in considerable additional hypoxaemia at high altitude. Studies at 4500 m (15 000 ft)[35] and at 6300 m (21 000 ft)[22] found nocturnal reductions in saturation of 8 per cent and 10 per cent respectively; in the former study this reduced median nocturnal saturation to just 50 per cent. The primary problem is an abnormality of respiratory control, with arousal occurring at the end of a period of apnoea, presumably secondary to hypoxia.[21] The severity of periodic breathing is related to the strength of the subject's hypoxic ventilatory drive,[26] and is seldom seen in high altitude residents who have a much attenuated hypoxic drive. The onset of sleep disturbance and severe nocturnal hypoxia may also contribute to the symptoms of acute mountain sickness; subjects developing HAPE have lower oxygen saturations during sleep.[35]

Treatment of altitude-induced illness

With any severe form of AMS, administration of oxygen and descent to a lower altitude are the first essentials. Without these simple interventions, there will be a high mortality in patients with cerebral oedema or HAPE. Nifedipine is now an established treatment for HAPE, and when used prophylactically prevents HAPE developing in susceptible individuals.[26,30] It is an effective drug for treating pulmonary hypertension, and the convenience of administration by oral or sublingual route makes it a popular choice for mountaineers.

People with milder degrees of AMS do not need to be removed from high altitude. With acclimatization, most symptoms of AMS will resolve but, if time is limited or symptoms interfere with planned activities, acetazolamide may be useful. This carbonic anhydrase inhibitor interferes with the transport of carbon dioxide out of cells, causing an intracellular acidosis that includes the cells of the medullary chemoreceptors and so drives respiration.[36] In effect, this accelerates acclimatization, and so may improve the arterial Po_2. Acetazolamide also improves sleep-induced periodic breathing, reducing the number and severity of episodes of apnoea, and thereby alleviates daytime symptoms.

Flying

Only a very small number of people will ever visit places of high enough altitude to induce any of the respiratory changes described in this chapter so far. However, a substantial proportion of the population will at some stage fly in commercial aircraft, so the final section deals with the respiratory effects of aviation.

Altitude exposure[37]

For reasons of fuel economy and avoidance of weather systems, commercial aircraft operate at between 9000 and 12 000 m (30 000 and 40 000 ft). The passenger cabin must therefore be pressurized, and a typical design aims for a cabin pressure equivalent to less than 2400 m (8000 ft), often referred to as the 'cabin altitude'.[38] Cabin pressure is maintained by indrawing and compression of external air while limiting cabin air outflow to maintain the desired pressure. In practice, a differential pressure is established which represents the absolute pressure difference between the outside and inside of the aircraft. Differential pressure is increased as the aircraft climbs, and *vice versa*. Thus cabin pressure changes in parallel with altitude, but to a much lesser degree than the external pressure. Maximum cabin differential pressures and normal operating cabin altitudes for common commercial aircraft are shown in Table 16.3. Peak cabin altitude measured on commercial aircraft is around 2000–2400 m (6200–7600 ft), newer aircraft tending to operate with *higher* cabin altitudes than older models.[38,39,40] Compressed external air is often obtained from the compression chamber of the engines, so cabin pressure may vary during flight according to engine performance. For example, when flying over high altitude terrain such as the Himalayas or the Andes, cabin altitude will be increased. This occurs partly as a result of increased cruise altitude but also because compressed air supply from the engine will be reduced to facilitate better engine performance at higher altitude (Personal communication, Dr M Bagshaw, British Airways, 1998).

Supersonic flight requires much higher operating altitude to reduce air resistance, so Concorde operates at up to 18 300 m (60 000 ft). The differential pressure must therefore be greater to sustain a normal cabin environment at this altitude (Table 16.3), which is facilitated in Concorde by the significantly more powerful engines from which compressed air is drawn. Military aircraft fly prolonged reconnaissance missions at an altitude of 22 400 m (73 500 ft), with the cockpit pressurized to an equivalent altitude of 9000 m (30 000 ft). Pilots must therefore breathe 100% oxygen by mask to maintain an inspired Po_2 close to sea level to facilitate the required mental performance. At this altitude, military pilots are also at risk of altitude decompression sickness, which is discussed on page 385.[41]

In theory, cabin altitudes of below 2400 m (8000 ft) should represent a minimal physiological challenge to healthy individuals resulting in a drop of only a few per cent in oxygen saturation. In practice, a study of healthy cabin crew during normal flight patterns revealed that over half had saturation drops to less than 90%.[38] The effects of this degree of hypoxia on performance are controversial, though impaired night vision or colour recognition may occur at this altitude (page 359).[38] To patients with respiratory disease, flying may present a significant problem, particularly if hypoxia already exists at sea level, and careful preflight assessment is required.[37] If baseline arterial Po_2 is below 9.3 kPa (70 mmHg), supplemental oxygen during the flight has been recommended.[39] In more complex respiratory failure, for example with hypercapnia, a simulation of flying conditions using hypoxic gas mixtures has been advocated (Table 16.3).[42]

Depressurization. Loss of cabin pressure at altitude either through equipment failure or accident is extremely rare. In the event of slow loss of cabin pressure, oxygen is provided for passengers as an interim measure until the aircraft can descend: 100% oxygen provides adequate protection from loss of consciousness up to an altitude of about 12 000 m (40 000 ft), where the atmospheric pressure is roughly equal to the sea level atmospheric Po_2. This covers the maximal cruising altitude of subsonic transports. Concorde, however, operates above the altitude at which oxygen would be effective, and has therefore been

Table 16.3 Cabin pressure characteristics of commercial aircraft

Aircraft	Differential pressure kPa	Cabin pressure at 10 700 m (35 000 ft)		Cabin 'altitude' at 10 700 m (35 000 ft)		Equivalent oxygen at sea level %
		mmHg	kPa	ft	m	
Boeing 727	59.3	623	83.0	5400	1650	17.0
Boeing 737	51.4	563	75.1	8000	2440	15.2
Boeing 747	61.4	638	85.1	4700	1430	17.4
Boeing 767	59.3	623	83.0	5400	1650	17.0
Boeing 777	60.5	631	84.2	5000	1520	17.2
DC8	60.5	631	84.2	5000	1520	17.2
DC9	53.5	579	77.2	7300	2220	15.7
DC10	59.3	623	83.0	5400	1650	17.0
Airbus A320	57.2	607	80.9	6000	1830	16.5
Concorde	73.8	731	97.5	1000	300	20.2
Concorde*	73.8	604	80.6	6500	1980	16.4

Differential pressure is the absolute pressure difference between the cabin and outside environments. Atmospheric pressure at 10 700 m (35 000 ft) is 23.7 kPa (178 mmHg). Concorde* data refer to Concorde at its usual cruise height of 18 300 m (60 000 ft) where atmospheric pressure is only 6.8 kPa (51 mmHg). (Data from reference 39, and Dr M Bagshaw, British Airways Medical Services, 1998.)

designed to minimize the rate at which accidental depressurization would be likely to occur in the event of, for example, a window breaking.[43] Precautions include the small size of the windows, reserve capacity for pressurization and pressure breathing equipment for the flight crew. This equipment supplies oxygen at 4 kPa (40 cmH$_2$O) and is essential for all pilots flying above 12 200 m (40 000 ft).

There are sporadic reports of stowaway passengers undertaking long-haul flights in the wheel well of modern aircraft.[44] This environment affords little protection against the cold and severe hypoxia of altitude levels well above that of Everest. That half of these stowaways die is not surprising, but it is remarkable that half of them survive. Severe hypothermia is believed to protect them against the effects of hypoxia.

Cabin air quality[37,40,45,46]

Aircraft ventilation systems deliver 400–600 l.min^{-1} per passenger of air during flight. However, compression and temperature regulation of fresh air from outside is expensive in energy terms, and more recent designs of aircraft incorporate cabin air recirculation systems. Total air delivered remains the same, but up to 50 per cent may be recirculated rather than fresh.

Carbon dioxide concentration in aircraft often exceeds the generally accepted 'comfort' level of 1000 ppm, and would be expected to be higher in aircraft with greater amounts of recirculation air-conditioning. Concentrations observed in aircraft are between 1200 and 1700 ppm.[45] Carbon dioxide itself does not cause respiratory problems at these levels, but is used more as a marker of the adequacy of ventilation.

Humidity is invariably low in aircraft, most studies finding relative humidity to be 15–25 per cent during flight compared with over 50 per cent in most sea level environments.

Ozone concentration in atmospheric air increases with greater altitude. At altitudes used by Concorde, outside ozone levels are approximately 4000 ppb, well in excess of thresholds known to cause respiratory problems (page 416). Fortunately, compression of outside air at this altitude involves heating the air to 400°C, which completely removes ozone by its conversion to oxygen, and cabin ozone concentrations remain very low.[43] Atmospheric ozone concentrations are much lower below 12000 m (40 000 ft), so other aircraft are generally unaffected,[45,47] though one study did find significant levels in Boeing 747s.[48]

Smoking during flight has now been banned by many airlines world-wide, possibly as a result of reduced fresh air ventilation coupled with the threat of legal challenge for passive smoking-related illness.[37,40] In fact, aircraft ventilation systems are highly effective at preventing the spread of tobacco smoke through the cabin. Nicotine and carbon monoxide levels are higher in the smoking compared with non-smoking sections of aircraft, but levels in the non-smoking areas are the same as on completely non-smoking flights.[45] On this basis, provided seating areas are separated, passive smoking is minimal.

With the exception of low humidity, there is therefore little evidence that the cabin air of aircraft poses any threat to passengers. Thus the numerous symptoms reported following air travel almost certainly have their origins in other activities associated with air travel, in particular the consumption of alcohol and differing time zones.

References

1. West JB, Hackett PH, Maret KH, Milledge JS, Peters RM, Pizzo CJ, Winslow RM. Pulmonary gas exchange on the summit of Mount Everest. *J Appl Physiol* 1983; **55**: 678–87.
2. Sutton JT, Reeves JT, Wagner PD, Groves BM, Cymerman A, Malconian MK et al. Operation Everest II: oxygen transport during exercise at extreme simulated altitude. *J Appl Physiol* 1988; **64**: 1309–21.
3. Houston CS, Sutton JR, Cymerman A, Reeves JT. Operation Everest II: man at extreme altitude. *J Appl Physiol* 1987; **63**: 877–82.
4. Bisgard GE, Forster HV. Ventilatory responses to acute and chronic hypoxia. In: Fregly MJ, Blatteis CM, eds. *Handbook of physiology, Section 4: Environmental physiology*. New York and Oxford: Oxford University Press, 1996; 1207–39.
5. Severinghaus JW. Respiratory control related to altitude and anesthesia. In: Stanley TH, Sperry RJ, eds. *Anesthesia and the lung*. Dordrecht: Kluwer, 1992; 101–16.
6. Rahn H, Otis AB. Man's respiratory response during and after acclimatization to high altitude. *Am J Physiol* 1949; **157**: 445–62.
7. Purkayastha SS, Ray US, Arora BS, Chhabra PC, Thakur L, Bandopadhyay P, Selvamurthy W. Acclimatization at high altitude in gradual and acute induction. *J Appl Physiol* 1995; **79**: 487–92.
8. Michel CC, Milledge JS. Respiratory regulation in man during acclimatization to high altitude. *J Physiol* 1963; **168**: 631–43.
9. Merwarth CR, Sieker HO. Acid–base changes in blood and cerebrospinal fluid during altered ventilation. *J Appl Physiol* 1961; **16**: 1016–18.
10. Severinghaus JW, Mitchell RA, Richardson BW, Singer MM. Respiratory control at high altitude suggesting active transport regulation of CSF pH. *J Appl Physiol* 1963; **18**: 1155–66.
11. Crawford RD, Severinghaus JW. CSF pH and ventilatory acclimatization to altitude. *J Appl Physiol* 1978; **45**: 275–83.
12. Fencl V, Gabel RA, Wolfe D. Composition of cerebral fluids in goats adapted to high altitude. *J Appl Physiol* 1979; **47**: 508–13.

13. Goldberg SV, Schoene RB, Haynor D, Trimble B, Swenson ER, Morrison JB, Banister EJ. Brain tissue pH and ventilatory acclimatization to high altitude. *J Appl Physiol* 1992; **72**: 58–63.

14. Tansley JG, Fatemian M, Howard LSGE, Poulin MJ, Robbins PA. Changes in respiratory control during and after 48 h of isocapnic and poikilocapnic hypoxia in humans. *J Appl Physiol* 1998; **85**: 2125–34.

15. Wagner PD, Sutton JT, Reeves JT, Cymerman A, Groves BM, Malconian MK. Operation Everest II: pulmonary gas exchange during a simulated ascent of Mt Everest. *J Appl Physiol* 1987; **63**: 2348–59.

16. Groves BM, Reeves JT, Sutton JT, Wagner PD, Cymerman A, Malconian MK et al. Operation Everest II: elevated high-altitude pulmonary resistance unresponsive to oxygen. *J Appl Physiol* 1987; **63**: 521–30.

17. Cymerman A, Reeves JT, Sutton JT, Rock PB, Groves BM, Malconian MK et al. Operation Everest II: maximal oxygen uptake at extreme altitude. *J Appl Physiol* 1989; **66**: 2446–53.

18. Ward MP, Milledge JS, West JB. *High altitude medicine and physiology.* London: Chapman and Hall, 1995.

19. West JB. Severe hypoxia: insights from extreme altitude. In: Stanley TH, Sperry RJ, eds. *Anesthesia and the lung.* Dordrecht: Kluwer, 1992; 97–100.

20. Ramirez G, Bittle PA, Rosen R, Rabb H, Pineda D. High altitude living: genetic and environmental adaptation. *Aviat Space Environ Med* 1999; **70**: 73–81.

21. Khoo MCK, Anholm JD, Ko S-W, Downey R, Powles ACP, Sutton JR, Houston CS. Dynamics of periodic breathing and arousal during sleep at extreme altitude. *Respir Physiol* 1996; **103**: 33–43.

22. West JB. Highest inhabitants in the world. *Nature* 1986; **324**: 517.

23. West JB. Oxygen enrichment of room air to relieve the hypoxia of high altitude. *Respir Physiol* 1995; **99**: 225–32.

24. West JB, Boyer SJ, Graber DJ, Hackett PH, Maret KH, Milledge JS et al. Maximal exercise at extreme altitudes on Mount Everest. *J Appl Physiol* 1983; **55**: 688–98.

25. Pugh LGCE, Gill MB, Lahiri S, Milledge JS, Ward MP, West JB. Muscular exercise at great altitudes. *J Appl Physiol* 1964; **19**: 431–40.

26. Pollard AJ, Murdoch DR. *The high altitude medicine handbook.* Oxford and New York: Radcliffe Medical Press, 1997.

27. Honigman B, Theis MK, Koziol-McLain J, Roach R, Yip R, Houston C, More LG. Acute mountain sickness in a general tourist population at moderate altitudes. *Ann Intern Med* 1993; **118**: 587–92.

28. Jerome EH, Severinghaus JW. High-altitude pulmonary edema. *N Engl J Med* 1996; **334**: 662–3.

29. Hultgren HN. High-altitude pulmonary edema: current concepts. *Annu Rev Med* 1996; **47**: 267–84.

30. Richalet J-P. High altitude pulmonary oedema: still a place for controversy. *Thorax* 1995; **50**: 923–9.

31. Scherrer U, Vollenweider L, Delabays A, Savcic M, Eichenberger V, Kleger G-R et al. Inhaled nitric oxide for high-altitude pulmonary edema. *N Engl J Med* 1996; **334**: 624–9.

32. West JB, Tsukimoto K, Mathieu-Costello O, Prediletto R. Stress failure in pulmonary capillaries. *J Appl Physiol* 1991; **70**: 1731–42.

33. Hornbein TH, Townes BD, Schoene RB, Sutton JR, Houston CS. The cost to the central nervous system of climbing to extremely high altitude. *N Engl J Med* 1989; **321**: 1714–19.

34. Barry PW, Mason NP, Riordan M, O'Callaghan C. Cough frequency and cough-receptor sensitivity are increased in man at altitude. *Clin Sci* 1997; **93**: 181–6.

35. Eichenberger U, Weiss E, Riemann D, Oelz O, Bärtsch P. Nocturnal periodic breathing and the development of acute high altitude illness. *Am J Respir Crit Care Med* 1996; **154**: 1748–54.

36. Milledge JS. Acute mountain sickness: pulmonary and cerebral oedema of high altitude. *Intensive Care Med* 1985; **11**: 110–15.

37. Harding RM, Mills FJ. *Aviation medicine.* London: BMJ Publishing, 1993.

38. Cottrell JJ, Lebovitz BL, Fennell RG, Kohn GM. Inflight arterial saturation: continuous monitoring by pulse oximetry. *Aviat Space Environ Med* 1995; **66**: 126–30.

39. Cottrell JJ. Altitude exposures during aircraft flight. *Chest* 1988; **92**: 81–4.

40. Smith T. Smoke-free flying. *BMJ* 1988; **297**: 1001.

41. Bendrick GA, Ainscough MJ, Pilmanis AA, Bisson RU. Prevalence of decompression sickness among U-2 pilots. *Aviat Space Environ Med* 1996; **67**: 199–206.

42. Gong H, Tashkin DP, Lee EY, Simmons MS. Hypoxia-altitude simulation test. *Am Rev Respir Dis* 1984; **130**: 980–6.

43. Mills FJ, Harding RM. Special forms of flight. III. Supersonic transport aircraft. *BMJ* 1983; **287**: 411–12.

44. Veronneau SJH, Mohler SR, Pennybaker AL, Wilcox BC, Sahiar F. Survival at high altitudes: wheel-well passengers. *Aviat Space Environ Med* 1996; **67**: 784–6.

45. Crawford WA, Holcomb LC. Environmental tobacco smoke (ETS) in airliners – a health hazard evaluation. *Aviat Space Environ Med* 1991; **62**: 580–6.

46. Rayman RB. Passenger safety, health, and comfort: a review. *Aviat Space Environ Med* 1997; **68**: 432–40.

47. Thibeault C. Cabin air quality. *Aviat Space Environ Med* 1997; **68**: 80–2.

48. Nastrom GD, Holdeman JD, Perkins PJ. Measurements of cabin and ambient ozone on B747 airplanes. *J Aircraft* 1980; **17**: 246–9.

Chapter 17

High pressure and diving

Humans have sojourned temporarily in high pressure environments since the introduction of the diving bell. The origin of this development is lost in antiquity but Alexander the Great was said to have been lowered to the sea bed in a diving bell.

The environment of the diver is often, but not invariably, aqueous. Saturation divers spend most of their time in a gaseous environment in chambers that are held at a pressure close to that of the depth of water at which they will be working. Tunnel and caisson workers may also be at high pressure in a gaseous environment. Those in an aqueous environment also have the additional effect of different gravitational forces applied to their trunks, which influence the mechanics of breathing and other systems of the body (page 378). Workers in both environments share the physiological problems associated with increased ambient pressures and partial pressures of respired gases. Further problems arise as a result of changes in gas density at high pressure and the necessity to breathe gases of composition different from air, which is standard practice at pressures of more than about 6 atmospheres.

In this field, as in others, we cannot escape from the multiplicity of units, and some of these are set out in Table 17.1. Note particularly that 'atmosphere gauge' is relative to ambient pressure. Thus 2 atmospheres absolute (ATA) equals 1 atmosphere gauge relative to sea level. Throughout this chapter, atmospheres of pressure mean absolute and not gauge.

Exchange of oxygen and carbon dioxide[1]

Oxygen consumption

The relationship between power output and oxygen consumption at pressures up to 66 ATA, whether under water or dry, is not significantly different from the relationship at normal pressure,[2,3] shown in Figure 14.1. Oxygen consumption is expressed under standard conditions of temperature and pressure, dry (STPD; see Appendix C) and therefore represents an absolute quantity of oxygen. However, this volume, when expressed at the diver's environmental pressure, is inversely related to the pressure. Thus, an oxygen consumption of $1 \, l.min^{-1}$ (STPD) at a pressure of 10 atmospheres would be only $100 \, ml.min^{-1}$ when expressed at the pressure to which the diver was exposed. Similar considerations apply to carbon dioxide output.

The ventilatory requirement for a given oxygen consumption at increased pressure is also not greatly different from the normal relationship shown in Figure 14.5, provided that

Table 17.1 Pressures and Po_2 values at various depths of sea water

Depth of sea water		Pressure (absolute)		Po_2 breathing air				Percentage oxygen to give sea level inspired Po_2
				inspired		alveolar		
metres	feet	atm	kPa	kPa	mmHg	kPa	mmHg	
0	0	1	101	19.9	149	13.9	104	20.9
10	32.8	2	203	41.2	309	35.2	264	10.1
20	65.6	3	304	62.3	467	56.3	422	6.69
50	164	6	608	126	945	120	900	3.31
Usual limit for breathing air								
100	328	11	1 110					1.80
200	656	21	2 130					0.94
Usual limit for saturation dives								
Threshold for high pressure nervous syndrome								
500	1640	51	5 170					0.39
1000	3280	101	10 200					0.20
Depth reached by sperm whale								
2000	6560	201	20 400					0.098
2500	8200	251	25 400					0.078
Pressure reached by non-aquatic mammals with pharmacological amelioration of high pressure nervous syndrome								

10 metres sea water = 1 atmosphere (gauge). Alveolar Po_2 is assumed to be 6 kPa (45 mmHg) less than inspired Po_2.

the oxygen consumption is expressed at STPD, and minute volume is expressed at body temperature, saturated with water vapour, and at the pressure to which the diver is exposed (BTPS; see Appendix C). Considerable confusion is possible as a result of the different methods of expressing gas volumes, and though the differences are trivial at sea level they become very important at high pressures.

Exercise.[4] Oxygen consumption may reach very high values during free swimming[5] and are of the order of 2–3 l.min^{-1} (STPD) for a swimming speed of only 2 km.h^{-1}. Maximal oxygen consumption ($\dot{V}o_{2max}$) during exercise is improved slightly at modest high pressures (<20 ATA), an observation that results from hyperoxia (0.3 ATA oxygen) normally used at this depth. With deeper dives, there is a progressive reduction in exercise capacity, irrespective of the oxygen pressure, as a result of respiratory limitation secondary to higher gas density. $\dot{V}o_{2max}$ in the range 2.4–3.3 l.min^{-1} has been attained at pressures of 66 atmospheres.[3]

Effect of pressure on alveolar Pco_2 and Po_2

Pressure has complicated and very important effects on Pco_2 and Po_2. The alveolar concentration of CO_2 equals its rate of production divided by the alveolar ventilation (page 234). However, both gas volumes must be measured under the same conditions of temperature and pressure. Alveolar CO_2 concentration at 10 ATA will be about one-tenth of sea level values – that is, 0.56% compared with 5.3% at sea level. When these concentrations are multiplied by pressure to give Pco_2, values are similar at sea level and 10 atmospheres. Thus, as a rough approximation, alveolar CO_2 concentration decreases inversely to the environmental pressure, but the PCO_2 remains near its sea level value.

Effects on the PO_2 are slightly more complicated but no less important. The difference between the inspired and alveolar oxygen *concentrations* equals the ratio of oxygen uptake to inspired alveolar ventilation (see the universal alveolar air equation, page 130). This fraction, like the alveolar concentration of CO_2, decreases inversely with the increased pressure. However, the corresponding *partial pressure* will remain close to the sea level value, as does the alveolar PCO_2. Therefore, the difference between the inspired and alveolar PO_2 will remain roughly constant, and the alveolar PO_2, to a first approximation, increases by the same amount as the inspired PO_2 (Figure 17.1). However, these considerations take into account only the direct effect of pressure on gas tensions. There are other and more subtle effects on respiratory mechanics and gas exchange, which must now be considered.

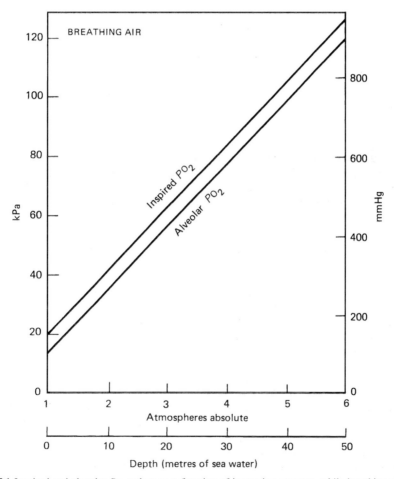

Figure 17.1 Inspired and alveolar PO_2 values as a function of increasing pressure, while breathing air at rest.

Effect on mechanics of breathing

Two main factors must be considered. First, there is the increased density of gases at pressure, although this can be reduced by changing the composition of the inspired gas. The second factor is the pressure of water on the body, which alters the gravitational effects to which the respiratory system is normally exposed.

Gas density is increased in direct proportion to pressure. Thus air at 10 atmospheres has ten times the density of air at sea level, which increases the resistance to turbulent gas flow (page 61). One study found that the maximal breathing capacity (MBC) of a subject breathing air was $200 \, l.min^{-1}$ at sea level, $100 \, l.min^{-1}$ at 5 atmospheres and $50 \, l.min^{-1}$ at 15 atmospheres.[5] In fact, it is usual to breathe a helium/oxygen mixture at pressures in excess of about 6 atmospheres because of nitrogen narcosis (see below). Helium has only one-seventh the density of air and so is easier to breathe. Furthermore, lower inspired oxygen concentrations are both permissible and indeed desirable as the pressure increases (see Table 16.1). Therefore, at 15 atmospheres it would be reasonable to breathe a mixture of 98% helium and 2% oxygen. This would more than double the MBC that the diver could attain while breathing air at that pressure.[5] Hydrogen has an even lower density than helium, and has been used in gas mixtures for dives to more than 500 metres deep.[4]

The effect of immersion is additional to any change in the density of the respired gases. In open-tube snorkel breathing, the alveolar gas is close to normal atmospheric pressure but the trunk is exposed to a pressure depending on the depth of the subject, which is limited by the length of the snorkel tube. This is equivalent to a standing subatmospheric pressure applied to the mouth, and it is difficult to inhale against a 'negative' pressure loading of more than about 5 kPa (50 cmH$_2$O). This corresponds to a mean depth of immersion of only 50 cm, and it is therefore virtually impossible to use a snorkel tube at a depth of 1 metre. However, the normal length of a snorkel tube ensures that the swimmer is barely more than awash, so these problems should not arise.

'Negative' pressure loading is prevented by supplying gas to the diver's airway at pressure that is close to the hydrostatic pressure surrounding the diver. This may be achieved by providing an excess flow of gas with a pressure-relief valve controlled by the surrounding water pressure. Such an arrangement was used for the traditional helmeted diver supplied by an air pump on the surface. Free-swimming divers carrying their own compressed gas supply rely on inspiratory demand valves, which are also balanced by the surrounding water pressure.

These arrangements supply gas that is close to the hydrostatic pressure surrounding the trunk. However, the precise 'static lung loading' depends on the location of the pressure-controlling device in relation to the geometry of the chest. Minor differences also result from the various postures that the diver may assume. Thus, if he is 'head-up' when using a valve at mouthpiece level, the pressure surrounding the trunk is higher than the airway pressure by a mean value of about 3 kPa (30 cmH$_2$O). If he is 'head-down', airway pressure is greater than the pressure to which the trunk is exposed. The head-down position thus corresponds to positive pressure breathing and the head-up position to negative pressure breathing.[2] The latter causes a reduction of functional residual capacity (FRC) of about 20–30 per cent but breathing is considered to be easier head-up than head-down.[1,5] Apart from these considerations, immersion has relatively little effect on respiratory function, and the additional respiratory work of moving extracorporeal water does not seem to add appreciably to the work of breathing.

Effect on efficiency of gas exchange

Dead space/tidal volume ratio in divers is increased from 35 per cent at sea level to 42 per cent at 47 and 66 atmospheres.[3] However, during exercise at depth, values remain close to 40 per cent, in contrast to a decrease to 20 per cent during exercise at sea level. Therefore, for the same minute volume, alveolar ventilation would be less at depth in comparison with sea level.

The best measure of the efficiency of oxygenation of the arterial blood is the alveolar/arterial P_{O_2} gradient. Measurement of arterial blood gas tensions presents formidable technical difficulties at high pressures. However, in 1984 Salzano et al.[3] reported arterial P_{O_2} values in the range 33–41 kPa (248–308 mmHg) at pressures of 47 and 66 atmospheres, both at rest and at work, when inspired oxygen tensions were in the range 47–50 kPa (353–375 mmHg). Intrapulmonary shunting did not thus appear to exceed about 5 per cent (Figure E.4).

Since it is customary to supply deep divers with an inspired oxygen tension of at least 0.5 atmosphere, arterial hypoxaemia is unlikely to occur either from hypoventilation or from maldistribution of pulmonary ventilation and perfusion in healthy subjects.[3] More elderly, unfit or obese divers, faced with a reduced FRC as described above, do however display some degree of hypoxaemia during diving as FRC approaches their closing volume causing airway closure and pulmonary shunting.[6]

The position as regards arterial P_{CO_2} is less clear. The study by Salzano and colleagues[3] found values within the normal range at pressures of 47 and 66 atmospheres when the subjects were at rest. During exercise, arterial P_{CO_2} remained normal in one of the subjects, but the remaining four subjects became hypercapnic at exercise levels ranging from 100 to 200 watts. Maximal values of arterial P_{CO_2} at exercise and pressure were in the range 6.2–8.3 kPa (46.7–62.2 mmHg). This cannot be regarded as satisfactory, because 9 kPa is approaching the level at which there may be some clouding of consciousness, and that is potentially dangerous at depth. It seems likely that the increased dead space during exercise at pressure compared with the value at sea level plays a significant role by reducing the alveolar ventilation. Hypercapnia is a well-recognized complication of diving, and divers are known to have a blunted P_{CO_2}/ventilation response, though the cause of this is unknown.[1]

Effects attributable to the composition of the inspired gas

Air

Until about 60 years ago, helmeted divers worked with pressures up to about 10 atmospheres breathing air. Nowadays with the increased use of helium, it is unusual to breathe air at pressures of more than 6 ATA (depths of 50 metres of sea water).

Oxygen. When breathing air at a pressure of 6 ATA, the inspired P_{O_2} will be about 126 kPa (945 mmHg) and the alveolar P_{O_2} about 120 kPa (900 mmHg). This is below the threshold for oxygen convulsions of about 2 ATA, but probably above the threshold for pulmonary oxygen toxicity if exposure is continued for more than a few hours[1] (see Chapter 25).

Nitrogen. It is actually nitrogen that limits the depth to which air should be breathed. It has three separate undesirable effects.

First, nitrogen is an anaesthetic and, in accord with its lipid solubility, can cause full surgical anaesthesia at a partial pressure of about 30 atmospheres. The narcotic effect of nitrogen is first detectable when breathing air at about 4 ATA and there is usually serious impairment of performance at 10 atmospheres.[7] This effect is known as nitrogen narcosis or 'the rapture of the deep'. It is a general rule that nitrogen narcosis precludes the use of air at depths greater than 100 metres of sea water (11 ATA pressure) and, in fact, air is not used today at pressures greater than 6 atmospheres. Helium is the preferred substitute at higher pressures and has no detectable narcotic properties up to at least 100 atmospheres.

The second problem attributable to nitrogen at high pressures is its density, which causes greatly increased hindrance to breathing at high pressure (see above). Helium has only one-seventh the density of nitrogen, and this is the second reason for its choice.

The third problem with nitrogen is its solubility in body tissues, with the resultant formation of bubbles on decompression. This is discussed in more detail below. Other inert gases, particularly helium, are less soluble in body tissues and this is the third reason for the use of helium at high pressures.

Helium/oxygen mixtures (Heliox)

For the three reasons outlined in the previous section, helium is the preferred diluent inert gas at pressures above about 6 atmospheres. The concentration of oxygen required to give the same inspired gas Po_2 as at sea level is shown in Table 17.1. In fact, it is usual practice to provide an inspired Po_2 of about 0.5 ATA (50 kPa or 375 mmHg) to give a safety margin in the event of error in gas mixing and to provide protection against hypoventilation or defective gas exchange. This level of Po_2 seems to be below the threshold for pulmonary oxygen toxicity, even during prolonged saturation dives.

With an inspired Po_2 of 0.5 ATA, the *concentration* of oxygen in the gas mixture is very low at high pressures (e.g. 2.5% oxygen at 20 atmospheres pressure). Clearly such a mixture would be lethal if breathed at sea level. Therefore, the inspired oxygen concentration must be monitored very carefully as it is changed during compression and decompression.

A special problem of helium is its very high thermal conductivity, which tends to cause hypothermia unless the diver's environment is heated. Heat loss from radiation and evaporation remain generally unchanged, but convective heat loss from the respiratory tract and skin is greatly increased.[4] It is usual for chambers to be maintained at temperatures as high as 30–32°C during saturation dives on helium/oxygen mixtures. The low density of helium causes a considerable increase in the pitch of the voice, sometimes resulting in difficulty in communication.

Helium/oxygen/nitrogen mixtures (Trimix)

The pressure that can be attained while breathing helium/oxygen mixtures is currently limited by the high pressure nervous syndrome (HPNS).[4,8] This is a hyperexcitable state of the central nervous system, which seems to be due to hydrostatic pressure *per se* and not to any changes in gas tensions. It becomes a serious problem for divers at pressures in excess of about 50 atmospheres, but is first apparent at about 20 atmospheres.

Various treatments can mitigate this effect and so increase the depth at which a diver can operate safely. The most practicable is the addition of 5–10% nitrogen to the helium/oxygen mixture. This in effect reverses HPNS with partial nitrogen narcosis, whilst the HPNS reverses the narcosis that would be caused by the nitrogen.[9] Trimix containing 5% nitrogen allows divers to function normally at depths of over 600 metres.[4]

Types of diving activity and their respiratory effects

Snorkelling is the simplest form of human diving but, as described above, respiratory effects limit the diver to the top 50 cm of water. Many other forms of diving have therefore evolved.

Breath-hold diving[10]

The simplest method of diving is by breath holding, and this is still used for collecting pearls, sponge and various edibles from the sea bed. After breathing air, breath-holding time is normally limited to 60–75 seconds; the changes in alveolar gas tensions are shown in Figure 5.11. Astonishingly, the depth record is 117 metres, requiring some minutes of submersion. Many remarkable mechanisms interact to make this possible.

Lung volume. As pressure increases, lung volume decreases by Boyle's law (page 644). Thus at 10 ATA, an initial lung volume of 6 litres would be reduced to about 600 ml, well below residual volume (RV), and with the loss of 5.4 kg of buoyancy. During descent a point is reached when the body attains neutral buoyancy and the body will sink below that depth.

Alveolar Po_2 increases with depth as the alveolar gas is compressed, providing a doubling of Po_2 at about 8 metres deep. More of the alveolar oxygen is therefore available at depth. Conversely, during ascent, alveolar Po_2 decreases, due partly to oxygen consumption but mainly to decreasing pressure. There is thus danger of hypoxia just before reaching the surface. However, when the alveolar Po_2 falls below the mixed venous Po_2, there is a paradoxical transfer of oxygen from mixed venous blood to alveolar gas, and the arterial Po_2 is maintained. This may be an important factor in preventing loss of consciousness in the final stages of ascent.

Alveolar Pco_2. By a similar mechanism, alveolar Pco_2 is greater during a breath-hold dive than during a simple breath hold at sea level. At an environmental pressure of only 12 kPa (90 mmHg) gauge, the alveolar Pco_2 will be increased above the mixed venous Pco_2, and there will be a paradoxical transfer of carbon dioxide from alveolus to arterial blood. Fortunately, there is a limited quantity of carbon dioxide in the alveolar gas, and the process is reversed during late descent and ascent. Duration of breath hold can be increased by previous hyperventilation, but this carries the danger of syncope from hypoxia before the breaking point is reached. Duration can be increased more safely by preliminary oxygen breathing, resulting in a record surface breath hold of 14 minutes, but only just over 3 minutes for a dive.

Adaptations in the diving mammals.[11] The diving mammals rely on breath holding for dives and have adaptations that permit remarkably long times under water and the attainment of great depths. Sperm whales, for example, can attain depths of 1000 metres.[8] Weddell seals can reach 500 metres and remain submerged for 70 minutes.[12] Such feats depend on a variety of biochemical and physiological adaptations. It seems likely that the lungs of the Weddell seal collapse completely at depths between 25 and 50 metres, thus preventing the partial pressure of nitrogen increasing above the level of 320 kPa (2400 mmHg), which has been recorded at depths between 40 and 80 metres.

Many diving mammals are believed to use the spleen as a reservoir for oxygenated blood during dives. In some diving species, the spleen represents over 10 per cent of body mass, and contains a much more muscular capsule than terrestrial animals. Splenic contraction is the probable cause of an increase of haemoglobin concentration from 15 to 25 g.dl^{-1} during long dives.[13] Furthermore, these animals have twice the blood volume per kilogram body weight relative to humans, so oxygen stored in blood for a dive is proportionately about three times that of humans.

During a dive the circulation is directed almost exclusively through heart and brain, which rely on the oxygen stores in the blood and, to a much smaller extent, the lungs. With a smaller brain, total cerebral oxygen consumption is much less than in humans. Intense vasoconstriction severely limits flow through other organs and also the voluntary muscles. Muscle contraction is based on myoglobin oxygen stores and anaerobic metabolism. There is extreme lactacidosis, which is confined to the muscle beds and so is not sensed by the peripheral chemoreceptors. After surfacing, the vasoconstriction is relaxed and there is generalized acidaemia. While on the surface, the excess lactate is metabolized and the arterial P_{CO_2} returns to normal.

Circulatory changes in response to submersion are collectively referred to as the diving reflex, which does exist in humans (page 402) but to a much lesser extent than in more specialized diving species.

Limited duration dives

Most dives are of relatively brief duration and involve a rapid descent to operating depth, a period spent at depth, followed by an ascent, the rate of which is governed by the requirement to avoid release of inert gas dissolved in the tissues. The profile and duration of the ascent are governed by the depth attained, the time spent at depth and the nature of the diluent inert gas.

The diving bell. The simplest and oldest technique was the diving bell. Air was trapped on the surface but the internal water level rose as the air was compressed at depth. Useful time at depth was generally no more than 20–30 minutes. Crude though this technology seems, it was used to recover most of the guns from the Wasa in Stockholm harbour in 1663 and 1664 from a depth of 34 metres. It seems unlikely that the salvage operators left the bell. At a later date, additional air was introduced into the bell under pressure from the surface and divers could leave the bell.

The helmeted diver. From about 1820 until recent times, the standard method of diving down to 100 metres has been by a helmeted diver supplied with air pumped from the surface into the helmet and escaping from a relief valve controlled by the water pressure. This gave much greater mobility than the old diving bell and permitted the execution of complex tasks. The system was used with helium/oxygen mixtures in 1939 for the salvage of the US submarine *Squalus* from a depth of 74 metres.

SCUBA diving.[14] There was for some years a desire to move towards free-swimming divers carrying their own gas supply (SCUBA – self-contained underwater breathing apparatus), first achieved in 1943 by Jacques Cousteau and Emile Gagnon. The system is based on a demand valve that is controlled by both the ambient pressure and the inspiration of the diver. Air-breathing SCUBA dives are usually restricted to depths of 30 metres. Greater depths are possible but special precautions must then be taken to prevent decompression sickness. SCUBA divers are far more mobile than helmeted divers and can work in almost any body position.

Caisson and tunnel working. Since 1839, tunnel and bridge foundations have been constructed by pressurizing the work environment to exclude water. The work environment is maintained at pressure, normally of less than 4 ATA, with staff entering and leaving by air locks. Entry is rapid but exit requires adherence to the appropriate decompression schedule if the working pressure is in excess of 2 ATA. Workers can be rapidly transferred from the working pressure to atmosphere and then, within 5 minutes, transferred to a separate chamber where they are rapidly recompressed to the working pressure and then follow the decompression schedule.[15] This process, known as decanting, has obvious logistic advantages.

Free submarine escape. It is possible to escape from a submarine by free ascent from depths down to about 100 metres. The submariner first enters an escape chamber which is then pressurized to equal the external water pressure. He then opens a hatch communicating with the exterior and leaves the chamber. His natural buoyancy is sufficient to take him to the surface but he may be helped with additional buoyancy or an apron that traps gas leaving the escape chamber. During the ascent, the gas in his lungs expands according to Boyle's law. It is therefore imperative that he keeps his glottis and mouth open, allowing gas to escape in a continuous stream. If gas is not allowed to escape, barotrauma is almost certain to occur (see below). Buoyancy is not changed by the loss of gas during ascent. In an uneventful escape, the time spent at pressure is too short for there to be any danger of decompression sickness. Thorough training is necessary and all submariners are trained in a vertical tank of 100 feet depth.

The maintenance of an adequate atmosphere in submarines is described on page 389.

Saturation dives[5]

When prolonged and repeated work is required at great depths, it is more convenient to hold the divers in a dry chamber, kept on board a ship or oil rig, and held at a pressure close to the pressure of their intended working depth. Divers transfer to a smaller chamber at the same pressure which is lowered to depth as and when required. The divers then leave the chamber for work, without any major change in pressure, but remaining linked to the chamber by an umbilical. On return to the chamber, they can be raised to the surface where they wait, still at pressure, until they are next required. A normal tour of duty is about three weeks, the whole of which is spent at operating pressure, currently up to about 20 atmospheres breathing helium/oxygen mixtures.

During the long period at pressure, tissues are fully saturated with inert gas at the chamber pressure and prolonged decompression is then required. which may last for several days.

Respiratory aspects of decompression illness

Returning to the surface after a dive is a hazardous procedure, and can give rise to a variety of complications variously known as 'bends', 'chokes' or caisson disease. In its mildest form, subjects have short-lived joint pain, but more serious presentations include pulmonary barotrauma or neurological deficit, which can result in permanent disability. In the late nineteenth century, before decompression illness was understood, the effects on caisson workers were severe. For example, of the 600 men involved in building the underwater foundations of the St Louis Bridge in the USA, 119 had serious decompression illness and 14 died.[16] Nowadays some form of decompression illness is thought to affect 1 in 5000–10 000 recreational dives and one in 500–1000 commercial dives.[16] Nomenclature of the many syndromes associated with decompression is confusing, but there are two main ways in which illness arises.

Barotrauma

Barotrauma as a result of change in pressure will affect any closed body space containing gas, and tends to occur during ascent when the gas expands. The ears and sinuses are the most commonly affected areas, but pulmonary barotrauma, although rare, is much more dangerous. Pulmonary barotrauma may occur during rapid ascent in untrained subjects, for example during submarine escape training (see above) when the subject forgets to exhale during ascent.[17] Some divers develop barotrauma during relatively shallow dives,[18] and efforts have been made to identify which divers are at risk.[19] In this case, barotrauma is believed to result from expansion of air trapped in the periphery of the lung by small airway closure. Subjects with reduced expiratory flow rates at low lung volume, including some asthmatics, are therefore at particular risk.[19] Barotrauma results in disruption of the airway or alveolar wall, and air may enter either the interstitial tissue or the pulmonary vessels. In the former, mediastinal or pleural air pockets continue to expand during ascent, until chest pain or breathing difficulties occur within a few minutes of surfacing. Air entering the pulmonary vessels will produce arterial gas embolism, and almost certainly result in decompression sickness.

Decompression sickness

Tissue bubble formation[1,16] occurs when tissues become 'supersaturated' with an inert gas, usually nitrogen. As decompression occurs, tissue P_{N_2} becomes greater than the ambient pressure and bubbles form, exactly as occurs when opening a carbonated drink. The increase in tissue P_{N_2} during descent and the decrease in P_{N_2} on ascent are both exponential curves, exactly as for the pharmacokinetics of inhaled general anaesthetics. Tissues poorly perfused with blood have the slowest half-time for both uptake and elimination, hence on decompression tissue P_{N_2} decreases most slowly in poorly perfused tissues such as cartilage, giving rise to the 'bends'.

Arterial gas embolism. Venous bubbles occur commonly during decompression, and the filtration provided by the lung is probably extremely effective. Overload of the filtration system may result in arterial gas embolism, but this is believed to be the case only in severe decompression sickness. There is an increasing body of evidence that arterial gas embolism follows shunting of blood containing air bubbles from the right to left sides of the heart, normally through an otherwise asymptomatic atrial septal defect.[20,21]

Whatever the origins, arterial gas embolism is believed to be the major factor causing the neurological deficits of decompression sickness, and may be contributing to long-term neurological damage in divers.[22]

Treatment of decompression sickness is best achieved by avoidance. Detailed and elaborate tables have been prepared to indicate the safe rate of decompression depending on the pressure and time of exposure. Administration of oxygen will reduce the blood P_{N_2} and so accelerate the resorption of bubbles in both blood and tissue. In severe cases, including all divers with neurological deficits, urgent recompression in a chamber is required, followed by slow decompression with oxygen and other therapeutic interventions.[23]

Altitude decompression sickness[24,25]

High altitude flying by military aircraft exposes the pilots to significant degrees of decompression, a cabin altitude of 9000 m (30 000 ft) being equivalent to about 0.3 ATA (see Chapter 16). During actual flights, symptoms of decompression sickness tend to be under-reported because these elite pilots may fear restrictions on their flying activities. However, during their careers, three-quarters of pilots experience problems, and almost 40 per cent of trainee pilots develop symptoms during hypobaric chamber testing to normal cabin altitudes. Joint pain is predictably the most common symptom, whilst the 'chokes' (substernal pain, cough and dyspnoea) occurs in 3 per cent of cases. Breathing oxygen prior to altitude exposure is likely to significantly ameliorate the symptoms seen, and is required by the US Air Force prior to altitude exposure in hypobaric chambers. Many pilots who have experienced decompression symptoms when flying previously are known to voluntarily increase their oxygen prebreathing time before subsequent flights. Accidental decompression of aircraft flying at altitudes above 8000 m (26 000 ft) is likely to cause decompression sickness, and one death from pulmonary barotrauma has been reported.[26]

Flying in the partially pressurized cabin (page 370) of commercial aircraft shortly after underwater diving also carries the theoretical risk of decompression sickness. There are few data available to quantify the risk but many tables and recommendations are published,[27] and a comprehensive study is currently in progress.[28] Over 24 hours between diving and flying is generally accepted as a suitable interval.

References

1. Lundgren CEG, Harabin A, Bennett PB, Van Liew HD, Thalmann ED. Gas physiology in diving. In: Fregly MJ, Blatteis CM, eds. *Handbook of physiology, Section 4: Environmental physiology*. New York and Oxford: Oxford University Press, 1996; 999–1019.
2. Lundgren CEG. Respiratory function during simulated wet dives. *Undersea Biomed Res* 1984; **11**: 139–45.
3. Salzano JV, Camporesi EM, Stolp BW, Moon RE. Physiological responses to exercise at 47 and 66 ATA. *J Appl Physiol* 1984; **57**: 1055–68.
4. Hong SK, Bennett PB, Shiraki K, Lin Y-C, Claybaugh JR. Mixed gas saturation diving. In: Fregly MJ, Blatteis CM, eds. *Handbook of physiology, Section 4: Environmental physiology*. New York and Oxford: Oxford University Press, 1996; 1023–45.
5. Lanphier EH, Camporesi EM. Respiration and exercise. In: Bennett PB, Elliott DH, eds. *The physiology and medicine of diving*. London: Baillière Tindall, 1982.
6. Prefaut C, Ramonatxo M, Boyer R, Chardon G. Human gas exchange during water immersion. *Respir Physiol* 1978; **34**: 307–18.
7. Bennett PB. Inert gas narcosis. In: Bennett PB, Elliott DH, eds. *The physiology and medicine of diving*. London: Baillière Tindall, 1982.
8. Halsey MJ. The effects of high pressure on the central nervous system. *Physiol Rev* 1982; **62**: 1341–77.
9. Halsey MJ, Wardley-Smith B, Green CJ. Pressure reversal of general anaesthesia – a multi-site expansion hypothesis. *Br J Anaesth* 1978; **50**: 1091–7.
10. Lin Y-C, Hong SK. Hyperbaria: breath-hold diving. In: Fregly MJ, Blatteis CM, eds. *Handbook of physiology, Section 4: Environmental physiology*. New York and Oxford: Oxford University Press, 1996; 979–95.
11. Butler PJ, Jones DR. Physiology of diving of birds and mammals. *Physiol Rev* 1997; **77**: 837–95.
12. Zapol WM. Diving adaptations of the Weddell seal. *Sci Am* 1987; **256**: 80–5.
13. Qvist J, Hill RD, Schneider RC, Falke KJ, Liggins GC, Guppy M et al. Hemoglobin concentrations and blood gas tensions of free-diving Weddell seals. *J Appl Physiol* 1986; **61**: 1560–9.

14. Lynch PR. Historical and basic perspectives of SCUBA diving. *Med Sci Sports Exerc* 1996; **28**: 570–2.
15. Walder DN. The compressed air environment. In: Bennett PB, Elliott DH, eds. *The physiology and medicine of diving*. London: Baillière Tindall, 1982.
16. Moon RE, Vann RD, Bennett PB. The physiology of decompression illness. *Sci Am* 1995; **273**: 54–61.
17. Broome CR, Jarvis LJ, Clark RJ. Pulmonary barotrauma in submarine escape training. *Thorax* 1994; **49**: 186–7.
18. Raymond LW. Pulmonary barotrauma and related events in divers. *Chest* 1995; **107**: 1648–52.
19. Bove AA. Pulmonary barotrauma in divers: can prospective pulmonary function testing identify those at risk? *Chest* 1997; **112**: 576–8.
20. Knauth M, Ries S, Pohimann S, Kerby T, Forsting M, Daffertshofer M et al. Cohort study of multiple brain lesions in sport divers: role of a patent foramen ovale. *BMJ* 1997; **314**; 701–5.
21. Wilmshurst P, Davidson C, O'Connell G, Byrne C. Role of cardiorespiratory abnormalities, smoking and dive characteristics in the manifestations of neurological decompression illness. *Clin Sci* 1994; **86**: 297–303.
22. Wilmshurst P. Brain damage in divers. *BMJ* 1997; **314**; 689–90.
23. Moon RE, Sheffield PJ. Guidelines for treatment of decompression illness. *Aviat Space Environ Med* 1997; **68**: 234–43.
24. Bendrick GA, Ainscough MJ, Pilmanis AA, Bisson RU. Prevalence of decompression sickness among U-2 pilots. *Aviat Space Environ Med* 1996; **67**: 199–206.
25. Ryles MT, Pilmanis AA. The initial signs and symptoms of altitude decompression sickness. *Aviat Space Environ Med* 1996; **67**: 983–9.
26. Neubauer JC, Dixon JP, Herndon CM. Fatal pulmonary decompression sickness: a case report. *Aviat Space Environ Med* 1988; **59**: 1181–4.
27. Harding RM, Mills FJ. *Aviation medicine*. London: BMJ Publishing, 1993.
28. Zorpette G. Flying and the bends. *Sci Am* 1997; **277**: 14–15.

Chapter 18

Respiration in closed environments and space

The fascination of the human race with exploration has taken humans well beyond the high altitude and underwater environments described in Chapters 16 and 17. Our ability to maintain life in space, the most hostile of environments yet explored, was developed as a result of techniques used to sustain breathing in other seemingly unrelated environments on Earth. All these environments share the problems common to maintaining respiration while separated from Earth's atmosphere.

Closed-system anaesthesia

This may not represent the most dramatic example of closed-environment breathing but it is by far the most common. Careful control of the composition of respiratory gas is the hallmark of inhalational anaesthesia. The anaesthetist must therefore maintain safe concentrations of oxygen and carbon dioxide in the patient's lungs, while controlling with great precision the dose of inhaled anaesthetic. It was recognized well over 100 years ago that anaesthesia could be prolonged by allowing patients to rebreathe some of their expired gas, including the anaesthetic vapour.[1] Provided oxygen is added and carbon dioxide removed, other gases can be circulated round a breathing system many times, providing beneficial effects such as warm and humid inspired gas. More recently, rebreathing systems have become popular as a method of reducing both the amount of anaesthetic used and the pollution of the operating theatre environment. Some recently introduced anaesthetic agents, such as xenon, are so expensive to produce that their widespread use is a practical proposition only if closed systems are used.[2]

A totally closed system during anaesthesia means that all expired gases are recirculated to the patient, with oxygen added only to replace that consumed and anaesthetic agent added to replace that absorbed by the patient's tissues. In practice, low-flow anaesthesia, in which over half the patient's expired gases are recirculated, is much more commonly used.[1] In each case, carbon dioxide is absorbed by chemical reaction with combinations of calcium, sodium, potassium or barium hydroxides, resulting in the formation of the respective carbonate and water. The reaction cannot be reversed, and the absorbent must be discarded after use. Circuit volume is typically 5–8 litres.

Widespread use of closed-circuit anaesthesia is limited by perceived difficulties with maintaining adequate circuit concentrations of gases that the patient is consuming, such as oxygen and anaesthetic agent.[1] Differences between fresh gas and circuit oxygen concentration become larger with lower fresh gas flow rate and, so, a greater proportion of gas rebreathing. The rate of change of circuit gas concentrations is affected by the same factors. However, gas-monitoring systems are now almost universally used with low-flow and closed circuit anaesthesia, allowing accurate control of circuit gas composition.

Accumulation of other gases in closed circuits

Closed-circuit systems with a constant inflow and consumption of oxygen will allow accumulation of other gases entering the circuit either with the fresh gas or from the patient. This affects the patient in two quite distinct ways. First, essentially inert gases such as nitrogen and argon may accumulate to such an extent that they dilute the oxygen in the system. Secondly, small concentrations of more toxic gases may arise in the breathing system.

Nitrogen enters the closed circuit from the patient at the start of anaesthesia. Body stores of dissolved nitrogen are small, but air present in the lungs may contain 2–3 litres of nitrogen which will be transferred to the circuit in the first few minutes. If nitrogen is not intended to be part of the closed-circuit gas mixture, the patient must 'denitrogenate' by breathing high concentrations of oxygen before being anaesthetized, or higher fresh gas flow rates must be used initially.

Argon is normally present in air at a concentration of 0.93%. Oxygen concentrators effectively remove nitrogen from air, and so concentrate argon in similar proportions to oxygen, resulting in argon concentrations of around 5%. In a study of closed-circuit breathing in volunteers using oxygen from an oxygen concentrator, argon levels in the circuit reached 40% after only 80 minutes.[3] Cylinders of medical grade oxygen and hospital supplies from liquid oxygen evaporators contain negligible argon, so the risk of significant accumulation is low. Even so, current recommendations to 'flush' the closed circuit at least every 2 hours seem prudent.

Methane is produced in the distal colon by anaerobic bacterial fermentation and is mostly excreted direct from the alimentary tract. Some methane is, however, absorbed into the blood, where it has low solubility so is rapidly excreted by the lung, following which it will accumulate in the closed circuit. There is a large variation between subjects in methane production and, therefore, the concentrations seen during closed-circuit anaesthesia. Mean levels in the circle system in healthy patients reached over 900 ppm, well below levels regarded as unacceptable in other closed environments (see below),[4] but sufficient to cause interference with standard anaesthetic gas concentration analysers.[5]

Acetone, ethanol and carbon monoxide all have high blood solubility, so concentrations in the closed circuit gas remain low, but rebreathing causes accumulation in the blood. Levels achieved are generally low,[4,5] but acetone accumulation may be associated with postoperative nausea.[6] Closed-circuit anaesthesia is not recommended in patients with increased excretion of acetone or alcohol, such as uncontrolled diabetes mellitus, recent alcohol ingestion or during prolonged starvation.[1]

Inhaled anaesthetic derivatives. Currently used volatile anaesthetics are remarkably stable compounds, mostly consisting of halogenated hydrocarbons, and their metabolism in the body is low. In certain circumstances these compounds can, however, produce toxic metabolites, and closed-circuit systems make this much more likely. Carbon monoxide may be produced when desflurane, enflurane or isoflurane react with barium hydroxide used for CO_2 absorption, and significant levels have been reported.[7] The reaction seems to occur only under dry conditions; once the CO_2 absorber has been used for a short period, generating water vapour, production of carbon monoxide becomes minimal.

Sevoflurane, a relatively new volatile anaesthetic agent, is degraded in closed-circuit anaesthesia to a derivative known as compound A, which has been associated with renal damage in animals.[1] Levels of compound A achieved in low-flow anaesthesia are variable, and sevoflurane is therefore not recommended for use in closed systems.

Submarines

Submersible ships have been used for almost 100 years, almost exclusively for military purposes until the last few decades when they have become more widespread for undersea exploration and industrial use. Atmospheric pressure in the submarine remains approximately the same as at surface level during a dive, the duration of which is limited by the maintenance of adequate oxygen and carbon dioxide levels for the crew in the ship.

Diesel powered

Submarines were used extensively during both world wars, and were powered by diesel engines like surface-based warships. Clearly, the oxygen requirement of the engines precluded them from use during dives and battery-powered engines were used, thus limiting the duration of dives to just a few hours. A more significant limitation to dive duration was atmospheric regulation. No attempt was made to control the internal atmosphere, and, after ventilation at the surface, the submarine dived with only the air contained within. After about 12 hours, the atmosphere contained 15% oxygen, 5% carbon dioxide and a multitude of odours and contaminants. The need to return to the surface was apparent when the submariners became short of breath and were unable to light their cigarettes because of low levels of oxygen.[8]

Nuclear powered

Short dive duration severely limited the use of submarines. The development of nuclear power allowed submarines to generate an ample supply of heat and electricity completely independent of oxygen supply, and so allowed prolonged activity underwater. Atmospheric regeneration was therefore needed. Current nuclear-powered submarines have a crew of up to 180, and routinely remain submerged for many weeks at considerable depths.

Atmosphere regeneration.[8,9] The plentiful supply of sea water and electricity make hydrolysis of water the obvious method for oxygen generation. Sea water must first have all electrolytes removed by a combination of evaporation and de-ionization. Physical, though not electrical, separation of the electrolysis electrodes allows the oxygen to be taken directly from the anode, thus removing the necessity to separate it from the hydrogen produced at the cathode. Theoretically, 1 litre of water can yield 620 litres of oxygen, so, even with less than 100 per cent efficient electrolysis, large volumes of oxygen are easily produced. Submarine atmosphere oxygen concentration is maintained at $21 \pm 2\%$.

Atmospheric carbon dioxide in submarines is absorbed by passage through mono-ethanolamine, which chemically combines with carbon dioxide to produce carbonates. When fully saturated, the absorber can either be replaced or be regenerated by heating with steam, when the carbon dioxide is given off in gaseous form to be vented into the sea. This method maintains the carbon dioxide concentration in submarines at 0.5–1.5%, and though further reduction is possible, the energy cost of doing so is prohibitive.

Atmospheric contamination during prolonged submarine patrols is well recognized, many hundreds of substances entering the atmosphere, originating from both machinery and crew.[8] These substances include volatile hydrocarbons such as benzene, oil droplets, carbon monoxide, cadmium and microbial organisms,[8] with varying concentrations in different parts of the submarine. Continuous monitoring of many compounds is now routine, and maximum allowable levels during prolonged patrols are defined.[4,10,11] Submarine air-conditioning units now include catalytic burners that oxidize carbon monoxide, hydrogen and other hydrocarbons to carbon dioxide and water, and charcoal absorbers to absorb any remaining contaminants. The health risks from submarine occupation are therefore believed to be extremely small.[8,10,12] To maintain crew morale, smoking continues to be permitted in most nuclear submarines, and passive smoking (page 413) is therefore inevitable. Carbon monoxide levels of 9 ppm have been reported, which is close to the recommended maximum level of 10 ppm for prolonged atmospheric exposure (Table 20.2) or 15 ppm for submarine personnel exposure.[11]

Physiological effects of prolonged hypercapnia[13]

Definition of a 'safe' level of atmospheric CO_2 over long periods has concerned submariners for some years. The respiratory response to inhalation of low concentrations of CO_2 (<3%) are similar to those at higher levels (page 95), but compensatory acid–base changes seem to be quite different.

Respiratory changes.[14,15] Atmospheric CO_2 levels of 1% cause an elevation of inspired P_{CO_2} of 1 kPa (7.5 mmHg), which results in an average increase in minute ventilation of 2–3 l.min^{-1}.[14,15] However, the degree of hyperventilation is highly variable between subjects, and presumably relates to their central chemoreceptor sensitivity to CO_2 (page 95). Measurements of arterial blood gases in submariners show that the elevated minute volume limits the increase in arterial P_{CO_2} to an average of only 0.14 kPa (1 mmHg). After a few days, the increase in ventilation declines and minute volume returns towards normal, allowing arterial P_{CO_2} to increase further to reflect the inspired P_{CO_2}. The time course of the decline in ventilation is too short to result from blood acid–base compensation (see below), and is believed to reflect a small attenuation of the central chemoreceptor response. On return to the surface, ventilation may be temporarily reduced following withdrawal of the CO_2 stimulus.

Lung volumes are unaffected by atmospheric CO_2 concentrations of 1.2% or below, though small changes in the CO-diffusing capacity have been described.[16] Similarly, there are no significant changes in the hypercapnic ventilatory response.[15]

Calcium metabolism.[13,14,17] Elevation of arterial P_{CO_2} causes a respiratory acidosis, which is normally, over the course of one or two days, compensated for by the retention of bicarbonate by the kidney (page 469). The changes in pH seen when breathing less than 3% CO_2 seem to be too small to stimulate renal compensation, and pH remains slightly lowered for some time. During this period, CO_2 is deposited in bone as calcium carbonate, and urinary and faecal calcium excretion is drastically reduced to facilitate this. Serum calcium levels also decrease, and recent work suggests a shift of extracellular calcium to the intracellular space.[17] After about three weeks, when bone stores of CO_2 are saturated, renal excretion of calcium and hydrogen ions begins to increase and pH tends to return to normal. Abnormalities of calcium metabolism have been demonstrated with inspired CO_2 concentrations as low as 0.5%.

Some other effects of low levels of atmospheric CO_2 during space travel are described below (page 393).

Space[9,18,19]

Space represents the most hostile environment into which humans have sojourned. At 80 km (50 miles) above Earth there is insufficient air to allow aerodynamic control of a vehicle, and at 200 km (125 miles) there is an almost total vacuum. True space begins above 700 km (435 miles), where particles become so scarce that the likelihood of a collision between two atoms becomes negligible. Even under these conditions, there are estimated to be 10^8 particles (mainly hydrogen) per cubic metre compared with 10^{25} on Earth's surface. Maintenance of a respirable atmosphere in these circumstances is challenging, and both US and Soviet space pioneers have lost their lives during the development of suitable technology. Current experience is based on relatively short periods (up to 1 year) in close proximity to Earth, usually involving Earth orbit or travel to the moon. This means that the raw materials for atmosphere regeneration can be repeatedly supplied from Earth.

Atmosphere composition

A summary of manned space missions and the atmospheres used is given in Table 18.1. Spacecraft have an almost totally sealed, closed-circuit system of atmospheric control, and early Soviet space vehicles aimed to be completely sealed environments. Their designers had such confidence in the structure that emergency stores of oxygen for leakage were considered unnecessary until Soyuz 11 depressurized on re-entry in 1971, tragically killing all three cosmonauts. US Apollo missions leaked approximately 1 kg of gas per day in space, even with a lower atmospheric pressure (Table 18.1).
    The use of a total pressure of 34.5 kPa (259 mmHg) in early US space vehicles required a high atmospheric oxygen concentration to provide an adequate inspired Po_2 (Table 18.1). Because of the tragic fire in 1967, the composition during launch was changed from 100% oxygen to 64% oxygen in 36% nitrogen at the same pressure, which still gave an inspired Po_2 in excess of the normal sea level value. Previous Soviet designs were all based on maintaining normal atmospheric pressure, and space vehicles in current use continue to do so with inspired oxygen concentrations of near 21%. Extravehicular activity in space presents a particular problem. Flexibility of the space suit in the vacuum of space requires an internal pressure of only 28 kPa (212 mmHg). This entails the use of 100% oxygen after careful decompression and denitrogenation.

Oxygen supply

Storage of oxygen and other gases in space presents significant problems. The weight of the containers used is critical during launch, and storage of significant quantities of oxygen requires high pressures and therefore strong, heavy tanks. Liquid oxygen presents

Table 18.1 Summary of manned space missions and their respiratory environments

Missions	Period of use	Number of crew	Habitable volume (m^3)	Maximum duration (days)	Cabin pressure kPa	Cabin pressure mmHg	Oxygen conc. (%)	O_2 supply	CO_2 removal
Vostok	1961–65	1	2.5	5	100	760	100	KO_2	KO_2
Mercury	1961–63	1	1.6	1.5	34	258	100	Pressurized O_2	LiOH
Gemini	1965–66	2	2.3	14	34	258	100	Liquid O_2	LiOH
Soyuz	1967–	2/3	–	17	100	760	22	KO_2	KO_2/LiOH
Apollo	1968–72	3	5.9	12	34	258	100†	Liquid O_2	LiOH
Salyut	1971–86	5	100	237	100	760	21	KO_2	KO_2/LiOH
Skylab	1973–74	3	361	84	34	258	72	Liquid O_2	Molecular sieve
Shuttle	1981–	7	74	10	100	760	21	Liquid O_2	LiOH
Mir	1986–	6	150	365	100	760	23	Electrolysis/Chemical	Molecular sieve

† Oxygen concentration reduced to 60% during launch to reduce fire risk.
All missions, except early Soyuz launches, carry emergency oxygen supplies as pressurized or liquid oxygen. (Data derived from references 9, 18 and 19.)

a greatly improved storage density, but the behaviour of stored liquids in weightless conditions is complex.

Chemical generation of oxygen has been used mainly by Soviet space missions. Potassium superoxide releases oxygen on exposure to moisture, a reaction that generates potassium hydroxide as an intermediate and so also absorbs carbon dioxide:

$$4KO_2 + 3H_2O + 2CO_2 \rightarrow 2K_2CO_3 + 3H_2O + 3O_2$$

One kilogram of KO_2 can release over 200 litres of oxygen, but the reaction is irreversible and the used canisters must be discarded. Sodium chlorate candles release oxygen when simply ignited, and were used for generating emergency oxygen on older submarines and in most Soviet space missions, including the current Mir space station.

Electrolysis of water, as used in submarines, is an efficient way to produce oxygen in space where solar panels provide the electricity supply. In contrast to submarines, water is scarce in space vehicles, again because of weight considerations at launch. The Mir space station generates oxygen by electrolysis using waste water generated by the occupants, though this alone does not produce sufficient oxygen for a reasonably active cosmonaut, and the electrolysis must be supplemented with stored water.

Carbon dioxide removal

Chemical absorption by lithium hydroxide has been the mainstay of the US space programme, whilst the Soviet program used KO_2 as described above. Reversible chemical reactions such as those used in submarines have been investigated for space use, and can be regenerated by exposure to the vacuum of space. These techniques are very effective, with atmospheric CO_2 concentration being maintained at less than 0.2% on Shuttle missions[20] – significantly lower than that accepted in submarines.

Molecular sieves allow CO_2 to be adsorbed into a chemical matrix without undergoing any chemical reaction. Water is also adsorbed, reducing the efficiency of the system, so the gas must be dried first. When saturated with CO_2, exposure to the space vacuum causes release of the adsorbed gas. Use of two- or four-bed molecular sieves allows continuous CO_2 removal by half the processors while the others are regenerated.

Maintenance of CO_2 levels below 0.2% on prolonged future space missions is likely to have unacceptable costs in terms of energy and consumables.[21] This fact recently led to three space agencies world-wide undertaking a joint research programme to study the effects of 1.2% and 0.7% atmospheric CO_2 on a wide range of physiological systems. The study involved normal volunteers spending 22 days in a closed mock 'space station' on the ground.[21] Some of the results have already been described above (page 390).[15,16,17] Effects at 0.7% atmospheric CO_2 were generally concluded to be minimal.[22] At 1.2%, however, changes in respiration and calcium metabolism were significant and, more important, mental performance was impaired with a loss of alertness and visuomotor performance.[23]

Atmospheric contamination

Chemical contamination in space vehicles is mainly from within the habitable area of the vehicle, external contamination from propellants etc. being very rare.[18] The greatest contribution to atmospheric contamination is the astronauts themselves, but the compounds released such as carbon monoxide, ammonia, methane and indole are easily dealt with by standard methods. More complex chemicals may be released into the atmosphere by a process called off-gassing. Almost any non-metallic substance, but particularly plastics, release small quantities of volatile chemicals for many months and years after manufacture. This is more likely to occur at low atmospheric pressure, as on the earlier space missions. In a closed environment, these chemicals may accumulate to toxic levels. Acidic compounds are absorbed by the hydroxide-based carbon dioxide absorbers. In addition, atmosphere regeneration systems include a catalytic oxidizer to convert hydrocarbons into carbon dioxide and water, and regenerable charcoal absorbers.

Long-term space travel

Manned space travel to planets more distant than the moon requires expeditions of years' duration with no access to supplies from Earth. Carriage of oxygen stores and non-regenerable carbon dioxide absorbents is therefore impractical. There has been much interest in finding ways of reversing the effects of animal metabolism on a closed atmosphere. Biological solutions are believed by many to be the only feasible option, and these are discussed below. Physicochemical methods are, however, now realistic options, and are likely to act as valuable back-up systems in the future.

CO_2 reduction reactions convert carbon dioxide back into oxygen, and two main methods are described.[24]
    The Sabatier reaction requires hydrogen to produce methane and water:

$$CO_2 + 4H_2 \rightarrow CH_4 + 2H_2O$$

Methane can then be converted to solid carbon and hydrogen gas, which re-enters the Sabatier reactor.
    The Bosch reaction produces solid carbon in one stage:

$$CO_2 + 2H_2 \rightarrow 2H_2O + \text{solid C}$$

Electrolysis of water generates oxygen and hydrogen gas, the latter enters the Bosch reaction and the water produced is recycled. Both reactions generate solid carbon, which must be removed from the reactors periodically. Use of catalysts has allowed the development of small, efficient reactors based on a combination of the two chemical processes. Current hardware can convert carbon dioxide into oxygen for 60 person-days before the carbon deposits must be emptied.[24]

Microgravity[25]

All bodies with mass exert gravitational forces on each other, so *zero* gravity is theoretically impossible. Once in space, away from the large mass of Earth or other planets, gravitational forces become negligible and are referred to as microgravity. Spacecraft in orbit around Earth are still subject to its considerable gravitational forces, but these are matched almost exactly by the centrifugal force from the high tangential velocity of the spaceship.[19] Occupants of orbiting spacecraft are normally subject to a gravitational force of about 10^{-6} times that on Earth's surface.
    Chapter 8 contains numerous references to the effect of gravity on the topography of the lung and the distribution of perfusion and ventilation. Microgravity may therefore be predicted to have significant effects on respiratory function.[26]

The first studies of short-term microgravity used a Lear jet flying in a series of keplerian arcs, which gave 20–25 seconds of weightlessness. Unfortunately, between each period of microgravity the subject is exposed to a similar duration of increased gravitational forces (2G) as the jet pulls out of the free-fall portion of the flight,[27] and this may influence the results of physiological studies. Sustained microgravity has now been studied in space. In June 1991 an extended series of investigations on seven subjects was undertaken in Spacelab SLS-1, which was carried into orbit by the space shuttle for a nine-day mission.

Lung volumes. Chest radiography in the sitting position during short-term microgravity revealed no striking changes other than a tendency for the diaphragm to be slightly higher in some of the subjects at functional residual capacity (FRC).[28] This accords with a 413 ml reduction in FRC also measured in keplerian arc studies on seated subjects.[27] Abdominal contribution to tidal excursion was increased at microgravity in the seated position, probably because of loss of postural tone in the abdominal muscles,[27] an observation recently confirmed in space studies.[29]

During sustained microgravity, subdivisions of lung volume were again found to be intermediate between the sitting and supine volumes at normal gravity, except for residual volume which was reduced below that seen in any position at 1G (Figure 18.1).[20] The FRC was reduced by 750 ml compared with preflight standing values. These changes in lung volume are ascribed to altered respiratory mechanics and increased thoracic blood volume.

Topographical inequality of ventilation and perfusion.[25] Early results in the Lear jet, using single-breath nitrogen washout (page 168), indicated a substantial reduction in topographical inequality of ventilation and perfusion during weightlessness, as expected.[30] However, the more detailed studies in Spacelab revealed that a surprising degree of residual inequality of blood flow[31] and ventilation[32] persisted despite the major improvement at zero gravity. Ventilatory inequality is believed to result from continued airway closure at low lung volume,[26,32] but currently available data cannot define in which areas of lung this occurs. Similarly, the cause of the continued small degree of perfusion

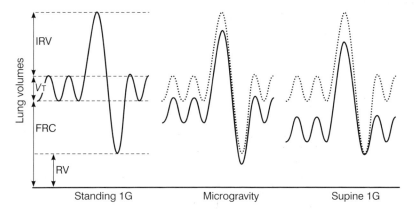

Figure 18.1 Static lung volumes during sustained microgravity for nine days in Earth orbit. Dotted line shows the normal standing values on Earth for comparison. Volumes at microgravity are generally intermediate between standing and supine values at 1G, except residual volume which is further reduced. FRC, functional residual capacity; IRV, inspiratory reserve volume; RV, residual volume; V_T, tidal volume.

inequality is uncertain.[31] A possible explanation is the presence of a slight peripheral to central perfusion gradient in each horizontal slice of lung, which is completely overshadowed at 1G by the large vertical perfusion gradient.[26] Early results from long-term missions in the Mir space station indicate that the changes in ventilation and perfusion may be associated with reduced arterial Po_2.[25]

Diffusing capacity. SLS-1 studies have shown progressive increases in CO_2-diffusing capacity, the membrane component and the pulmonary capillary blood volume (page 212) – all reaching 33 per cent more than control by the ninth day in orbit.[33]

Biospheres[19]

A biosphere is defined as 'a closed space of two or more connected ecosystems in equilibrium with their environment'.[34] Only energy enters and leaves the biosphere. Earth is the largest and most successful known biosphere, though the equilibrium between its ecosystems is almost certainly changing (see Chapter 1). Attempts to create smaller biospheres have mostly been driven by the prospect of long-term space travel.[35] Physicochemical methods of sustaining life, as described above, have many limitations whereas a biological system has numerous advantages. Plants perform the complex CO_2-reduction chemistry using chlorophyll, and at the same time, rather than generating carbon, they produce varying amounts of food.[36] Plants also act as efficient water-purification systems via transpiration. It has been estimated that plants transpire 300 grams of water vapour for each gram of CO_2 used.[19]

Small-scale biological atmospheric regeneration

The first report of prolonged biological atmosphere regeneration was described in 1961 when a single mouse was maintained in a closed chamber for 66 days.[37] Air from the chamber was circulated through a second chamber containing 4 litres of *Chlorella* alga solution illuminated with artificial light. Over the course of the experiment, oxygen concentration in the chamber increased from 21% to 53%, and carbon dioxide concentrations remained below 0.2%. Subsequent experiments by both US and Soviet researchers demonstrated the feasibility of human life support by *Chlorella*, culminating in the 30-day closure of a single researcher in a 4.5 m³ room, maintained by just 30 litres of alga solution. Algae alone are unsuitable for long-term life support.[19] Their excellent atmospheric regeneration properties result from a very fast rate of growth but *Chlorella* is generally regarded as inedible, and so presents a significant disposal problem in a totally closed system. In addition, if the algal solution becomes acidic for any reason, algae produce carbon monoxide in unacceptable quantities.

Unknown to the scientific community at large, from 1963 the Soviet Union ran a 'Bios' research centre at the Institute of Biophysics in Krasnoyarsk, Siberia.[19,38] A whole series of progressively more complex biospheres were constructed, but details of this work remain scarce. In 1983, two researchers successfully spent five months in a biosphere (Bios 3), which provided all their atmospheric regeneration needs and over three-quarters of their food.[38] In these studies, plants were grown hydroponically – that is, without soil but with their roots bathed in carefully controlled nutrient solution. Light was provided with continuous xenon lighting to maximize growth, to such an extent that, under these conditions, wheat can be harvested six times per year. An estimated $13\,m^2$ of planted area will then produce enough oxygen for one human, though over $30\,m^2$ is probably required to produce almost enough food as well. Beds of *Chlorella* algae were also used to maximize oxygen production and, along with larger planted areas, resulted in excess oxygen. This was reduced by incineration of the non-edible portion of the plants, and so enabled the researchers to exercise some control over the balance between oxygen and carbon dioxide concentration in the biosphere. In this way, levels of carbon dioxide in Bios 3 were maintained at between 0.03% and 0.14%.[19]

American research of controlled ecological life support systems (CELSS) began in 1977 and has focused on basic plant physiology.[19] Plant species, light, humidity, nutrients and atmospheric gas concentrations all have profound effects on the design of a CELSS. Atmospheric regeneration is usually the easiest problem to overcome, whilst the plant species used has important implications for the dietary intake and psychological well-being of the CELSS inhabitants.[36,38]

Biosphere 2[19]

Small-scale biosphere experiments never attained a totally closed system, particularly with respect to food supplies and waste disposal. In addition, biodiversity in these systems was low, with very few species of plant, animal, insect or microbes contained within. Finally, build-up of toxic atmospheric compounds was significant, with the requirement for extensive physicochemical methods of removal similar to those used in the closed systems of submarines and space. With these problems in mind, an ambitious series of biosphere experiments were established in Arizona, USA, culminating in the Biosphere 2 project in 1991.

A totally sealed complex, covering 3.15 acres (1.3 hectares) and containing $204\,000\,m^3$ (7.2 million ft^3) of atmosphere, was purpose built with a stainless steel underground lining and principally glass cover. Two flexible walls, or 'lungs', were included to minimize pressure changes in the complex with expansion and contraction of the atmosphere. A two-year closure was carried out commencing in September 1991, the complex containing a wide range of flora and fauna, including eight humans, other mammals, fish and insects. The biosphere was divided into seven smaller ecosystems: rain forest, savannah, desert, ocean, saltmarsh, intensive agriculture area and a human/animal habitat. Soil was chosen as the growing medium for all plants in preference to hydroponic techniques used previously. This was to facilitate air purification by soil bed reactors, in which atmospheric air is pumped through the soil where bacterial action provides an adaptable and efficient purification system.[19] A CO_2-recycling system was included in biosphere 2 to control atmospheric CO_2 levels, particularly during winter when shorter days reduce photosynthetic activity. Also, the amount of O_2-consuming biomass relative to atmosphere volume was known to be high, and therefore small increases in CO_2 levels were anticipated. Extensive monitoring and computer systems were used to control the interplay between the ecosystems in the biosphere.

Biosphere 2 aimed, wherever possible, to use ecological engineering. By the inclusion of large numbers of species (3800 in total), it was hoped that there would be sufficient flexibility between systems to respond to changes in the environment. In particular, microbial diversity is believed to be extremely important in maintaining biosphere 1 (Earth), and the multiple habitats were established to facilitate this type of diversity in biosphere 2.

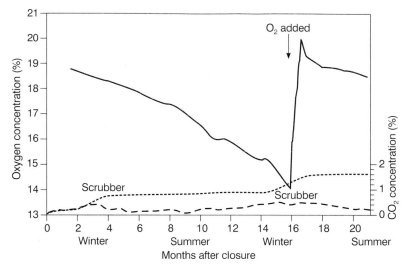

Figure 18.2 Changes in atmospheric concentrations of oxygen (solid line) and carbon dioxide (dashed line) during the two-year closure of biosphere 2. Less daylight during winter months reduces photosynthesis, causing increased levels of CO_2. Carbon dioxide was therefore removed using a CO_2 'scrubber' system, during the periods shown. Even when CO_2 absorption by the scrubbers is taken into account (dotted line), it can clearly be seen that the reduction in O_2 concentration exceeds the increase in CO_2 concentration; after 16 months, O_2 had to be added to the biosphere. See text for details. (Data from references 19 and 40.)

Outcome from the two-year closure. Concentrations of oxygen and carbon dioxide in biosphere 2 were very unstable (Figure 18.2) and, after 16 months, oxygen concentration had fallen to only 14%. Extensive symptoms were reported by the inhabitants,[34] including significantly reduced work capacity, which was crucial for controlling plant growth. External oxygen therefore had to be added to the atmosphere. Carbon dioxide levels did increase slightly during winter months (Figure 18.2) when it was removed by the recycling system. It was never expected that all species introduced into biosphere 2 would survive, and extinction of some species was seen as a natural response to stabilization of the ecosystem. However, after two years, extinct species were numerous, including 19 of 25 vertebrates and most insects, including all pollinators.[39] In contrast, ants and cockroaches thrived.

The success of biosphere 2 as a closed ecosystem was therefore limited, and, in contrast to the smaller biospheres previously used, basic atmospheric regeneration was a significant problem. Any increase in CO_2 concentration should be matched by an equivalent decrease in O_2 concentration, as biological reactions between CO_2 and O_2 are generally equimolar. Even when the CO_2 removed by the recycling system is taken into account, it can clearly be seen from Figure 18.2 that oxygen losses were much greater. The explanation for this is believed to be twofold.[40] First, oxygen depletion occurred due to respiration in the biosphere proceeding faster than photosynthesis, most likely as a result of microbial activity in the soil. Secondly, much of the CO_2 produced by this respiration was lost from the atmosphere by chemical reaction with the concrete from which the biosphere complex was built.

We therefore remain some way away from being able to establish a long-term habitable atmosphere away from Earth.

References

1. Baum JA, Aitkenhead AR. Low-flow anaesthesia. *Anaesthesia* 1995; **50** (Supp): 37–44
2. Nunn JF, Halsey MJ. Xenon in anaesthesia. *Lancet* 1990; **336**: 112–13.
3. Parker CJR, Snowdon SL. Predicted and measured oxygen concentrations in the circle system using low fresh gas flows with oxygen supplied by an oxygen concentrator. *Br J Anaesth* 1988; **61**: 397–402.
4. Baumgarten RK, Reynolds WJ. Much ado about nothing: trace gaseous metabolites in the closed circuit. *Anesth Analg* 1985; **64**: 1029–38.
5. Versichelen L, Rolly G, Vermeulen H. Accumulation of foreign gases during closed-system anaesthesia. *Br J Anaesth* 1996; **76**: 668–72.
6. Strauß JM, Hausdörfer J. Accumulation of acetone in blood during long-term anaesthesia with closed systems. *Br J Anaesth* 1993; **70**: 363–4.
7. Kharasch ED. Keep the blood red . . . the right way. *Anesthesiology* 1997; **87**: 202–3.
8. Knight DR, Tappan DV, Bowman JS, O'Neill HJ, Gordon SM. Submarine atmospheres. *Toxicol Lett* 1989; **49**: 243–51.
9. Wieland PO. *Designing for human presence in space: An introduction to environmental control and life support systems*, NASA Reference Publication 1324. Washington DC: National Aeronautics and Space Administration, 1994.
10. Dean MR. Benzene exposure in Royal Naval submarines. *J R Soc Med* 1996; **89**: 286P–8P.
11. Seufert KT, Kiser WR. End-expiratory carbon monoxide levels as an estimate of passive smoking exposure aboard a nuclear-powered submarine. *South Med J* 1996; **89**: 1181–3.
12. Lambert RJW. Environmental problems in nuclear submarines. *Proc R Soc Med* 1972; **65**: 795–6.
13. Schaefer KE. Effects of increased ambient CO_2 levels on human and animal health. *Experientia* 1982; **38**: 1163–8.
14. Pingree BJW. Acid–base and respiratory changes after prolonged exposure to 1% carbon dioxide. *Clin Sci Mol Med* 1977; **52**: 67–74.
15. Elliott AR, Prisk GK, Schöllmann C, Hoffmann U. Hypercapnic ventilatory response in humans before, during, and after 23 days of low level CO_2 exposure. *Aviat Space Environ Med* 1998; **69**: 391–6.
16. Sexton J, Mueller K, Elliott A, Gerzer D, Strohl KP. Low level CO_2 effects on pulmonary function in humans. *Aviat Space Environ Med* 1998; **69**: 387–90.
17. Drummer C, Friedel V, Börger A, Störmer I, Wolter S, Zitterman A et al. Effects of elevated carbon dioxide environment on calcium metabolism in humans. *Aviat Space Environ Med* 1998; **69**: 291–8.
18. Nicogossian AE, Huntoon CL, Pool SL. *Space physiology and medicine*, 3rd edn. Philadelphia PA: Lea & Febiger, 1994.
19. Churchill SE. *Fundamentals of space life sciences*. Malabar FL: Krieger Publishing, 1997.
20. Elliott AR, Prisk GK, Guy HJB, West JB. Lung volumes during sustained microgravity on Spacelab SLS-1. *J Appl Physiol* 1994; **77**: 2005–14.
21. Wenzel J, Luks N, Plath G, Wilke D, Gerzer R. The influence of CO_2 in a space-like environment: study design. *Aviat Space Environ Med* 1998; **69**: 285–90.
22. Frey MAB, Sulzman FM, Oser H, Ruyters G. The effects of moderately elevated ambient carbon dioxide levels on human physiology and performance: a joint NASA–ESA–DARA study – overview. *Aviat Space Environ Med* 1998; **69**: 282–4.
23. Manzey D, Lorenz B. Effects of chronically elevated CO_2 on mental performance during 26 days of confinement. *Aviat Space Environ Med* 1998; **69**: 506–14.
24. Noyes GP. Carbon dioxide reduction processes for spacecraft ECLSS: a comprehensive review. *Proceedings of the 18th intersociety conference on environmental systems*, July 1988, San Francisco, paper 881042. Warrendale, USA: Society of Automotive Engineers, 1989.
25. West JB, Guy HJB, Elliott AR, Prisk GK. Respiratory system in microgravity. In: Fregly MJ, Blatteis CM eds. *Handbook of physiology, Section 4: Environmental physiology*. New York and Oxford: Oxford University Press, 1996; 675–89.
26. Linnarsson D. Pulmonary function and cardiopulmonary interactions at microgravity. *Med Sci Sports Exerc* 1996; **28**: S14–17.
27. Paiva M, Estenne M, Engel LA. Lung volumes, chest wall configuration, and pattern of breathing in microgravity. *J Appl Physiol* 1989; **67**: 1542–50.

28. Michels DB, Friedman PJ, West JB. Radiographic comparison of human lung shape during normal gravity and weightlessness. *J Appl Physiol* 1979; **47**: 851–7.

29. Wantier M, Estenne M, Verbanck S, Prisk GK, Paiva M. Chest wall mechanics in sustained microgravity. *J Appl Physiol* 1998; **84**: 2060–5.

30. Michels DB, West JB. Distribution of pulmonary ventilation and perfusion during short periods of weightlessness. *J Appl Physiol* 1978; **45**: 987–98.

31. Prisk GK, Guy HJB, Elliott AR, West JB. Inhomogeneity of pulmonary perfusion during sustained microgravity on SLS-1. *J Appl Physiol* 1994; **76**: 1730–8.

32. Guy HJB, Prisk GK, Elliott AR, Deutschman III RA, West JB. Inhomogeneity of pulmonary ventilation during sustained microgravity as determined by single breath washouts. *J Appl Physiol* 1994; **76**: 1719–29.

33. Prisk GK, Guy HJB, Elliott AR, Deutschman III RA, West JB. Pulmonary diffusing capacity, capillary blood volume, and cardiac output during sustained microgravity. *J Appl Physiol* 1993; **75**: 15–26.

34. Walford RL, Bechtel R, MacCallum T, Paglia DE, Weber LJ. 'Biospheric medicine' as viewed from the two-year first closure of biosphere 2. *Aviat Space Environ Med* 1996; **67**: 609–17.

35. Schwartzkopf SH. Human life support for advanced space exploration. *Adv Space Biol Med* 1997; **6**: 231–53.

36. Mitchell CA. Bioregenerative life-support systems. *Am J Clin Nutr* 1994; **60**: 820S–4S.

37. Bowman RO, Thomae FW. Long-term nontoxic support of animal life with algae. *Science* 1961; **134**: 55–6.

38. Ivanov B, Zubareva O. To Mars and back again on board Bios. *Soviet Life* April 1985; 22–5.

39. Cohen JE, Tilman D. Biosphere 2 and biodiversity: the lessons so far. *Science* 1996; **274**: 1150–1.

40. Severinghaus JP, Broecker WS, Dempster WF, MacCallum T, Wahlen M. Oxygen loss in biosphere 2. *EOS* 1994; **75**: 33–40.

Chapter 19

Drowning

In several countries, drowning is a major cause of accidental death, many victims being children. In the USA nearly half the victims of drowning are under 4 years old,[1] and in most developed countries drowning is the second commonest cause of accidental death in children, exceeded only by road traffic accidents.[2,3] In adults, men are drowned more commonly than women and alcohol is a major aetiological factor.[3,4] For each victim of death by drowning, there are estimated to be between 6 and 10 cases of 'near-drowning' that are severe enough to require hospital admission,[2] and probably hundreds of other less severe incidents.[3] Death from pulmonary complications ('secondary drowning') may occur a considerable time after the accident, in patients who were initially normal. Permanent neurological damage occurs in more than 20 per cent of children who required cardiopulmonary resuscitation for near-drowning.[5]

The essential feature of drowning is asphyxia, but many of the physiological responses depend on whether aspiration of water occurs and on the substances that are dissolved or suspended in the water. The temperature of the water is crucially important, and hypothermia following drowning in very cold water is a major factor influencing survival, though the mechanism underlying this observation remains controversial.

Physiology of immersion[3]

The hydrostatic pressure exerted on the body during immersion can be substantial. As a result, there is a huge increase in venous return, causing increased pulmonary blood volume, cardiac output and, soon afterwards, a significant diuresis. Cephalad displacement of the diaphragm from raised abdominal pressure coupled with direct chest compression increases the work of breathing by about 65 per cent. Three reflexes affect the respiratory system and come into play in drowning, as outlined below.

Airway irritant reflexes play a major part in drowning. Aspiration of water into the mouth initially stimulates swallowing followed by coughing, glottic closure and laryngospasm. If water penetrates deeper into the respiratory tract, below the vocal folds, bronchospasm results.

Cold shock describes a combination of several cardiovascular and respiratory reflexes that occur in response to sudden total-body immersion in cold water.[6] Sudden immersion in water below 25°C is a potent stimulant to respiration and causes an initial large gasp followed by substantial hyperventilation. The stimulus is increased with colder temperatures, reaching a maximum at 10°C.[3] Functional residual capacity is acutely increased, and individuals may find themselves breathing almost at total lung capacity, giving a sensation of dyspnoea. Breath-hold time is severely reduced, often to less than 10 seconds, which impairs the ability of victims to escape from a confined space underwater or to orientate themselves before seeking safety.

Diving reflex. In response to cold water stimulation of the face and eyes, the diving reflex produces bradycardia, peripheral vasoconstriction and apnoea in most mammals. It is particularly well developed in diving mammals, to reduce oxygen consumption and facilitate long duration dives. The reflex is present in humans,[7] though of small magnitude compared with other species, and is believed to be more significant in infants than in adults.[3]

Physiological mechanisms of drowning

Glottic closure from inhaled water, pulmonary aspiration, cold shock and the diving response all influence the course of events following submersion in water; the relative importance of each depends, among many other factors, on the age of the victim and the temperature of the water. Conflicting influences on the heart from activation of both the parasympathetic (diving reflex) and sympathetic (cold shock response) systems are believed to contribute to death from cardiac dysrhythmia in some victims.[3]

Drowning without aspiration of water

This occurs in less than 10 per cent of drowning victims.[8] In thermoneutral water, when cold-stimulated reflexes will be minimal, the larynx is firmly closed during submersion and some victims will lose consciousness before water is aspirated.[9] Because of the difference in alveolar/mixed venous gas tension gradients, arterial Po_2 falls initially at almost ten times the rate of rise of arterial Pco_2. The subsequent rate of decrease depends mainly on the lung volume and the oxygen consumption. Oxygen stored in the alveolar gas after a maximal inspiration is unlikely to exceed 1 litre, and an oxygen consumption of $2\,l.min^{-1}$ would not be unusual in a subject either swimming or struggling (see Figure 14.1). Loss of consciousness from decreased alveolar Po_2 usually occurs very suddenly and without warning. The critical level is probably in the range 4–6 kPa (30–45 mmHg).

In cold water, hypoxia secondary to glottic closure may still occur. In addition, the cold shock and diving reflexes both leave the victim vulnerable to cardiovascular complications such as arrhythmias and sudden circulatory failure, leading to death before aspiration can occur. This is likely to be more common in elderly individuals.

Drowning with aspiration of water

Almost 90 per cent of drowning victims have aspirated significant volumes of water. Following sudden immersion in cold water the cold shock response is believed to be more common than the diving reflex, and hyperventilation rapidly leads to aspiration. In thermoneutral water, glottic closure may either be overcome by the conscious victim or will eventually subside due to hypoxia, and in both circumstances aspiration is likely to continue. Once aspiration occurs, reflex bronchospasm quickly follows, further worsening respiratory function.

Fresh water. Aspiration of fresh water further down the bronchial tree causes rapid and profound changes to the alveolar surfactant, leading to loss of the normal elastic properties of the alveoli and a disturbed ventilation/perfusion ratio. In fresh water drowning, alveolar water is quickly absorbed, resulting in alveolar collapse and a pulmonary shunt, this being in addition to the changes resulting from dilution of surfactant. A significant shunt is therefore quickly established, with resultant hypoxia. Some studies indicate that neurogenic pulmonary oedema due to cerebral hypoxia might coexist with alveolar flooding from aspirated water.[10,11] The distinction would clearly be difficult. One report cited a patient with severe pulmonary oedema thought to be a near-drowned victim but who, on careful enquiry, was found to have fractured his skull in a misjudged dive without having actually entered the water.[9] The pulmonary changes caused by immersion seem to be quickly reversible,[11] with good prospects of return to normal pulmonary function in those who survive near-drowning.[12]

Absorption of fresh water from the lungs results in haemodilution. This becomes significant when the aspirated water approaches 800 ml for a 70 kg man.[13] However, redistribution rapidly corrects the blood volume and there may even be hypovolaemia if pulmonary oedema supervenes. Haemodilution can theoretically result in haemolysis but dangerous changes in plasma electrolytes and the appearance of free haemoglobin are unusual, probably because most human victims inhale only small quantities of water.[10] Nevertheless, profound hyponatraemia (less than $100 \, \text{mmol.l}^{-1}$) may occur in infants drowned in fresh water.

Sea water. Sea water is hypertonic, having more than three times the osmolarity of blood. Consequently, sea water in the lungs is not initially absorbed and, on the contrary, draws fluid from the circulation into the alveoli. Thus, in laboratory animals that have aspirated sea water, it is possible to recover from the lungs 50 per cent more than the original volume that was inhaled.[14] This clearly maintains the proportion of flooded alveoli and results in a persistent shunt with reduction in arterial Po_2. However, surprisingly, sea water has less effect than fresh water on the surfactant that remains.[15]

Other material contaminating the lungs

It is not unusual for a drowning person to swallow large quantities of water and then to regurgitate or vomit. Material aspirated into the lungs may then be contaminated with gastric contents and the drowning syndrome complicated with features of the acid-aspiration syndrome. Aspiration of solid foreign bodies is a frequent complication of near-drowning in shallow rivers and lakes.

Post-mortem tests of drowning

There seems to be no conclusive test for aspiration of either fresh or sea water. One report reviewed and dismissed the use of tests based on differences in specific gravity and chloride content of plasma from the right and left chambers of the heart.[9] The demonstration of diatoms in bone marrow tissue is also controversial.[9] Recent work has shown the accuracy of the diatom test to be greatly improved if the type and size of diatoms found in the bone marrow are compared with those in a sample of the water in which the victim allegedly drowned.[16]

The role of hypothermia[3]

Some degree of hypothermia is usual in near-drowned victims, and body temperature is usually in the range 33–36°C.[17] Hypothermia-induced reduction in cerebral metabolism is protective during hypoxia and is believed to contribute to the numerous reports of survival after prolonged immersion in cold water. There have been reports of survival of near-drowned children trapped for periods as long as 40 minutes beneath ice. However, for the reasons outlined above, arterial hypoxia is believed to develop very quickly, and there is controversy surrounding how body temperature can decrease quickly enough to provide any degree of cerebral protection. Surface cooling is not believed to allow a rapid enough fall in temperature, as normal physiological responses to cold such as peripheral vasoconstriction and shivering limit the decline in temperature. Absorption of cold water either from the lungs or stomach will contribute to hypothermia during prolonged immersion, but quantitatively the volumes required are unlikely to be absorbed, particularly in sea water. Heat loss from the flushing of cold water in and out of the respiratory tract, without absorption occurring, is another possible explanation. Recent animal studies have shown that airway flushing with cold water reduces carotid artery blood temperature by several degrees within a few minutes,[18] which is sufficient to produce a useful reduction in cerebral oxygen requirement.

In spite of these potential benefits, hypothermia in most drowning victims probably does more harm than good. Consciousness is lost at around 32°C, making further aspiration almost inevitable, and ventricular fibrillation or asystole commonly occur at temperatures below 28°C. Once rescued, near-drowned patients should not be allowed to cool further before transport to hospital. Current practice is to rewarm the patient over a few hours and then to maintain normal temperature, except when hypothermia is indicated for treatment of brain damage.

Principles of treatment of near-drowning

There is a high measure of agreement on general principles of treatment.[3,8,10,16]

Immediate treatment

At the scene of the drowning, it can be very difficult to determine whether there has been cardiac or even respiratory arrest. However, there are many records of apparently dead victims who have recovered without evidence of brain damage after long periods of total immersion. It is therefore essential that cardiopulmonary resuscitation be undertaken in all victims until fully assessed in hospital, no matter how hopeless the outlook may appear.

Early treatment of near-drowning is crucial and this requires efficient instruction in resuscitation for people who may be available in locations where drowning is likely to occur. The normal priorities of airway clearance, artificial ventilation and chest compression (cardiac massage) should be observed. Out of hospital, mouth-to-mouth ventilation is the method of choice, but high inflation pressures are usually required when there has been flooding of the lungs. In sea water drowning it may be possible to drain water from the lungs by gravity but this is less important than the prompt institution of ventilation. Abdominal thrust (the Heimlich manoeuvre) may expel some water from the lungs, but is not generally recommended because of the risk of squeezing swallowed water out of the stomach, which may then be inhaled. Even without this manoeuvre, vomiting occurs in over 50 per cent of resuscitation procedures. Oxygen is clearly valuable if available and should be continued until hospital is reached. Most survivors will breathe spontaneously within 1–5 minutes after removal from the water. The decision to discontinue resuscitation should not be taken until assessment in hospital, particularly if the state of consciousness is confused by hypothermia.

Circulatory failure and loss of consciousness may occur when a victim is lifted from the water in a vertical position, as for example by a helicopter winch. This is probably due to the loss of water pressure resulting in relative redistribution of blood volume into the legs.

Hospital treatment

On arrival at the accident and emergency department of a hospital, victims should be triaged into the following categories:

1. Awake.
2. Blunted (but conscious).
3. Comatose.

There should be better than 90 per cent survival in the first two categories, but victims should still be admitted for observation and followed up after discharge. People who are comatose or hypoxic will require admission to intensive care. Treatment follows the general principles for hypoxic cerebral damage and aspiration lung injury. There may be late deterioration of pulmonary function – known as 'secondary drowning' – which is a form of the acute lung injury (see Chapter 30). If spontaneous breathing does not result in satisfactory levels of Po_2 and Pco_2, continuous positive airway pressure (CPAP) may be tried and is frequently useful. If this is unsuccessful, or in a patient with neurological impairment, artificial ventilation is required with or without positive end-expiratory pressure (PEEP).

References

1. Orlowski JP. Drowning, near-drowning and ice-water submersions. *Pediatr Clin North Am* 1987; **34**: 75–92.
2. Carey VF. Childhood drownings: who is responsible? *BMJ* 1993; **307**: 1086–7.
3. Golden FStC, Tipton MJ, Scott RC. Immersion, near-drowning and drowning. *Br J Anaesth* 1997; **79**: 214–25.
4. Howland J, Hingson R, Mangione TW, Bell N, Bak S. Why are most drowning victims men? Sex differences in aquatic skills and behaviors. *Am J Public Health* 1996; **86**: 93–6.
5. Wintemute GJ. Childhood drowning and near-drowning in the United States. *Am J Dis Child* 1990; **144**: 663–9.
6. Tipton MJ. The initial responses to cold water immersion in man. *Clin Sci* 1989; **77**: 581–8.
7. Schagatay E, Holm B. Effects of water and ambient air temperatures on human diving bradycardia. *Eur J Appl Physiol* 1996; **73**: 1–6.
8. Modell JH. Drowning. *N Engl J Med* 1993; **328**: 253–6.
9. Modell JH. Drowning. In: Staub NC, Taylor AE, eds. *Edema*. New York: Raven Press, 1984; 679.
10. Modell JH, Spohr RW. Drowning and near-drowning. In: Nunn JF, Utting JE, Brown BR, eds. *General anaesthesia*, 5th edn. London: Butterworths, 1989.
11. Rumbak MJ. The etiology of pulmonary edema in fresh water near drowning. *Am J Emerg Med* 1996; **14**: 176–9.
12. Butt MP, Jalowayski A, Modell JH, Giammona ST. Pulmonary function after resuscitation from near drowning. *Anesthesiology* 1970; **32**: 275–7.

13. Modell JH, Moya F. Effects of volume of aspirated fluid during chlorinated fresh water drowning. *Anesthesiology* 1966; **27**: 662–72.
14. Modell JH, Calderwood HW, Ruiz BC, Downs JB, Chapman R. Effects of ventilatory patterns on arterial oxygenation after near-drowning in sea water. *Anesthesiology* 1974; **40**: 376–84.
15. Giammona ST, Modell JH. Drowning by total immersion. Effects on pulmonary surfactant of distilled water, isotonic saline and sea water. *Am J Dis Child* 1967; **114**: 612–16.
16. Pollanen MS. The diagnostic value of the diatom test for drowning. II. Validity: analysis of diatoms in bone marrow and drowning medium. *J Forensic Sci* 1997; **42**: 286–90.
17. Pearn J. The management of near drowning. *BMJ* 1985; **291**: 1447–52.
18. Conn AW, Miyassaka K, Katayama M, Fujita M, Orima H, Barker G, Bohn D. A canine study of cold water drowning in fresh versus salt water. *Crit Care Med* 1995; **23**: 2029–36.

Chapter 20

Smoking and air pollution

The air we breathe is rarely a simple mixture of oxygen, nitrogen and water vapour. For much of the world's population air also contains a highly varied collection of other, more noxious, gases and particles. In addition, a substantial proportion of people choose to further contaminate the air they breathe with cigarette smoke.

Tobacco

In the Americas tobacco was used for medicinal purposes for many centuries before being introduced from the New World into Europe in the sixteenth century. Through his acquaintance with Queen Elizabeth I, Sir Walter Raleigh made smoking tobacco an essential fashionable activity of every gentleman. Thereafter the practice steadily increased in popularity until the explosive growth of the habit following the First World War (1914–1918). Particularly in the Second World War (1939–1945), large numbers of women adopted the habit.

There have always been those opposed to smoking, and King James I (1603–1625) described it as 'a custom loathsome to the eye, hateful to the nose, harmful to the brain and dangerous to the lungs'. However, firm evidence to support his last conclusion was delayed by some 350 years. Only relatively recently did it become clear that smokers had a higher mortality and that the causes of the excess mortality included lung cancer, chronic bronchitis, emphysema and cor pulmonale.[1,2,3] The proportion of the population who smoke has generally declined since evidence of serious health consequences emerged. Unfortunately, the proportion of young smokers has remained constant for some time, with currently 7 per cent of 15- to 16-year-olds in the UK regularly smoking more than 10 cigarettes a day.[4]

Constituents of tobacco smoke

More than 2000 potentially noxious constituents have been identified in tobacco smoke, some in the gaseous phase and others in the particulate or tar phase. The particulate phase is defined as the fraction eliminated by passing smoke through a Cambridge filter of pore size 0.1 μm. This is not to be confused with the 'filter tip', which allows passage of considerable quantities of particulate matter.

There is great variation in the yields of the different constituents between different brands and different types of cigarettes. This is achieved by using leaves of different species of plants, by varying the conditions of curing and cultivation and by using filter tips. Ventilated filters have a ring of small holes in the paper between the filter tip and the tobacco. These holes admit air during a puff and dilute all constituents of the smoke. By these means, it is possible to have wide variations in the different constituents of smoke, which do not bear a fixed relationship to one another. Quantities of constituents retained by the smoker are also influenced by the pattern of smoking (see below).

The gaseous phase. Carbon monoxide is present in cigarette smoke at a yield of between 15 and 25 mg (12 and 20 ml) per cigarette,[5] but levels as low as 1.8 mg have been achieved. The concentration issuing from the butt of the cigarette during a puff is in the range 1–5%, which is far into the toxic range. A better indication of the extent of carbon monoxide exposure is the percentage of carboxyhaemoglobin in blood. For non-smokers, the value is normally less than 1.5% but is influenced by exposure to air pollution and other people's cigarette smoke (see below). Typical values for smokers range from 2% to 12%. The value is influenced by the number of cigarettes smoked, the type of cigarette and the pattern of inhalation of smoke. Nevertheless, it remains the most reliable objective indication of smoke exposure and correlates well with most of the harmful effects of smoking (see below).

Tobacco smoke also contains very high concentrations (about 400 ppm) of the potential free radical nitric oxide[6] (page 499) and trace concentrations of nitrogen dioxide, the former being slowly oxidized to the latter in the presence of oxygen. The toxicity of these compounds is well known. Nitrogen dioxide hydrates in alveolar lining fluid to form an equimolecular mixture of nitrous and nitric acids. In addition, the nitrite ion converts haemoglobin to methaemoglobin.

Other constituents of the gaseous phase include hydrocyanic acid, cyanogen, aldehydes, ketones and volatile polynuclear aromatic hydrocarbons and nitrosamines.

The particulate phase. The material removed by a Cambridge filter is known as the 'total particulate matter', with aerosol particle size in the range 0.2–1 μm. The particulate phase comprises water, nicotine and 'tar'. Nicotine ranges from 0.05 to 2.5 mg per cigarette and 'tar' from 0.5 to 35 mg per cigarette. Yields of the main constituents of cigarette smoke are currently classified in the UK as set out in Table 20.1.

Individual smoke exposure

Individual smoke exposure is a complex function of the quantity of cigarettes that are smoked and the pattern of inhalation.

Table 20.1 Classification of tar content of British cigarettes (yields in mg per cigarette)

	Tar	Nicotine	Carbon monoxide
Low tar	<4–10	<0.3–1	<3–14
Low to medium tar	11–16	0.6–1.6	10–19
Medium tar	17–23	1.1–1.9	10–19
Medium to high tar	24–26	1.3–2.6	14–19

The quantity of cigarettes smoked

Exposure is usually quantified in 'pack years'. This equals the product of the number of packs (20 cigarettes) smoked per day, multiplied by the number of years that that pattern was maintained. The totals for each period are then summated for the lifetime of the subject.

There is good evidence that the habituated smoker adjusts his smoking pattern to maintain a particular blood level of nicotine.[7] For example, after changing to a brand with a lower nicotine yield, it is common practice to modify the pattern of inhalation to maximize nicotine absorption.

The pattern of inhalation

There are very wide variations in patterns of smoking. Air is normally drawn through the cigarette in a series of 'puffs' with a volume of about 25–50 ml per puff. The puff may be simply drawn into the mouth and rapidly expelled without appreciable inhalation. However, the habituated smoker will either inhale the puff directly into the lungs or, more commonly, pass the puff from the mouth to the lungs by inhaling air either through the mouth or else through the nose while passing the smoke from the mouth into the pharynx by apposing the tongue against the palate and so obliterating the gas space in the mouth. The inspiration is often especially deep, to flush into the lung any smoke remaining in the dead space.

It will be clear that the quantity of nicotine, tar and carbon monoxide obtainable from a single cigarette is highly variable, and the number and type of cigarettes smoked are not the sole determinants of effective exposure. Furthermore, retention by the lung is different for different constituents, being about 60% for carbon monoxide but as much as 90% for nicotine.

Respiratory effects of smoking

Cigarette smoking has extensive effects on respiratory function and is clearly implicated in the aetiology of a number of respiratory diseases, particularly emphysema, chronic bronchitis and bronchial carcinoma. The progress of emphysema is usually accelerated in smokers, who also have an increased susceptibility to respiratory infection.

Airway mucosa

Airway reflexes[8] are more sensitive in smokers when measured using either mechanical stimulation or inhalation of small concentrations of ammonia vapour. This increased sensitivity almost certainly contributes to the 'smoker's cough', and is believed to contribute to anaesthetic complications in smokers. Sensitivity takes several days to resolve following smoking abstinence. The concentration of inhaled histamine required to reduce specific airway conductance by 35% is, in smokers, less than 40% of that required in non-smokers.[9]

Ciliary function is inhibited by both particulate and gas phase compounds *in vitro*, but *in vivo* studies have given contradictory results, some studies showing increased ciliary activity in response to cigarette smoke.[10]

Mucus production[10] is increased in chronic smokers, who have hyperplasia of submucosal glands and increased numbers of goblet cells even when asymptomatic. In spite of the inconsistent findings regarding ciliary activity, mucus clearance is universally found to be impaired in smokers, which, coupled with increased mucus production and airway sensitivity, gives rise to the normally productive 'smoker's cough'. Three months after smoking cessation, many of these changes are reversed except in patients who have developed airway damage from chronic bronchitis.

Airway diameter

Airway diameter is reduced acutely with smoking as a result of reflex bronchoconstriction in response to inhaled particles and the increased production of mucus already described. Airway narrowing is greatest in subjects with known bronchial hypersensitivity, such as asthmatics. The long-term impact on the mucosa of small airways causes chronic airway narrowing that has a multitude of effects on lung function. Airway narrowing promotes premature airway closure during expiration, which results in an increase in closing volume and disturbed ventilation/perfusion relationships. Distribution of inspired gas as indicated by the single-breath nitrogen test (page 168) is therefore often abnormal in smokers. Small airway narrowing over many years gives rise to a progressive reduction in the forced expiratory volume in one second (FEV_1) described below. Many of these changes are at an advanced stage before smokers develop respiratory symptoms.

Ventilatory capacity[11]

FEV_1 normally reaches a peak in early adulthood, remains constant for some years and then declines steadily as the subject grows older (Figure 20.1). Longitudinal studies of FEV_1 in smokers reveal a very different picture, illustrated in Figure 20.1. Most smokers begin smoking in early adulthood, and the rate of increase of FEV_1 immediately slows, resulting in a delayed and lower plateau. The plateau in FEV_1 is also shorter, before a more rapid decline begins. Smoking cessation is followed by a small improvement in FEV_1, followed by a return to the normal rate of decline, but rarely demonstrates a return to non-smoker values. Similar pictures almost certainly exist for other measures of expiratory lung function such as mean expiratory flow rate at 25 per cent of a forced vital capacity. Eventually, this decline in lung function results in lung pathology, with one in every five smokers developing chronic obstructive pulmonary disease. The Report of the US Surgeon General (1984) concluded that cigarette smoking was the major cause of morbidity in chronic obstructive pulmonary disease in the USA, and that 80–90 per cent of cases were attributable to cigarette smoking.

Alveolar/capillary barrier function

The integrity of the alveolar/capillary barrier is impaired by smoking. The most sensitive indication of impaired respiratory function in smokers is the clearance of ^{99m}Tc-DTPA from the alveoli into the blood.[12] The mean half-time of clearance was 59 minutes in non-smokers but only 20 minutes in smokers, with almost total separation of the two groups. This change occurs in all smokers, including young and asymptomatic smokers in whom all other pulmonary function tests are normal. Clearance is increased within days of starting smoking and returns to a plateau value about 70 per cent of normal within a week of stopping smoking.[13]

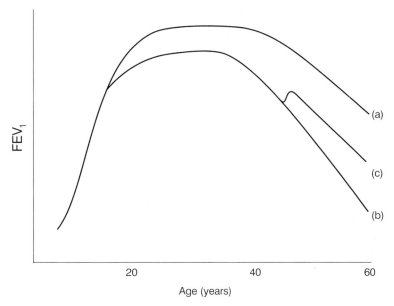

Figure 20.1 Schematic diagram showing the effects of smoking on normal lifelong changes in the forced expiratory volume in one second (FEV_1). (a) Normal changes; (b) smoking begins at age 16 years; (c) smoking stopped at 45 years of age. See text for details.

Other effects on respiratory function

Smokers have a significantly increased V_D/V_T ratio, with values of 37 per cent (upright) and 32 per cent (supine), compared with 29 per cent (upright) and 26 per cent (supine) for non-smokers.[14] Smokers were evenly distributed among their age groups. Carbon monoxide-diffusing capacity is slightly reduced in heavy smokers.[15]

In view of the presence of nitric oxide in cigarette smoke, an effect on pulmonary blood vessels would be expected. A study of a single subject showed that cigarette smoke does indeed reverse hypoxic pulmonary vasoconstriction, to a similar degree as 80 ppm of inhaled nitric oxide (page 584).[16]

Mechanisms of smoking-related lung damage

Many of the compounds present in cigarette smoke have direct irritant and toxic effects on the lungs. There are three other mechanisms by which lung damage occurs.

Oxidative injury[6,17,18]

There is compelling evidence for believing that oxidative injury, including peroxidation of membrane lipids, is an important component of the pulmonary damage caused by cigarette smoking.

Direct oxidative damage. The tar phase contains quinone, the semiquinone free radical and hydroquinone in a polymeric matrix, and the gas phase contains nitric oxide. These compounds can reduce oxygen in the body, to yield the superoxide free radical and thence the highly damaging hydroxyl free radical (see Figure 25.3).[6]

Cell-mediated oxidative damage results from smoking-induced activation of, or enhancement of, neutrophil and macrophage activity in the respiratory tract. Broncho-alveolar lavage in humans has shown that smokers have larger numbers of intra-alveolar macrophages and also significant numbers of neutrophils that are not normally present in non-smokers.[19] It is the particulate component of smoke that is responsible for the recruitment and activation of neutrophils in the alveoli. This suggests that the interaction of particulate matter and alveolar macrophages releases a neutrophil chemattractant and that neutrophils are subsequently activated to release either proteases or oxygen-derived free radicals. This activation may be a direct response to cigarette smoke or may represent excessive free radical production in response to minor infective challenge in smokers.

Evidence of *in vivo* oxidative stress in smokers' lungs is based mainly on measures of antioxidant activity. Compared with non-smokers, human smokers have reduced levels of vitamin E in alveolar fluid, reduced plasma concentrations of vitamin C, and greatly increased superoxide dismutase and catalase activity in alveolar macrophages.

Carcinogenesis[20]

Smoking contributes to the development of cancer in many organs, but the respiratory tract clearly receives substantial exposure to tobacco smoke carcinogens. There are two groups of compounds with carcinogenic activity, found mostly in the tar of the particulate phase. Some hydrocarbons, in particular polynuclear aromatic hydrocarbons (PAH), are carcinogenic, whilst others such as aromatic phenols (phenol, indole and catechol) are co-carcinogens and tumour promoters, without which the carcinogenic compounds are relatively innocuous. Tobacco-related nitrosamines and nicotine derivatives are also carcinogenic and, because of their ease of absorption into the blood, are responsible for cancer formation not only in the respiratory tract and oesophagus but also in more distant organs such as the pancreas. Knowledge about these carcinogens has led to many attempts to reduce their concentration in smoke by modifying the cigarette, and tar levels in cigarettes have declined almost threefold since 1955. Cellulose in filter tips reduces nitrosamine yields, and the addition of nitrate to tobacco reduces PAH yield but unfortunately increases nitrosamine levels. The filter-tip cigarette reduces particulate matter, and is particularly effective when provided with air holes to dilute all constituents of the smoke. Although smokers modify their smoking pattern to account for this,[7] prolonged use of 'low-tar' cigarettes does reduce an individual's cancer risk.

Smoking cessation remains the best way of preventing smoking-related cancers. For people who cannot achieve this goal, some early (mostly animal) research has identified several strategies which may reduce cancer risk, including ingestion of beta-carotene and a reduction in dietary fat.[20]

Immunological activation[21]

Smokers have elevated serum IgE levels compared with non-smokers, the cause of which is uncertain but may be twofold. Direct toxicity and oxidative cell damage result in greater airway mucosal cell permeability, allowing better access for allergens to underlying immunologically active cells. Smoking also increases the activity of some T-lymphocyte subsets that are responsible for producing interleukin-4, a cytokine well known for stimulating IgE production.

These observations thus raise the possibility that an 'allergic' mechanism is responsible for smoking-related changes in lung function, such as small airway narrowing. An association between IgE levels and impaired lung function is well established in asthma, but has been less consistently seen in non-asthmatic smokers except in older subjects. Thus causality between smoking and an IgE-mediated mechanism is far from established. It is possible that smoking sensitizes the airway to 'new' allergens, and that this contributes to the development of chronic airways disease seen in some smokers.

Passive smoking

The non-smoker is exposed to all constituents of smoke when indoors in the presence of smokers. Exposure varies with many factors, including size and ventilation of the room, number of people smoking and absorption of smoke constituents on soft furnishings and clothing. Carbon monoxide concentrations of 20 ppm have been reported, which is above the recommended environmental concentration (see below). It has been estimated that non-smokers are exposed to quantities of 'tar' ranging from zero to 14 mg per day.[22] 'Side-stream' smoke from a smouldering cigarette stub produces greater quantities of potentially noxious substances than 'main-stream' smoke produced when a cigarette burns in a stream of air drawn through it during a puff. On average, 'side-stream' smoke is generated during 58 seconds in each minute of cigarette smoking, and this is not included in the measured yield of a cigarette.

The respiratory effects of passive smoking begin *in utero*.[23] In addition to lower birth weight, infants born to mothers who smoked during pregnancy have increased levels of IgE[24] and reduced expiratory flows,[25] even before leaving hospital, when exposure to cigarette smoke begins.[26] Up to 2 years of age, infants with smoking parents have more respiratory tract illnesses; when older, they have reduced lung volumes, higher carboxyhaemoglobin levels and a greater likelihood of developing asthma.[11,27,28] Recent studies indicate that maternal smoking during pregnancy may be mainly responsible for these differences throughout childhood.[29]

Evidence for respiratory effects of passive smoking in adults is much less clear, but the increased risk of passive smokers developing lung cancer is now undisputed.[30]

Smoking and perioperative complications[31]

The increased sensitivity of the airway to inhaled irritants seen in smokers causes a greater incidence of adverse events such as cough, breath hold or laryngospasm on induction of general anaesthesia, even in passive smokers.[32] These complications are not necessarily associated with decreases in oxygen saturation, although episodes of desaturation in the recovery period may be more common in smokers, or even in passively smoking children.[28] It is worth noting once again that commercially available pulse oximeters record carboxyhaemoglobin as if it were oxyhaemoglobin (page 297), and so will consistently overestimate oxygen saturation in recent smokers.

There is ample evidence that smokers have an increased incidence of postoperative respiratory complications, which are between two and six times more common in smokers, depending on the definitions used and type of surgery undertaken.[33,34] This is attributable both to increased secretion and impaired clearance of mucus and to small airway narrowing. Almost all studies of the perioperative effects of smoking have been undertaken in patients having major surgery, usually coronary artery revascularization or upper abdominal surgery. The high incidence of respiratory complications in this group makes them an ideal study population, but there remains little information regarding the respiratory effects of perioperative smoking and more minor surgery.

Preoperative smoking cessation is vital.[33,34] Nicotine, which is responsible for many untoward cardiovascular changes, has a half-life of only 30 minutes, whilst carboxyhaemoglobin has a half-life of 4 hours when breathing air. A smoking fast of just a few hours will therefore effectively remove the risks associated with carbon monoxide and nicotine. Airway reflexes take a few days to return to normal.[8] The incidence of respiratory complications after major surgery is reduced to that of non-smokers only by over eight weeks' abstinence. Furthermore, there is some evidence that surgery performed within this eight-week period is associated with a greater complication rate than if the patient had continued to smoke until 12 hours before the operation.[33]

Air pollution[35]

Fossil fuels have formed the major source of energy for society for many centuries, and continue to do so today. Detrimental effects of air pollution were first recognized in the thirteenth century, though it is only in the last 50 years that effective control of pollution has been achieved. In spite of these controls, increased overall energy requirements and the internal combustion engine have ensured that air pollution remains a problem. Production of carbon dioxide is not considered as pollution; its effects on the atmosphere are discussed in Chapter 1.

Sources of pollutants

Primary pollutants are substances that are released into the atmosphere directly from the polluting source, and are mostly derived from the combustion of fossil fuels. Petrol engines that ignite the fuel in an oxygen-restricted environment produce varying quantities of carbon monoxide, nitrogen oxides and hydrocarbons such as benzene and polycyclic aromatic compounds. All of these pollutants are reduced by the use of a catalytic converter. In contrast, diesel engines burn fuel with an excess of oxygen and so produce little carbon monoxide but more nitrogen oxides and particulate matter. Burning of coal and oil is now restricted almost entirely to power generation, and the pollutants produced depend on the type of fuel used and the amount of effort expended on 'cleaning' the emissions. However, particulates and nitrogen oxides are invariably produced, and power generation remains the major source of sulphur dioxide.

Secondary pollutants are formed in the atmosphere from chemical changes to primary pollutants. Nitric oxide produced from vehicle engines is quickly converted to nitrogen dioxide, and in doing so may react with ozone, reducing the atmospheric concentration of the latter. Alternatively, when exposed to sunlight in the lower atmosphere, both nitric oxide and nitrogen dioxide react with oxygen to produce ozone (O_3).[36]

Meteorological conditions have an enormous influence on air pollution. In conditions of strong wind, pollutants are quickly dispersed; in cloudy weather the development of secondary pollutants is unlikely. Ground level pollution in urban areas is exacerbated by clear, calm weather, when 'temperature inversion' can occur. On a clear night, heat is lost from the ground to the atmosphere by radiation and the ground level air cools dramatically (Figure 20.2a). At dawn the ground is quickly heated by the sun's radiation and warms the

(a)
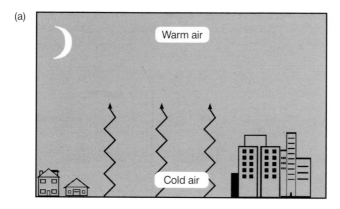

(b)
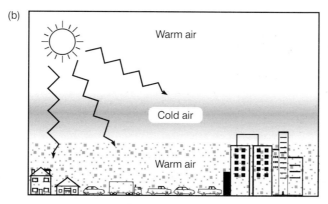

Figure 20.2 Temperature inversion producing pollution in the morning rush hour. (a) At night the ground loses heat to the atmosphere by radiation, and ground level air cools. (b) In the morning, with strong sun and still conditions, the ground heats up quickly and displaces the blanket of cold air upwards, so preventing effective air mixing and trapping vehicular pollution at ground level.

air, which lifts a blanket of cool air to about 50–100 m high. Because in still conditions mixing of air masses is slow to occur, the relatively cold air sits on top of the warm air below. In the meantime, the morning rush hour produces large amounts of pollutants that are unable to disperse and become trapped near the ground (Figure 20.2b)

Respiratory effects of pollutants[35,36,37,38]

Recommended maximum levels of common pollutants are listed in Table 20.2. The extent to which these levels are achieved varies greatly between different countries and from year to year. Almost 20 million residents of the USA are thought to be regularly exposed to pollutant levels greater than the nationally agreed maxima.[37] Air pollution is now believed to be a significant public health problem, a recent report indicating that between 12 000 and 24 000 deaths per year in the UK are attributable to pollution.[35]

Carbon monoxide. Carbon monoxide is found in trace concentrations in the blood of patients, partly as a result of its production in the body but mainly as a result of smoking

Table 20.2 Recommended air quality standards

Pollutant	Duration of exposure		
	Short (≤ 1 hour)	Moderate (8–24 hours)	Annual
Ozone	76–110 ppb	50–60 ppb	
Particulates (PM_{10})		150 µg.m^{-3}	50 µg.m^{-3}
Sulphur dioxide	175 ppb	45 ppb	17 ppb
Nitrogen dioxide	110 ppb	80 ppb	21 ppb
Carbon monoxide	25–87 ppm	10 ppm	

Figures are derived from World Health Organization air quality guidelines, except those for particulates which are from the National Ambient Air Quality Standards in the USA.[35,37] ppb, parts per billion; ppm, parts per million.

and air pollution. One study reported carboxyhaemoglobin levels of 0.4–9.7% in London taxi drivers but the highest level in a non-smoking driver was 3%.[39] Maternal smoking results in appreciable levels of carboxyhaemoglobin in fetal blood,[40] and smoking prior to blood donation may result in levels of carboxyhaemoglobin up to 10% in the blood that seem to persist throughout the usual three weeks of storage.[41] Carboxyhaemoglobin levels greater than 3% impair exercise capacity in subjects with ischaemic heart disease, and levels over 5% limit exercise in healthy subjects and impair vigilance.

The amount of carboxyhaemoglobin formed when breathing air polluted with carbon monoxide will depend on the subject's minute volume. The recommended levels shown in Table 20.2 are calculated to result in a carboxyhaemoglobin concentration of less than 2.5% even during moderate exercise. Carbon monoxide levels similar to those seen in smokers are likely to occur only during episodes of severe pollution.

Nitrogen dioxide is mainly a primary pollutant, but a small amount is produced from nitric oxide. In the UK, about half of atmospheric nitrogen dioxide is derived from vehicles. Indoor levels of nitrogen dioxide commonly exceed outdoor levels, and the respiratory effects of nitrogen dioxide are therefore described in the next section.

Ozone is a secondary pollutant formed by the action of sunlight on nitrogen oxides, and therefore highest levels tend to occur in rural areas downwind from cities and roads. In all areas, the dependence on sunlight means that ozone levels slowly increase throughout the day, reaching peak levels shortly after the evening rush hour. Ozone is toxic to the respiratory tract, with effects being dependent on both concentration and duration of exposure. Exposure to concentrations of 80–100 ppb for just a few hours commonly causes throat irritation, chest discomfort and cough, presumably through stimulation of irritant receptors in the airway. Bronchoconstriction may occur accompanied by a decrease in FEV_1, and exercise capacity is limited. Repeated daily exposure to ozone (200 ppb), which is common in susceptible areas, causes a gradual reduction in the response.[42] There is also large variability between individuals in their spirometric response to ozone, with about 10 per cent of subjects having a severe response. It is interesting that laboratory studies have failed to demonstrate that asthmatic subjects are more susceptible to ozone-induced pulmonary symptoms. Even so, there is good evidence that high concentrations of atmospheric ozone are associated with increased hospital attendance and admission rates for respiratory problems. Ozone therefore seems to present a respiratory challenge to some subjects, with or without asthma, even at modest atmospheric levels.

Sulphur dioxide. Declining use of coal has substantially reduced the production of sulphur dioxide over recent years, and two-thirds of production in the UK now originates from oil-burning power stations. Normal atmospheric levels have no short-term effect on healthy subjects, but asthmatic patients may develop bronchoconstriction at between 100 and 250 ppb.

Particulate matter consists of a mixture of soot, liquid droplets, recondensed metallic vapours and organic debris. Only particles of less than 10 μm diameter are considered to be 'inhalable' into the lung, so particulate pollution is measured as the concentration of particles less than this diameter, known as PM_{10}. The disparate nature of particulate pollution reflects its very varied origins, but in the urban environment, diesel engines are a major source. Acute effects of particles on lung function again include airway irritation and small reductions in lung volumes such as FVC.[43] It is, however, associations between PM_{10} levels and overall mortality that have been the focus of much recent research. Even when smoking habits are taken into account, particulate pollution is associated with an increased risk of death from lung cancer or other cardiopulmonary diseases.[44]

Indoor air pollution[45]

Energy-efficient homes have become the norm in recent years, with effective heating systems and extensive insulation. This has led to dramatic changes in indoor air quality, including warmer temperatures, higher humidity levels and reduced ventilation. Indoor air quality still generally reflects that of the outdoor air except that ozone levels are invariably low indoors owing to the rapid reaction of ozone with the synthetic materials that make up much of the indoor environment. In addition to pollutants from outside, there are two specific indoor pollutants.

Allergens. Warm moist air, poor ventilation and extensive floor coverings provide ideal conditions for house dust mite infestation and the retention of numerous other allergens. This is believed to contribute to the recent upsurge in the prevalence of atopic diseases such as asthma, and is discussed in Chapter 27.

Nitrogen dioxide. Gas-fired cookers, stoves and boilers all produce NO_2, the amount being dependent on the arrangements for waste gas exclusion. In this respect, gas cookers are the worst culprits, as they are rarely associated with chimneys and flues and normally discharge their waste gases directly into the kitchen atmosphere. During cooking, NO_2 levels may reach over 400 ppb, which is well in excess of outdoor pollution targets (Table 20.2). Mild airway irritant reactions are seen at levels of around 300 ppb in asthmatic subjects, or at 1000 ppb in non-asthmatic subjects,[35] so significant reactions are probably uncommon. However, animal studies have revealed that, at higher concentrations of NO_2, pulmonary epithelial integrity may be breached and the susceptibility of the lung to infection increased.[46] One epidemiological study did find an association between use of gas cookers and reduced FEV_1, but only in women.[47] In addition, the decline in lung function was greater in atopic women, indicating that NO_2 may mediate part of its effects on lung function via an immunological mechanism similar to that recently suggested for smoking (page 412).

References

1. Doll R, Peto M. Mortality in relation to smoking: 20 years' observations on male British doctors. *BMJ* 1976; **2**: 1525–36.
2. Doll R, Hill AB. Smoking and carcinoma of the lung. *BMJ* 1950; **2**: 739–48.
3. Anderson DO, Ferris BG. Role of tobacco smoking in the causation of chronic respiratory disease. *N Engl J Med* 1962; **267**: 787–94.
4. Miller PMcC, Plant M. Drinking, smoking, and illicit drug use among 15 and 16 year olds in the United Kingdom. *BMJ* 1996; **313**: 394–7.
5. Borland C, Chamberlain A, Higenbottam T, Shipley M, Rose G. Carbon monoxide yield of cigarettes and its relation to cardiorespiratory disease. *BMJ* 1983; **287**: 1583–6.
6. Church DF, Pryor WA. The oxidative stress placed on the lung by cigarette smoke. In: Crystal RG, West JB, eds. *The lung: scientific foundations.* New York: Raven, 1991; 1975–9.
7. Ashton H, Stepney R, Thompson PW. Self-titration by cigarette smokers. *BMJ* 1979; **2**: 357–60.
8. Erskine RJ, Murphy PJ, Langton JA. Sensitivity of upper airway reflexes in cigarette smokers: effect of abstinence. *Br J Anaesth* 1994; **73**: 298–302.
9. Gerrard JW, Cockcroft DW, Mink JT, Cotton DJ, Poonawala R, Dosman JA. Increased nonspecific bronchial reactivity in cigarette smokers with normal lung function. *Am Rev Respir Dis* 1980; **122**: 577–81.
10. Wanner A, Salathe M, O'Riordan TG. Mucociliary clearance in the airways. *Am J Respir Crit Care Med* 1996; **154**: 1868–902.
11. Samet JM, Lange P. Longitudinal studies of active and passive smoking. *Am J Respir Crit Care Med* 1996; **154**: S257–65.
12. Jones JG, Minty BD, Lawler P, Hulands G, Crawley JCW, Veall N. Increased alveolar epithelial permeability in cigarette smokers. *Lancet* 1980; **1**: 66–7.
13. Minty BD, Jordan C, Jones JG. Rapid improvement in abnormal pulmonary epithelial permeability after stopping cigarettes. *BMJ* 1981; **282**: 1183–6.
14. Craig DB, Wahba WM, Don HF, Couture JG, Becklake MR. 'Closing volume' and its relationship to gas exchange in seated and supine positions. *J Appl Physiol* 1971; **31**: 717–21.
15. Tockman M, Menkes H, Cohen B, Permutt S, Benjamin J, Ball WC, Tonascia J. A comparison of pulmonary function in male smokers and non-smokers. *Am Rev Respir Dis* 1976; **114**: 711–22.
16. Dupuy PM, Lançon J-P, Françoise M, Frostell CG. Inhaled cigarette smoke selectively reverses human hypoxic vasoconstriction. *Intensive Care Med* 1995; **21**: 941–4.
17. Chow CK. Cigarette smoking and oxidative damage in the lung. *Ann N Y Acad Sci* 1993; **686**: 289–98.
18. McCusker K. Mechanisms of respiratory tissue injury from cigarette smoking. *Am J Med* 1992; **93** (Supp 1A): 18S–21S.
19. Hunninghake GW, Crystal RG. Cigarette smoking and lung destruction. Accumulation of neutrophils in the lungs of cigarette smokers. *Am Rev Respir Dis* 1983; **128**: 833–8.
20. Hoffman D, Rivenson A, Chung F-L, Wynder EL. Potential inhibitors of tobacco carcinogenesis. *Ann N Y Acad Sci* 1993; **686**: 140–60.
21. Villar MTA, Holgate ST. IgE, smoking and lung function. *Clin Exp Allergy* 1995; **25**: 206–9.
22. Rapace JL, Lowrey AH. Tobacco smoke, ventilation and indoor air quality. *Am Soc Heating, Refrigerating and Air-conditioning Engineers, Inc Trans* 1982; **88**: 895.
23. Morgan WJ, Martinez FD. Maternal smoking and infant lung function: Further evidence for an *in utero* effect. *Am J Respir Crit Care Med* 1998; **158**: 689–90.
24. Magnusson CGM. Maternal smoking influences cord serum IgE and IgD levels and increases the risk for subsequent infant allergy. *J Allergy Clin Immunol* 1986; **78**: 898–904.
25. Hanrahan JP, Tager IB, Segal MR, Tosteson TD, Castile RG, Van Vunakis H et al. The effect of maternal smoking during pregnancy on early infant lung function. *Am Rev Respir Dis* 1992; **145**: 1129–35.
26. Hoo AF, Henschen M, Dezateux C, Costeloe K, Stocks J. Respiratory function among preterm infants whose mothers smoked during pregnancy. *Am J Respir Crit Care Med* 1998; **158**: 700–5.
27. Gidding SJ, Morgan W, Perry C, Isabel-Jones J, Bricker JT. Active and passive tobacco exposure: a serious pediatric health problem. *Circulation* 1994; **90**: 2581–90.
28. Lyons B, Frizelle H, Kirby F, Casey W. The effect of passive smoking on the incidence of airway complications in children undergoing general anaesthesia. *Anaesthesia* 1996; **51**: 324–6.

29. Cunningham J, Dockery DW, Speizer FE. Maternal smoking during pregnancy as a predictor of lung function in children. *Am J Epidemiol* 1994; **139**: 1139–52.
30. Trichopoulos D, Mollo F, Tomatis L, Agapitos E, Delsedime L, Zavitsanos X et al. Active and passive smoking and pathological indicators of lung cancer risk in an autopsy study. *JAMA* 1992; **268**: 1697–701.
31. Nel MR, Morgan M. Smoking and anaesthesia revisited. *Anaesthesia* 1996; **51**: 309–11.
32. Dennis A, Curran J, Sherriff J, Kinnear W. Effects of passive and active smoking on induction of anaesthesia. *Br J Anaesth* 1994; **73**: 450–2.
33. Egan TD, Wong KC. Perioperative smoking cessation and anesthesia: a review. *J Clin Anesth* 1992; **4**: 63–72.
34. Pearce AC, Jones RM. Smoking and anesthesia: preoperative abstinence and perioperative morbidity. *Anesthesiology* 1984; **61**: 576–84.
35. Committee on the Medical Effects of Air Pollutants. *Handbook on air pollution and health.* London: Stationery Office, 1997.
36. Tattersfield AE. Air pollution: brown skies research. *Thorax* 1996; **51**: 13–22.
37. Committee of the environmental and occupational health assembly of the American Thoracic Society. Health effects of outdoor air pollution. *Am J Respir Crit Care Med* 1996; **153**: 3–50.
38. Committee on the Medical Effects of Air Pollution. *The quantification of the effects of air pollution on health in the United Kingdom.* London: Stationery Office, 1998.
39. Jones RD, Commins BT, Cernik AA. Blood lead and carboxyhaemoglobin levels in London taxi drivers. *Lancet* 1972; **2**: 302–3.
40. Longo LD. Carbon monoxide in the pregnant mother and fetus and its exchange across the placenta. *Ann N Y Acad Sci* 1970; **174**: 313–41.
41. Millar RA, Gregory IC. Reduced oxygen content in equilibrated fresh heparinised and ACD-stored blood from cigarette smokers. *Br J Anaesth* 1972; **44**: 1015–19.
42. Christian DL, Chen LL, Scannell CH, Ferrando RE, Welch BS, Balmes JR. Ozone-induced inflammation is attenuated with multiday exposure. *Am J Respir Crit Care Med* 1998; **158**: 532–7.
43. Scarlett JF, Abbott KJ, Peacock JL, Strachan DP, Anderson HR. Acute effects of summer air pollution on respiratory function in primary school children in southern England. *Thorax* 1996; **51**: 1109–14.
44. Dockery DW, Pope CA, Xu X, Spengler JD, Ware JH, Fay ME et al. An association between air pollution and mortality in six US cities. *N Engl J Med* 1993; **329**: 1753–9.
45. Alberts WM. Indoor air pollution: NO, NO_2, CO, and CO_2. *J Allergy Clin Immunol* 1994; **94**: 289–95.
46. Fuhlbrigge A, Weiss S. Domestic gas appliances and lung disease. *Thorax* 1997; **52** (Supp 3): S58–62.
47. Jarvis D, Chinn S, Luczynska C, Burney P. Association of respiratory symptoms and lung function in young adults with use of domestic gas appliances. *Lancet* 1996; **347**: 426–31.

Chapter 21

Anaesthesia

Only 12 years after the first successful public demonstration of general anaesthesia in 1846, John Snow reported the pronounced changes that occur in respiration during the inhalation of chloroform.[1] Subsequent observations have confirmed that anaesthesia has profound effects on the respiratory system. However, these effects are diverse and highly specific, some aspects of respiratory function being profoundly modified while others are scarcely affected at all.

Control of breathing[2]

Unstimulated ventilation

It has long been known that anaesthesia may diminish pulmonary ventilation, and hypercapnia is commonplace if spontaneous breathing is preserved. Reduced minute volume is due partly to a reduction in metabolic demand but mainly to interference with the chemical control of breathing, in particular a reduced sensitivity to CO_2 as described below. In an uncomplicated anaesthetic, there should not be sufficient resistance to breathing to affect the minute volume. However, the minute volume may be much decreased if there is overt respiratory obstruction.

At lower concentrations of inhaled anaesthetics, minute volume may remain unchanged, but smaller tidal volumes with higher respiratory frequency often occur, resulting in reduced alveolar ventilation and an increase in $P\text{CO}_2$. With higher concentrations of anaesthetic breathing becomes slower and spontaneous minute volume may decrease to very low levels, particularly in the absence of surgical stimulation. This will inevitably result in hypercapnia, and end-expiratory $P\text{CO}_2$ commonly rises to 10 kPa (75 mmHg). Clearly there is no limit to the rise that may occur if the anaesthetist is prepared to tolerate gross hypoventilation, and one study reported arterial $P\text{CO}_2$ values up to 20 kPa (150 mmHg) during closed-circuit halothane anaesthesia (not administered by the authors!).[3]

There are anaesthetists in many parts of the world, including the UK, who do not believe that temporary hypercapnia during anaesthesia is harmful to a healthy patient. In normal circumstances, arterial $P\text{CO}_2$ rapidly returns to normal in the postoperative period.[4] Many hundreds of millions of patients must have been subjected to this transient physiological trespass since 1846, and there seems to be no convincing evidence of harm resulting from it – except perhaps increased bleeding from the incision. In other parts of the world, particularly the USA, the departure from physiological normality is regarded with concern and it is usual either to assist spontaneous respiration by manual compression of the reservoir bag or, more commonly, to paralyse and ventilate artificially as a routine.

Quite different conditions apply during anaesthesia with artificial ventilation. The minute volume can then be set at any level that seems appropriate to the anaesthetist; in the past there was a tendency to hyperventilate patients, resulting in hypocapnia. Routine monitoring of end-expiratory P_{CO_2} has radically altered the control of minute volume during anaesthesia. Artificial ventilation can very easily be adjusted to maintain the target P_{CO_2} selected by the anaesthetist. This is more satisfactory than monitoring ventilatory volumes, because the patient's metabolic rate and dead space are not usually known.

Effect on P_{CO_2}/ventilation response curve (see page 95)

Progressive increases in the alveolar concentration of all inhalational anaesthetic agents decrease the slope of the P_{CO_2}/ventilation response curve and, at deep levels of anaesthesia, there may be no response at all to P_{CO_2}. Furthermore, the anaesthetized patient, as opposed to the awake subject, always becomes apnoeic if the P_{CO_2} is reduced below this intercept, which is known as the apnoeic threshold P_{CO_2} (page 96). In Figure 21.1, the flat curve rising to the left represents the starting points for various P_{CO_2}/ventilation response curves. Without added carbon dioxide in the inspired gas, deepening anaesthesia is associated with a decreasing ventilation and a rising P_{CO_2}, points moving progressively down and to the right. At intervals along this curve are

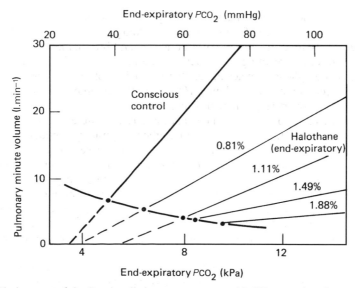

Figure 21.1 Displacement of the P_{CO_2}/ventilation response curve with different end-expiratory concentrations of halothane. The curve sloping down to the right indicates the pathway of P_{CO_2} and ventilation change resulting from depression without the challenge of exogenous carbon dioxide. The broken lines indicate extrapolation to apnoeic threshold P_{CO_2}. (The curves have been constructed from the data of reference 5.)

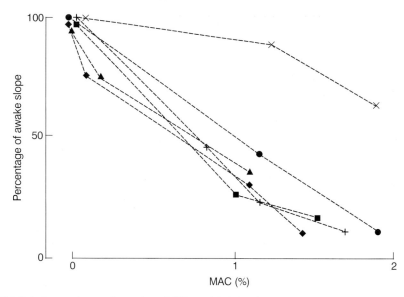

Figure 21.2 Relative respiratory depression of different inhalational anaesthetics as a function of minimum alveolar concentration (MAC). ●, halothane; ▲, enflurane; ■, isoflurane; ◆, sevoflurane; +, desflurane; ×, diethylether. (Data from references 6, 7 and 8.)

shown P_{CO_2}/ventilation response curves resulting from adding carbon dioxide to the inspired gas.

Anaesthetics differ quantitatively in their capacity to depress the response of ventilation to P_{CO_2}. This is conveniently shown by plotting the slope of the P_{CO_2}/ventilation response curve against equi-anaesthetic concentrations of different anaesthetics (Figure 21.2), shown as multiples of minimum alveolar concentration (MAC), although the validity of using MAC multiples in this way has been questioned. The halogenated agents do not differ greatly from one another but diethyl ether is exceptional in having little effect up to 1 MAC. Thereafter the effect increases markedly with increasing concentrations until, at 2.5 MAC, the extrapolated value seems to be comparable to the halogenated agents. Anaesthesia with diethyl ether causes an increase in the level of circulating catecholamines, which may counteract the depressant effect of the anaesthetic.

Surgical stimulation antagonizes the effect of anaesthesia on the P_{CO_2}/ventilation response curve (Figure 21.3). It may easily be observed that a surgical incision increases the ventilation, whatever the depth of anaesthesia, provided that spontaneous breathing is still present. During prolonged anaesthesia without surgical stimulation, there is no progressive change in the response curve for up to 3 hours, but some return towards the preanaesthetic position has been reported after 6 hours.[9] With the exception of ketamine, intravenous anaesthetics have effects on ventilation similar to those of the inhalational anaesthetics.

Ventilatory response to metabolic acidaemia. The ventilatory response to non-respiratory changes in arterial pH has been described on page 97. This response is also obtunded by anaesthesia and possibly even by subanaesthetic concentrations of anaesthetics.[11]

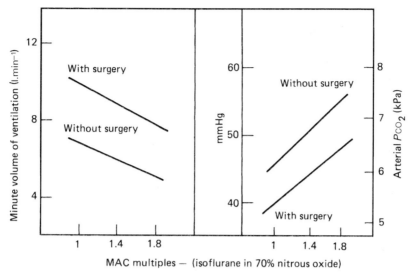

Figure 21.3 Respiratory depression by isoflurane with and without surgery at different multiples of minimum alveolar concentration (MAC) required for anaesthesia. (Drawn from data of reference 10.)

Effect on P_{O_2}/ventilation response curve

The normal relationship between P_{O_2} and ventilation has been described on pages 96 *et seq*. It was long believed that this reflex was the *ultima moriens* and, unlike the P_{CO_2}/ventilation response curve, unaffected by anaesthesia. This doctrine was a source of comfort to many generations of anaesthetists in the past. Little attention was given to the observation of Gordh in 1945 that ether anaesthesia nearly abolished the ventilatory response to hypoxaemia while the response to carbon dioxide was still present.[12]

Over 30 years later, halothane anaesthesia was shown to reduce the acute hypoxic ventilatory response (AHVR) in humans.[13] Shortly afterwards in 1978, Knill and Gelb[14] showed that not only was the hypoxic response affected by inhalational anaesthetics but it was also, in fact, exquisitely sensitive (Figure 21.4). Hypoxic drive was markedly attenuated at 0.1 MAC, a level of anaesthesia that would not be reached for a considerable time during recovery from anaesthesia. Similar effects with isoflurane,[15] enflurane[16] and nitrous oxide[17] were subsequently demonstrated by the same group. Recent work has also shown depression of AHVR with the newer volatile anaesthetic agents sevoflurane[18] and desflurane,[19] and with the intravenous anaesthetic propofol.[20]

These findings were widely accepted for some years, until a study by Temp and colleagues[21] in 1992 showed that AHVR was diminished only in hypercapnic conditions. This study initiated an extensive debate on the topic[22] but, more important, also initiated a great deal of further research. A summary of the findings of these and previous studies are shown in Figure 21.5. The most notable feature of these results is their diversity, with, for example, different studies of similar concentrations of isoflurane, particularly at sedative levels, obtaining completely opposite results. However, for the other agents there does seem to be a generally dose-dependent depression of the hypoxic ventilatory response, though at 0.1 MAC considerable variation remains. There are many possible explanations for these results, mostly relating to methodological differences between studies.

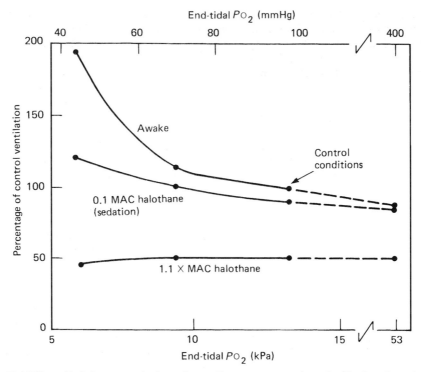

Figure 21.4 Effect of halothane anaesthesia on the ventilatory response to hypoxia. The data shown in this figure has now been challenged; see text for details. (Drawn from data of reference 14.)

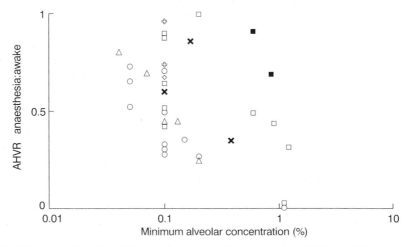

Figure 21.5 Summary of studies of the acute hypoxic ventilatory response (AHVR) and inhalational anaesthesia or sedation. The ordinate is the ratio of the increase in minute volume with hypoxia during anaesthesia or sedation and the awake (control) response. Thus a ratio of unity represents no depression of the response and zero represents a completely abolished response. All studies were performed under isocapnic conditions except the two solid squares which used poikilocapnia. See text for details. O, halothane; △, enflurane; □, isoflurane; ◇, sevoflurane; ×, nitrous oxide; ⊕, desflurane. (Derived from references quoted in the text and references 20, 23, 24, 25, 26, 27 and 28.)

Hypoxic challenge. The rate of onset, degree and duration of hypoxia will all affect the ventilatory response, which is normally biphasic with hypoxic ventilatory decline (HVD) occurring a few minutes after the onset of hypoxia (see Figure 5.8). Recent studies used rapid 'step' changes into hypoxic conditions,[29] whilst earlier studies used a 'ramp' onset of hypoxia over 8–10 minutes.[15] In the latter situation, the response under study will be a combination of AHVR and HVD.[21] A study addressing different patterns of hypoxic onset on AHVR has found no difference between the two.[30] Hypoxic ventilatory decline seems to be uninfluenced by anaesthesia.[21,29,31,32,33]

Sleep. The degree of arousal of subjects is known to affect the AHVR. Studies of hypoxic response at 'sedative' levels of anaesthesia (0.2 MAC or less) have differed in the amount of stimulation provided, some forcing the subjects to remain awake[21] and others leaving subjects undisturbed. One study comparing awake and asleep subjects with 0.1 MAC isoflurane found no depression of the hypoxic response in the awake group.[34]

Subject selection. The magnitude of the AHVR differs greatly between individuals (page 100). Some studies have been performed using only subjects found to have a 'brisk' ventilatory response to hypoxia,[29] and these results cannot therefore be extrapolated to a broader range of individuals.

Carbon dioxide concentration may be maintained at normal, prehypoxic, levels (isocapnia) or allowed to find its own level (poikilocapnia). This has a large effect in the awake subject, with the hypoxic response being greatly attenuated during poikilocapnia (Figure 5.8). During anaesthesia with up to 0.85 MAC isoflurane, the hypoxic ventilatory response in the presence of poikilocapnia is essentially maintained[35,36] – that is, the increase in ventilation with hypoxic challenge is the same when asleep as when awake. This has led some workers in this field to suggest that anaesthesia has less effect on the hypoxic ventilatory response itself, but may reduce the normally additive interaction between the ventilatory responses to hypoxia and hypercapnia[21,36] (see Figure 5.9).

It is generally agreed that the effect of anaesthetics on AHVR is on the peripheral chemoreceptors,[37] possibly exclusively so at sedative levels.[38] Anaesthesia also impairs the ventilatory response to doxapram, which acts on the peripheral chemoreceptors.[14,33]

There are four important practical implications of the attenuation of AHVR by anaesthesia. First, the patient cannot act as his own hypoxia alarm by responding with hyperventilation. Secondly, the patient who has already lost his sensitivity to P_{CO_2} (e.g. some patients with chronic respiratory failure) may stop breathing after induction of anaesthesia has abolished his hypoxic drive. Thirdly, anaesthesia may be dangerous at very high altitude or in other situations where survival depends on hyperventilation in response to hypoxia (Chapter 16). Finally, because the hypoxic drive is obtunded at subanaesthetic concentrations, this effect will persist into the early postoperative period after the patient has regained consciousness and is apparently able to fend for himself.

Recent uncertainty about the effect of subanaesthetic concentrations on AHVR has cast doubt on the validity of extrapolating the results of earlier studies to patients recovering from anaesthesia. The degree of stimulation of individual patients is likely to affect their AHVR response, which will therefore be affected by many factors such as pain control and the amount of activity in their surroundings. A patient should behave like a poikilocapnic subject, and so some studies suggest that depression of

AHVR will be minimal.[35,36] Finally, patients recovering from an anaesthetic will frequently be hypercapnic secondary to opiate administration sometimes compounded by airway obstruction. In these circumstances the ventilatory response to the combination of hypoxia and hypercapnia is almost certainly reduced to less than that seen when awake.

There is little doubt that more research is needed to understand the complex effects of anaesthesia on ventilatory responses.[39,40] Although recent work may have cast some doubt on the earlier studies of Knill and colleagues[14] (Figure 21.4), there remains ample evidence that a sleeping patient in the recovery room is at risk of failing to mount a suitable ventilatory response to hypoxia.

Pattern of contraction of respiratory muscles

One of the most remarkable examples of the specificity of anaesthetic actions is on the muscles associated with respiration. Many of these effects could hardly have been predicted but, nevertheless, have great clinical importance and underlie many of the secondary effects described later in this chapter.

The pharynx

Anaesthesia usually causes obstruction of the pharyngeal airway unless measures are taken for its protection. Figure 21.6 shows changes in the sagittal geometry of the pharynx immediately after induction of anaesthesia in the supine position.[41] The soft palate falls against the posterior pharyngeal wall, occluding the nasopharynx in almost every patient, presumably owing to interference with the action of some or all of tensor palati, palatoglossus or palatopharyngeus (page 113). There is considerable posterior movement of tongue and epiglottis, but usually not sufficient to occlude the oral or hypopharyngeal airway. In the cat, there is marked interference with genioglossus activity during anaesthesia,[42] and human observations have shown that thiopentone decreases the electromyographic (EMG) activity of genioglossus and the strap muscles.[43] Nevertheless, Nandi et al.[41] showed that the posterior movement of the palate was not caused by pressure from the tongue. The changes shown in Figure 21.6 are very similar to those observed with anaesthesia and paralysis.[44]

Secondary changes occur when the patient attempts to breathe. Upstream obstruction then often causes major passive downstream collapse of the entire pharynx (Figure 21.7), a mechanism with features in common with obstructive sleep apnoea (page 348). This secondary collapse of the pharynx is due to interference with the normal action of pharyngeal dilator muscles, particularly genioglossus. The epiglottis may be involved in hypopharyngeal obstruction during anaesthesia,[45] and posterior movement is clearly shown in Figures 21.6 and 21.7.

Protection of the pharyngeal airway. The changes described above are countered most effectively by the use of a tracheal tube, which requires the use of either 'deep' anaesthesia or muscle relaxants. However, there are effective alternatives to tracheal intubation that are useful for relatively minor procedures, particularly when spontaneous breathing is preserved. Extension of the neck moves the origin of genioglossus anteriorly by 1–2 cm and usually clears the hypopharyngeal airway.[44] Protrusion of the mandible moves the origin of genioglossus still further forward and was proposed by Heiberg in 1874.[46] The use of a pharyngeal airway, such as that of Guedel, is frequently helpful, but the tip may

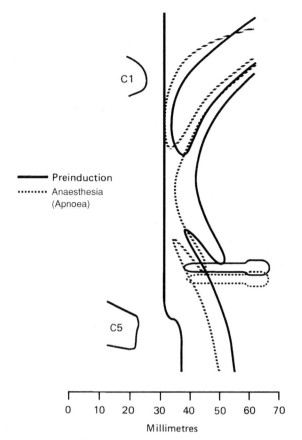

C1

■ Preinduction
•••••••• Anaesthesia
(Apnoea)

C5

```
┌──┬──┬──┬──┬──┬──┬──┬──┐
0   10  20  30  40  50  60  70
```
Millimetres

Figure 21.6 Median sagittal section of the pharynx to show changes between the conscious state (continuous lines) and following induction of anaesthesia (broken lines). The most consistent change was occlusion of the nasopharynx. (Reproduced from reference 41 by permission of the Editors and publishers of the *British Journal of Anaesthesia*.)

become lodged in the valecula, or the tongue may be pushed downwards and backwards to obstruct the tip of the airway.[47] The laryngeal mask is a relatively new approach to airway management, introduced in 1983.[48] This device provides an airtight seal around the laryngeal perimeter, allowing spontaneous ventilation. The laryngeal mask does not prevent regurgitated gastric contents gaining access to the larynx, and occasionally allows air leakage out of the mouth or into the oesophagus and stomach, particularly when airway pressure is increased.[49] Use of the laryngeal mask for intermittent positive pressure ventilation (IPPV) is therefore more controversial, but seems to be acceptable in patients with normal lungs who do not require high inflation pressures.[50] Radiographic appearances of normal and abnormal anatomical locations of the mask have been described.[51]

The inspiratory muscles[2,52]

John Snow's early observations of respiration during anaesthesia clearly describe that a decrease in thoracic respiratory excursion may be used as a sign of deepening anaesthesia.

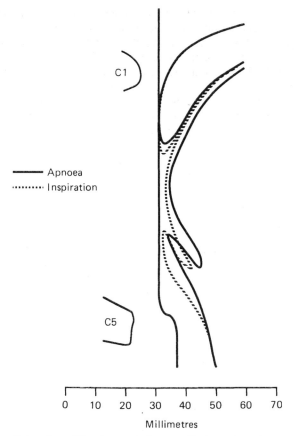

——— Apnoea
·········· Inspiration

0   10   20   30   40   50   60   70

Millimetres

Figure 21.7 Median sagittal section of the pharynx during anaesthesia to show changes between the apnoeic state (continuous lines, corresponding to the broken lines in Figure 21.6) and following attempted inspiration (broken lines). Upstream obstruction in the nasopharynx results in downstream collapse of the oro- and hypopharynx. (Reproduced from reference 41 by permission of the Editors and publishers of the *British Journal of Anaesthesia*.)

The effect was quantified by Miller in 1925[53] and more precisely related to depth of anaesthesia with halothane in 1979.[54] Selective depression of some inspiratory ribcage muscles does occur. Electromyography of the parasternal intercostal muscles in humans shows their activity to be consistently abolished by 1 MAC of anaesthesia, and absent in some subjects at just 0.2 MAC.[55,56] Thiopentone decreases the EMG activity of sternothyroid, sternohyoid and the scalene muscles.[43] In contrast, diaphragmatic function seems to be well preserved during anaesthesia, particularly phasic EMG activity during inspiration. This combination of changes in muscle activity commonly gives rise to paradoxical inspiratory movements whereby diaphragmatic contraction causes expansion of the lower ribcage and abdomen whilst the upper ribcage is drawn in owing to the negative intrathoracic pressure and a lack of support from upper ribcage respiratory muscles (page 116). This pattern of breathing is more marked in children, who have a more compliant chest wall than adults, and in adults when respiratory resistance is increased causing a greater decrease in intrathoracic pressure. Some studies have, however, found no reduction in ribcage movement with, for example, isoflurane at minimum alveolar concentration for anaesthesia (MAC = 1),[57] methohexitone[58] or ketamine.[59] It is possible that changes in spinal curvature during anaesthesia have caused earlier studies of ribcage movement to overestimate the changes.[55,60] Also, spontaneous ventilation via a tracheal tube is associated with greater airway resistance than other methods such as a laryngeal mask, which may contribute to less ribcage expansion during anaesthesia.[61] Thus earlier descriptions of selective depression of ribcage movement should not be regarded as an invariable feature of anaesthesia with spontaneous ventilation, particularly at the depth of anaesthesia used clinically and with a low-resistance, unobstructed airway. There is certainly an increased thoracic component of ventilation during IPPV of the anaesthetized paralysed patient.[62]

The resting position and dimensions of the ribcage and diaphragm during anaesthesia are described below.

The expiratory muscles

General anaesthesia causes expiratory phasic activity of the abdominal muscles, which are normally silent in the conscious supine subject. This activity begins in some subjects at only 0.2 MAC of halothane,[55] and is very difficult to abolish as long as spontaneous breathing continues.[63] Activation of expiratory muscles seems to serve no useful purpose and does not appear to have any significant effect on the change in functional residual capacity.[64]

Respiratory muscle coordination often becomes disturbed during anaesthesia with spontaneous ventilation.[57,61] Paradoxical movements as described above are accompanied

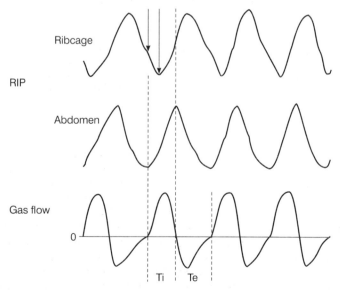

Figure 21.8 Respiratory inductance plethysmography (RIP) tracings of ribcage and abdominal movements during 1.5 MAC halothane anaesthesia, and the accompanying respiratory gas flows. Note the phase delay between abdominal and ribcage movements, indicated by solid arrows, which in the example shown is approximately 30 per cent of the inspiratory time. Ti, inspiratory time; Te, expiratory time. (Redrawn from reference 9 by permission of the authors and the publishers of *Anesthesiology*.)

by changes in respiratory timing between inspiratory and expiratory muscle groups. These are believed to originate in selective effects of anaesthesia on different respiratory neuronal groups in the central pattern generator,[56] and are more marked when airway resistance is higher.[61] The most usual pattern seen is a phase delay between abdominal and ribcage movement, as illustrated in Figure 21.8.

Change in functional residual capacity[65]

Bergman in 1963 was the first to report a decrease of functional residual capacity (FRC) during anaesthesia.[66] This was followed by many studies, which have established the following characteristics of the change:[58,64,67,68,69,70]

1. FRC is reduced during anaesthesia with all anaesthetic drugs that have been investigated, by a mean value of about 16–20 per cent of the FRC (in the supine position). However, there is considerable individual variation and changes range from about +19 per cent to −50 per cent.
2. FRC is reduced immediately on induction of anaesthesia, reaches its final value within the first few minutes and does not seem to fall progressively throughout anaesthesia. It does not return to normal until some hours after the end of anaesthesia.
3. FRC is reduced to the same extent during anaesthesia whether the patient is paralysed or not. In one study using spontaneous respiration with barbiturate anaesthesia, FRC was reduced only when subjects were intubated, there being no change in the group breathing via a facemask.[58]
4. The reduction in FRC has a weak but significant correlation with the age of the patient.

The cause of the reduction in FRC

The search for a mechanism to explain FRC changes during anaesthesia has involved several groups of researchers over many years, and no definitive answer has been reached. There is, however, some agreement that there are three possible contributory factors, as follows.

Chest shape. Earlier studies that measured anteroposterior and lateral diameters, or the circumference, of the external chest wall gave conflicting results regarding changes in internal chest volume with anaesthesia. However, the introduction of fast computed tomography (CT) scanners led to general agreement that there is a reduction in the cross-sectional area of the ribcage corresponding to a decrease in lung volume of about 200 ml.[71,72] Current technology involves a dynamic spatial reconstructor (DSR), which allows scans of half the chest to be obtained in just 0.3 seconds, following which a three-dimensional picture of all chest structures can be generated and analysed.[55] This has confirmed that changes in chest wall shape account for a reduction in FRC of about 200 ml.

There is less agreement about why the chest wall changes shape, possible explanations including the changes in ribcage muscle activity already described, diaphragmatic position and activity, or spinal curvature.

Diaphragm position. In the conscious subject in the supine position, Muller et al.[73] found evidence for residual end-expiratory tone in the diaphragm, which was believed to prevent the weight of the viscera pushing the diaphragm too far into the chest in the supine position. They showed that this diaphragmatic end-expiratory tone was lost during anaesthesia with halothane. Such a change would result in the diaphragm moving cephalad during anaesthesia, which was reported in early studies.[72,74] However, other investigators found no consistent cephalad movement of the diaphragm during anaesthesia. Studies using DSR and fast computed tomography have provided good evidence that diaphragm *shape* alters during anaesthesia.[55,75,76] Although there is a large variation between subjects, these studies have consistently shown a cephalad movement of the dependent regions of the diaphragm, with little or no movement of the non-dependent regions.[55] One recent study found a significantly greater cephalad shift of the diaphragm in patients who were paralysed,[75] though this had not been observed in earlier studies. The change in FRC that can be ascribed to changes in diaphragm shape is on average less than 30 ml.[55] A summary of the changes in chest wall and diaphragm positions during anaesthesia is shown in Figure 21.9.

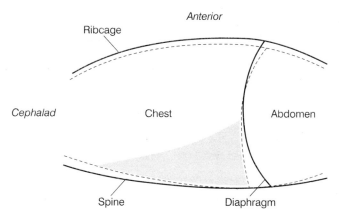

Figure 21.9 Schematic diagram showing a mid-sagittal section of the chest wall and diaphragm awake (solid line) and during anaesthesia (dashed line). Note the reduction in ribcage volume, increased spinal curvature and change in diaphragmatic position. The shaded area shows where atelectasis usually occurs during anaesthesia. (Redrawn from reference 68 by permission of the authors and the publishers of *Anesthesiology*.)

Thoracic blood volume. A shift of blood from the peripheral circulation into the chest during anaesthesia has been postulated as a cause of reduced FRC,[64] and one CT study seemed to demonstrate this.[77] However, this observation has not been confirmed,[55,72,78] and is currently regarded as an unlikely contributory factor to the reduced FRC.

Atelectasis during anaesthesia[79,80]

Hedenstierna's group in Sweden were the first to demonstrate pulmonary opacities on CT scans of subjects during anaesthesia. These opacities occurred commonly in the dependent areas of lung just above the diaphragm and were termed 'compression atelectasis'(Figure 21.10). Their extent correlated very strongly with the calculated intrapulmonary shunt.[71] Animal studies showed that the areas of opacity had a typical histological appearance of total collapse with only moderate vascular congestion and no clear interstitial oedema.[78] 'Miliary atelectasis' was first proposed by Bendixen and colleagues in 1963 as an

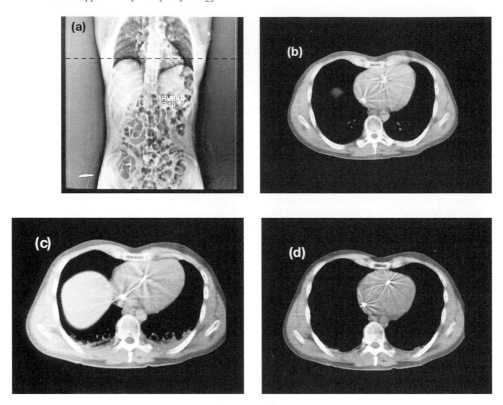

Figure 21.10 Computed tomography of transverse sections of the thoracic cage (supine position) at the level shown in the scout view (a). (b) Control (awake) view. (c) Anaesthesia with zero end-expiratory pressure. Note the development of atelectasis in the dependent region of lung and some ascent of the right dome of the diaphragm. (d) The same patient with positive end-expiratory pressure, which causes the atelectasis to disappear. (Scans (a) and (b) are reproduced from reference 82 with the permission of the authors and the Editors and publishers of *Acta Anaesthesiologica Scandinavica*. I am indebted to the authors for supplying the other two scans.)

explanation of the increased alveolar/arterial Po_2 difference during anaesthesia.[81] Conventional radiography, however, failed to show any appreciable areas of collapse, presumably because most atelectasis was behind the diaphragm on anteroposterior radiographs (see below).

Atelectasis occurs in between 75 and 90 per cent of healthy individuals having general anaesthesia with muscle paralysis,[68,83] and is most commonly found in dependent lung regions, becoming less pronounced at the cephalad end of the chest (Figure 21.9).[68] A recent study using the DSR found the average volume of atelectasis to be 29 ± 10 ml,[68] though atelectasis may represent up to 10 per cent of lung tissue.[80]

Causes of atelectasis

Three mechanisms are involved, all closely interrelated, and it is likely that all are involved in the formation of atelectasis *in vivo*.

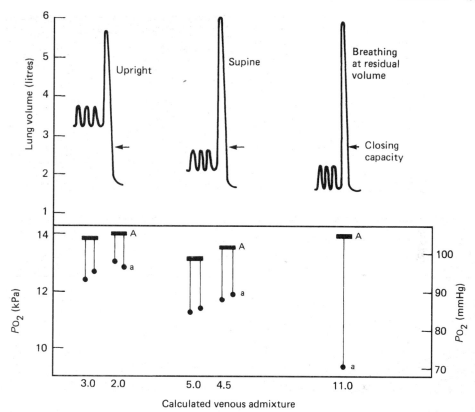

Figure 21.11 Changes in tidal excursion relative to vital capacity in Dr Nunn when aged 45; arrows indicate the closing capacity. Ideal alveolar (A) Po_2 is shown by the horizontal bar and arterial (a) Po_2 by the black circles. Venous admixture was calculated on the assumption of an arterial/mixed venous oxygen content difference of 5 ml.dl[-1]. (Reproduced from reference 86 by permission of the Editors of *Acta Anaesthesiologica Scandinavica*.)

Airway closure as a result of the reduced FRC may lead to atelectasis. In the supine position, the expiratory reserve volume has a mean value of approximately 1 litre in males and 600 ml in females. Therefore, the reduction in FRC following the induction of anaesthesia will bring the lung volume close to residual volume. This will tend to reduce the end-expiratory lung volume below the closing capacity, particularly in older patients (see Figure 3.11), and so result in airway closure and lung collapse. Pulmonary atelectasis can easily be demonstrated in conscious subjects who voluntarily breathe oxygen close to residual volume,[84] and Figure 21.11 shows the effect on arterial Po_2 of simulating the reduction in lung volume that occurs during anaesthesia. Even if lung collapse does not occur, for example in younger patients, the airway narrowing caused by reduced lung volume creates areas with low $\dot{V}/\dot{Q}$ ratios that contribute to impaired gas exchange.[85]

An important aspect of this problem is whether closing capacity (CC) remains constant during anaesthesia or changes with FRC. Earlier studies by Hedenstierna and colleagues suggested that CC remained constant.[87] However, two other studies provided convincing evidence that FRC and CC are both reduced in parallel following the induction of anaesthesia.[88,89] It is possible that bronchodilatation caused by the anaesthetic counteracts the reduction in airway calibre that would be expected to result from the reduction in FRC (see below). The results of the last two studies suggest that there should be no increased tendency towards airway closure during anaesthesia, but this is clearly at variance with Hedenstierna's work.[85]

Compression atelectasis may occur because of changes in chest wall and diaphragm position, which lead to the transmission of high intra-abdominal pressure to the chest and compression of areas of lung. As shown in Figure 21.9, the predominantly caudal distribution of atelectasis also points to a role for changes in the position of the dependent regions of the diaphragm.

Absorption atelectasis[90] develops when an airway becomes partially or totally closed and the gas contained in the pulmonary units distal to the airway is absorbed into the blood. Absorption of gas does not in itself cause atelectasis, but in effect accelerates collapse if airway closure occurs from either of the preceding mechanisms. The rapid uptake of oxygen or nitrous oxide into the blood makes these important contributors to the development of absorption atelectasis (page 560), though the role of absorption in anaesthesia-induced atelectasis is disputed.[90]

Prevention and re-expansion of atelectasis[80]

Recognition of atelectasis during anaesthesia has led to great interest in ways to prevent its occurrence. Several interesting findings have emerged.

Gas composition. Administration of high concentrations of oxygen during anaesthesia would be expected to promote atelectasis, and there is some evidence for this. Earlier studies found no association between gas composition and atelectasis,[91] but three recent studies by the same group have challenged this finding. Breathing 100% oxygen immediately before the induction of anaesthesia leads to significantly more atelectasis than in patients breathing either 30% oxygen[92] or air[93] during induction. Similarly, following re-expansion of atelectasis during anaesthesia, a high inspired oxygen concentration causes a more rapid recurrence of atelectasis.[94]

Positive end-expiratory pressure (PEEP) has been known for some time to cause the CT opacities to disappear (Figure 21.10), though high levels of PEEP may be required.[91] Also, resolution of atelectasis is not complete, collapse recurring within minutes when PEEP is discontinued.[95] In addition, PEEP causes significant changes to ventilation/perfusion ($\dot{V}/\dot{Q}$) relationships in the lung (see below) and so does not improve oxygenation of the patient.[80]

Hyperinflation may be used to re-expand collapsed lung. Two methods have been described, and are shown in Figure 21.12. The first involves a series of hyperinflation manoeuvres consisting of three breaths to an airway pressure of 30 cmH$_2$O followed by a final breath to 40 cmH$_2$O, each sustained for 15 seconds (Figure 21.12a).[96] Between these large breaths normal intermittent positive pressure ventilation is continued for 3–5 minutes. Computed tomography assessment during this manoeuvre shows that the first hyperinflation of 30 cmH$_2$O reduces the area of atelectasis by half, and the subsequent

(a)

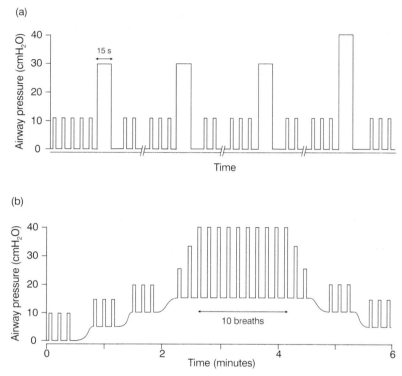

Figure 21.12 Schematic representation of proposed manoeuvres to re-expand collapsed lung during anaesthesia. (a) Method of Rothen et al.,[96] involving three large breaths sufficient to achieve airway pressures of 30 cmH$_2$O followed by a single breath to 40 cmH$_2$O, each sustained for 15 seconds. The breaks on the abscissa represent 3–5 minutes of intermittent positive pressure ventilation with normal tidal volume. (b) Method of Tusman et al.,[97] showing progressive application of positive end-expiratory pressure up to 15 cmH$_2$O, followed by increased tidal volume until a peak airway pressure of 40 cmH$_2$O or tidal volume of 18 ml.kg^{-1} is achieved, which is then maintained for 10 breaths. (Reproduced from references 96 and 97 by permission of the authors and the publishers of *British Journal of Anaesthesia*.)

inflations to 30 cmH$_2$O have little additional effect, but the final breath to 40 cmH$_2$O completely re-expands the atelectasis. The second study used increasing levels of PEEP up to 15 cmH$_2$O, in conjunction with large tidal volumes, until airway pressures of 40 cmH$_2$O were again achieved (Figure 21.12b).[97] This study did not use CT assessment but inferred re-expansion of atelectasis from improved arterial P_{O_2}.

An airway pressure of 40 cmH$_2$O equates to administering a vital capacity breath. This is not without risk during anaesthesia, including the possibility of cardiovascular disturbances and pulmonary barotrauma (Chapter 31). Atelectasis reforms within 5 minutes if the inspired oxygen concentration is 100%, but with 60% nitrogen beneficial effects are seen for up to 40 minutes.[94,98] In a similar fashion to PEEP, these recruitment manoeuvres reduce intrapulmonary shunt, but increase $\dot{V}/\dot{Q}$ mismatch such that there is usually only a small improvement in oxygenation (see below).[96,97] Obese patients develop greater amounts of atelectasis during anaesthesia, and hyperinflation is particularly effective in this situation, often leading to a sustained improvement in oxygenation.[98]

Respiratory mechanics[99]

Calibre of the lower airways[100]

Effect of reduced FRC. Figures 4.5 and 21.13 both show the hyperbolic relationship between lung volume and airway resistance. Figure 21.13 clearly shows that the curve is steep in the region of FRC in the supine position and therefore the reduction in FRC that occurs during anaesthesia might be expected to result in a marked increase in airway resistance. However, most anaesthetics are bronchodilators, as outlined in the following paragraphs, and, at least with halothane, this effect almost exactly offsets the effect of reduction in lung volume.[101] Thus total respiratory system resistance during anaesthesia is only slightly greater than in the awake supine subject, most of the change occurring in the lung/airway components rather than the chest wall (Table 21.1).[102] As would be expected, resistance increases with increasing flow rate and decreases with increasing inflation volume during anaesthesia.[103]

Inhalational anaesthetics. All inhalational anaesthetics investigated have shown bronchodilator effects. Suppression of airway vagal reflexes, direct relaxation of airway smooth

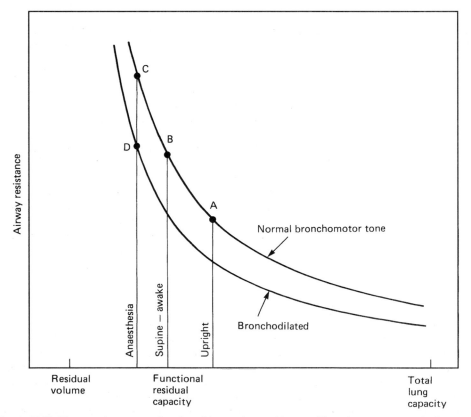

Figure 21.13 Airway resistance as a function of lung volume with normal bronchomotor tone and when bronchodilated. A = upright and awake; B = supine and awake; C = supine and anaesthetized without bronchodilatation; D = supine, anaesthetized and with the degree of bronchodilatation that normally occurs during anaesthesia. Note that the airway resistance is similar at B and D, bronchodilatation approximately compensating for the decrease in FRC.

Table 21.1 Respiratory mechanics during anaesthesia

Compliance (static)	Anaesthetized		Awake normal range	
	$l.kPa^{-1}$	$ml.cmH_2O^{-1}$	$l.kPa^{-1}$	$ml.cmH_2O^{-1}$
Respiratory system	0.81	81	0.5–1.9	47–190
Lungs	1.5	150	0.9–4.0	90–400
Chest wall	2.0	203	1.0–3.5	100–350
Resistance	$kPa.l^{-1}.s$	$cmH_2O.l^{-1}.s$	$kPa.l^{-1}.s$	$cmH_2O.l^{-1}.s$
Respiratory system	0.48	4.8	0.12–0.44	1.2–4.4
Lung tissue/airway	0.35	3.5	0.07–0.24	0.7–2.4
Chest wall	0.13	1.3	0.05–0.20	0.5–2.0

(Data during anaesthesia are in the supine position from reference 102.)

muscle and inhibition of release of bronchoconstrictor mediators combine to cause an increase in specific airway conductance.[104,105] In clinical concentrations, halothane reduces the amount of acetylcholine released from nerve terminals in response to nerve stimulation,[106] and suppresses the increase in both airway and tissue resistance following vagal stimulation.[101] This seems to be more important than the direct effect of clinical concentrations of halothane on airway smooth muscle or histamine release from mast cells.[100] Diethyl ether has been used in the treatment of status asthmaticus.

Other anaesthetic agents. Deep barbiturate anaesthesia has generally similar effects to those of inhalational anaesthetics. However, there are many older reports of bronchospasm occurring in relation to the use of thiopentone, although others have found no such association.[100] Undoubtedly some instances were reflex bronchospasm due to stimuli such as the presence of a tracheal tube, with barbiturate doses too low to provide adequate protection. Ketamine has bronchodilator effects that seem to be largely due to catecholamine release and stimulation of β_2-adrenoreceptors on airway smooth muscle. Some older neuromuscular blocking drugs and opiates may cause bronchoconstriction in asthmatic patients, due to histamine release, but have little effect on normal lungs.

Other sites of increased airway resistance

Breathing systems. Excessive resistance or obstruction may arise in apparatus such as breathing systems, valves, connectors and tracheal tubes. The tubes may be kinked, the lumen may be blocked or the cuff may herniate and obstruct the lower end, which may also abut against the carina or the side wall of the trachea. A reduction in diameter of a tracheal tube greatly increases its resistance, the pattern of flow being intermediate between laminar and turbulent for the conditions shown in Figure 21.14.

Resistance imposed by a laryngeal mask airway is less than that of a corresponding size of tracheal tube.[107]

The pharynx and larynx. The pharynx is commonly obstructed during anaesthesia by the mechanisms described earlier in this chapter, unless active steps are taken to preserve

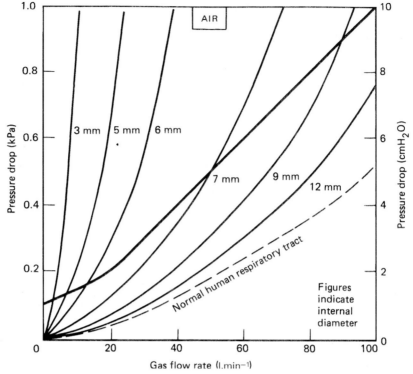

Figure 21.14 Flow rate/pressure drop plots of a range of tracheal tubes, with their connectors and catheter mounts. The heavy line is the author's suggested upper limit of acceptable resistance for an adult. Pressure drop does not quite increase according to the fourth power of the radius because the catheter mount offered the same resistance throughout the range of tubes. With 70% N_2O/30% O_2, the pressure drop is about 40 per cent greater for the same gas flow rate when flow is turbulent, but little different when the flow is chiefly laminar.

patency. Reflex laryngospasm is still possible at depths of anaesthesia that suppress other airway protective reflexes. The resulting obstruction is usually total and may be life-threatening. In most cases the spasm eventually resolves spontaneously, but is most reliably terminated by neuromuscular blockade.

Compliance

Total respiratory system compliance is reduced during anaesthesia to a figure approaching the lower end of the normal range (Table 21.1).[102,108] Both static and dynamic measurements (page 54) are reduced compared with the awake state.[103] The effects of different inspiratory flow rates and volumes have been studied in terms of the spring and dashpot model (see Figure 4.4).[103] Compliance seems to be reduced very early in anaesthesia and the change is not progressive.

Figure 21.15 summarizes the effect of anaesthesia on the pressure/volume relationships of the lung and chest wall. The diagram shows the major differences between the conscious state and anaesthesia. There are only minor differences between anaesthesia

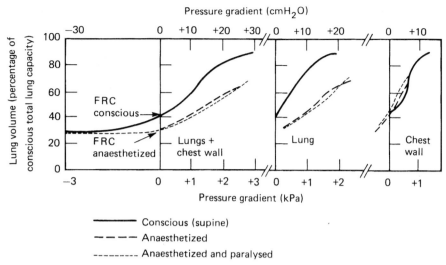

Figure 21.15 Pressure/volume relationships in supine volunteers before and after the induction of anaesthesia and paralysis. The first section shows the relationship for lungs plus chest wall where the relevant pressure gradient is alveolar minus ambient. The second section represents lungs alone where the pressure gradient is alveolar minus intrathoracic (transmural). The third section relates to chest wall alone for which the pressure gradient is intrathoracic minus ambient. There are only insignificant differences between observations during anaesthesia with and without paralysis. There are, however, major differences in pressure/volume relationships of the lung and total respiratory system following the induction of anaesthesia. Arrows indicate the FRC which, during anaesthesia, is only slightly greater than the residual volume. (Redrawn from data of reference 109, except that the subatmospheric extensions of the curves for the lungs plus chest wall have been derived from other sources.)

with and without paralysis. The left-hand section shows the relationship for the whole respiratory system comprising lungs plus chest wall. The curves obtained during anaesthesia clearly show the reduction in FRC (lung volume with zero pressure gradient from alveoli to ambient). The subatmospheric section of the curve also shows the very small volume change that can be achieved by application of a subatmospheric pressure to the airway of an anaesthetized patient. This implies a very low expiratory reserve volume. Application of a positive pressure as high as 3 kPa (30 cmH$_2$O) to the airways expands the lungs to barely 70 per cent of the preoperative total lung capacity, which implies a reduced overall compliance. The two sections of Figure 21.15 on the right and Table 21.1 show that the major changes are in the lung rather than the chest wall.

Cause of the reduced compliance. The change seems to be mainly due to a reduction in pulmonary compliance, the cause of which has been difficult to explain. There is no convincing evidence that anaesthesia affects pulmonary surfactant in humans at clinically used concentrations. A more likely explanation is that the reduced lung compliance is simply the consequence of breathing at reduced lung volume.[110] Strapping the chest of volunteers, thereby decreasing their lung volume, results in a decrease in pulmonary compliance that can be restored to normal by taking a maximal inspiration.[111] This suggests that partial pulmonary atelectasis is the explanation, and the demonstration of atelectasis during anaesthesia makes this the most likely cause of the reduced compliance.

Gas exchange

Every factor influencing gas exchange may be altered during anaesthesia, and many of the changes must be considered as normal features of the anaesthetized state. These 'normal' changes usually pose no threat to the patient, as their effects can easily be overcome by such simple means as increasing the concentration of oxygen in the inspired gas and the minute volume. The 'normal' changes may be contrasted with a range of pathological alterations in gas exchange that may arise during anaesthesia from such circumstances as airway obstruction, apnoea, bronchospasm or tension pneumothorax. These may be life threatening and require urgent action for their correction.

The major changes that adversely affect gas exchange during anaesthesia are reduced minute volume of ventilation (described above), increased dead space and shunt (considered in terms of the three-compartment model) and altered distribution of ventilation and perfusion in relation to ventilation/perfusion ratios.

The three-compartment model of gas exchange has been described on pages 173 *et seq.* In essence it presents the lung as though it comprised three compartments – ideally perfused and ventilated alveoli, alveolar dead space and shunt. Physiological (= anatomical + alveolar) dead space is quantified by the Bohr equation (page 177) and shunt by the shunt equation (page 182), with or without direct measurement of the mixed venous oxygen content. It is obviously not a true representation of the lung during anaesthesia but, *as a model*, it has the following very cogent advantages:

1. The model is simple to understand.
2. It is a valid model to explain changes in arterial P_{CO_2} and P_{O_2} during anaesthesia with inspired oxygen concentrations in the range 30–100%.
3. The parameters of dysfunction (dead space and shunt) can be measured with facilities available in most hospitals.
4. These parameters offer clear quantitative guidance for optimizing minute volume of ventilation and inspired oxygen concentration.

Physiological dead space (see page 175)

The increase in physiological dead space during anaesthesia was first observed in 1958[112] and subsequently confirmed in many studies. With allowance for the apparatus dead space of the tracheal tube and its connections, the dead space/tidal volume ratio *from carina downwards* averages 32 per cent during anaesthesia with either spontaneous or artificial ventilation.[113] This is approximately equal to the ratio for the normal conscious subject *including trachea, pharynx and mouth* (approx. 70 ml). Physiological dead space equals the sum of its anatomical and alveolar components, and the subcarinal anatomical dead space is not normally increased. Therefore, the increase in subcarinal physiological dead space during anaesthesia must be in the alveolar component.[113] There is no measurable difference between physiological and anatomical dead space in the normal conscious subject and therefore the alveolar dead space is negligible.

Anatomical dead space. In the study of Nunn and Hill[113] (Figure 21.16), subcarinal anatomical dead space was always significantly less than physiological, reaching a maximum of about 70 ml at tidal volumes above 350 ml. This roughly accords with the expected geometric dimensions of the lower respiratory tract. At smaller tidal volumes, the anatomical dead space was less than the expected geometric volume. Values of less

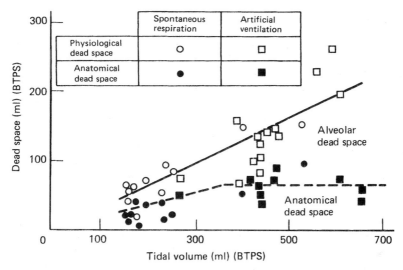

Figure 21.16 Data and regression lines for physiological and anatomical dead space (the difference indicating alveolar dead space) as a function of tidal volume. There were no significant differences between anaesthesia with and without paralysis. Note the range over which physiological dead space seemed to be a constant fraction of tidal volume. Anatomical dead space was constant above a tidal volume of 350 ml, resulting in increased alveolar dead space. (Modified from reference 113 by permission of the Editor and publishers of the *Journal of Applied Physiology*.)

than 30 ml were recorded in some patients with a tidal volume less than 250 ml. This is attributed to axial streaming and the mixing effect of the heart beat, and is clearly an important and beneficial factor in patients with depressed breathing.

Alveolar dead space increases with tidal volume, so the sum of anatomical and alveolar (= physiological) dead space remains about 32 per cent of tidal volume (Figure 21.16). The cause of the increase in alveolar dead space during anaesthesia is not immediately obvious. There is no evidence that it is due to pulmonary hypotension causing development of a zone 1 (page 147), and the reduced vertical height of the lung in the supine position would militate against this. The alternative explanation is maldistribution with overventilation of *relatively* underperfused alveoli. Studies of ventilation/perfusion relationships outlined below give some support to this view, but such patterns of maldistribution have not invariably been observed during anaesthesia.

Apparatus dead space. For practical purposes the apparatus dead space of the tracheal tube and its connections must be included for the purpose of calculating alveolar ventilation during anaesthesia. The total dead space then increases to a mean of 50 per cent of tidal volume (Figure 21.17). If the trachea is not intubated, it is necessary to add the volume of the facemask and its connections to the physiological dead space, which now includes trachea, pharynx and mouth. The total dead space then amounts to about two-thirds of the tidal volume.[114] Thus, a seemingly adequate minute volume of 6 l.min^{-1} might be expected to result in an alveolar ventilation of only 2 l.min^{-1}, which would almost inevitably result in hypercapnia.

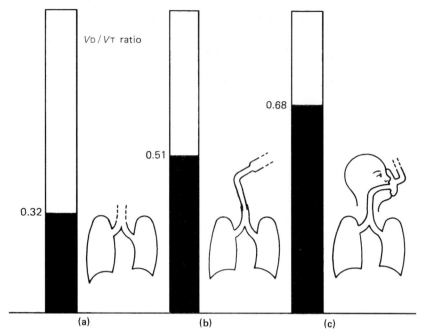

Figure 21.17 Physiological plus apparatus dead space (where applicable) as a fraction of tidal volume in anaesthetized patients: (a) from carina downwards; (b) including tracheal tube and connector; and (c) including upper airway, facemask and connector.

Compensation for increased dead space may be made by increasing the minute volume to maintain the alveolar ventilation. In practice, the problem hardly exists. The artificially ventilated anaesthetized patient may have a large dead space, but the high minute volumes commonly selected usually provide more than adequate compensation. Thus the alveolar ventilation is almost always greater than necessary for carbon dioxide homoeostasis. With monitoring of end-expiratory P_{CO_2}, there is very seldom any difficulty in maintaining a value in the range 4–5 kPa (30–37.5 mmHg). However, the existence of an alveolar dead space means that the arterial P_{CO_2} during anaesthesia is usually 0.5–1 kPa (3.8–7.5 mmHg) greater than the end-expiratory P_{CO_2}.

In the case of the hypoventilating patient who is allowed to breathe spontaneously during anaesthesia, the reduction in dead space at smaller tidal volumes shown in Figure 21.16 prevents some of the alveolar hypoventilation that would be expected if the *volume* of the dead space remained constant. This, together with the reduced metabolic rate, results in the hypercapnia being much less than the values for minute volume sometimes observed during anaesthesia might lead one to expect. No doubt, over the years, many patients have owed their lives to these factors.

Shunt

Magnitude of the change during anaesthesia. In the conscious healthy subject, the shunt or venous admixture amounts to only 1–2 per cent of cardiac output (page 183). This results in an alveolar/arterial P_{O_2} gradient of less than 1 kPa (7.5 mmHg) in the young healthy subject breathing air, but the gradient increases with age. During anaesthesia, the

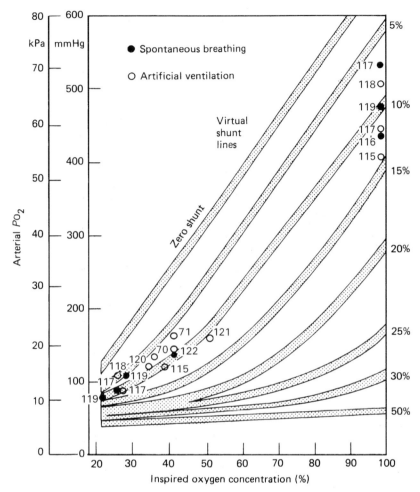

Figure 21.18 Mean values for arterial P_{O_2} are plotted against inspired oxygen concentrations for 10 published studies of anaesthetized patients, using the same coordinates as in Figure 8.12.

alveolar/arterial P_{O_2} difference is usually increased to a value that corresponds to an average shunt of about 10 per cent. Figure 21.18 shows the mean values for shunt, taken from a large number of different studies, plotted on the iso-shunt diagram which is explained on page 185. Throughout the range of inspired oxygen concentrations, the means for the studies are grouped along the 10% shunt line. Formal measurements of pulmonary venous admixture, taking into account the mixed venous oxygen content, have also been made and these concur with shunts being of the order of 10%. This provides an acceptable basis for predicting arterial P_{O_2} during an uncomplicated anaesthetic and also permits calculation of the concentration of oxygen in the inspired gas that will provide an acceptable arterial P_{O_2}. Some 30–40% inspired oxygen is usually adequate in an uncomplicated anaesthetic.

The cause of the venous admixture during anaesthesia was long debated but it is now clear that about half is true shunt through the areas of atelectasis described above. There is a very strong correlation between the shunt (measured as perfusion of alveoli with a ventilation/perfusion ($\dot{V}/\dot{Q}$) ratio of less than 0.005) and the area or volume of atelectasis seen on CT scans.[68,71] Recent studies using isotope techniques have demonstrated intrapulmonary shunting in the same areas of lung where atelectasis is seen on CT scans.[123] However, the venous admixture during anaesthesia also contains components due to dispersion of the $\dot{V}/\dot{Q}$ distribution, and to perfusion of alveoli with low $\dot{V}/\dot{Q}$ ratios (0.005–0.1). The effect of age is complex and is considered below.

Ventilation/perfusion relationships[124]

The three-compartment model of the lung provides a definition of lung function in terms of dead space and shunt, parameters that are easily measured, reproducible and provide a basis for corrective therapy. Nevertheless, it does not pretend to provide a true picture of what is going on in the lung. A far more sophisticated approach is provided by the analysis of the distribution of pulmonary ventilation and perfusion in terms of $\dot{V}/\dot{Q}$ ratios by the multiple inert gas elimination technique (page 191), and many studies during anaesthesia have now been reported.[71,85,124]

During general anaesthesia and paralysis, both ventilation and perfusion are found to be distributed to a wider range of $\dot{V}/\dot{Q}$ ratios than when awake (Figure 21.19).[92,125] Other studies have also found substantial $\dot{V}/\dot{Q}$ mismatch during anaesthesia and paralysis, ventilation being preferentially distributed to ventral areas and *vice versa* for perfusion.[123] In the healthy young subject shown in Figure 21.19, the true intrapulmonary shunt had a mean value of less than 1% during anaesthesia, but the alveolar/arterial P_{O_2} gradient was

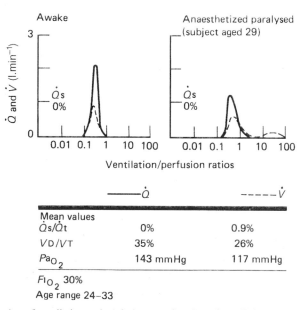

Mean values	$\dot{Q}$	$\dot{V}$
$\dot{Q}s/\dot{Q}t$	0%	0.9%
V_D/V_T	35%	26%
Pa_{O_2}	143 mmHg	117 mmHg

$F_{I_{O_2}}$ 30%
Age range 24–33

Figure 21.19 Distribution of ventilation and perfusion as a function of ventilation/perfusion ratios in the awake and anaesthetized paralysed subject. (Adapted from reference 125 and reproduced from reference 126 by permission of the publishers.)

slightly increased and this was attributed to the increased spread of the distribution of perfusion to areas of poorer ventilation (lower $\dot{V}/\dot{Q}$ ratio). Anatomical dead space was reduced, largely because of tracheal intubation, but alveolar dead space was increased, partly due to increased spread of distribution of ventilation to areas of poorer perfusion (higher $\dot{V}/\dot{Q}$ ratio).

Effect of age on $\dot{V}/\dot{Q}$ ratios during anaesthesia. In awake subjects, increasing age causes a widening of the distribution of $\dot{V}/\dot{Q}$ ratios, and the distribution widens still further with anaesthesia.[71] It would thus be expected that intrapulmonary shunt during anaesthesia would also increase with age, but studies of this effect have produced conflicting results. One study involving typical surgical patients with ages ranging from 37 to 64 years found that the true intrapulmonary shunt was increased during anaesthesia.[122] However, the shunt calculated from the alveolar/arterial P_{O_2} gradient according to the three-compartment lung model would be larger still, and the difference would be due to perfusion of areas of low $\dot{V}/\dot{Q}$ ratio. A second study of older patients (mean age 60) who all had some deterioration in pulmonary function showed wide variations in pulmonary shunt.[127] The results of this study can most easily be appreciated by considering the patients in three groups (Figure 21.20). In the first, there was only a small increase in the true shunt following the induction of anaesthesia but there seemed to be a 'shelf' of perfusion of regions of very low $\dot{V}/\dot{Q}$ ratios in the range 0.01–0.1. In the second group, this 'shelf' was less prominent but there was a substantial increase in true shunt. Finally, in the

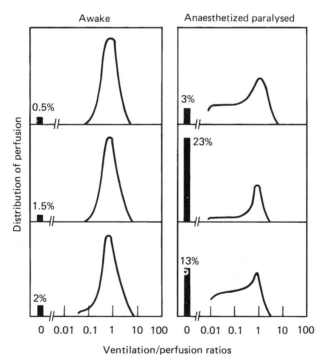

Figure 21.20 Changes in pulmonary perfusion as a function of ventilation/perfusion ratios following induction of anaesthesia in elderly patients. Numbers to the left of each block indicate the shunt. (Adapted from reference 127 and reproduced from reference 126 by permission of the publishers.)

third group, there was both a 'shelf' and an increase in true shunt. All of these changes are compatible with a decrease in FRC below closing capacity.

Finally, the most recent study by Gunnarsson et al. in 1991[71] involved 45 patients of age range 23–69 years. They reached the surprising conclusion that atelectasis (as seen with CT) and true intrapulmonary shunt (determined by multiple inert gas elimination technique as alveoli with $\dot{V}/\dot{Q}$ ratio less than 0.005) did not relate to age. However, both were substantially increased during anaesthesia and correlated with each other. It is difficult to reconcile the lack of correlation between age and shunt with the striking differences seen in previous studies. Nevertheless, Gunnarsson confirmed the enhanced decline in arterial P_{O_2} with increasing age during anaesthesia, and venous admixture (calculated as for the Riley three-compartment model) was increased significantly, from a mean value of 5.5 per cent of cardiac output before anaesthesia to 9.2 per cent during anaesthesia. Venous admixture increased steeply with age (0.17 per cent per year), and this

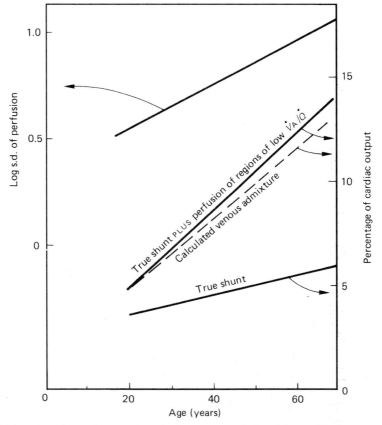

Figure 21.21 Age dependence of various factors influencing alveolar/arterial P_{O_2} difference during anaesthesia.[71] The logarithm of standard deviation of distribution of perfusion is significantly greater during anaesthesia (shown) than when awake (not shown) and has a significant regression against age in both circumstances. True shunt is significantly increased almost tenfold compared with before anaesthesia, but the correlation with age is not significant. Perfusion of areas of poorly ventilated regions ($0.005 < \dot{V}/\dot{Q} < 0.1$) was significantly increased compared with before anaesthesia and correlated with age in both circumstances. Venous admixture here refers to the value obtained from the shunt equation (page 182) and agrees well with the sum of shunt and perfusion of regions of low $\dot{V}/\dot{Q}$.

was attributed to an age-dependent increase in the spread of $\dot{V}/\dot{Q}$ ratios (Figure 21.21) and to greater perfusion of alveoli with low $\dot{V}/\dot{Q}$ ratios (0.005–0.1).

Effect of PEEP. It has long been known that, in contrast to the situation in intensive care, PEEP does little to improve the arterial P_{O_2} during anaesthesia.[118] As already described, the application of PEEP leads to a re-expansion of atelectasis and intrapulmonary shunt fraction is substantially reduced, but there are two reasons why these changes are not associated with improved oxygenation. First, the decrease in the cardiac output associated with PEEP reduces the saturation of the blood traversing the remaining shunt and so reduces arterial P_{O_2}.[122] Secondly, PEEP increases ventilation of alveoli with high $\dot{V}/\dot{Q}$ ratio, so further increasing overall $\dot{V}/\dot{Q}$ mismatch. The essential difference from the patient undergoing intensive care is probably the lack of protection of intrathoracic blood vessels from raised airway pressure that is afforded by stiff lungs in most patients requiring intensive care.

Other factors affecting $\dot{V}/\dot{Q}$ ratio during anaesthesia. Hypoxic pulmonary vasoconstriction (HPV) contributes to maintaining a normal $\dot{V}/\dot{Q}$ ratio by reducing perfusion to underventilated alveoli (see Chapter 7, pages 151 *et seq.*). Inhalational anaesthetics inhibit HPV (see below) and so may worsen $\dot{V}/\dot{Q}$ mismatch during anaesthesia. There is some evidence from animal studies that this is the case,[124] and one human study of anaesthesia with intravenous barbiturates, which are believed to have less effect on HPV, demonstrated only a small amount of intrapulmonary shunting.[128] High concentrations of inspired oxygen will inhibit HPV by maintaining alveolar P_{O_2} at a high level even in poorly ventilated alveoli. Some work has shown that lower inspired oxygen concentrations during anaesthesia (30%) are associated with less $\dot{V}/\dot{Q}$ scatter than when breathing 100% oxygen.[92]

Summary

These studies of $\dot{V}/\dot{Q}$ relationships during anaesthesia complement one another and give us greatly increased insight into the effect of anaesthesia on gas exchange. We are now in a position to summarize the effect of anaesthesia on gas exchange as follows:

1. Uniformity of distribution of ventilation and perfusion is decreased by anaesthesia. The magnitude of the change is age-related and may be affected by the anaesthetic agents used and inspired oxygen concentration.
2. The increase in alveolar dead space seems to be due to increased distribution of ventilation to areas of high (but not usually infinite) $\dot{V}/\dot{Q}$ ratios.
3. Venous admixture is increased in anaesthesia to a mean value of about 10 per cent, but the change is markedly affected by age, being minimal in the young.
4 The increased venous admixture during anaesthesia is due partly to an increase in true intrapulmonary shunt (due to atelectasis), and partly to increased distribution of perfusion to areas of low (but not zero) $\dot{V}/\dot{Q}$ ratios. The latter component increases with age.
5. The major differences are between the awake and the anaesthetized states. Paralysis and artificial ventilation do not greatly alter the parameters of gas exchange in spite of the different spatial distribution of ventilation.
6. Both PEEP and lung hyperinflation manoeuvres reduce the shunt, but the beneficial effect on arterial P_{O_2} is offset by greater $\dot{V}/\dot{Q}$ mismatch and a decrease in cardiac output, which reduces the mixed venous oxygen content.

Typical values for the various factors discussed are shown in Table 21.2.

Table 21.2 Changes in factors influencing gas exchange after induction of anaesthesia

	Awake	Anaesthetized		
		Spontaneous ventilation	IPPV	IPPV + PEEP
$F_{I_{O_2}}$	0.21	0.4	0.4	0.4
$\dot{Q}s/\dot{Q}t$ (%)	1.6	6.2	8.6	4.1
V_D/V_T (%)	30	35	38	44
Cardiac output (l.min^{-1})	6.1	5.0	4.5	3.7
Pa_{O_2} (kPa)	10.5	17.6	18.8	20.5
Pa_{O_2} (mmHg)	79	132	141	153
$\dot{V}$ – mean $\dot{V}/\dot{Q}$	0.81	1.3	2.20	3.03
$\dot{Q}$ – mean $\dot{V}/\dot{Q}$	0.47	0.51	0.83	0.55

(Adapted from reference 122 and reproduced from reference 126 by permission of the publishers.)

Other effects of general anaesthesia on the respiratory system

Response to added resistance

The preceding sections would lead one to expect that anaesthesia would cause grave impairment of the ability of patients to increase their work of breathing in the face of added resistance. Surprisingly, this is not the case and anaesthetized patients preserve a remarkable ability to overcome added resistance.[129,130] The anaesthetized patient responds to inspiratory loading in two phases. First, there is an instant augmentation of the force of contraction of the inspiratory muscles, mainly the diaphragm, during the first loaded breath.[73] This has the appearance of a typical spindle reflex, and the same authors have reported the existence of spindles in the human diaphragm. Detection of the inspiratory resistance may be mediated by either airway or lung receptors, and is only slightly inhibited by anaesthesia.[131] The second response is much slower and overshoots when the loading is removed, and the time course suggests that this is mediated by an increase in P_{CO_2}.[129] In combination, these two mechanisms enable the anaesthetized patient to achieve good compensation with inspiratory loading up to about 0.8 kPa (8 cmH$_2$O). Even more remarkable is the preservation of the elaborate response to expiratory resistance (see Figure 4.8), with a large *increase* in minute volume occurring with expiratory resistive loading during enflurane anaesthesia.[132]

Metabolic rate

During anaesthesia, the metabolic rate is reduced about 15 per cent below basal according to the conventional standards developed over 70 years ago.[133] However, these standards do not stipulate sedation or any period of rest. In 1952, new standards were proposed for metabolic rate,[134] based on three hours' rest, with or without sedation. These values are about 15 per cent below the conventional standards and so correspond fairly closely to those of the anaesthetized patient.[135] Table 21.3 lists expected values for oxygen consumption and carbon dioxide output during uncomplicated anaesthesia at normal body temperature (mean 36.5°C). In comparison with the conscious subject, there are major reductions in cerebral and cardiac oxygen consumption during anaesthesia.

Table 21.3 Predicted values for oxygen consumption and carbon dioxide output during uncomplicated anaesthesia (ml.min^{-1}, STPD)

Age	Oxygen consumption			Carbon dioxide production		
	Small patient	Average patient	Large patient	Small patient	Average patient	Large patient
Male						
14–15		190			152	
16–17		200			160	
18–19	168	210	252	134	168	202
20–29	162	203	243	130	162	194
30–39	162	203	243	130	162	194
40–49	158	198	237	126	158	190
50–59	155	194	233	124	155	186
60–69	150	187	224	120	149	179
Female						
14–15		174			139	
16–17		188			150	
18–19	156	194	233	125	155	186
20–29	152	190	228	122	152	182
30–39	150	187	224	120	150	179
40–49	148	184	221	118	147	177
50–59	144	180	216	115	144	173
60–69	140	175	210	112	140	168

Values for CO_2 output will apply only in a steady respiratory state.
Values are probably about 6 per cent lower during artificial ventilation.
Figures are based on 85 per cent of basal according to the data of reference 133.

Hypoxic pulmonary vasoconstriction[136,137]

The contribution to $\dot{V}/\dot{Q}$ mismatch of disturbed HPV during anaesthesia has already been described above, but the effects of anaesthesia on HPV merit further discussion. Early animal studies using isolated lungs found that several inhalational anaesthetics inhibit HPV,[138] but no such effect was found with intravenous anaesthetics.[139] Although *in vitro* studies gave clear evidence that inhalational anaesthetics depressed HPV, *in vivo* studies were inconsistent. Some studies showed that inhalational anaesthetics increased the pulmonary blood flow through hypoxic areas of lung (i.e. reduction of HPV), whereas others showed no change or even a slight increase. This was resolved in 1985 by Marshall and Marshall,[136] who analysed a large number of studies and showed that the confusing factor was concomitant depression of cardiac output by inhalational anaesthetics. In Chapter 7 it was explained how hypoxia influences pulmonary vascular resistance not only by the alveolar Po_2 but also, in part, by the mixed venous Po_2. A reduction in cardiac output must decrease the mixed venous Po_2 if oxygen consumption remains unchanged, and this would intensify pulmonary vasoconstriction. Thus, on the one hand, an inhalational anaesthetic will inhibit HPV by direct action while, on the other hand, it may intensify HPV by reducing mixed venous Po_2 as a result of decreasing cardiac output. Thus Marshall and Marshall[136] showed that most investigators' results are consistent with the view that inhalational anaesthetics depress HPV provided that allowance is made for the effect of concomitant changes of cardiac output.

Quantitative effect of inhalational anaesthetics Suppression of HPV by inhalational anaesthetics follows a typical sigmoid dose/response curve with an effective dose (50%; ED_{50}) of slightly less than twice MAC, and an ED_{90} of 3 MAC.[140] Thus, during a typical anaesthetic at 1.3 MAC, HPV is attenuated by only about 30 per cent. There are no major differences between the volatile anaesthetics. Nitrous oxide (0.3 MAC) has a slight but significant effect.

Special conditions arising during anaesthesia

Patient position

Lateral. In Chapter 8 it was explained that, in the lateral position, there is preferential distribution of inspired gas to the lower lung (see Table 8.1) and this accords approximately with the distribution of pulmonary blood flow. This favourable distribution of inspired gas is disturbed by anaesthesia whether respiration is spontaneous or artificial in the paralysed patient,[141] with preferential ventilation of the non-dependent (upper) lung and continued preferential perfusion of the dependent lung. This predictably leads to a greater spread of $\dot{V}/\dot{Q}$ ratios and a further fall in Po_2 compared with the supine position.[142] Atelectasis seen on CT scanning forms only in the dependent lung, but the overall amount of atelectasis and the intrapulmonary shunt are similar to those seen in anaesthetized and paralysed subjects when supine.[142]

Prone. A patient anaesthetized in the prone position should have the upper chest and pelvis supported, to allow free movement of the abdomen and lower chest. In subjects anaesthetized and paralysed in this position, respiratory mechanics are only minimally affected, and both FRC and arterial Po_2 are greater than when supine.[102] A study using the DSR showed that, with anaesthesia in the prone position, motion of non-dependent areas of the diaphragm predominates, leading the authors to suggest a difference in the anatomical structure between dorsal and ventral areas of the diaphragm.[76] Other explanations for improved oxygenation when prone include more uniform lung perfusion and less ventilation of, or atelectasis formation in, dependent areas of lung that are reduced in volume by the presence of the mediastinum and heart.[102]

Lithotomy. In awake subjects the lithotomy position has little effect on FRC, $\dot{V}/\dot{Q}$ relationships or shunt, although some overweight subjects in lithotomy position with an epidural anaesthetic may develop atelectasis or increased shunt.[143]

Thoracotomy

In the early days of thoracic surgery it was commonplace to maintain spontaneous respiration. This resulted in pendulum breathing between the two lungs, and routine arterial Pco_2 values were recorded in excess of 30 kPa (225 mmHg) – apparently without evidence of overt harm to the patients.[144] Spontaneous respiration with an open chest but without pendulum breathing can be achieved by collapse of the exposed lung, but at the cost of severe shunting. It took many years to realize that the solution to the open chest was IPPV. However, when one side of the chest is opened, the exposed lung may receive a very large proportion of the total ventilation during IPPV. Because the patient is commonly in the lateral position, there will then be a gross mismatch between the overventilated upper and exposed lung and the overperfused lower lung. Ventilation of the upper lung should therefore be avoided.

One-lung anaesthesia. The surgeon may find his task is simplified by total collapse of the upper (exposed) lung. This is usually achieved by the use of a double-lumen tracheal tube, with the lumen connecting to the exposed lung left open to atmosphere. Although pulmonary blood flow through the collapsed lung is reduced, it is not zero and there is still usually a substantial shunt, usually in the range 30–50%. There is seldom difficulty in maintaining a satisfactory P_{CO_2} but oxygenation is usually compromised.

Hypoxia may be minimized by restricting the duration of one-lung anaesthesia and by increasing the inspired oxygen concentration. However, the use of even 99% oxygen does not always guarantee a normal arterial P_{O_2}, and measures may be required to reduce blood flow through the non-ventilated lung. Adequate collapse of the lung should be ensured; in an inflated but non-ventilated lung, pulmonary vessels are dilated by the elastic forces in the lung (see Figure 7.4), causing a huge shunt. If surgery involves resection of part or the whole of the lung, efforts should be taken to expedite surgical ligation of the pulmonary vessels. In the non-ventilated lung, HPV should contribute to reducing shunt. Anaesthetic techniques that avoid inhalational agents, such as a propofol infusion, may therefore cause less severe reductions in oxygenation.[145,146] Apnoeic oxygenation of the non-ventilated lung often improves P_{O_2}, presumably by oxygenating blood flowing through the non-ventilated lung, in spite of the possibility of this abolishing HPV and so increasing shunt. PEEP applied to the ventilated lung may improve oxygenation, but the pressure used is crucial, increasing levels of PEEP usually reducing arterial P_{O_2} by diverting more blood to the non-ventilated lung and reducing cardiac output. A compromise PEEP value must therefore be used, which is believed to be about $5\,cmH_2O$ and referred to as 'best' PEEP.[147]

If one-lung anaesthesia is used in the supine position, the beneficial effect of gravity on the diversion of pulmonary blood flow to the ventilated lung is lost, and oxygenation may be harder to maintain.

Regional anaesthesia

Epidural or spinal anaesthesia may be expected to influence the respiratory system, either by a central effect of drugs absorbed from the spinal canal or by affecting the pattern or strength of contraction of respiratory muscle groups. These affects are generally small, but of great importance in view of the tendency to use regional anaesthetic techniques in patients with respiratory disease or in obstetric practice when respiratory function is already abnormal (Chapter 13).

Control of breathing has been investigated during epidural anaesthesia. Thoracic epidural anaesthesia may cause a small reduction in resting tidal volume as a result of reduced ribcage movement.[148,149,150,151] Predictably, this does not occur following lumbar epidural anaesthesia.[152] Studies of hypercapnic and hypoxic ventilatory responses during epidural anaesthesia have produced conflicting results. One study of thoracic epidurals demonstrated a reduced response to hypercapnia, ascribed to reduced intercostal muscle contribution to stimulated ventilation,[148] whilst a more recent study of elderly patients found no change.[150] Lumbar epidurals may result in an *increased* response to hypercapnia,[150,153] which is believed to be stimulated by anxiety (the study was performed immediately before surgery),[150] or because of a direct stimulant effect of lignocaine on the respiratory centre.[153] The acute hypoxic ventilatory response is unaffected by thoracic epidural anaesthesia, but lumbar epidurals may increase ventilation in response to hypoxia, by a poorly understood mechanism.[150,151]

Respiratory muscle function has recently been studied extensively using EMGs and the DSR during high lumbar (block up to T1 dermatome) epidural anaesthesia.[154] This study confirmed the reduced contribution of the ribcage to resting ventilation. Functional residual capacity was increased by 300 ml as a result of both caudad movement of the diaphragm and reduced thoracic blood volume. In spite of these changes, most respiratory function measurements remain essentially unchanged during epidural anaesthesia, with only small changes in forced vital capacity and peak expiratory flow rate.[155] The situation is quite different in late pregnancy, when regional anaesthesia is commonly employed. Significant reductions in forced vital capacity and peak expiratory flow rate have been reported after spinal anaesthesia,[156] with lesser changes following epidural anaesthesia.[157] Peak expiratory pressure, a measure of abdominal muscle activity, was also decreased after lumbar epidural for caesarean section, particularly when bupivacaine was used.[158]

Oxygenation during epidural anaesthesia is largely unaffected. In a recent study by Hedenstierna's group, lumbar epidural anaesthesia produced no changes in $\dot{V}/\dot{Q}$ relationships or pulmonary shunt, and no CT evidence of atelectasis except in one subject with a higher than normal body mass index in the lithotomy position.[143]

Respiratory function in the postoperative period[159]

Early postanaesthetic recovery

In the first few minutes of recovery, alveolar P_{O_2} may be reduced by elimination of nitrous oxide, which dilutes alveolar oxygen (diffusion hypoxia) and carbon dioxide, but this effect is usually transient. Desaturation is very common during transfer to the recovery room when monitoring is often interrupted.[160] Airway obstruction, often associated with residual muscle paralysis, is a common potential cause of hypoxia shortly after anaesthesia. This may be compounded by the residual effects of anaesthetic agents on ventilatory control that have been described above. Both reduced FRC and the increased alveolar/arterial P_{O_2} gradient observed during anaesthesia usually return to normal during the first few hours after minor operations.[4]

Late postoperative respiratory changes

After major surgery, the restoration of a normal alveolar/arterial P_{O_2} gradient may take several days, and episodes of hypoxia are common. There are several contributory factors.

Lung volume and atelectasis. There is a continued reduction in FRC, usually reaching its lowest value 1–2 days postoperatively, before slowly returning to normal values within a week.[161] Reduction of the FRC is greatest in patients having surgery near the diaphragm – that is, upper abdominal or thoracic incisions[162] – but is less following laparoscopic surgery in the upper abdomen.[163] Atelectasis seen on CT scans during anaesthesia persists for at least 24 hours in patients having major surgery.[164] The effects of these changes on $\dot{V}/\dot{Q}$ relationships and oxygenation will be similar to those seen during anaesthesia, but the provision of adequate inspired oxygen concentration is now far less reliable.

Effort-dependent lung function tests such as FVC, FEV_1 and PEF are all reduced significantly following surgery, particularly if pain control is inadequate. Laparoscopic surgery is again associated with lesser, but still significant, reductions in lung function, and the degree of change is again related to the site of surgery.[162]

Sleep. During sleep, particularly in a patient receiving opioid analgesics, there are often episodes of obstructive apnoea. These episodes were originally described as occurring during the first postoperative night,[165] but may continue for at least three nights, particularly in association with rapid eye movement (REM) sleep, which is usually absent on the first postoperative night. Morphine abolishes REM sleep but induces obstructive apnoea in the absence of REM sleep.[159]

Respiratory muscles.[166] Diaphragmatic dysfunction is a term that has been used to describe changes in the pattern of contraction of respiratory muscles in patients following major surgery. Impairment of diaphragmatic contraction is believed to result from reflex inhibition of phrenic nerve output in response to surgical trauma. Changes are independent of the level of pain control, and are improved only by thoracic epidural, which is believed to result in neural blockade of the inhibitory reflex.[161] The existence of diaphragmatic dysfunction has been challenged, mainly on the grounds that methods used to study diaphragm function are largely indirect and greatly affected by changes in other respiratory muscle groups.[166] For example, there are well-described increases in expiratory abdominal muscle activity following surgery[167] that might be interpreted as changes in diaphragm activity.

Sputum retention occurs in many patients after surgery. General anaesthesia, particularly with a tracheal tube, causes impairment of mucociliary transport in the airways,[168] an effect that may persist into the postoperative period. This, coupled with reduced FRC, residual atelectasis and an ineffective cough, is likely to contribute to the development of chest infections, including pneumonia. Many of these factors are more pronounced in smokers, who are known to be more susceptible to chest complications after major surgery (page 413).

References

1. Snow J. *On chloroform and other anaesthetics: their action and administration.* London: Churchill, 1858.
2. Nunn JF. Effects of anaesthesia on respiration. *Br J Anaesth* 1990; **65**: 54–62.
3. Birt C, Cole P. Some physiological effects of closed circuit halothane anaesthesia. *Anaesthesia* 1965; **20**: 258–68.
4. Nunn JF, Payne JP. Hypoxaemia after general anaesthesia. *Lancet* 1962; **2**: 631–2.
5. Munson ES, Larson CP, Babad AA, Regan MJ, Buechel DR, Eger EI. The effects of halothane, fluroxene and cyclopropane on ventilation: a comparative study in man. *Anesthesiology* 1966; **27**: 716–28.
6. Eger EI. Isoflurane: a review. *Anesthesiology* 1981; **55**: 559–76.
7. Lockhart SH, Rampil IJ, Yasuda N, Eger EI, Weiskopf RB. Depression of ventilation by desflurane in humans. *Anesthesiology* 1991; **74**: 484–8.
8. Doi M, Ikeda K. Respiratory effects of sevoflurane. *Anesth Analg* 1987; **66**: 241–4.
9. Fourcade HE, Larson CP, Hickey RF, Bahlman SH, Eger EI. Effects of time on ventilation during halothane and cyclopropane anesthesia. *Anesthesiology* 1972; **36**: 83–8.
10. Eger EI, Dolan WM, Stevens WC, Miller RD, Way WL. Surgical stimulation antagonizes the respiratory depression produced by Forane. *Anesthesiology* 1972; **36**: 544–9.
11. Knill RL, Clement JL. Ventilatory responses to acute metabolic acidemia in humans awake, sedated and anesthetized with halothane. *Anesthesiology* 1985; **62**: 745–53.
12. Gordh T. Postural circulatory and respiratory changes during ether and intravenous anesthesia. *Acta Chir Scand* 1945; **92** (Suppl 102): 26.
13. Duffin J, Triscott A, Whitwam JG. The effect of halothane and thiopentone on ventilatory responses mediated by the peripheral chemoreceptors in man. *Br J Anaesth* 1976; **48**: 975–81.

14. Knill RL, Gelb AW. Ventilatory responses to hypoxia and hypercapnia during halothane sedation and anesthesia in man. *Anesthesiology* 1978; **49**: 244–51.
15. Knill RL, Kieraszewicz HT, Dodgson BG, Clement JL. Chemical regulation of ventilation during isoflurane sedation and anaesthesia in humans. *Can Anaesth Soc J* 1983; **30**: 607–14.
16. Knill RL, Manninen PH, Clement JL. Ventilation and chemoreflexes during enflurane sedation and anaesthesia in man. *Can Anaesth Soc J* 1979; **26**: 353–60.
17. Knill RL, Clement JL. Variable effects of anaesthetics on the ventilatory response to hypoxaemia in man. *Can Anaesth Soc J* 1982; **29**: 93–9.
18. Sarton E, Dahan A, Teppema L, van den Elsen M, Olofsen E, Berkenbosch A, van Kleef J. Acute pain and central nervous system arousal do not restore impaired hypoxic ventilatory response during sevoflurane sedation. *Anesthesiology* 1996; **85**: 295–303.
19. Dahan A, Sarton E, van den Elsen M, van Kleef J, Teppema L, Berkenbosch A. Ventilatory response to hypoxia in humans: influences of subanesthetic desflurane. *Anesthesiology* 1996; **85**: 60–8.
20. Nagyova B, Dorrington KL, Gill EW, Robbins PA. Comparison of the effects of sub-hypnotic concentrations of propofol and halothane on the acute ventilatory response to hypoxia. *Br J Anaesth* 1995; **75**: 713–18.
21. Temp JA, Henson LC, Ward DS. Does a subanaesthetic concentration of isoflurane blunt the ventilatory response to hypoxia. *Anesthesiology* 1992; **77**: 1116–24.
22. Knill RL. Subanaesthetic isoflurane and the ventilatory response to hypoxaemia. *Anesthesiology* 1993; **78**: 1189–91.
23. Nagyova B, Dorrington KL, Robbins PA. Effect of low-dose enflurane on the ventilatory response to hypoxia in humans. *Br J Anaesth* 1994; **72**: 509–14.
24. Gelb AW, Knill RL. Subanaesthetic halothane: its effect on regulation of ventilation and relevance to the recovery room. *Can Anaesth Soc J* 1978; **25**: 488–94.
25. Dahan A, van den Elsen MJLJ, Berkenbosch A, DeGoede J, Olievier ICW, van Kleef JW, Bovill JG. Effects of subanesthetic halothane on the ventilatory response to hypercapnia and acute hypoxia in healthy volunteers. *Anesthesiology* 1994; **80**: 727–38.
26. Solevi A, Lindahl SGE. Hypoxic and hypercapnic ventilatory response during isoflurane sedation and anaesthesia in women. *Acta Anaesthesiol Scand* 1995; **39**: 931–8.
27. Dahan A, Ward DS. Effects of 20% nitrous oxide on the ventilatory response to hypercapnia and sustained isocapnic hypoxia in man. *Br J Anaesth* 1994; **72**: 17–20.
28. Yacoub O, Doell D, Kryger MH, Anthonisen NR. Depression of hypoxic ventilatory response by nitrous oxide. *Anesthesiology* 1976; **45**: 385–9.
29. Young CH, Drummond GB, Warren PM. Effect of a sub-anaesthetic concentration of halothane on the ventilatory response to sustained hypoxia in healthy humans. *Br J Anaesth* 1993; **71**: 642–7.
30. Temp JA, Henson LC, Ward DS. Effect of a subanesthetic minimum alveolar concentration of isoflurane on two tests of the hypoxic ventilatory response. *Anesthesiology* 1994; **80**: 739–50
31. Nagyova B, Dorrington KL, Poulin MJ, Robbins PA. Influence of 0.2 minimum alveolar concentration of enflurane on the ventilatory response to sustained hypoxia in humans. *Br J Anaesth* 1997; **78**: 707–13.
32. Foo IT, Martin SE, Lee RJ, Drummond GB, Warren PM. Interaction of the effects of domperidone and sub-anaesthetic concentrations of isoflurane on the immediate and sustained hypoxic ventilatory response in humans. *Br J Anaesth* 1995; **74**: 134–40.
33. Dahan A, van den Elsen MJLJ, Berkenbosch A, DeGoede J, Olievier ICW, Burm AGL, van Kleef JW. Influence of a subanesthetic concentration of halothane on the ventilatory response to step changes into and out of sustained isocapnic hypoxia in healthy volunteers. *Anesthesiology* 1994; **81**: 850–9.
34. van den Elsen MJLJ, Dahan A, Berkenbosch A, DeGoede J, van Kleef JW, Olievier ICW. Does subanesthetic isoflurane affect the ventilatory response to acute isocapnic hypoxia in healthy volunteers. *Anesthesiology* 1994; **81**: 860–7.
35. Sjögren D, Sollevi A, Ebberyd A, Lindahl SGE. Poikilocapnic hypoxic ventilatory response in humans during 0.85 MAC isoflurane anesthesia. *Acta Anaesthesiol Scand* 1994; **38**: 149–55.
36. Sjögren D, Sollevi A, Ebberyd A, Lindahl SGE. Isoflurane anesthesia (0.6 MAC) and hypoxic ventilatory response in humans. *Acta Anaesthesiol Scand* 1995; **39**: 17–22.
37. Knill RL, Clement JL. Site of selective action of halothane on the peripheral chemoreflex pathway in humans. *Anesthesiology* 1984; **61**: 121–6.

38. van den Elsen M, Sarton E, Teppema L, Berkenbosch A, Dahan A. Influence of 0.1 minimum alveolar concentration of sevoflurane, desflurane and isoflurane on dynamic ventilatory response to hypercapnia in humans. *Br J Anaesth* 1998; **80**: 174–82.
39. Goodman NW. Volatile agents and the ventilatory response to hypoxia. *Br J Anaesth* 1994; **72**: 503–5
40. Robotham JL. Do low dose inhalational anesthetic agents alter ventilatory control. *Anesthesiology* 1994; **80**: 723–6.
41. Nandi PR, Charlesworth CH, Taylor SJ, Nunn JF, Dorè CJ. Effect of general anaesthesia on the pharynx. *Br J Anaesth* 1991; **66**: 157–62.
42. Ochiai R, Guthrie RD, Motoyama EK. Effects of varying concentrations of halothane on the activity of the genioglossus, intercostals, and diaphragm in cats: an electromyographic study. *Anesthesiology* 1989; **70**: 812–16.
43. Drummond GB. Influence of thiopentone on upper airway muscles. *Br J Anaesth* 1989; **63**: 12–21.
44. Morikawa S, Safar P, DeCarlo J. Influence of the head–jaw position upon upper airway patency. *Anesthesiology* 1961; **22**: 265–70.
45. Boidin MP. Airway patency in the unconscious patient. *Br J Anaesth* 1985; **57**: 306–10.
46. Heiberg J. A new expedient in administering chloroform. *Medical Times and Gazette* 1874; 10 Jan: 36.
47. Marsh AM, Nunn JF, Taylor SJ, Charlesworth CH. Airway obstruction associated with the use of the Guedel airway. *Br J Anaesth* 1991; **67**: 517–23.
48. Brain AIJ. The laryngeal mask: a new concept in airway management. *Br J Anaesth* 1983; **55**: 801–5.
49. Weiler N, Latorre F, Eberle B, Goedecke R, Heinrichs W. Respiratory mechanics, gastric insufflation pressure, and air leakage of the laryngeal mask airway. *Anesth Analg* 1997; **84**: 1025–8.
50. Devitt JH, Wenstone R, Noel AG, O'Donnell MP. The laryngeal mask airway and positive pressure ventilation. *Anesthesiology* 1994; **80**: 550–5.
51. Nandi PR, Nunn JF, Charlesworth CH, Taylor SJ. Radiological study of the laryngeal mask. *Eur J Anaesthesiol Supp* 1991; **4**: 33–9.
52. Drummond GB. Chest wall movements in anaesthesia. *Eur J Anaesthesiol* 1989; **6**: 161–96.
53. Miller AH. Ascending respiratory paralysis under general anaesthesia. *JAMA* 1925; **84**: 201–2.
54. Jones JG, Faithfull D, Jordan C, Minty B. Rib cage movement during halothane anaesthesia in man. *Br J Anaesth* 1979; **51**: 399–407.
55. Warner DO, Warner MA, Ritman EL. Human chest wall function while awake and during halothane anesthesia. I. Quiet breathing. *Anesthesiology* 1995; **82**: 6–19.
56. Warner DO, Warner MA, Joyner MJ, Ritman EL. The effect of nitrous oxide on chest wall function in humans and dogs. *Anesth Analg* 1998; **86**: 1058–64.
57. Lumb AB, Petros AJ, Nunn JF. Rib cage contribution to resting and carbon dioxide stimulated ventilation during 1 MAC isoflurane anaesthesia. *Br J Anaesth* 1991; **67**: 712–21.
58. Bickler PE, Dueck R, Prutow RJ. Effects of barbiturate anesthesia on functional residual capacity and ribcage/diaphragm contributions to ventilation. *Anesthesiology* 1987; **66**: 147–52.
59. Mankikian B, Cantineau JP, Sartene R, Clergue F, Viars P. Ventilatory pattern and chest wall mechanics during ketamine anesthesia in humans. *Anesthesiology* 1986; **65**: 492–9.
60. Morton CPJ, Drummond GB. Change in chest wall dimensions on induction of anaesthesia: a reappraisal. *Br J Anaesth* 1994; **73**: 135–9.
61. Reigner J, Ameur MB, Ecoffey C. Spontaneous ventilation with halothane in children: a comparative study between endotracheal tube and laryngeal mask airway. *Anesthesiology* 1995; **83**: 674–8.
62. Vellody VPS, Nassery M, Balasaraswathi K, Goldberg NG, Sharp JT. Compliances of human rib cage and diaphragm–abdomen pathways in relaxed versus paralysed states. *Am Rev Respir Dis* 1978; **118**: 479–91.
63. Kaul SU, Heath JR, Nunn JF. Factors influencing the development of expiratory muscle activity during anaesthesia. *Br J Anaesth* 1973; **45**: 1013–18.
64. Hewlett AM, Hulands GH, Nunn JF, Heath JR. Functional residual capacity. II. Spontaneous respiration. *Br J Anaesth* 1974; **46**: 486–94.
65. Wahba RWM. Perioperative functional residual capacity. *Can J Anaesth* 1991; **38**: 384–400.
66. Bergman NA. Distribution of inspired gas during anesthesia and artificial ventilation. *J Appl Physiol* 1963; **18**: 1085–9.
67. Rutherford JS, Logan MR, Drummond GB. Changes in end-expiratory lung volume on induction of anaesthesia with thiopentone or propofol. *Br J Anaesth* 1994; **73**: 579–82.

68. Warner DO, Warner MA, Ritman EL. Atelectasis and chest wall shape during halothane anesthesia. *Anesthesiology* 1996; **85**: 49–59.
69. Don HF, Wahba WM, Craig DB. Airway closure, gas trapping, and the functional residual capacity during anesthesia. *Anesthesiology* 1970; **36**: 533–9.
70. Hewlett AM, Hulands GH, Nunn JF, Milledge JS. Functional residual capacity. III. Artificial ventilation. *Br J Anaesth* 1974; **46**: 495–503.
71. Gunnarsson L, Tokics L, Gustavsson H, Hedenstierna G. Influence of age on atelectasis formation and gas exchange impairment during general anaesthesia. *Br J Anaesth* 1991; **66**: 423–32.
72. Hedenstierna G, Strandberg A, Brismar B, Lundquist H, Svensson L, Tokics L. Functional residual capacity, thoracoabdominal dimensions and central blood volume during general anesthesia with muscle paralysis and mechanical ventilation. *Anesthesiology* 1985; **62**: 247–54.
73. Muller N, Volgyesi G, Becker L, Bryan MH, Bryan AC. Diaphragmatic muscle tone. *J Appl Physiol* 1979; **47**: 279–84.
74. Froese AB, Bryan AC. Effects of anesthesia and paralysis on diaphragmatic mechanics in man. *Anesthesiology* 1974; **41**: 242–55.
75. Reber A, Nylund U, Hedenstierna G. Position and shape of the diaphragm: implications for atelectasis formation. *Anaesthesia* 1998; **53**: 1054–61.
76. Krayer S, Rehder K, Vettermann J, Didier P, Ritman EL. Position and motion of the human diaphragm during anesthesia-paralysis. *Anesthesiology* 1989; **70**: 891–8.
77. Krayer S, Rehder K, Beck KC, Cameron PD, Didier EP, Hoffman EA. Quantification of thoracic volumes by three-dimensional imaging. *J Appl Physiol* 1987; **62**: 591–8.
78. Hedenstierna G, Lundquist H, Undh B, Tokics L, Strandberg A, Brismar B, Frostell C. Pulmonary densities during anaesthesia. *Eur Respir J* 1989; **2**: 528–32.
79. Hedenstierna G. Gas exchange during anaesthesia. *Br J Anaesth* 1990; **64**: 507–14.
80. Hedenstierna G. Atelectasis and its prevention during anaesthesia. *Eur J Anaesthesiol* 1998; **15**: 387–90.
81. Bendixen HH, Hedley-Whyte J, Laver MB. Impaired oxygenation in surgical patients during general anesthesia with controlled ventilation. *N Engl J Med* 1963; **269**: 991–6.
82. Hedenstierna G, Tokics L, Strandberg A, Lundquist H, Brismar B. Correlation of gas exchange impairment to development of atelectasis during anaesthesia and muscle paralysis. *Acta Anaesthesiol Scand* 1986; **30**: 183–91.
83. Lundquist H, Hedenstierna G, Strandberg A, Tokics L, Brismar B. CT assessment of dependent lung densities in man during general anaesthesia. *Acta Radiol* 1995; **36**: 626–32.
84. Nunn JF, Williams IP, Jones JG, Hewlett AM, Hulands GH, Minty BD. Detection and reversal of pulmonary absorption collapse. *Br J Anaesth* 1978; **50**: 91–100.
85. Rothen HU, Sporre B, Engberg G, Wegenius G, Hedenstierna G. Airway closure, atelectasis and gas exchange during general anaesthesia. *Br J Anaesth* 1998; **81**: 681–6.
86. Nunn JF. Measurement of closing volume. *Acta Anaesthiol Scand Supp* 1978; **70**: 154–60.
87. Hedenstierna G, McCarthy G, Bergström M. Airway closure during mechanical ventilation. *Anesthesiology* 1976; **44**: 114–23.
88. Juno P, Marsh M, Knopp TJ, Rehder K. Closing capacity in awake and anesthetized-paralyzed man. *J Appl Physiol* 1978; **44**: 238–44.
89. Bergman NA, Tien YK. Contribution of the closure of pulmonary units to impaired oxygenation during anesthesia. *Anesthesiology* 1983; **59**: 395–401.
90. Joyce CJ, Baker AB. What is the role of absorption atelectasis in the genesis of perioperative pulmonary collapse? *Anaesth Intensive Care* 1995; **23**: 691–6.
91. Brismar B, Hedenstierna G, Lundquist H, Strandberg A, Svensson L, Tokics L. Pulmonary densities during anaesthesia with muscle relaxation – a proposal of atelectasis. *Anesthesiology* 1985; **62**: 422–8.
92. Rothen HU, Sporre B, Engberg G, Wegenius G, Reber A, Hedenstierna G. Prevention of atelectasis during general anaesthesia. *Lancet* 1996; **345**: 1387–91.
93. Reber A, Engberg G, Wegenius G, Hedenstierna G. Lung aeration: the effect of pre-oxygenation and hyperoxygenation during total intravenous anaesthesia. *Anaesthesia* 1996; **51**: 733–7.
94. Rothen HU, Sporre B, Engberg G, Wegenius G, Högman M, Hedenstierna G. Influence of gas composition on recurrence of atelectasis after a re-expansion maneuver during general anesthesia. *Anesthesiology* 1995; **82**: 832–42.

95. Hedenstierna G, Tokics L, Lundquist H, Andersson T, Strandberg A, Brismar B. Phrenic nerve stimulation during halothane anaesthesia. Effects on atelectasis. *Anesthesiology* 1994; **80**: 751–60.

96. Rothen HU, Sporre B, Engberg G, Wegenius G, Hedenstierna G. Re-expansion of atelectasis during general anaesthesia: a computed tomography study. *Br J Anaesth* 1993; **71**: 788–95.

97. Tusman G, Böhm SH, Vazquez de Anda GF, do Campo JL, Lachmann B. 'Alveolar recruitment strategy' improves arterial oxygenation during general anaesthesia. *Br J Anaesth* 1999; **82**: 8–13.

98. Rothen HU, Sporre HU, Engberg G, Wegenius G, Hedenstierna G. Reexpansion of atelectasis during general anaesthesia may have a prolonged effect. *Acta Anaesthesiol Scand* 1995; **39**: 118–25.

99. Milic-Emili J, Robatto FM, Bates JHT. Respiratory mechanics in anaesthesia. *Br J Anaesth* 1990; **65**: 4–12.

100. Hirshman CA, Bergman NA. Factors influencing intrapulmonary airway calibre during anaesthesia. *Br J Anaesth* 1990; **65**: 30–42.

101. Joyner MJ, Warner DO, Rehder K. Halothane changes the relationships between lung resistances and lung volume. *Anesthesiology* 1992; **76**: 229–35.

102. Pelosi P, Croci M, Calappi E, Cerisara M, Mulazzi D, Vicardi P, Gattinoni L. The prone position during general anesthesia minimally affects respiratory mechanics while improving functional residual capacity and increasing oxygen tension. *Anesth Analg* 1995; **80**: 955–60.

103. D'Angelo E, Robatto FM, Calderini E, Tavola M, Bono D, Torri G, Milic-Emili J. Pulmonary and chest wall mechanics in anesthetized paralyzed humans. *J Appl Physiol* 1991; **70**: 2602–10.

104. Lehane JR, Jordan C, Jones JG. Influence of halothane and enflurane on respiratory airflow resistance and specific conductance in anaesthetized man. *Br J Anaesth* 1980; **52**: 773–81.

105. Heneghan CPH, Bergman NA, Jones JG. Changes in lung volume and (P_{AO_2} – Pa_{O_2}) during anaesthesia. *Br J Anaesth* 1986; **56**: 437–45.

106. Korenaga S, Takeda K, Ito Y. Differential effects of halothane on airway nerves and muscle. *Anesthesiology* 1984; **60**: 309–18.

107. Bhatt SB, Kendall AP, Lin ES, Oh TE. Resistance and additional inspiratory work imposed by the laryngeal mask airway: a comparison with tracheal tubes. *Anaesthesia* 1992; **47**: 343–7.

108. Rehder K, Sessler AD, Marsh HM. General anesthesia and the lung. *Am Rev Respir Dis* 1975; **112**: 541–63.

109. Westbrook PR, Stubbs SE, Sessler AD, Rehder K, Hyatt RE. Effects of anesthesia and muscle paralysis on respiratory mechanics in normal man. *J Appl Physiol* 1973; **34**: 81–6.

110. Schmid ER, Rehder K. General anesthesia and the chest wall. *Anesthesiology* 1981; **55**: 668–75.

111. Scheidt M, Hyatt RE, Rehder K. Effects of rib cage or abdominal restriction on lung mechanics. *J Appl Physiol* 1981; **51**: 1115–21.

112. Campbell EJM, Nunn JF, Peckett BW. A comparison of artificial ventilation and spontaneous respiration with particular reference to ventilation/blood-flow relationships. *Br J Anaesth* 1958; **30**: 166–75.

113. Nunn JF, Hill DW. Respiratory dead space and arterial to end-tidal CO_2 tension difference in anesthetized man. *J Appl Physiol* 1960; **15**: 383–9.

114. Kain ML, Panday J, Nunn JF. The effect of intubation on the dead space during halothane anaesthesia. *Br J Anaesth* 1969; **41**: 94–102.

115. Michenfelder JD, Fowler WS, Theye RA. CO_2 levels and pulmonary shunting in anesthetized man. *J Appl Physiol* 1966; **21**: 1471–6.

116. Marshall BE, Cohen PJ, Klingenmaier CH, Aukberg S. Pulmonary venous admixture before, during, and after halothane:oxygen anesthesia in man. *J Appl Physiol* 1969; **27**: 653–7.

117. Price HL, Cooperman LH, Warden JC, Morris JJ, Smith TC. Pulmonary hemodynamics during general anesthesia in man. *Anesthesiology* 1969; **30**: 629–36.

118. Nunn JF, Bergman NA, Coleman AJ. Factors influencing the arterial oxygen tension during anaesthesia with artificial ventilation. *Br J Anaesth* 1965; **37**: 898–914.

119. Nunn JF. Factors influencing the arterial oxygen tension during halothane anaesthesia with spontaneous respiration. *Br J Anaesth* 1964; **36**: 327–41.

120. Theye RA, Touhy GF. Oxygen uptake during light halothane anesthesia in man. *Anesthesiology* 1964; **25**: 627–33.

121. Gold MI, Helrich M. Ventilation and blood gases in anaesthetized patients. *Can Anaesth Soc J* 1967; **14**: 424–34.

122. Bindslev L, Hedenstierna G, Santesson J, Gottlieb I, Carvallhas A. Ventilation/perfusion distribution during inhalation anaesthesia. *Acta Anaesthesiol Scand* 1981; **25**: 360–71.

123. Tokics L, Hedenstierna G, Svensson L, Brismar B, Cederlund T, Lundquist H, Strandberg A. V̇/Q̇ distribution and correlation to atelectasis in anesthetized paralyzed humans. *J Appl Physiol* 1996; **81**: 1822–33.

124. Hedenstierna G. Contribution of the multiple inert gas elimination technique to pulmonary medicine. 6. Ventilation/perfusion relationships during anaesthesia. *Thorax* 1995; **50**: 85–91.

125. Rehder K, Knopp TJ, Sessler AD, Didier EP. Ventilation/perfusion relationship in young healthy awake and anesthetized-paralyzed man. *J Appl Physiol* 1979; **47**: 745–53.

126. Nunn JF. Oxygen – friend and foe. *J R Soc Med* 1985; **78**: 618–22.

127. Dueck R, Young I, Clausen J, Wagner PD. Altered distribution of pulmonary ventilation and blood flow following induction of inhalational anesthesia. *Anesthesiology* 1980; **52**: 113–25.

128. Anjou-Lindskog E, Broman L, Broman M, Holmgren A, Settergren G, Öhqvist G. Effects of intravenous anesthesia on V̇A/Q̇ distribution: a study performed during ventilation with air and with 50% oxygen, supine and in the lateral position. *Anesthesiology* 1985; **62**: 485–92.

129. Nunn JF, Ezi-Ashi TI. The respiratory effects of resistance to breathing in anesthetized man. *Anesthesiology* 1961; **22**: 174–85.

130. Moote CA, Knill RL, Clement J. Ventilatory compensation for continuous inspiratory resistive and elastic loads during halothane anesthesia in humans. *Anesthesiology* 1986; **64**: 582–9.

131. Drummond GB, Cullen JP. Detection of inspiratory resistive loads after anaesthesia for minor surgery. *Br J Anaesth* 1997; **78**: 308–10.

132. Isono S, Nishino T, Sugimori K, Mizuguchi T. Respiratory effects of expiratory flow-resistive loading in conscious and anesthetized humans. *Anesth Analg* 1990; **70**: 594–9.

133. Boothby WM, Sandiford I. Basal metabolism. *Physiol Rev* 1924; **18**: 1085.

134. Roberston JD, Reid DD. Standards for the basal metabolism of normal people in Britain. *Lancet* 1952; **1**: 940–3.

135. Nunn JF, Matthews RL. Gaseous exchange during halothane anaesthesia: the steady respiratory state. *Br J Anaesth* 1959; **31**: 330–40.

136. Marshall BE, Marshall C. Anesthesia and the pulmonary circulation. In: Covino BG, Fozzard HA, Rehder K, Strichartz G, eds. *Effects of anesthesia.* Bethesda MD: American Physiological Society, 1985.

137. Eisenkraft JB. Effects of anaesthetics on the pulmonary circulation. *Br J Anaesth* 1990; **65**: 63–78.

138. Sykes MK, Loh L, Seed RF, Kafer ER, Chakrabarti MK. The effect of inhalational anaesthetics on hypoxic pulmonary vasoconstriction and pulmonary vascular resistance in the perfused lungs of the dog and cat. *Br J Anaesth* 1972; **44**: 776–88.

139. Bjertnæs LJ. Hypoxia-induced vasoconstriction in isolated perfused lungs exposed to injectable or inhalation anaesthetics. *Acta Anaesthesiol Scand* 1977; **21**: 133–47.

140. Marshall BE. Pulmonary blood flow and oxygenation. In: Marshall BE, Longnecker DE, Fairley HB, eds. *Anesthesia for thoracic procedures.* Oxford: Blackwell Scientific, 1988.

141. Rehder K, Hatch DJ, Sessler AD, Fowler WS. The function of each lung of anesthetized and paralyzed man during mechanical ventilation. *Anesthesiology* 1972; **37**: 16–26.

142. Klingstedt C, Hedenstierna G, Baehrendtz S, Lundqvist H, Strandberg A, Tokics L, Brismar B. Ventilation–perfusion relationships and atelectasis formation in the supine and lateral positions during conventional mechanical and differential ventilation. *Acta Anaesthesiol Scand* 1990; **34**: 421–9.

143. Reber A, Bein T, Högman M, Khan ZP, Nilsson S, Hedenstierna G. Lung aeration and pulmonary gas exchange during lumbar epidural anaesthesia and in the lithotomy position in elderly patients. *Anaesthesia* 1998; **53**: 854–61.

144. Ellison RG, Ellison LT, Hamilton WF. Analysis of respiratory acidosis during anesthesia. *Ann Surg* 1955; **141**: 375–82.

145. Benumof JL, Augustine SD, Gibbons JA. Halothane and isoflurane only slightly impair arterial oxygenation during one-lung ventilation in patients undergoing thoracotomy. *Anesthesiology* 1987; **67**: 910–15.

146. Abe K, Shimizu T, Takashina M, Shiozaki H, Yoshiya I. The effects of propofol, isoflurane, and sevoflurane on oxygenation and shunt fraction during one-lung ventilation. *Anesth Analg* 1998; **87**: 1164–9.

147. Inomata S, Nishikawa T, Saito S, Kihara S. 'Best' PEEP during one-lung ventilation. *Br J Anaesth* 1997; **78**: 754–6.

148. Kochi T, Sako S, Nishino T, Mizuguchi T. Effect of high thoracic extradural anaesthesia on ventilatory response to hypercapnia in normal volunteers. *Br J Anaesth* 1989; **62**: 362–7.

149. Takasaki M, Takahashi T. Respiratory function during cervical and thoracic extradural analgesia in patients with normal lungs. *Br J Anaesth* 1980; **52**: 1271–6.

150. Sakura S, Saito Y, Kosaka Y. The effects of epidural anesthesia on ventilatory response to hypercapnia and hypoxia in elderly patients. *Anesth Analg* 1996; **82**: 306–11.

151. Sakura S, Saito Y, Kosaka Y. Effect of extradural anaesthesia on the ventilatory response to hypoxaemia. *Anaesthesia* 1993; **48**: 205–9.

152. Sakura S, Saito Y, Kosaka Y. Effect of lumbar epidural anesthesia on ventilatory response to hypercapnia in young and elderly patients. *J Clin Anesth* 1993; **5**: 109–13.

153. Labaille T, Clergue F, Samii K, Ecoffey C, Berdeaux A. Ventilatory response to CO_2 following intravenous and epidural lidocaine. *Anesthesiology* 1985; **63**: 179–85.

154. Warner DO, Warner MA, Ritman EL. Human chest wall function during epidural anesthesia. *Anesthesiology* 1996; **85**: 761–73.

155. Moir DD. Ventilatory function during epidural analgesia. *Br J Anaesth* 1963; **35**: 3–7.

156. Kelly MC, Fitzpatrick KTJ, Hill DA. Respiratory effects of spinal anaesthesia for caesarean section. *Anaesthesia* 1996; **51**: 1120–2.

157. Gamil M. Serial peak expiratory flow rates in mothers during caesarean section under extradural anaesthesia. *Br J Anaesth* 1989; **62**: 415–18.

158. Yun E, Topulos GP, Body SC, Datta S, Bader AM. Pulmonary function changes during epidural anesthesia for cesarean delivery. *Anesth Analg* 1996; **82**: 750–3.

159. Jones JG, Sapsford DJ, Wheatley RG. Postoperative hypoxaemia: mechanisms and time course. *Anaesthesia* 1990; **45**: 566–73.

160. Moller JT, Johannessen NW, Berg H, Espersen K, Larsen LE. Hypoxaemia during anaesthesia – an observer study. *Br J Anaesth* 1991; **66**: 437–44.

161. Liu S, Carpenter RL, Neal JM. Epidural anesthesia and analgesia: their role in postoperative outcome. *Anesthesiology* 1995; **82**: 1474–506.

162. McKeague H, Cunningham AJ. Postoperative respiratory dysfunction: is the site of surgery crucial. *Br J Anaesth* 1997; **79**: 415–16.

163. Couture JD, Chartrand D, Gagner M, Bellemare F. Diaphragmatic and abdominal muscle activity after endoscopic cholecystectomy. *Anesth Analg* 1994; **78**: 733–9.

164. Strandberg A, Tokics L, Brismar B, Lundquist H, Hedenstierna G. Atelectasis during anaesthesia and in the postoperative period. *Acta Anaesthesiol Scand* 1986; **30**: 154–8.

165. Catley DM, Thornton C, Jordan C, Lehane JR, Royston D, Jones JG. Pronounced, episodic oxygen desaturation in the postoperative period: its association with ventilatory pattern and analgesic regime. *Anesthesiology* 1985; **63**: 20–8.

166. Drummond GB. Diaphragmatic dysfunction: an outmoded concept. *Br J Anaesth* 1998; **80**: 277–80.

167. Nimmo AF, Drummond GB. Respiratory mechanics after abdominal surgery measured with continuous analysis of pressure, flow and volume signals. *Br J Anaesth* 1996; **77**: 317–26.

168. Keller C, Brimacombe J. Bronchial mucus transport velocity in paralyzed anesthetized patients: a comparison of the laryngeal mask airway and cuffed tracheal tube. *Anesth Analg* 1998; **86**: 1280–2.

Chapter 22

Changes in the carbon dioxide tension

The effects of changes in P_{CO_2} were a matter of grave concern some 40 years ago, when there were no convenient techniques for monitoring or measuring P_{CO_2} in the clinical environment. Gross departures from normality were relatively common, and hypercapnia was an appreciable cause of mortality. All of this has changed with routine monitoring of end-expiratory P_{CO_2} and the ease of direct measurement of arterial P_{CO_2}. It should now be possible to prevent both hypo- and hypercapnia in almost all clinical circumstances.

Renewed interest in hypercapnia has occurred in the 1990s, for two reasons. First, changes in the approach to artificial ventilation in severe lung injury have led to the use of 'permissive hypercapnia' (page 581). In order to minimize pulmonary damage, minute volume of ventilation is maintained deliberately low, and the arterial P_{CO_2} is allowed to increase. Secondly, a massive expansion of laparoscopic surgical techniques, mostly using carbon dioxide for abdominal insufflation, has led to the anaesthetist having to control arterial P_{CO_2} under conditions of significantly increased pulmonary carbon dioxide output.

Before describing the effects of carbon dioxide on various physiological systems, this chapter briefly outlines the causes of changes in arterial P_{CO_2}.

Causes of hypocapnia

Hypocapnia can result only from an alveolar ventilation that is excessive in relation to carbon dioxide production. Low values of arterial P_{CO_2} are commonly found, resulting from artificial ventilation with a generous minute volume or from voluntary hyperventilation due to psychological disturbance such as hysteria. A low arterial P_{CO_2} may also result simply from hyperventilation when an arterial sample is drawn. Persistently low values may be due to an excessive respiratory drive resulting from one or more of the following causes.

Hypoxaemia is a common cause of hypocapnia, occurring in congenital heart disease with right-to-left shunting, residence at high altitude, pulmonary collapse or consolidation and any other condition that reduces the arterial P_{O_2} below about 8 kPa (60 mmHg). Hypocapnia, secondary to hypoxaemia, opposes the ventilatory response to the hypoxaemia (page 100).

Metabolic acidosis produces a compensatory hyperventilation (air hunger), which minimizes the fall in pH that would otherwise occur. This is a pronounced feature of diabetic ketoacidosis and severe haemorrhagic shock. Arterial P_{CO_2} values below 3 kPa (22.5 mmHg) are not uncommon in severe metabolic acidosis. This is a vital compensatory mechanism. Failure to maintain the required hyperventilation, either from fatigue or inadequate ventilation following tracheal intubation, leads to a rapid life-threatening decrease in arterial pH.

Mechanical abnormalities of the lung may drive respiration through the vagus, resulting in moderate reduction of the P_{CO_2}. Thus conditions such as pulmonary fibrosis and asthma are usually associated with a low to normal P_{CO_2} until the patient passes into type 2 respiratory failure (page 513).

Neurological disorders may result in hyperventilation and hypocapnia. This is seen most commonly in conditions that lead to the presence of blood in the cerebrospinal fluid, such as occurs following head injury or subarachnoid haemorrhage.

Causes of hypercapnia

It is uncommon to encounter an arterial P_{CO_2} above the normal range in a healthy subject. Any value of more than 6.1 kPa (46 mmHg) should be considered abnormal, but values up to 6.7 kPa (50 mmHg) may be attained by breath holding. It is difficult for the healthy subject to exceed this level by any respiratory manoeuvre other than by breathing mixtures of carbon dioxide in oxygen.

   When a patient is hypercapnic, there are only four possible causes. These should be considered systematically, as follows.

Increased concentration of carbon dioxide in the inspired gas

This iatrogenic cause of hypercapnia is very uncommon but it is dangerous and differs fundamentally from the other causes listed below. It should therefore be excluded at the outset in any patient unexpectedly found to be hypercapnic when breathing from or being ventilated by external equipment. The carbon dioxide may be endogenous or exogenous, the former resulting from rebreathing while the latter is usually therapeutic or accidental. The only essential difference between the two is the rate at which the P_{CO_2} can increase. If all the carbon dioxide produced by metabolism is retained and distributed in the body stores, arterial P_{CO_2} can increase no faster than about 0.4–0.8 kPa.min^{-1} (3–6 mmHg.min^{-1}). This limits the rate of increase of P_{CO_2} during rebreathing. In contrast, the P_{CO_2} may rise extremely rapidly when exogenous carbon dioxide is inhaled.

Increased carbon dioxide production

If the pulmonary minute volume is fixed by artificial ventilation and the production of carbon dioxide is increased by, for example, malignant hyperpyrexia, hypercapnia is inevitable. Like the previous category, this is a rare but dangerous cause of hypercapnia, which should be excluded when there is no other obvious explanation for an increasing P_{CO_2}. A less dramatic, but very common, reason for increased carbon dioxide production is sepsis leading to pyrexia, which often results in hypercapnia in ventilated patients in intensive care.

Though not strictly an increase in production, absorption of carbon dioxide from the peritoneum during laparoscopic surgery has the same respiratory effects.[1] Absorption of gas from the peritoneal cavity depends on the partial pressure of gas present and its solubility in peritoneal tissue. Gas mixtures are rarely used, so the partial pressure is normally equal to the insufflation pressure. Insoluble gases such as helium or nitrogen would be absorbed to a much smaller extent, but would also be more disastrous during the rare complication of gas embolus. Air, oxygen and nitrous oxide all support combustion, so preclude the use of diathermy which is fundamental to laparoscopic surgery. Thus carbon dioxide remains the usual gas used for the erroneously named 'pneumo-peritoneum'. The recent development of surgical techniques for complex and major abdominal procedures has led to the use of prolonged insufflation with carbon dioxide at higher intra-abdominal pressures than were used previously. Carbon dioxide absorption during laparoscopy is estimated at between 15 and 50 ml.min^{-1}, and requires a significant increase in minute ventilation if hypercapnia is to be prevented. Changes in the cardiovascular system during laparoscopy may, however, reduce the efficiency of the lungs in removing carbon dioxide and allow its accumulation in spite of normal end-expiratory concentrations. Thus, even when minute volume is increased, alterations in body stores of carbon dioxide will still occur during prolonged surgery[2] and may be predicted to take several hours to return to normal postoperatively (see Figure 10.9).

Hypoventilation

An inadequate pulmonary minute volume is by far the commonest cause of hypocapnia. Pathological causes of hypoventilation leading to hypercapnia are considered in Chapter 26. In respiratory medicine, the commonest cause of long-standing hypercapnia is chronic bronchitis. The type of patient known as the 'blue bloater' has reduced ventilatory capacity combined with reduced ventilatory response to carbon dioxide. There are many other possible causes (see Figure 26.2), including medullary depression by drugs, neuromuscular blockade, respiratory obstruction and restriction of the lungs or chest wall.

Increased dead space

This very rare cause of hypercapnia is usually diagnosed by a process of exclusion when a patient has a high $P\text{co}_2$, with a normal minute volume and no evidence of a hypermetabolic state or inhaled carbon dioxide. The cause may be incorrectly configured breathing apparatus or an excessively large alveolar dead space (page 179). This might be due to pulmonary embolism or a cyst communicating with the tracheobronchial tree and receiving preferential ventilation.

Effects of carbon dioxide on the nervous system

A number of special difficulties hinder an understanding of the effects of changes in $P\text{co}_2$ on any physiological system. First, there is the problem of species difference, which is a formidable obstacle to the interpretation of animal studies in this as in other fields. The second difficulty arises from the fact that carbon dioxide can exert its effect either directly or in consequence of (respiratory) acidosis. The third difficulty arises from the fact that carbon dioxide acts at many different sites in the body, sometimes producing opposing effects on a particular function, such as blood pressure (see below).

Carbon dioxide has at least five major effects on the brain:

1. It is a major factor governing cerebral blood flow.
2. It influences the CSF pressure through changes in cerebral blood flow.
3. It is the main factor influencing the intracellular pH, which is known to have important effects on the metabolism, and therefore function, of the cell.
4. It may be presumed to exert the inert gas narcotic effect in accord with its physical properties, which are similar to those of nitrous oxide.
5. It influences the excitability of certain neurones, particularly relevant in the case of the reticuloactivating system.

The interplay of these effects is difficult to understand, although the gross changes produced are well established.

Effects on consciousness

Carbon dioxide has long been known to cause unconsciousness in dogs entering the Grotto del Cane in Italy, where carbon dioxide issuing from a fumarole forms a layer near the ground. It was used as an anaesthetic in animals by Henry Hill Hickman in 1824,[3] and has been widely used as a routine anaesthetic agent for very short procedures in small laboratory animals. Inhalation of 30% carbon dioxide is sufficient to produce anaesthesia in humans, but is complicated by the frequent occurrence of convulsions.[4] In patients with ventilatory failure, carbon dioxide narcosis occurs when the P_{CO_2} rises above 12–16 kPa (90–120 mmHg).[5]

Narcosis by carbon dioxide is probably not due primarily to its inert gas narcotic effects, because its oil solubility predicts a very much weaker narcotic than it seems to be. It is likely that the major effect on the central nervous system is by alteration of the intracellular pH, with consequent derangements of metabolic processes. In 1967 Eisele and colleagues showed that the narcotic effect in dogs correlated better with cerebrospinal fluid pH than with arterial P_{CO_2}.[6]

Cerebral blood flow[7]

Cerebral blood flow (CBF) increases with arterial P_{CO_2} at a rate of about 7–15 ml.100 g^{-1}.min^{-1} for each kPa increase in P_{CO_2} (1–2 ml.100 g^{-1}.min^{-1}.mmHg^{-1}) within the approximate range 3–10 kPa (20–80 mmHg). The full response curve is S-shaped (Figure 22.1). The response at very low P_{CO_2} is probably limited by the vasodilator effect of tissue hypoxia, and the response above 16 kPa (120 mmHg) seems to represent maximal vasodilatation. The changes shown in Figure 22.1 represent the brain as a whole and it is not possible to generalize about regional changes. There is some evidence that considerable regional variations in carbon dioxide responsiveness exist within the human central nervous system.[8]

Mechanisms. In the intact animal, CBF is increased in response to P_{CO_2} by a combination of vasodilatation of cerebral blood vessels and an increase in blood pressure (see below). Changes in P_{CO_2} lead to a complex series of events that bring about vasodilatation of cerebral blood vessels.[7] In adults, the effect is initiated by changes in the extracellular pH in the region of the arterioles, which alters intracellular calcium levels both directly and indirectly via nitric oxide production and the formation of cyclic GMP. With prolonged hypocapnia, and to a lesser extent hypercapnia, changes in CBF return towards baseline after a few hours,[7,9] an effect thought to result from changes in cerebrospinal fluid pH

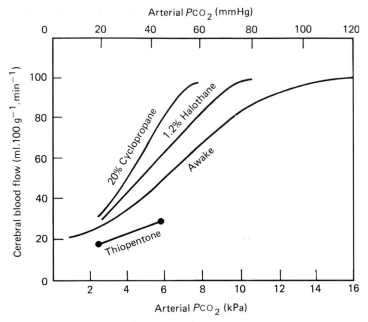

Figure 22.1 Relationship of cerebral blood flow to arterial P_{CO_2} in awake and anaesthetized patients.

correcting the extracellular acidosis. Hypercapnic cerebral vasodilatation in neonates is believed to operate by a quite different mechanism involving the production of prostaglandins and cyclic AMP.

Pathological effects. Sensitivity to carbon dioxide may be lost in a variety of pathological circumstances such as cerebral tumour, infarction or trauma. There is commonly a fixed vasodilatation in these areas, giving rise to so-called luxury perfusion;[10] far from being luxurious, though, if widespread it may cause dangerous increases in intracranial pressure. Areas of brain with luxury perfusion may respond to altered P_{CO_2} in the opposite direction to normal. For example, a high P_{CO_2} may increase blood flow through normal brain tissue and actually decrease perfusion through ischaemic areas that have lost their response to carbon dioxide, an effect referred to as intracerebral steal. The reverse phenomenon may occur when P_{CO_2} is lowered in patients with an area of luxury perfusion. Vasoconstriction in the surrounding normal tissue may divert blood flow towards the abnormal area of luxury perfusion, which has no ability to respond to lowered P_{CO_2} – an effect known as the inverse steal.

Anaesthesia. All inhalational anaesthetics have a direct cerebral vasodilator effect and increase normocapnic CBF considerably.[11,12,13,14] They also accentuate the response to both hypocapnia and hypercapnia; that is, they increase the slope of the relationship between P_{CO_2} and CBF (Figure 22.1). In spite of the increased slope during hypocapnia, global CBF during anaesthesia with hyperventilation is normally still greater than when awake.[7] Intravenous anaesthetics such as thiopentone[15] and propofol[16] reduce CBF at normal P_{CO_2}, in accordance with the reduced cerebral oxygen consumption (Table 22.1). Vasoconstriction in response to hyperventilation continues to occur (Figure 22.1), but at

Table 22.1 Effects of hyperventilation and anaesthesia on cerebral blood flow and oxygenation in humans

State of patient or subject	Cerebral oxygen consumption $(ml.100\,g^{-1}.min^{-1})$	Cerebral blood flow $(ml.100g^{-1}.min^{-1})$	Internal jugular venous P_{O_2}	
			kPa	mmHg
Conscious				
Arterial P_{CO_2} 5.3 kPa (40 mmHg)	3.0	44.0	4.7–5.3	35–40
Arterial P_{CO_2} 2.7 kPa (20 mmHg)	3.0	22.0	–	–
Anaesthetized				
Thiopentone				
Arterial P_{CO_2} 5.9 kPa (44 mmHg)	1.5	27.6	4.7	35
Arterial P_{CO_2} 2.4 kPa (18 mmHg)	1.7	16.4	2.4	18
Halothane 1.0%				
Arterial P_{CO_2} 5.5 kPa (41 mmHg)	2.2	54.4	–	–

(Data from references 12, 15 and 17.)

deeper levels of anaesthesia the response is reduced compared with when awake.[7] Even so, hyperventilation during deep thiopentone anaesthesia has been shown to reduce jugular venous oxygen P_{O_2}, indicating a significant reduction in CBF (Table 22.1).

Intracranial pressure (ICP) tends to rise with increasing P_{CO_2}, probably as a result of cerebral vasodilatation. Hyperventilation was used for many years as a standard method of acutely reducing ICP after head injury,[18] but the reduction in ICP may only be shortlived and the effects on cerebral blood flow are variable. The possibility of *increased* cerebral blood flow as a result of lowered ICP must be offset against *reduced* cerebral blood flow from hypocapnic vasoconstriction. It is therefore preferable to monitor ICP, an invasive technique not available in many units dealing with head-injured patients. Recent recommendations on the management of head injury therefore advise that hyperventilation should be used to reduce intracranial pressure only when other therapeutic approaches have failed.[19]

Effects on the autonomic and endocrine systems

Survival in severe hypercapnia is, to a large extent, dependent on the autonomic response. A great many of the effects of carbon dioxide on other systems are due wholly or in part to the autonomic response to carbon dioxide.

In 1960, Millar[20] clearly showed the increase in plasma levels of both adrenaline and noradrenaline, caused by an elevation of P_{CO_2} during apnoeic mass-movement oxygenation (Figure 22.2). In moderate hypercapnia there is a proportionate rise of adrenaline and noradrenaline, but in gross hypercapnia (P_{CO_2} more than 27 kPa or 200 mmHg) there is an abrupt rise of adrenaline. Similar, though very variable, changes have been obtained over a lower range of P_{CO_2} in human volunteers inhaling carbon dioxide mixtures.[21,22] The increase in catecholamine levels is markedly attenuated by either epidural anaesthesia or the administration of clonidine.[23]

The effect of an increased level of circulating catecholamines is, to a certain extent, offset by a decreased sensitivity of target organs when the pH is reduced. This is additional

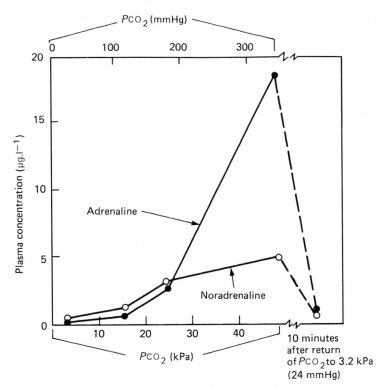

Figure 22.2 This graph shows the changes in plasma catecholamine levels in the dog during the rise of P_{CO_2} from 2.9 to 45 kPa (22 to 338 mmHg) in the course of 1 hour of apnoeic oxygenation. After 10 minutes of ventilation with oxygen, P_{CO_2} returned to 3.2 kPa (24 mmHg). Catecholamines were almost back to control values but the adrenaline remained higher than noradrenaline. (From data in reference 20.)

to the general depressant direct effect of carbon dioxide on target organs. There is also evidence that the anterior pituitary is stimulated by carbon dioxide, resulting in increased secretion of ACTH.[24] Acetylcholine hydrolysis is reduced at low pH and therefore certain parasympathetic effects may be enhanced during hypercapnia.

Effects on the respiratory system

Chapter 5 describes the role of carbon dioxide in the control of breathing, and this is not discussed further here.

Pulmonary circulation

A raised P_{CO_2} causes vasoconstriction in the pulmonary circulation (page 153) but the effect is less marked than that of hypoxia.[25] Nevertheless, in healthy subjects an end-expiratory P_{CO_2} of 7 kPa (52 mmHg) increased pulmonary vascular resistance by 32 per cent, which, along with elevated cardiac output, led to a 60 per cent increase in mean pulmonary arterial pressure.[26] Though regional variations in blood flow have not been demonstrated, this effect is believed to act in a similar fashion to hypoxic pulmonary vasoconstriction (HPV, page 151), tending to divert blood away from underventilated alveoli. Hypocapnia significantly attenuates HPV in dogs, though this has not been described in humans. There is evidence from both animal[27] and human[28] studies that pH is the factor responsible for CO_2-mediated changes in the pulmonary vasculature, rather than P_{CO_2} per se.

Effects on oxygenation of the blood

Quite apart from its effect on ventilation, carbon dioxide exerts three other important effects that influence the oxygenation of the blood. First, if the concentration of nitrogen (or other 'inert' gas) remains constant, the concentration of carbon dioxide in the alveolar gas can increase only at the expense of oxygen, which must be displaced. Secondly, an increase in P_{CO_2} causes a displacement of the oxygen dissociation curve to the right (page 267). Finally, in animals, changes in P_{CO_2} are known to affect the distribution of ventilation/perfusion ratios as measured by the multiple inert gas elimination technique (page 191). This results from changes in pH influencing pulmonary vessels, as described in the previous section, as well as causing changes in the size of small-diameter bronchi.[27]

Effects on the circulatory system[29]

The effects of carbon dioxide on the circulation are complicated by the alternative modes of action on the different components of the system (Figure 22.3). Many actions are in opposition to each other and, under different circumstances, the overall effect of carbon dioxide on certain circulatory functions can be entirely reversed.

Myocardial contractility and heart rate

Both contractility and heart rate are diminished by elevated P_{CO_2} in the isolated preparation, probably as a result of change in pH. However, in the intact subject the direct depressant effect of carbon dioxide is overshadowed by the stimulant effect mediated through the sympathetic system. In artificially ventilated humans, increased P_{CO_2} raises cardiac output and slightly reduces total peripheral resistance,[22] and blood pressure therefore tends to be increased. Awake healthy subjects studied with non-invasive Doppler echocardiography show similar changes.[26] With an end-expiratory P_{CO_2} of 7 kPa (52 mmHg), cardiac output was increased by about 1 l.min^{-1} as a result of increases in both heart rate and stroke volume, and accompanied by a small rise in blood pressure. Measurements of left ventricular systolic and diastolic function were unchanged, confirming the dominance of catecholamine stimulation compared with direct depressant effects on the heart. The response of cardiac output to hypercapnia is diminished by most anaesthetics.[22]

Arrhythmias

Arrhythmias have been reported in awake humans during acute hypercapnia, but seldom seem to be of serious import. One study of normal subjects with modest degrees of hypercapnia did, however, demonstrate an increase in QT dispersion of the electrocardiogram during hypercapnia.[26] This finding reflects regional repolarization abnormalities of the ventricles and, under other circumstances such as ischaemic heart disease, indicates a propensity to develop life-threatening arrhythmias.

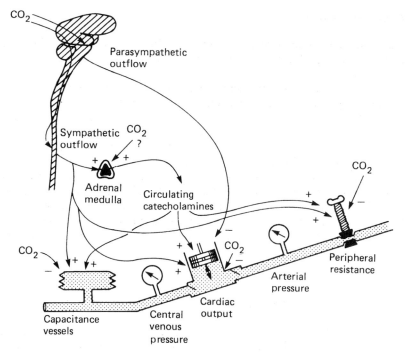

Figure 22.3 The complexity of the mechanisms by which carbon dioxide may influence the circulatory system. The overall effect in the anaesthetized patient is an increase in cardiac output that is roughly proportional to the arterial $P\text{co}_2$. The rise in cardiac output exceeds the rise in blood pressure, indicating a reduction in systemic vascular resistance. In spite of the rise in cardiac output, there is an increase in central venous pressure. This implies that capacitance vessels are contracted to cause a rise in filling pressure with which the increased cardiac output does not keep pace. In the absence of sympathetic nervous system activity, the direct effect of carbon dioxide on the myocardium causes a fall of cardiac output.

The use of some older inhalational anaesthetic agents is also associated with hypercapnia-induced arrhythmias. With cyclopropane and halothane, it seems that arrhythmias will always occur above a '$P\text{co}_2$ arrhythmic threshold' of around 10–12 kPa (75–90 mmHg). Multifocal ventricular extrasystoles have been reported and the danger of ventricular fibrillation cannot be discounted. These arrhythmias occurred at catecholamine levels that were above normal, but not high enough to cause arrhythmias by themselves.

Blood pressure

The effect of $P\text{co}_2$ is the result of the interaction of a great many individual actions, some tending to increase and some to decrease the blood pressure. In fact, pressure is generally raised, as $P\text{co}_2$ increases in both conscious and anaesthetized patients. However, the response is variable and certainly cannot be relied on as an infallible diagnostic sign of hypercapnia. Hypotension accompanies an elevation of $P\text{co}_2$ if there is blockade of the sympathetic system by ganglioplegic drugs or spinal blockade. There is general agreement that hypotension follows a sudden fall of an elevated $P\text{co}_2$.

Effect on the kidney

Renal blood flow and glomerular filtration rate are little influenced by minor changes of $P\text{CO}_2$. However, at high levels of $P\text{CO}_2$ there is constriction of the glomerular afferent arterioles, leading to anuria.

Chronic hypercapnia results in increased resorption of bicarbonate by the kidneys, further raising the plasma bicarbonate level, and constituting a secondary or compensatory metabolic alkalosis. Chronic hypocapnia decreases renal bicarbonate resorption, resulting in a further fall of plasma bicarbonate and producing a secondary or compensatory 'metabolic acidosis'. In each case the arterial pH returns towards the normal value but the bicarbonate ion concentration departs even further from normality.

Although acute changes of $P\text{CO}_2$ do not produce a true metabolic acid–base change, the interpolation technique of Siggaard-Andersen et al.[30] indicates an apparent base deficit of about 2 mmol.l^{-1} when the $P\text{CO}_2$ of a normal patient is acutely raised from 5.3 to 10.7 kPa (40 to 80 mmHg). Similarly, a base excess of about 2 mmol.l^{-1} appears when the $P\text{CO}_2$ is rapidly lowered to 2.7 kPa (20 mmHg) The explanation of this artefact is to be found above (page 231).

Effect on blood electrolyte levels

Hypercapnia is accompanied by a leakage of potassium ions from the cells into the plasma.[31] Hepatectomy has demonstrated that most of the potassium comes from the liver, probably in association with glucose that is mobilized in response to the rise in plasma catecholamine levels.[32] Because it takes an appreciable time for the potassium ions to be transported back into the intracellular compartment, repeated bouts of hypercapnia at short intervals result in a stepwise rise in plasma potassium.

A reduction in the ionized fraction of the total calcium has, in the past, been thought to be the cause of the tetany that accompanies severe hypocapnia. However, the changes that occur are too small to account for tetany, which occurs only in parathyroid disease when there has been a fairly gross reduction of ionized calcium.[33] Hyperexcitability affects all nerves, and spontaneous activity ultimately occurs. The spasms probably result from activity in proprioceptive fibres, causing reflex muscle contraction.

Gross hypercapnia in clinical practice

Relatively few cases of gross hypercapnia are documented, but there are sufficient to indicate that complete recovery from gross hypercapnia without hypoxia is possible and may even be the rule.[34] Inhaled concentrations of about 30% were formerly used in psychiatry for abreaction, apparently without ill effect. During anaesthesia, gross hypercapnia has been reported,[35] particularly in relation to thoracotomy without artificial ventilation (page 450). Arterial $P\text{CO}_2$ values in excess of 30 kPa (225 mmHg) were apparently not unusual. A report from 1990[36] detailed five instances of hypercapnia without hypoxia in children with arterial $P\text{CO}_2$ values in the range 21–36 kPa (155–269 mmHg). All were comatose or stuperose but recovered. A recent single case report of massive grain aspiration reported survival following a $P\text{CO}_2$ of 66.8 kPa (501 mmHg).[37] These cases, along with a review of earlier literature,[35] indicated that, *of the reported cases*, full recovery was the usual outcome. In spite of the cardiac changes described above, arrhythmias did not seem to be a problem in these patients. In general, hypoxia seems to be much more dangerous than hypercapnia.

Bedside recognition of hypercapnia

Hyperventilation is the cardinal sign of hypercapnia due to an increased concentration of carbon dioxide in the inspired gas, whether it be endogenous or exogenous. However, this sign will be absent in the paralysed patient and also in those in whom hypercapnia is the result of hypoventilation. Such patients, including those with chronic obstructive airway disease, constitute the great majority of those with hypercapnia.

Dyspnoea may or may not be present. In patients with central failure of respiratory drive (including 'blue bloaters'), dyspnoea may be entirely absent. On the other hand, when hypoventilation results from mechanical failure in the respiratory system (airway obstruction, pneumothorax, pulmonary fibrosis, etc.), dyspnoea is usually obvious. This problem is discussed further on page 515 in relation to Figure 26.2.

In patients with chronic bronchitis, hypercapnia is usually associated with a flushed skin and a full and bounding pulse with occasional extrasystoles. The blood pressure is often raised but this is not a reliable sign. Muscle twitchings and a characteristic flap of the hands may be observed when coma is imminent. Convulsions may occur. The patient will become comatose when the Pco_2 is in the range 12–16 kPa (90–120 mmHg) (see above). Hypercapnia should always be considered in cases of unexplained coma.

Hypercapnia cannot be reliably diagnosed on clinical examination. This is particularly true when there is a neurological basis for hypoventilation. Now that it has become so simple to measure the arterial Pco_2, an arterial sample should be taken in all cases of doubt.

References

1. Sharma KC, Brandstetter RD, Brensilver JM, Jung LD. Cardiopulmonary physiology and pathophysiology as a consequence of laparoscopic surgery. *Chest* 1996; **110**: 810–15.
2. Wahba RWM, Mamazza J. Ventilatory requirements during laparoscopic cholecystectomy. *Can J Anaesth* 1993; **40**: 206–10.
3. Rushman GB, Davies NJH, Atkinson RS. *A short history of anaesthesia: the first 150 years.* Oxford: Butterworth-Heinemann, 1996.
4. Leake CD, Waters RM. The anesthetic properties of carbon dioxide. *J Pharmacol Exp Ther* 1928; **33**: 280–1.
5. Refsum HE. Relationship between state of consciousness and arterial hypoxaemia and hypercapnia in patients with pulmonary insufficiency, breathing air. *Clin Sci* 1963; **25**: 361–7.
6. Eisele JH, Eger EI, Muallem M. Narcotic properties of carbon dioxide in the dog. *Anesthesiology* 1967; **28**: 856–65.
7. Brian JE. Carbon dioxide and the cerebral circulation. *Anesthesiology* 1998; **88**: 1365–86.
8. Wilkinson IMS, Browne DRG. The influence of anaesthesia and of arterial hypocapnia on regional blood flow in the normal human cerebral hemisphere. *Br J Anaesth* 1970; **42**: 472–82.
9. Raichle ME, Posner JB, Plum F. Cerebral blood flow during and after hyperventilation. *Arch Neurol* 1970; **23**: 394–403.
10. Lassen NA. The luxury-perfusion syndrome and its possible relation to acute metabolic acidosis localised within the brain. *Lancet* 1966; **2**: 1113–5.
11. Strebel S, Kaufmann M, Baggi M, Zenklusen U. Cerebrovascular carbon dioxide reactivity during exposure to equipotent isoflurane and isoflurane in nitrous oxide anaesthesia. *Br J Anaesth* 1993; **71**: 272–6.

12. Christensen MS, Hoedt-Rasmussen K, Lassen NA. Cerebral vasodilatation by halothane anaesthesia in man and its potentiation by hypotension and hypercapnia. *Br J* Anaesth 1967; **39**: 927–34.

13. Ornstein E, Young WL, Fleischer LH, Ostapkovich N. Desflurane and isoflurane have similar effects on cerebral blood flow in patients with intracranial mass lesions. *Anesthesiology* 1993; **79**: 498–502.

14. Cho S, Kujigaki T, Uchiyama Y, Fukusai M, Shibata O, Somikawa K. Effects of sevoflurane with and without nitrous oxide on human cerebral circulation. *Anesthesiology* 1996; **85**: 755–60.

15. Pierce EC, Lambertson CJ, Deutsch S, Chase PE, Linde HW, Dripps RD, Price HL. Cerebral circulation and metabolism during thiopental anesthesia and hyperventilation in man. *J Clin Invest* 1962; **41**: 1664–71.

16. Eng C, Lam AM, Mayberg TS, Lee C, Mathisen T. The influence of propofol with and without nitrous oxide on cerebral blood flow velocity and CO_2 reactivity in humans. *Anesthesiology* 1992; **77**: 872–9.

17. Smith AL, Wollman H. Cerebral blood flow and metabolism. *Anesthesiology* 1972; **36**: 378–400.

18. Shenkin HA, Bouzarth WF. Clinical methods of reducing intracranial pressure. *N Engl J Med* 1970; **282**: 1465–71.

19. Yundt KD, Diringer MN. The use of hyperventilation and its impact on cerebral ischaemia in the treatment of traumatic brain injury. *Crit Care Clin* 1997; **13**: 163–84.

20. Millar RA. Plasma adrenaline and noradrenaline during diffusion respiration. *J Physiol* 1960; **150**: 79–90.

21. Sechzer PH, Egbert LD, Linde HW, Cooper DY, Dripps RD, Price HL. Effect of CO_2 inhalation on arterial pressure ECG and plasma catecholamines and 17-OH corticosteroids in normal man. *J Appl Physiol* 1960; **15**: 454–8.

22. Cullen DJ, Eger EI. Cardiovascular effects of carbon dioxide in man. *Anesthesiology* 1974; **41**: 345–9.

23. Nishikawa T, Naito H. Clonidine modulation of hemodynamic and catecholamine responses associated with hypoxia or hypercapnia in dogs. *Anesthesiology* 1996; **84**: 672–85.

24. Tenney SM. The effect of carbon dioxide on neurohumeral and endocrine mechanisms. *Anesthesiology* 1960; **21**: 674–85.

25. Barer GR, Howard P, McCurrie JR. The effect of carbon dioxide and changes in blood pH on pulmonary vascular resistance in cats. *Clin Sci* 1967; **32**: 361–76.

26. Kiely DG, Cargill RI, Lipworth BJ. Effects of hypercapnia on hemodynamic, inotropic, lusitropic, and electrophysiological indices in humans. *Chest* 1996; **109**: 1215–21.

27. Domino KB, Swenson ER, Hlastala MP. Hypocapnia-induced ventilation/perfusion mismatch: a direct CO_2 or pH-mediated effect. *Am J Respir Crit Care Med* 1995; **152**: 1534–9.

28. Loeppky JA, Scotto P, Riedel CE, Roach RC, Chick TW. Effects of acid–base status on acute hypoxic pulmonary vasoconstriction and gas exchange. *J Appl Physiol* 1992; **72**: 1787–97.

29. Foëx P. Effects of carbon dioxide on the systemic circulation. In: Prys-Roberts C, ed. *The circulation in anaesthesia.* Oxford: Blackwell Scientific, 1980.

30. Siggaard-Andersen O, Engel K, Jorgensen K, Astrup P. A micro method for determination of pH, carbon dioxide tension, base excess and standard bicarbonate in capillary blood. *Scand J Clin Lab Invest* 1960; **12**: 172–6.

31. Clowes GHA, Hopkins AL, Simeone FA. A comparison of physiological effects of hypercapnia and hypoxia in the production of cardiac arrest. *Ann Surg* 1955; **142**: 446–60.

32. Fenn WO, Asano T. Effects of carbon dioxide inhalation on potassium liberation from the liver. *Am J Physiol* 1956; **185**: 567–9.

33. Tenney SM, Lamb TW. Physiological consequences of hypoventilation and hyperventilation. *Handbk Physiol Sect. 3* 1965; **2**: 979.

34. Potkin RT, Swenson ER. Resuscitation from severe acute hypercapnia. Determinants of tolerance and survival. *Chest* 1992; **102**: 1742–5.

35. Prys-Roberts C, Smith WDA, Nunn JF. Accidental severe hypercapnia during anaesthesia. *Br J Anaesth* 1967; **39**: 257–67.

36. Goldstein B, Shannon DC, Todres ID. Supercarbia in children: clinical course and outcome. *Crit Care Med* 1990; **18**: 166–8.

37. Slinger P, Blundell PE, Metcalf IR. Management of massive grain aspiration. *Anesthesiology* 1997; **87**: 993–5.

Chapter 23

Hypoxia

Chapter 1 explained how all but the simplest forms of life have evolved to exploit the immense advantages of oxidative metabolism. The price they have paid is to become dependent on oxygen for their survival. The essential feature of hypoxia is the cessation of oxidative phosphorylation (page 280) when the mitochondrial P_{O_2} falls below a critical level. Anaerobic pathways, in particular the glycolytic pathway (see Figure 11.14), then come into play. These trigger a complex series of cellular changes leading first to reduced cellular function and ultimately to cell death.

Biochemical changes in hypoxia

Depletion of high energy compounds

Anaerobic metabolism produces only one-nineteenth of the yield of the high energy phosphate compound adenosine triphosphate (ATP) per mole of glucose, when compared with aerobic metabolism (page 282). In organs with a high metabolic rate such as the brain, it is impossible to increase glucose transport sufficiently to maintain the normal level of ATP production. Therefore, during hypoxia, the ATP/ADP ratio falls and there is a rapid decline in the level of all high energy compounds (Figure 23.1). Very similar changes occur in response to arterial hypotension. These changes will rapidly block cerebral function, but organs with a lower energy requirement will continue to function for a longer time and are thus more resistant to hypoxia (see below).

Under hypoxic conditions, there are two ways in which reductions in ATP levels may be minimized, both of which are effective for only a short time. First, the high energy phosphate bond in phosphocreatine may be used to create ATP,[2] and initially this slows the rate of reduction of ATP (Figure 23.1). Secondly, two molecules of ADP may combine to form one of ATP and one of AMP (the adenylate kinase reaction). This reaction is driven forward by the removal of AMP (adenosine monophosphate), which is converted to adenosine (a potent vasodilator) and thence to inosine, hypoxanthine, xanthine and uric acid, with irreversible loss of adenine nucleotides.[3] The implications for production of free radicals are discussed on page 500.

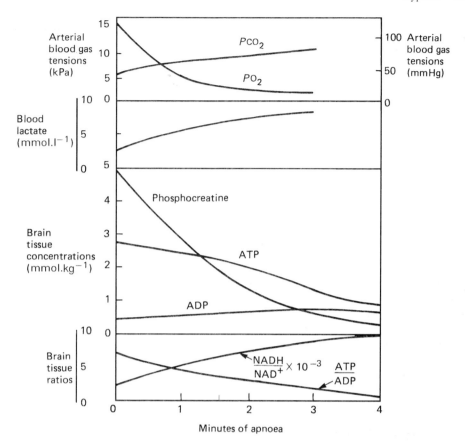

Figure 23.1 Biochemical changes during 4 minutes of respiratory arrest in rats previously breathing 30% oxygen. Recovery of all values, except blood lactate, was complete within 5 minutes of restarting pulmonary ventilation. (Drawn from the data of reference 1.)

End-products of metabolism

The end-products of aerobic metabolism are carbon dioxide and water, both of which are easily diffusible and lost from the body. The main anaerobic pathway produces hydrogen and lactate ions which, from most of the body, escape into the circulation, where they may be conveniently quantified in terms of the base deficit, excess lactate or lactate/pyruvate ratio. However, the blood–brain barrier is relatively impermeable to charged ions, and therefore hydrogen and lactate ions are retained in the neurones of the hypoxic brain. Lactacidosis can occur only when circulation is maintained to provide the large quantities of glucose required for conversion to lactic acid.

   In severe cerebral hypoxia, a major part of the dysfunction and damage is due to intracellular acidosis rather than simply depletion of high energy compounds (see below). Gross hypoperfusion is more damaging than total ischaemia, because the latter limits glucose supply and therefore the formation of lactic acid.[3] Similarly, patients who have an episode of cerebral ischaemia while hyperglycaemic (e.g. a stroke) have been found to have more severe brain injury than those with normal or low blood glucose levels at the time of the hypoxic event.[4]

Initiation of glycolysis[5]

The enzyme 6-phosphofructokinase (PFK) is the rate-limiting step of the glycolytic pathway (see Figure 11.14). Activity of PFK is enhanced by the presence of ADP, AMP and phosphate, which will rapidly accumulate during hypoxia, thus accelerating glycolysis. PFK is, however, inhibited by acidosis, which will therefore quickly limit the formation of ATP from glucose, and may even result in hyperglycaemia. The intracellular production of phosphate from ATP breakdown also promotes the activity of glycogen phosphorylase, which cleaves glycogen molecules to produce fructose-1,6-diphosphate. This enters the glycolytic pathway below the rate-limiting PFK reaction, and also avoids the expenditure of two molecules of ATP in its derivation from glucose. Therefore four molecules of ATP are produced from one of fructose-1,6-diphosphate in comparison with two from one molecule of glucose. There is no subsequent stage in the glycolytic pathway that is significantly rate-limited by acidosis. Provided glycogen is available within the cell, this second pathway therefore provides a valuable reserve for the production of ATP.

Mechanisms of hypoxic cell damage

Many mechanisms contribute to cell damage or death from hypoxia. The precise role of each remains unclear, but there is general agreement that different tissues respond to hypoxia in quite varied ways. Also, the nature of the hypoxic insult has a large effect, with differing speed of onset, degree of hypoxia, blood flow, blood glucose concentration and tissue metabolic activity all influencing the resulting tissue dysfunction. Because of the dramatic clinical consequences of nervous system damage, neuronal cells are the most widely studied and therefore form the basis for the mechanisms described in this section.[2]

Changes in the transmembrane potential of a hypoxic neurone are shown in Figure 23.2, along with the major physiological changes that occur. At the onset of anoxia, CNS cells immediately become either slightly hyperpolarized (as shown in the Figure) or depolarized, depending on the cell type. This is followed by a gradual reduction in membrane potential until a 'threshold' value is reached, when a spontaneous rapid depolarization occurs. At this stage there are gross abnormalities in ion channel function and the normal intracellular and extracellular ionic gradients are abolished, leading to cell death.

Potassium and sodium flux

Hypoxia has a direct effect on potassium channels, increasing transmembrane K^+ conductance and causing the immediate hyperpolarization. Potassium begins to leak out from the cell, increasing the extracellular K^+ concentration and thus tending to depolarize the cell membrane. Potassium leakage, along with sodium influx, is accelerated when falling ATP levels cause failure of the Na/K ATPase pump. Following rapid depolarization, sodium and potassium channels probably simply remain open, allowing free passage of ions across the cell membrane, leading to cellular destruction.

Calcium

Intracellular calcium concentration increases shortly after the onset of anoxia as a result of release from intracellular stores such as endoplasmic reticulum and mitochondria.[6]

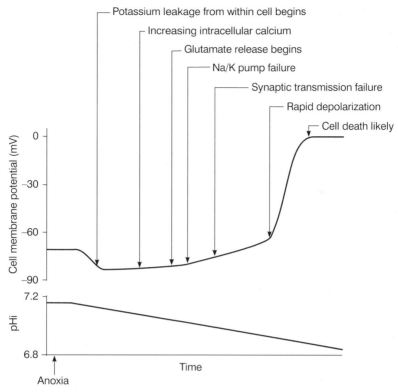

Figure 23.2 Changes in transmembrane potential and intracellular pH (pHi) in a neuronal cell following the sudden onset of anoxia. Significant physiological events in the course of the hypoxic insult are shown. Once membrane potential reaches zero, cell death is almost inevitable (see text for details). The time between anoxia and rapid depolarization is highly variable, between about 4 minutes with complete ischaemia to almost an hour with hypoxia and preserved blood flow. (Derived from reference 2.)

Intracellular calcium is increased further by the failure of ATP-driven calcium pumps.[7] The increase in intracellular calcium is generally harmful, causing the activation of ATPase enzymes just when ATP may be critically low, the activation of proteases to damage sarcolemma and the cytoskeleton, and the uncontrolled release of neurotransmitters (see below). At this stage, the cell has probably not been irretrievably damaged by spontaneous depolarization, but derangement of calcium channel function effectively prevents normal synaptic transmission and therefore cellular function. Extracellular adenosine, formed from the degradation of AMP, is also believed to play a role in blocking calcium channels during anoxia.[2]

Excitatory amino acid release[8]

The excitatory amino acids glutamate and aspartate are released from many neurones at concentrations two to five times normal early in the course of a hypoxic insult followed by further dramatic increases after rapid depolarization. Glutamate reuptake mechanisms also fail, and extracellular concentrations quickly reach neurotoxic levels,[8,9] acting via the N-methyl-D-aspartate (NMDA) receptor.

Delayed cellular damage following hypoxia

Animal studies have found that some areas of brain, particularly the hippocampus, are peculiarly susceptible to late injury following only transient hypoxia. A similar effect is almost certainly present in humans, in whom brain injury, as evidenced by cerebral oedema, often continues to develop for some hours after the initial insult. There are many possible explanations for this delayed neuronal damage, but the following two closely related mechanisms have recently been implicated.

Excitatory amino acid release described above has been implicated in delayed cell damage.[8,9] Cells with depleted energy stores are particularly susceptible,[10] but the mechanism by which glutamate and aspartate bring about cell damage is currently unknown.

Nitric oxide (NO) formation is increased in the area surrounding focal ischaemia in animals.[11,12] This occurs via the production of inducible nitric oxide synthase (page 150) in glial cells, probably stimulated by inflammatory cytokines released at the time of injury. Nitric oxide may be toxic to cells in many ways, including the formation of reactive oxygen species described in Chapter 25, but in this case nitric oxide is believed to act via sensitization of neuronal cells to enhance the toxic effects of glutamate and aspartate via an effect on the NMDA receptor.

Clearly, the mechanisms of delayed neuronal damage following hypoxia are as yet poorly understood, particularly in humans. However, there is a huge therapeutic potential in hypoxic injury for NMDA receptor blockade or selective nitric oxide synthase inhibition, and early results in animals seem promising.[13]

Po_2 levels at which hypoxia occurs

Cellular Po_2

'Critical Po_2' refers to the oxygen tension below which oxidative cellular metabolism fails. For isolated mitochondria, this is known to be below 0.13 kPa (1 mmHg), and possibly as low as 0.01 kPa (0.1 mmHg) in muscle cells[5] despite their large oxygen consumption. Venous Po_2 approximates to end-capillary Po_2, and though highly variable this is usually in excess of 3 kPa ($\approx$20 mmHg) even in maximally working skeletal muscle. Thus with the minimal Po_2 in the nearby capillary being about 200 times greater than that required by the mitochondria, it is difficult to envisage how cellular hypoxia can occur in any but the most extreme situations. There are reasons why this is not the case *in vivo*.

Measurement of intracellular Po_2 is difficult. The most widely used technique is applicable only to muscle cells and involves measurement of myoglobin saturation, from which Po_2 may be determined. These studies have indicated that intracellular Po_2 is in the range 0.5–2 kPa (3–15 mmHg), depending on cell activity.[5] Many studies have also indicated a minimal difference between the Po_2 in extracellular fluid and in cells.[14] This would indicate a possibly substantial barrier to oxygen diffusion between the capillary and extracellular fluid. Finally, diffusion of oxygen in cells is believed to be slow because of the proteinaceous nature of the cytoplasm, and therefore large variations in intracellular Po_2 are likely to exist. Thus in intact cells, as opposed to isolated mitochondria, critical Po_2 is more likely to be of the order of 0.5–1.3 kPa (3–10 mmHg), much closer to the end-capillary value.[15]

Venous P_{O_2} was for many years thought to reflect the P_{O_2} at the cell surface, but as indicated in the previous paragraph this is no longer believed to be so. However, the factors that alter P_{O_2} between capillary and tissue probably remain fairly constant, so venous P_{O_2} remains a useful and practicable measure of the functional state of oxygenation of an organ. For example, consciousness is usually lost when the internal jugular venous P_{O_2} falls below about 2.7 kPa (20 mmHg), whatever the cause.

Critical arterial P_{O_2} for cerebral function

The minimal safe level of arterial P_{O_2} is that which will maintain a safe tissue P_{O_2}. This depends on many factors besides arterial P_{O_2}, including haemoglobin concentration, tissue perfusion and tissue oxygen consumption. These factors accord with Barcroft's classification of 'anoxia' into anoxic, anaemic and stagnant (page 284), which has previously been shown as a Venn diagram (see Figure 11.17).

This argument may be extended to consider in which circumstances the venous P_{O_2} (and by implication tissue P_{O_2}) may fall below its critical level corresponding, in normal blood, to 32% saturation and oxygen content of 6.4 ml.dl^{-1}. If the brain has a mean oxygen consumption of 46 ml.min^{-1} and a blood flow of 620 ml.min^{-1}, the arterial/venous oxygen content difference will be 7.4 ml.dl^{-1}. Therefore, *with normal cerebral perfusion, haemoglobin concentration, pH, etc.*, this would correspond to a critical arterial oxygen content of 13.8 ml.dl^{-1}, saturation 68% and P_{O_2} 4.8 kPa (36 mmHg). This calculation and others under various different conditions are set out in Table 23.1.

However, the other factors in italics (above) will probably not be normal. They may be unfavourable as a result of multiple disability in the patient (e.g. anaemia or a decreased cerebral blood flow). Alternatively, there may be favourable factors, including compensatory mechanisms such as polycythaemia in chronic arterial hypoxaemia and increased blood flow in anaemia and hypoxia. Cerebral vascular resistance is diminished by reduced arterial blood pressure and arterial hypoxaemia. Cerebral oxygen requirements are reduced by hypothermia and anaesthesia. The possible combinations of circumstances are so great that it is not feasible to consider every possible situation. Instead, certain important examples have been selected that illustrate the fundamentals of the problem, and are shown in Table 23.1.

A twofold increase of cerebral blood flow would allow the arterial P_{O_2} to decrease further from 4.8 to 3.6 kPa (36 to 27 mmHg) before the cerebral venous P_{O_2} reached 2.7 kPa (20 mmHg). This is important, as an increase in cerebral blood flow may be expected to follow severe hypoxia. Polycythaemia (e.g. a haemoglobin concentration of 18 g.dl^{-1}) does not confer the same degree of benefit, and the critical arterial P_{O_2} would then be 4.3 kPa (32 mmHg). Alkalosis, which may be expected to result from the hypoxic drive to respiration, confers no advantage at all. Considerable advantage derives from hypothermia, due to the reduction in cerebral metabolism but not to the shift of the dissociation curve.

Uncompensated ischaemia is dangerous and, with a 45 per cent reduction in cerebral blood flow, any reduction of arterial P_{O_2} exposes the brain to risk of hypoxia. Uncompensated anaemia is almost equally dangerous, although an increase in cerebral blood flow restores a satisfactory safety margin. In the example in Table 23.1, a 40 per cent reduction of blood oxygen-carrying capacity and a 40 per cent increase of cerebral blood flow permits the arterial P_{O_2} to fall to 5.3 kPa (40 mmHg) without the cerebral venous P_{O_2} falling below 2.7 kPa (20 mmHg). The last line in Table 23.1 shows the very dangerous combination of anaemia (haemoglobin concentration 11 g.dl^{-1}) and cerebral blood flow three-quarters of normal. Neither abnormality is very serious considered

Table 23.1 Lowest arterial oxygen levels compatible with a cerebral venous Po_2 of 2.7 kPa (20 mmHg) under various conditions

	Blood O_2 capacity ml.dl^{-1}	Brain O_2 consump. ml.min^{-1}	Cerebral blood flow ml.min^{-1}	Cerebral venous blood			Art./ven. O_2 content difference ml.dl^{-1}	Arterial blood			
				Po_2 kPa	Po_2 mmHg	Sat. %	O_2 content ml.dl^{-1}		O_2 content ml.dl^{-1}	Sat. %	Po_2 kPa	Po_2 mmHg
Normal values	20	46	620	4.4	33	63	12.6	7.4	20.0	98	13	100
Uncompensated arterial hypoxaemia	20	46	620	2.7	20	32	6.4	7.4	13.8	68	4.8	36
Arterial hypoxaemia with increased cerebral blood flow	20	46	1240	2.7	20	32	6.4	3.7	10.1	50	3.6	27
Arterial hypoxaemia with polycythaemia	25	46	620	2.7	20	32	8.0	7.4	15.4	61	4.3	32
Arterial hypoxaemia with alkalosis*	20	46	620	2.7	20	46	9.2	7.4	16.6	82	4.9	37
Arterial hypoxaemia with hypothermia†	20	23	620	2.7	20	57	11.4	3.7	15.1	75	3.6	27
Uncompensated cerebral ischaemia	20	46	340	2.7	20	32	6.4	13.5	19.9	98	15	112
Uncompensated anaemia	12	46	620	2.7	20	32	3.8	7.4	11.2	93	8.9	67
Anaemia with increased cerebral blood flow	12	46	870	2.7	20	32	3.8	5.3	9.1	75	5.3	40
Combined anaemia and ischaemia	15	46	460	2.7	20	32	4.8	10.0	14.8	97	12	92

*pH 7.6.
† temperature 30°C; cerebral O_2 consumption reduced to half normal.

separately, but in combination the arterial P_{O_2} cannot be reduced below its normal value without the risk of cerebral hypoxia.

Table 23.1 is not be taken too literally, because there are many minor factors that have not been considered. However, it is a general rule that maximal cerebral vasodilatation may be expected to occur in any condition (other than cerebral ischaemia) that threatens cerebral oxygenation. Also, there are circumstances in which the critical organ is not the brain but the heart, liver or kidney.

The most important message of this discussion is that there is no simple answer to the question 'What is the safe lower limit of arterial P_{O_2}?'. Acclimatized mountaineers have remained conscious during exercise at high altitude with arterial P_{O_2} values as low as 2.7 kPa (20 mmHg) (Chapter 16). Patients presenting with severe respiratory disease tend to remain conscious down to the same level of arterial P_{O_2}.[16] However, both acclimatized mountaineers and patients with chronic respiratory disease have compensatory poly-cythaemia and maximal cerebral vasodilatation. Uncompensated subjects who are rapidly exposed to hypoxia are unlikely to remain conscious with an arterial P_{O_2} of less than about 3.6 kPa (27 mmHg), but considerable individual variation must be expected.

Organ survival times *in vivo*

Lack of oxygen stops the machine and then wrecks the machinery. The time of circulatory arrest up to the first event (survival time) must be distinguished from the duration of anoxia which results in the second event (revival time), the latter being defined as the time beyond which no recovery of function is possible. Incomplete recovery of function may follow anoxia lasting more than the survival time but less than the revival time. Revival times tend to be about four times as long as survival times.

From the complex sequence of cellular events already described it will be clear that tissue survival times depend on many factors. There is a very large difference between different organs, ranging from less than 1 minute for the cerebral cortex to about 2 hours for skeletal muscle. Heart is intermediate with a survival time of about 5 minutes, liver and kidney probably being about 10 minutes. Similarly, survival time is also influenced by oxygen consumption and oxygen stores in the tissue concerned. An inactive organ (such as a heart in asystole or the brain in hypothermia) has increased resistance to hypoxia, and there is a small but definite increase in survival time when tissue P_{O_2} has been increased by hyperbaric oxygenation. Hypothermia both decreases oxygen demand and increases the solubility of oxygen in the tissue.

Effects of hypoxia

Hypoxia presents a serious threat to the body, and compensatory mechanisms usually take priority over other changes. Thus, for example, in hypoxia with concomitant hypocapnia, hyperventilation and an increase in cerebral blood flow occur in spite of the decreased P_{CO_2}. Certain compensatory mechanisms will come into play whatever the reason for the hypoxia, although their effectiveness will depend to a large extent on the cause. For example, hyperventilation will be largely ineffective in stagnant or anaemic hypoxia, because hyperventilation while breathing air can do little to increase the oxygen content of arterial blood, and usually nothing to increase perfusion.

Hyperventilation results from a decreased arterial P_{O_2} but the response is non-linear (see Figure 5.9). There is little effect until arterial P_{O_2} is reduced to about 7 kPa (52.5 mmHg):

maximal response is at 4 kPa (30 mmHg). The interrelationship between hypoxia and other factors in the control of breathing is discussed in Chapter 5.

Pulmonary distribution of blood flow is improved by hypoxia as a result of increase in pulmonary arterial pressure (page 151).

Cardiac output is increased by hypoxia and results in improved regional blood flow to almost every major organ, particularly the brain.

The sympathetic system is concerned in many of the responses to hypoxia, particularly the increase in organ perfusion. The immediate response is reflex and is initiated by chemoreceptor stimulation: it occurs before there is any measurable increase in circulating catecholamines, although this does occur in due course. Reduction of cerebral and probably myocardial vascular resistance is not dependent on the autonomic system but depends on local responses in the vicinity of the vessels themselves. With the single exception of pulmonary arterioles, hypoxia causes vasodilatation of blood vessels almost everywhere in the body. This results mainly from a direct effect of adenosine and other metabolites generated by hypoxia.

Haemoglobin concentration is not increased in acute hypoxia in humans (unlike the seal, page 381), but is increased in chronic hypoxia due to residence at altitude and chronic respiratory disease.

The dissociation curve is displaced to the right by an increase in 2,3-DPG and by acidosis that may also be present. This tends to increase tissue Po_2 (see Figure 11.10).

Anaerobic metabolism is increased in severe hypoxia in an attempt to maintain the level of ATP (see above).

References

1. Kaasik AE, Nilsson L, Siesjö BK. The effect of asphyxia upon the lactate, pyruvate and bicarbonate concentrations of brain tissue and cisternal CSF, and upon the tissue concentrations of phosphocreatine and adenine nucleotides in anesthetized rats. *Acta Physiol Scand* 1970; **78**: 433–47.
2. Martin RL, Lloyd HGE, Cowan AI. The early events of oxygen and glucose deprivation: setting the scene for neuronal death? *Trends Neurosci* 1994; **17**: 251–6.
3. Gutierrez G. Cellular effects of hypoxaemia and ischaemia. In: Crystal RG, West JB, eds. *The lung: scientific foundations.* New York: Raven, 1991; 1525.
4. Candelise L, Landi G, Orazio EN, Boccardi E. Prognostic significance of hyperglycaemia in acute stroke. *Arch Neurol* 1985; **42**: 661–3.
5. Connett RJ, Honig CR, Gayeski TEJ, Brooks GA. Defining hypoxia: a systems view of Vo_2, glycolysis, energetics, and intracellular Po_2. *J Appl Physiol* 1990; **68**: 833–42.
6. Katchman AN, Hershkowitz N. Early anoxia-induced vesicular glutamate release results from mobilization of calcium from intracellular stores. *J Neurophysiol* 1993; **70**: 1–7.
7. Cheung JY, Bonventre JV, Malis CD, Leaf A. Calcium and ischemic injury. *N Engl J Med* 1986; **314**: 1670–6.
8. Choi DW. Cerebral hypoxia: some new approaches and unanswered questions. *J Neurosci* 1990; **10**: 2493–501.
9. Ohmori T, Hirashima Y, Kurimoto M, Endo S, Takaku A. In vitro hypoxia of cortical and hippocampal CA1 neurons: glutamate, nitric oxide, and platelet activating factor participate in the mechanism of selective neural death in CA1 neurons. *Brain Res* 1996; **743**: 109–15.

10. Novelli A, Reilly JA, Lysko PG, Henneberry RC. Glutamate becomes neurotoxic via the *N*-methyl-D-aspartate receptor when intracellular energy levels are reduced. *Brain Res* 1988; **451**: 205–12.
11. Hewett SJ, Muir JK, Lobner D, Symons A, Choi DW. Potentiation of oxygen-glucose deprivation-induced neuronal death after induction of iNOS. *Stroke* 1996; **27**: 1586–91.
12. Huang Z, Huang PL, Panahian N, Dalkara T, Fishman MC, Moskowitz MA. Effects of cerebral ischemia in mice deficient in neuronal nitric oxide synthase. *Science* 1994; **265**: 1883–5.
13. Iadecola C, Zhang F, Xu X. Inhibition of inducible nitric oxide synthase ameliorates cerebral ischemic damage. *Am J Physiol* 1995; **268**: R286–92.
14. Rumsey WL, Wilson DF. Tissue capacity for mitochondrial oxidative phosphorylation and its adaptation to stress. In: Fregly MJ, Blatteis CM, eds. *Handbook of physiology, Section 4: Environmental physiology.* New York and Oxford: Oxford University Press, 1996; 1095–114.
15. Epstein FH, Agmon Y, Brezis M. Physiology of renal hypoxia. *Ann N Y Acad Sci* 1995; **718**: 72–81.
16. McNicol MW, Campbell EJM. Severity of respiratory failure. *Lancet* 1965; **1**: 336–8.

Chapter 24

Anaemia

Anaemia is a widespread pathophysiological disorder that interferes with oxygen transport to the tissues. In developed countries it has a varied aetiology, including iron deficiency, chronic haemorrhage, loss of erythropoietin in end-stage renal failure and depletion of vitamin B_{12}. However, in the third world it is endemic, major factors including malnutrition and infestation with various parasites such as hook worm and Bilharzia. In many countries, haemoglobin concentrations within the range $6–10 \, g.dl^{-1}$ are regarded as normal.

Anaemia *per se* has no major direct effects on pulmonary function. Arterial P_{O_2} and saturation should remain within the normal range in uncomplicated anaemia, and the crucial effect is on the arterial oxygen content and therefore oxygen delivery. Important compensatory changes are increases in cardiac output, greater oxygen extraction from the arterial blood and to a lesser extent the small rightward displacement of the oxyhaemoglobin dissociation curve. However, there are limits to these adaptations, which define the minimal tolerable haemoglobin concentration, and also the exercise limits attainable at various levels of severity of anaemia.

Physiological aspects of blood transfusion and blood substitutes are discussed on page 274 *et seq.*

Pulmonary function

Gas exchange

Alveolar P_{O_2} is determined by dry barometric pressure, inspired oxygen concentration and the ratio of oxygen consumption to alveolar ventilation (page 251). Assuming that the first two are unchanged, and there being good evidence that the last two factors are unaffected in the resting state by anaemia down to a haemoglobin concentration of at least $5 \, g.dl^{-1}$ (see below), there is no reason why alveolar P_{O_2} or P_{CO_2} should be affected by uncomplicated anaemia.

The increased cardiac output (see below) will cause a small reduction in pulmonary capillary transit time which, together with the reduced mass of haemoglobin in the pulmonary capillaries, causes a modest decrease in diffusing capacity or transfer factor (page 210). However, such is the reserve in the capacity of pulmonary capillary blood to reach equilibrium with the alveolar gas (see Figure 9.2) that it is highly unlikely that this would have any measurable effect on the alveolar/end-pulmonary capillary P_{O_2}

gradient, which in the normal subject is now believed to be of the order of only 10^{-6} mmHg. Thus pulmonary end-capillary Po_2 should also be normal in uncomplicated anaemia.

Continuing down the cascade of oxygen partial pressures from ambient air to the site of use in the tissues, the next step is the gradient in Po_2 between pulmonary end-capillary blood and mixed arterial blood. The Po_2 gradient at this stage is caused by shunting and the perfusion of relatively underventilated alveoli. There is no evidence that these factors are altered in anaemia, and arterial Po_2 should therefore be normal. Because the peripheral chemoreceptors are stimulated by reduction in arterial Po_2 and not arterial oxygen content (page 97), there should be no stimulation of respiration unless the degree of hypoxia is sufficient to cause anaerobic metabolism and lactacidosis.

The haemoglobin dissociation curve

It is well established that intraerythrocytic 2,3-diphosphoglycerate is increased in anaemia (page 271), typical changes being from a normal value of 5 to 7 mmol.l^{-1} at a haemoglobin concentration of 6 g.dl^{-1}.[1] This results in an increase in P_{50} from 3.6 to 4 kPa (27 to 30 mmHg). This rightward shift of the dissociation curve would have a negligible effect on arterial saturation, which has indeed been reported to be normal in anaemia. The rightward shift will, however, increase the Po_2 at which oxygen is unloaded in the tissues, mitigating to a certain extent the effects of reduction in oxygen delivery so far as tissue Po_2 is concerned.

Arterial oxygen content

Although the arterial oxygen saturation usually remains normal in anaemia, the oxygen content of the arterial blood will be reduced in approximate proportion to the decrease in haemoglobin concentration. Arterial oxygen content can be expressed as follows:

$$Ca_{O_2} = ([Hb] \times Sa_{O_2} \times 1.31) + 0.3 \qquad \ldots(1)$$
$$\text{ml.dl}^{-1} \quad \text{g.dl}^{-1} \quad \%/100 \quad \text{ml.g}^{-1} \quad \text{ml.dl}^{-1}$$

e.g.
$$19 = (14.7 \times 0.97 \times 1.31) + 0.3$$

where Ca_{O_2} is arterial oxygen content, [Hb] is haemoglobin concentration, Sa_{O_2} is arterial oxygen saturation, 1.31 is the combining power of haemoglobin with oxygen (page 264) and 0.3 is dissolved oxygen at normal arterial Po_2.

Oxygen delivery

The important concept of oxygen delivery ($\dot{D}o_2$) is considered in detail on page 283. It is defined as the product of cardiac output ($\dot{Q}$) and Ca_{O_2}.

$$\dot{D}o_2 = \dot{Q} \times Ca_{O_2} \qquad \ldots(2)$$
$$\text{ml.min}^{-1} \quad \text{l.min}^{-1} \quad \text{ml.dl}^{-1}$$

e.g.
$$1000 = 5.25 \times 19$$

(the right-hand side is multiplied by a scaling factor of 10 to account for the differing units of volume).

Combining equations (1) and (2):

$$\dot{D}o_2 = \dot{Q} \times \{([Hb] \times Sa_{O_2} \times 1.31) + 0.3\} \qquad \ldots(3)$$
$$\text{ml.min}^{-1} \quad \text{l.min}^{-1} \quad \text{g.dl}^{-1} \quad \%/100 \quad \text{ml.g}^{-1} \quad \text{ml.dl}^{-1}$$

e.g. $1000 = 5.25 \times \{(14.7 \times 0.97 \times 1.31) + 0.3\}$

(the right-hand side is again multiplied by a scaling factor of 10).

Normal values give an oxygen delivery of approximately $1000 \, \text{ml.min}^{-1}$, which is about four times the normal resting oxygen consumption of $250 \, \text{ml.min}^{-1}$. Extraction of oxygen from the arterial blood is thus 25 per cent and this accords with an arterial saturation of 97% and mixed venous saturation of 72%.

If the small quantity of dissolved oxygen ($0.3 \, \text{ml.dl}^{-1}$) is ignored, oxygen delivery is seen to be proportional to the product of cardiac output, haemoglobin concentration and arterial oxygen saturation. There is, of course, negligible scope for any compensatory increase in saturation in a patient with uncomplicated anaemia at sea level.

Effect of anaemia on cardiac output

Equation (3) shows that, if other factors remain the same, a reduction in haemoglobin concentration will result in a proportionate reduction in oxygen delivery. Thus a haemoglobin concentration of $7.5 \, \text{g.dl}^{-1}$ with unchanged cardiac output would halve delivery to give a resting value of $500 \, \text{ml.min}^{-1}$, which would be approaching the likely critical value. However, patients with quite severe anaemia usually show little evidence of hypoxia at rest and, furthermore, achieve surprisingly good levels of exercise. Because arterial saturation cannot be increased, full compensation can be achieved only by a reciprocal relationship between cardiac output and haemoglobin concentration. Thus, if haemoglobin concentration is halved, maintenance of normal delivery will require a doubling of cardiac output. Full compensation does not normally occur, but fortunately a reduction in haemoglobin concentration is usually accompanied by some increase in cardiac output.

Duke and Abelmann in 1969[2] measured cardiac output in 15 patients before and after treatment of uncomplicated anaemia, and demonstrated that cardiac output was significantly greater before they increased their patients' haemoglobin concentration from 5.9 to $10.9 \, \text{g.dl}^{-1}$. Their results are represented by the lower curve in the upper part of Figure 24.1, for which it is assumed that the mean surface area of their patients was $1.7 \, \text{m}^2$. They did, however, show a negative correlation between age and cardiac index in the anaemic state, reflecting the relative inability of the older patient to compensate. Woodson and his colleagues[3] carried out an important study in volunteers whose haemoglobin concentration was isovolaemically reduced from a mean control value of 15.3 to $10 \, \text{g.dl}^{-1}$ by replacement of blood with the same volume of albumin solution: anaemia was then maintained at the same level for 14 days. Immediately after induction of anaemia there was a marked increase in cardiac output (55.5 per cent), but this decreased to only 14 per cent above control levels after 14 days of sustained anaemia (Figure 24.1).

More dramatic effects have been demonstrated in dogs. The effect of haematocrit (packed cell volume, PCV) on cardiac output was first studied in normovolaemic anaesthetized dogs in 1959,[4] which demonstrated a linear negative relationship between haematocrit and cardiac output. This extended from haematocrit (packed cell volume) values of 20%, through the normal to polycythaemic values of 70%. Circulatory measurements were made within minutes of establishing values for haematocrit. The

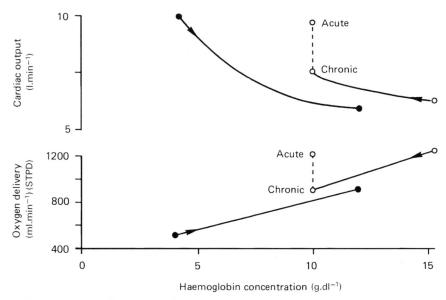

Figure 24.1 Changes in cardiac output and oxygen delivery as a function of haemoglobin concentration. The right-hand curves (open symbols; from reference 3) show the effect of induced anaemia in volunteers. The left-hand curves (closed symbols; from reference 2) show the effect of treatment of anaemic patients.

normal value for cardiac output was 100 ml.kg^{-1}.min^{-1}, increasing to 160 at a haematocrit of 20% and decreasing to 30 at a haematocrit of 70%. Subsequent studies gave similar results in dogs following acute isovolaemic haemodilution with dextran.[5]

The mechanism underlying the increase in cardiac output is not clear, but is mainly due to increased stroke volume, heart rate becoming elevated only when haematocrit is below 25%. These changes result from reduced cardiac afterload due to lowered blood viscosity and from increased preload due to greater venous return secondary to increased tone in capacitance vessels.[6]

The influence of cardiac output on oxygen delivery

The interaction of haemoglobin concentration and cardiac output on oxygen delivery (equation 3) is shown for the human studies in the lower part of Figure 24.1. Following the acute reduction of haemoglobin concentration to about 65% of control value in volunteers, cardiac output increased sufficiently to maintain normal or near-normal oxygen delivery. However, in sustained anaemia, the increase in cardiac output (only 14 per cent) was insufficient to maintain oxygen delivery, which decreased to 25 per cent below control values. Similarly, in the anaemic patients studied by Duke and Abelmann,[2] delivery was reduced in proportion to the degree of anaemia. Extrapolation of the curves in the lower part of Figure 24.1 suggests that a critical oxygen delivery (probably about 500 ml.min^{-1}) would be reached at a haemoglobin concentration of about 3 g.dl^{-1}, which is close to the minimum level compatible with life. At this point cardiac output would be about double the normal value and mixed venous saturation would be reduced from the normal value of 72% down to about 50%.

Without an increase in cardiac output, it is likely that a haemoglobin concentration of 6–8 g.dl^{-1} would be the minimum level compatible with life. It is clear that the ability of the cardiovascular system to respond to anaemia with an increase in cardiac output is an essential aspect of accommodation to anaemia, and this is less effective in the elderly or other subjects with reduced cardiac reserve.

Relationship between oxygen delivery and consumption

The relationship between oxygen delivery and consumption has been considered on pages 285 *et seq.* When oxygen delivery is reduced, for whatever reason, oxygen consumption is at first maintained at its normal value, but with increasing oxygen extraction and therefore decreasing mixed venous saturation. Below a 'critical' value for oxygen delivery, oxygen consumption decreases as a function of delivery, and is usually accompanied by evidence of hypoxia, such as increased lactate in peripheral blood. Values for critical oxygen delivery depend on the pathophysiological state of the patient and vary from one condition to another.

The critical level of oxygen delivery in chronic uncomplicated anaemia in humans has not been clearly established. However, in Woodson's study of volunteers[3] maintained at a haemoglobin concentration of 10 g.dl for 14 days, oxygen delivery decreased from about 1200 to 900 ml.min^{-1} while oxygen consumption remained virtually unchanged (Figure 24.2). Duke and Abelmann[2] found no increase in oxygen consumption in a group of 15 anaemic patients when haemoglobin concentration was increased from a mean value of 5.9 to 10.9 g.dl^{-1}. The corresponding change in oxygen delivery would have been from 600 to 900 ml.min^{-1}. Thus these patients and subjects all remained above the critical value for oxygen delivery down to haemoglobin values of about 6 g.dl^{-1}. This accords with

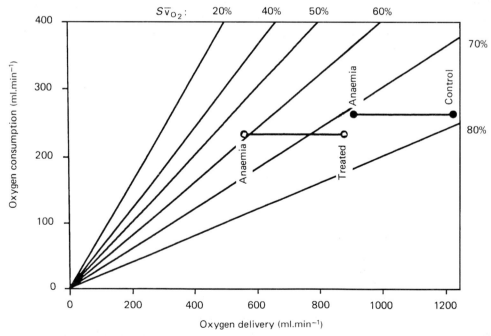

Figure 24.2 Relationship between oxygen delivery and consumption in studies of anaemia. Oxygen consumption remained above the critical value in experimental isovolaemic anaemia (open symbols; reference 3) and also in treated anaemic patients (closed symbols; reference 2).

animal data showing that critical oxygen delivery in uncomplicated anaemia is about half the normal value.

Anaemia and exercise

Figure 24.2 shows that, in patients with moderately severe anaemia, oxygen consumption is maintained constant in the face of reduction in delivery. This is achieved at the expense of reduction in mixed venous saturation, as a result of increased extraction of oxygen from the arterial blood. In the study described above[3] of chronic isovolaemic anaemic volunteers, the resting mixed venous saturation was reduced from 78% to 70%. This curtails the ability of the anaemic patient to encroach on his reserve of mixed venous oxygen saturation, which is an important response to exercise. Reduction of haemoglobin to $10\,g.dl^{-1}$ resulted in a curtailment of oxygen consumption attained at maximal exercise from the control values of $3.01\,l.min^{-1}$ (normalized to $70\,kg$ body weight) down to $2.53\,l.min^{-1}$ in the acute stage, and $2.15\,l.min^{-1}$ after 14 days of sustained anaemia (Figure 24.3).[3] The increase in cardiac output required for the same increase in oxygen consumption was greater in the anaemic state, and cardiac output at maximal oxygen consumption was slightly less than under control conditions. Maximal exercise in the anaemic state resulted in a reduction of mixed venous oxygen saturation to the exceptionally low value of 12%, compared with control values of 23% during maximal exercise with a normal haemoglobin concentration.

Brisk walking on level ground normally requires an oxygen consumption of about $1\,l.min^{-1}$ and a cardiac output of the order of $10\,l.min^{-1}$. At a haemoglobin level of $5\,g.dl^{-1}$, this would require a cardiac output of about $20\,l.min^{-1}$ to permit an oxygen consumption of $1\,l.min^{-1}$ with a satisfactory residual level of mixed venous oxygen saturation. It will be clear that, at this degree of anaemia, cardiac function is a critical factor determining the mobility of a patient.

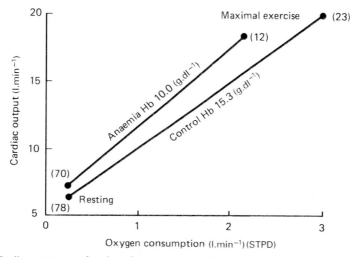

Figure 24.3 Cardiac output as a function of oxygen consumption during rest and maximal exercise under control and isovolaemic anaemic conditions. Numbers in parentheses indicate mean mixed venous saturation. (Redrawn from reference 3 on the assumption that mean weight of the subjects was 70 kg, by permission of the author, and the Editors and publishers of *Journal of Applied Physiology*.)

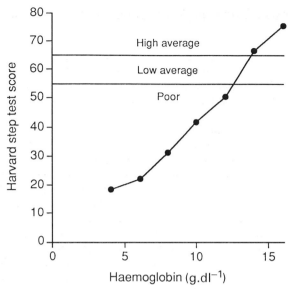

Figure 24.4 Relationship between capacity for exercise and haemoglobin concentration. (Redrawn from reference 7 by permission of the authors, and the Editor and publishers of *Clinics in Haematology.*)

Exercise tolerance may be limited by either respiratory or circulatory capacity. In uncomplicated anaemia, there is no reason to implicate respiratory limitation, and exercise tolerance is therefore, to a first approximation, governed by the remaining factors in the oxygen delivery equation (3) (above). On the assumption that the maximal sustainable cardiac output is only marginally affected by anaemia, it is to be expected that exercise tolerance will be reduced in direct proportion to the haemoglobin concentration. Available evidence supports this hypothesis (Figure 24.4).

Using haemoglobin to enhance athletic performance. The corollary of the preceding description is the question of improving athletic performance by increasing haemoglobin concentration above the normal range. This used to be achieved by removal of blood for replacement of red cells after a few weeks when the subject has already partially restored his haemoglobin concentration, a procedure known as blood doping. The same effect is now much more conveniently achieved by the administration of erythropoietin. Studies of trained athletes in this area are notoriously difficult, and it is easy to confuse the effects of changes in blood volume and haemoglobin concentration. Furthermore, blood doping involves the subject continuing his training after removal of blood while he is anaemic. This may well make his training more effective, as is the case when training is undertaken at altitude. In the pioneer study of Ekblom and colleagues in 1972,[8] it was reported that, following reinfusion of blood (resulting in an increase in haemoglobin concentration from 13.2 to 14.9 g.dl[-1]), maximal oxygen consumption was increased from 4.40 to 4.79 l.min[-1], and time to exhaustion during uphill treadmill running was extended from 5.43 to 6.67 minutes. Oxygen cost of the exercise task was unaltered. These findings were challenged in subsequent studies, but confirmed in a well-controlled study of highly trained runners,[9] in which a mean haemoglobin concentration of 16.7 g.dl[-1] was attained with significant increases in maximal oxygen uptake from 4.85 to 5.10 l.min[-1]. Differences of this magnitude are critically important in the arena of modern athletic competition.

What is the optimal haemoglobin concentration in the clinical setting?[10]

Evolution has resulted in a haemoglobin concentration of $13–16 \, g.dl^{-1}$ presumably for sound biological reasons, and this value must represent the best compromise between oxygen carriage, cardiac output and blood viscosity. However, blood transfusion has always been, and currently remains, a hazardous procedure and a haemoglobin concentration of over $10 \, g.dl^{-1}$ has for many years been regarded as acceptable.[11] At this level, increases in cardiac output are modest and though exercise tolerance may be reduced this is unlikely to trouble the patient. There is some evidence that lower values will be acceptable in some circumstances. Jehovah's Witnesses, whose religious beliefs prevent them from consenting to blood transfusion, frequently undergo major surgery and survival is reported following haemoglobin values of under $3 \, g.dl^{-1}$, albeit with substantial cardiovascular and respiratory support.[12] Studies of these patients[13] indicate that perioperative death is uncommon if haemoglobin concentration remains above $5 \, g.dl^{-1}$. There is also a suggestion that low haemoglobin values may actually be beneficial, lowered blood viscosity improving blood flow through diseased vessels and so increasing tissue oxygenation, though evidence for a clinically relevant effect is lacking. A target haemoglobin concentration of $10 \, g.dl^{-1}$ may therefore be too conservative[14] in fit healthy patients, or those with chronic anaemia. A recent review suggests that haemoglobin values of $7 \, g.dl^{-1}$ are acceptable in these groups.[10] This view was confirmed in a recent randomized controlled trial of intensive care patients in whom haemoglobin values of $7–9 \, g.dl^{-1}$ were associated with improved outcome compared with those in whom haemoglobin was maintained at over $10 \, g.dl^{-1}$.[15] The benefits were most pronounced in patients under 55 years old who were less acutely ill and did not have significant cardiac disease.

The organ that limits the acceptable degree of anaemia is the heart, where oxygen extraction is normally in excess of 50 per cent. Increased oxygen extraction as a compensatory mechanism is therefore limited and coronary blood flow must increase to facilitate the greater oxygen requirement of a raised cardiac output. Thus any patient with ischaemic heart disease will be considerably less tolerant of anaemia than those with normal coronary arteries, as shown in the study of intensive care patients already described.[15] For these patients, particularly in the postoperative period when cardiac output is elevated, the optimal haemoglobin may be as high as $12.8 \, g.dl^{-1}$.[16]

Chronic renal failure leads to a lack of renal erythropoietin release and chronic severe anaemia results, patients commonly having haemoglobin values of less than $8 \, g.dl^{-1}$. The availability of recombinant human erythropoietin has allowed partial correction of anaemia in many patients, leading to a substantial improvement in quality of life for most. There is, however, debate about the target haemoglobin concentration to aim for.[17] Aside from cost implications, there is also some evidence that correction of haemoglobin to normal values is associated with increased cardiac complications in these patients, and that a value of $10–12 \, g.dl^{-1}$ is therefore still recommended.[17]

References

1. Torrance J, Jacobs P, Restrepo A, Eschbach J, Lenfant C, Finch CA. Intraerythrocytic adaptation to anemia. *N Engl J Med* 1970; **283**: 165–9.
2. Duke M, Abelmann WH. The hemodynamic response to chronic anemia. *Circulation* 1969; **39**: 503–15.
3. Woodson RD, Wills RE, Lenfant C. Effect of acute and established anemia on O$_2$ transport at rest, submaximal and maximal work. *J Appl Physiol* 1978; **44**: 36–43.

4. Richardson TQ, Guyton AC. Effects of polycythemia and anemia on cardiac output and other circulatory factors. *Am J Physiol* 1959; **197**: 1167–70.

5. Cain SM. Oxygen delivery and uptake in dogs during anemic and hypoxic hypoxia. *J Appl Physiol* 1977; **42**: 228–34.

6. Chapler CK, Cain SM. The physiologic reserve in oxygen carrying capacity: studies in experimental haemodilution. *Can J Physiol Pharmacol* 1986; **64**: 7–12.

7. Viteri FE, Torun B. Anaemia and physical work capacity. *Clinics Hematol* 1974; **3**: 609–626.

8. Ekblom B, Goldbarg AN, Gullbring B. Response to exercise after blood loss and reinfusion. *J Appl Physiol* 1972; **33**: 175–80.

9. Buick FJ, Gledhill N, Froese AB, Spriet L, Meyers EC. Effect of induced erythrocythemia on aerobic work capacity. *J Appl Physiol* 1980; **48**: 636–42.

10. Wedgwood JJ, Thomas JG. Peri-operative haemoglobin: an overview of current opinion regarding the acceptable level of haemoglobin in the peri-operative period. *Eur J Anaesthesiol* 1996; **13**: 316–24.

11. Adams RC, Lundy JS. Anaesthesia in cases of poor surgical risk. *Surg Gynecol Obstet* 1942; **74**: 1011–19.

12. Olugbenga A, Akingbola A, Custer JR, Bunchman TE, Sedman A. Management of severe anemia without transfusion in a pediatric Jehovah's Witness patient. *Crit Care Med* 1994; **22**: 524–8.

13. Viele MK, Weiskopf RB. What can we learn about the need for transfusion from patients who refuse blood? The experience with Jehovah's Witnesses. *Transfusion* 1994; **34**: 396–401.

14. Welch HG, Meehan KR, Goodnough LT. Prudent strategies for elective red blood cell transfusion. *Ann Intern Med* 1992; **116**: 393–402.

15. Hébert PC, Wells G, Blajchman MA, Marshall J, Martin C, Pagliarello G et al. A multicenter, randomized, controlled clinical trial of transfusion requirements in critical care. *N Engl J Med* 1999; **340**: 409–17.

16. Kettler D. 'Permissive anaemia' compared with blood transfusion in patients with cardiac disease: another point of view. *Curr Opin Anaesthesiol* 1994; **7**: 908–18.

17. Ritz E, Amann K. Optimal haemoglobin during treatment with recombinant human erythropoietin. *Nephrol Dial Transplant* 1998; **13** (Supp 2): 16–22.

Chapter 25

Hyperoxia and oxygen toxicity

Chapter 23 described the disastrous consequences of lack of oxygen for life forms that depend on it, but for most organisms hypoxia is an infrequent event. However, oxygen itself also has toxic effects at the cellular level, which organisms have had to oppose by the development of complex antioxidant systems. Indeed, toxic derivatives of oxygen have now become so well controlled by animals that they are used to kill other invading organisms such as bacteria. The activity of toxic oxygen derivatives and antioxidant systems is perfectly balanced for most of the time. Nevertheless, there is a strengthening opinion that over many years oxidative mechanisms predominate, and are responsible for the generalized deterioration in function associated with ageing.[1] In a variety of diseases, or when exposed to extra oxygen, the balance is radically disturbed and oxidative tissue damage results.

Hyperoxia

Hyperventilation, while breathing air, can raise the arterial Po_2 to about 16 kPa (120 mmHg). Higher levels can be obtained only by oxygen enrichment of the inspired gas and/or by elevation of the ambient pressure. Although the arterial Po_2 can be raised to very high levels, the increase in arterial oxygen content is usually relatively small (Table 25.1). The arterial oxygen saturation is normally close to 95% and, apart from raising saturation to 100%, additional oxygen can be carried only in physical solution. Provided that the arterial/mixed venous oxygen content difference remains constant, it follows that venous oxygen content will rise by the same value as the arterial oxygen content. The consequences in terms of venous Po_2 (Table 25.1) are important because minimum tissue Po_2 approximates more closely to venous than to arterial Po_2. The rise in venous Po_2 is trivial when breathing 100% oxygen at normal barometric pressure, and it is necessary to breathe oxygen at 3 atmospheres absolute (ATA) pressure before there is a large increase in venous and therefore tissue Po_2. This is because most of the body requirement can then be met by dissolved oxygen, and the saturation of capillary and venous blood remains close to 100%.

   It is convenient to consider two degrees of hyperoxia. The first applies to the inhalation of oxygen-enriched gas at normal pressure, while the second involves inhaling oxygen at raised pressure and is termed hyperbaric oxygenation. The inhalation of air at raised pressures results in hyperoxia and an air-breathing diver at a depth of 50 metres of sea water (6 ATA) would have an arterial Po_2 comparable to that of a man breathing oxygen at sea level.

Table 25.1 Oxygen levels attained in the normal subject by changes in the oxygen tension of the inspired gas

	At normal barometric pressure		At 2 ATA	At 3 ATA
Inspired gas	Air	Oxygen	Oxygen	Oxygen
Inspired gas P_{O_2} (humidified)				
(kPa)	20	95	190	285
(mmHg)	150	713	1425	2138
Arterial P_{O_2}*				
(kPa)	13	80	175	270
(mmHg)	98	600	1313	2025
Arterial oxygen content†				
(ml.dl^{-1})	19.3	21.3	23.4	25.5
Arterial/venous oxygen content difference				
(ml.dl^{-1})	5.0	5.0	5.0	5.0
Venous oxygen content				
(ml.dl^{-1})	14.3	16.3	18.4	20.5
Venous P_{O_2}				
(kPa)	5.2	6.4	9.1	48.0
(mmHg)	39	48	68	360

Oxygen-induced vasoconstriction means that tissue perfusion may be reduced by elevation of P_{O_2}. This tends to increase the arterial/venous oxygen content difference, which will limit the rise in venous P_{O_2}. The increases in venous P_{O_2} shown in this Table are therefore likely to be greater than *in vivo*.
* Reasonable values have been assumed for P_{CO_2} and alveolar/arterial P_{O_2} difference.
† Normal values assumed for Hb, pH, etc.

Hyperoxia at normal atmospheric pressure

The commonest indications for oxygen enrichment of the inspired gas are the prevention of arterial hypoxaemia ('anoxic anoxia') caused either by hypoventilation (page 522) or by venous admixture (page 181). Oxygen enrichment of the inspired gas may also be used to mitigate the effects of hypoperfusion ('stagnant hypoxia'). The data in Table 25.1 show that there will be only marginal improvement in oxygen flux (page 283), but it may be critical in certain situations. 'Anaemic anoxia' will be only partially relieved by oxygen therapy but, because the combined oxygen is less than in a subject with normal haemoglobin concentration, the effect of additional oxygen carried in solution will be relatively more important.

Clearance of gas loculi in the body may be greatly accelerated by the inhalation of oxygen, which greatly reduces the *total* tension of the dissolved gases in the venous blood (Table 25.2). This results in the capillary blood having additional capacity to carry away gas dissolved from the loculi. Total gas tensions in venous blood are always slightly less than atmospheric, and this is of critical importance in preventing the accumulation of air in potential spaces such as the pleural cavity, where the pressure is subatmospheric (page 42). Oxygen is useful in the treatment of air embolus and pneumothorax, and has also been used to relieve intestinal distension.[2]

Carbon monoxide poisoning has long been recognized as an indication for oxygen therapy. Not only is the oxygen content of the arterial blood improved, but also the rate of dissociation of carboxyhaemoglobin is increased.[3] This is discussed below.

Table 25.2 Normal arterial and mixed venous blood gas tensions

	kPa		mmHg	
	Arterial blood	*Venous blood*	*Arterial blood*	*Venous blood*
Breathing air				
P_{O_2}	13.3	5.3	100	40
P_{CO_2}	5.3	6.1	40	46
P_{N_2}	76.0	76.0	570	570
Total gas tension	94.6	87.4	710	656
Breathing oxygen				
P_{O_2}	80.0	6.7	600	50*
P_{CO_2}	5.3	6.1	40	46
P_{N_2}	0	0	0	0
Total gas tension	85.3	12.8	640	96

* See Table 25.1.

Hyperbaric oxygenation

Mechanisms of benefit

Effect on P_{O_2}. Hyperbaric oxygenation is the only means by which arterial P_{O_2} values in excess of 90 kPa (675 mmHg) may be obtained. However, it is easy to be deluded into thinking that the tissues will be exposed to much the same P_{O_2} as applies in the chamber. Terms such as 'drenching the tissues with oxygen' have been used but are meaningless. In fact, the simple calculations shown in Table 25.1, supported by experimental observations, show that large increases in venous and presumably therefore minimum tissue P_{O_2} do not occur until the P_{O_2} of the arterial blood is of the order of 270 kPa (2025 mmHg), when the whole of the tissue oxygen requirements can be met from the dissolved oxygen. However, the relationship between arterial and tissue P_{O_2} is highly variable (page 250), and hyperoxia-induced vasoconstriction in the brain and other tissues limits the rise in venous and tissue P_{O_2}. Direct access of ambient oxygen will increase P_{O_2} in superficial tissues, particularly when the skin is breached.

Effect on P_{CO_2}. An increased haemoglobin saturation of venous blood reduces its buffering power and carbamino carriage of carbon dioxide, possibly resulting in carbon dioxide retention. In fact, the increase in tissue P_{CO_2} from this cause is unlikely to exceed 1 kPa (7.5 mmHg). However, in the brain this might result in a significant increase in cerebral blood flow, causing a secondary rise in tissue P_{O_2}.

Vasoconstriction, due to increase in P_{O_2}, may be valuable for reduction of oedema in the reperfusion of ischaemic limbs and in burns (see below).

Angiogenesis, the growth of new blood vessels, is improved when oxygen is increased to more than 1 ATA pressure.[4] There seems to be no effect with 100% oxygen at 1 ATA,[5] and the mechanism by which angiogenesis is promoted is unknown. With normoxia, macrophages are responsible for stimulating the growth of new capillaries at the interface between oxygenated and unoxygenated tissue, and the high lactate concentration in unperfused areas may be the trigger. Increased macrophage stimulation therefore seems an unlikely mechanism during hyperbaric oxygenation.

Antibacterial effect. Oxygen plays a major role in bacterial killing by the formation of free radicals and derived species, particularly in polymorphs and macrophages (see below). Apart from its direct effect, relief of hypoxia improves the performance of polymorphs.[6]

Boyle's law effect. The volume of gas spaces in the body is reduced inversely to the absolute pressure according to Boyle's law (page 644). This effect is additional to that resulting from reduction of the total tension of gases in venous blood (see above).

Clinical applications of hyperbaric oxygenation[7,8]

In practice, hyperbaric oxygen treatment means placing a patient into a chamber at 2–3 ATA and providing apparatus to allow them to breathe 100% oxygen, normally a tight fitting facemask. Treatment is usually for about 1–2 hours, and repeated daily for up to 30 days. Around 1960 it seemed that hyperbaric oxygenation would become a most important and widespread form of therapy. Since then, enthusiasm has waxed and waned, but its use is still confined to relatively few centres. Clear indications of its value have been slow to emerge from controlled trials, which are admittedly very difficult to conduct in the conditions for which benefit is claimed. In particular, a proper 'control' group of patients must undergo a sham treatment in a hyperbaric chamber, which has been used in very few trials. The most commonly accepted indications are as follows.

Infection is the most enduring field of application of hyperbaric oxygenation, particularly anaerobic bacterial infections. High partial pressures of oxygen increase the production of oxygen-derived free radicals, which are cidal not only to anaerobes but also to aerobes. The strongest indications are for clostridial myonecrosis (gas gangrene), refractory osteomyelitis and necrotizing soft tissue infections, including cutaneous ulcers.

Gas embolus and decompression sickness are unequivocal indications for hyperbaric therapy; the rationale of treatment is considered above and in Chapter 17.

Carbon monoxide poisoning has been an indication for hyperbaric oxygenation since the pioneer work of Sharp, Ledingham and Norman in 1962.[3] In spite of the exploitation of natural gas, there remains a high incidence of carbon monoxide poisoning from automobile exhaust and from fires. Carbon monoxide poisoning associated with loss of consciousness is generally regarded as an indication for hyperbaric oxygenation, but demonstration of clinical benefit remains controversial in this area.[7,9,10] The rationale of therapy – increased rate of dissociation of carboxyhaemoglobin (COHb) – seems simple when the half-life of COHb is 4–5 hours while breathing air and only 20 minutes with hyperbaric oxygen. However, breathing 100% oxygen at normal pressure reduces the half-life of COHb to just 40 minutes, and therefore in many cases, by the time transport to a hyperbaric chamber is achieved, COHb levels will already be considerably reduced. Other potential benefits of hyperbaric oxygen are believed to derive from minimizing the effects of carbon monoxide on cytochrome c oxidase[11] and neutrophil function.[12]

Tissue hypoxia as a result of hypoperfusion can be relieved by hyperbaric oxygenation when the perfusion is only marginally inadequate. The small increase in oxygen content of the arterial blood clearly cannot compensate for gross failure of perfusion but under some specific circumstances is believed to be helpful. These include compromised tissue transfer in plastic surgery and crush injury or other forms of traumatic ischaemia.

Severe anaemia following blood loss in patients who refuse transfusion (page 489) has been successfully treated using hyperbaric oxygenation to enhance oxygen carriage until the haemoglobin concentration recovers.

Burns. There is experimental evidence that in thermal burns hyperbaric oxygen causes vasoconstriction, reduces oedema, improves phagocytic killing of bacteria, improves angiogenesis and encourages collagen formation. Earlier studies reported many clinical benefits from these theoretical advantages. Recent advances in the general treatment of burns have, however, led to the publication of studies that failed to find any beneficial outcome from the use of hyperbaric oxygen.[7]

Wound healing is improved by hyperbaric oxygenation, even when used intermittently. It is particularly useful when ischaemia contributes to ineffective healing – for example, in diabetes mellitus or peripheral vascular disease. The mechanisms are similar to those for burns, and, in both cases, improved levels of tissue oxygen probably result from direct diffusion of oxygen into the affected superficial tissues.

Sports injuries. Hyperbaric oxygen is believed to expedite recovery from soft-tissue injuries and fractures incurred during competitive sports. Early treatment (within 8 hours) is most effective, indicating a probable effect on neutrophil activity at the site of injury.[13]

Multiple sclerosis. In the early 1980s there was great interest in the therapeutic value of hyperbaric oxygenation in multiple sclerosis. A study in 1983 reported a favourable response after 12 months in a double-blind controlled clinical trial of 40 patients, in which the treated group received 2 ATA oxygen, while the placebo group inhaled 10% oxygen in nitrogen, also at 2 atmospheres.[14] Unfortunately, these findings were not confirmed in subsequent studies, and a recent review of 14 controlled trials concluded that hyperbaric oxygen cannot be recommended for the treatment of multiple sclerosis.[15]

The toxicity of hyperbaric oxygen is considered below.

Oxygen toxicity
The oxygen molecule and derived species[16,17,18]

Although ground state oxygen (dioxygen) is a powerful oxidizing agent, the molecule is stable and has an indefinite half-life. However, the oxygen molecule can be transformed into a range of free radicals and other highly toxic substances, most of which are far more reactive than oxygen itself.

The dioxygen molecule (Figure 25.1) is unusual in having two unpaired electrons in the outer (2P) shell. Thus dioxygen itself qualifies as a 'double' free radical, but stability is conferred by the fact that the orbits of the two unpaired electrons are parallel. The two unpaired electrons also confer the property of paramagnetism, which has been exploited as a method of gas analysis that is almost specific for oxygen.

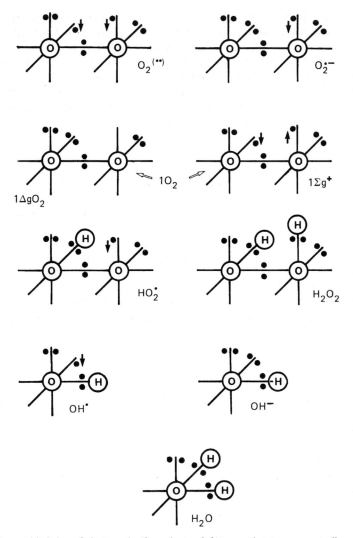

Figure 25.1 Outer orbital ring of electrons in (from the top left): ground state oxygen or dioxygen (O_2); superoxide anion ($O_2^{\cdot-}$); two forms of singlet oxygen ($1O_2$); hydroperoxyl radical ($HO_2^{\cdot}$); hydrogen peroxide (H_2O_2); hydroxyl free radical ($OH^{\cdot}$); hydroxyl ion (OH^-); and water. The arrows indicate the direction of rotation of unpaired electrons. See text for properties and interrelationships.

Singlet oxygen. Internal rearrangements of the unpaired electrons of dioxygen result in the formation of two highly reactive species, both known as singlet oxygen ($1O_2$). In $1\Delta gO_2$ one unpaired electron is transferred to the orbit of the other (Figure 25.1), imparting an energy level 22.4 kcal.mol^{-1} above the ground state. There being no remaining unpaired electron, $1\Delta gO_2$ is not a free radical. In $1\Sigma g^+$, the rotation of one unpaired electron is reversed, which imparts an energy level 37.5 kcal.mol^{-1} above the ground state and this species is still a free radical. $1\Sigma g^+$ is extremely reactive, and rapidly decays to the $1\Delta gO_2$ form, which is particularly relevant in biological systems and especially to lipid peroxidation.

Superoxide anion. In a wide range of circumstances, considered below, the oxygen molecule may be partially reduced by receiving a single electron, which pairs with one of the unpaired electrons forming the superoxide anion ($O_2^{\bullet-}$ in Figure 25.1), which is both an anion and a free radical. It is the first and crucial stage in the production of a series of toxic oxygen-derived free radicals and other compounds. The superoxide anion is relatively stable in aqueous solution at body pH, but has a rapid biological decay owing to the ubiquitous presence of superoxide dismutase (see below). Being charged, superoxide anion does not readily cross cell membranes.

Hydroperoxyl radical. Superoxide anion may acquire a hydrogen ion to form the hydroperoxyl radical thus:

$$O_2^{\bullet-} + H^+ = HO_2^{\bullet}$$

The reaction is pH dependent with a pK of 4.8, so the equilibrium is far to the left in biological systems.

Hydrogen peroxide. Superoxide dismutase (SOD) catalyses the transfer of an electron from one molecule of the superoxide anion to another. The donor molecule becomes dioxygen while the recipient rapidly combines with two hydrogen ions to form hydrogen peroxide (Figure 25.1). Although hydrogen peroxide is not a free radical, it is a powerful and toxic oxidizing agent that plays an important role in oxygen toxicity. The overall reaction is as follows:

$$2O_2^{\bullet-} + 2H^+ \rightarrow H_2O_2 + O_2$$

Reduction of hydrogen peroxide to water. Hydrogen peroxide is continuously generated by the dismutation and other reactions in the body. Two enzymes ensure its rapid removal. Catalase is a highly specific enzyme active against only hydrogen, methyl and ethyl peroxides. Hydrogen peroxide is reduced to water thus:

$$2H_2O_2 \rightarrow 2H_2O + O_2$$

Glutathione peroxidase acts against a much wider range of peroxides (R—OOH), which react with glutathione (G—SH) thus:

$$R—OOH + 2G—SH \rightarrow R—OH + G—S—S—G + H_2O$$

Deficiency of catalase or glutathione peroxidase has been reported in humans, and obligatory anaerobes are normally without catalase.

Three-stage reduction of oxygen. Figure 25.2 summarizes the three-stage reduction of oxygen to water, which is the fully reduced and stable state. This contrasts with the more familiar single-stage reduction of oxygen to water that occurs in the terminal cytochrome (page 281). Unlike the single-stage reduction of oxygen, the three-stage reaction shown in Figure 25.2 is not inhibited by cyanide.

Secondary derivatives of the products of dioxygen reduction

The Fenton reaction. Although both the superoxide anion and hydrogen peroxide have direct toxic effects, they interact to produce even more dangerous species. To the right of Figure 25.3 is shown the Fenton or Haber–Weiss reaction, which results in the formation

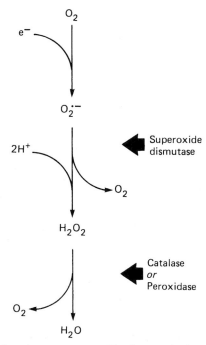

Figure 25.2 Three-stage reduction of oxygen to water. The first reaction is a single electron reduction to form the superoxide anion free radical. In the second stage the first products of the dismutation reaction are dioxygen and a short-lived intermediate which then receives two protons to form hydrogen peroxide. The final stage forms water, the fully reduced form of oxygen.

of the harmless hydroxyl ion together with two extremely reactive species, the hydroxyl free radical $(OH^{\bullet})$ and singlet oxygen $(1O_2)$.

$$O_2^{\bullet-} + H_2O_2 \rightarrow OH^- + OH^{\bullet} + 1O_2$$

The hydroxyl free radical is much the most dangerous species derived from oxygen. The Fenton reaction is more likely than the Haber–Weiss reaction to take place under biological circumstances and it is catalysed by metals, particularly ferrous iron (Fe^{2+}).

The myeloperoxidase reaction.[20] To the left of Figure 25.3 is shown the reaction of hydrogen peroxide with chloride ion to form hypochlorous acid. This occurs in the phagocytic vesicle of the neutrophil and plays a major role in bacterial killing. The reaction is accelerated by the enzyme myeloperoxidase which comprises some 7 per cent of the dried weight of a neutrophil. Hypochlorite has long been known as an effective antibacterial agent, and was used in the First World War as Dakin's solution. The myeloperoxidase reaction also occurs immediately after fertilization of the ovum, and hypochlorous acid so formed causes polymerization of proteins to form the membrane that prevents the further entry of sperms.

Relationship to ionizing radiation. The changes described above have many features in common with those caused by ionizing radiation, the hydroxyl free radical $(OH^{\bullet})$ being the most dangerous product in both cases. Gerschman et al. in 1954[21] were the first to draw the comparison, and to suggest that oxygen-derived free radicals were responsible

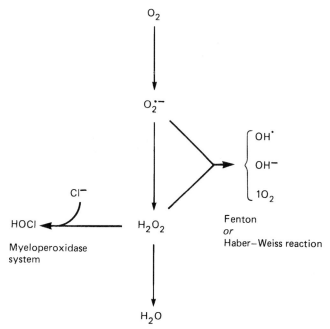

Figure 25.3 Interaction of superoxide anion and hydrogen peroxide in the Fenton or Haber–Weiss reaction to form hydroxyl free radical, hydroxyl ion and singlet oxygen. Hypochlorous acid is formed from hydrogen peroxide by the myeloperoxidase system. (Reproduced from reference 19 by courtesy of the Editor of the *Journal of the Royal Society of Medicine*.)

for the pathophysiology of oxygen poisoning. It is hardly surprising that the effect of radiation is increased by high partial pressures of oxygen, to which reference was made above. As tissue Po_2 is reduced below about 2 kPa (15 mmHg), there is progressively increased resistance to radiation damage until, at zero Po_2, resistance is increased threefold. This unfortunate effect promotes resistance to radiotherapy of malignant cells in hypoxic areas of tumours.

Nitric oxide may behave as a free radical by reacting with the superoxide anion to produce peroxynitrite ($ONOO^-$).[17] This molecule can either rearrange itself into relatively harmless nitrite or nitrate (page 274), or give rise to derivatives with similar biological activity to the hydroxyl radical. Conversely, nitric oxide may act as an antioxidant, binding to ferrous iron molecules and preventing them from contributing to the formation of superoxide anion (see below) or the Fenton reaction. The *in vivo* role of nitric oxide as a free radical or antioxidant therefore remains very unclear at present. In rats, administration of a nitric oxide antagonist caused significant worsening of oxygen-induced pulmonary injury, suggesting that in this model nitric oxide has an overall protective effect.[22]

Sources of electrons for the reduction of oxygen to superoxide anion

Figure 25.3 shows the superoxide anion as the starting point for the production of more toxic free radicals and related species. The first stage reduction of dioxygen to the superoxide anion is therefore critically important in oxygen toxicity.

Mitochondrial NADH dehydrogenase produces some superoxide anion radicals during normal oxidative respiration.[17] Animal studies suggest that this may account for almost 8 per cent of total oxygen consumption, indicating the importance of the highly efficient mitochondrial form of SOD (see below).

The NADPH oxidase system is the major electron donor in neutrophils and macrophages. The electron is donated from NADPH by the enzyme NADPH oxidase, which is located in the membrane of the phagocytic vesicle. This mechanism is activated during phagocytosis and is accompanied by an enormous increase in the oxygen consumption of the cells, a process known to be cyanide resistant. This is the so-called respiratory burst, and occurs in all phagocytic cells in response to a wide range of stimuli, including bacterial endotoxin, immunoglobulins and interleukins. Superoxide anion is released into the phagocytic vesicle, where it is reduced to hydrogen peroxide which then reacts with chloride ions to form hypochlorous acid in the myeloperoxidase reaction (Figure 25.3). NADPH oxidase is absent in chronic granulomatous disease, which results in a serious disability to contend with infection.

Although the NADPH oxidase system has extremely important biological advantages, there seems little doubt that its inappropriate activation in marginated neutrophils can damage the endothelium of the lung, and it may well play a part in the production of acute lung injury (Chapter 30).

Xanthine oxidase and reperfusion injury. The existence of the superoxide anion was first deduced by McCord and Fridovich in 1968[23] from a reaction in which the electron was donated by the conversion of xanthine to uric acid by the enzyme xanthine oxidase (Figure 25.4). Xanthine oxidase catalyses the conversion both of hypoxanthine to xanthine and of xanthine to uric acid, and under normal conditions occurs in its 'D form' as xanthine dehydrogenase. In this form, the enzyme uses NADH as a cofactor. In ischaemic or hypoxic tissue large quantities of hypoxanthine accumulate from ATP degeneration and xanthine oxidase is converted from the D form to the 'O form'. This form of xanthine oxidase cannot use NADH;[17] when oxygen is restored to the cell the production of uric acid proceeds quickly with dioxygen as the cofactor, resulting in the production of superoxide anion (Figure 25.4). Thus, during reperfusion there may be extensive production of oxygen-derived free radicals. It seems probable that, in certain circumstances, this mechanism may play a role in reperfusion tissue damage or postischaemic shock.[24]

A similar mechanism underlies the cytotoxic effects of tumour necrosis factor (TNF).[25] Binding to receptors on the cell wall initiates many intracellular biochemical pathways, which include the conversion of xanthine dehydrogenase (D form) to xanthine oxidase (O form), and thereby the formation of superoxide anion (Figure 25.5).

Ferrous iron loses an electron during conversion to the ferric state. This is an important aspect of the toxicity of ferrous iron and has been proposed as a mechanism of rheumatoid arthritis.[26] A similar reaction also occurs during the spontaneous oxidation of haemoglobin to methaemoglobin (page 272). It is for this reason that large quantities of SOD, catalase and other protective agents are present in the young erythrocyte. Their depletion may well determine the life of the cell. Apart from ferrous iron acting as an electron donor, it is a catalyst in the Fenton reaction (see above).

High P_{O_2}. Whatever other factors may apply, the production of oxygen-derived free radicals is increased at high levels of P_{O_2} by the law of mass action.[27] It would seem that

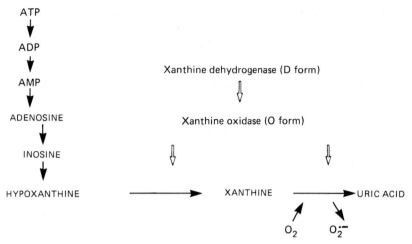

Figure 25.4 Generation of superoxide anion from oxygen by the activity of xanthine oxidase. Also shown are the pathways from ATP to hypoxanthine and the conversion of xanthine dehydrogenase (xanthine oxidase D form) to xanthine oxidase (O form), both of which occur in hypoxia.

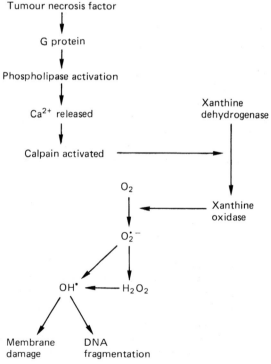

Figure 25.5 Sequence of events in the cytotoxic effects of tumour necrosis factor (TNF). Conversion of xanthine dehydrogenase to xanthine oxidase results in the formation of superoxide anion (see Figure 25.4), which then proceeds to the formation of other free radical species by the Fenton reaction (see Figure 25.3).

the normal tissue defences against free radicals (discussed below) are usually effective only up to a tissue Po_2 of about 60 kPa (450 mmHg). This accords with the development of clinical oxygen toxicity as discussed below. There is also evidence that generation of oxygen-derived free radicals is increased when normal oxygen usage is increased, for example during exercise.[28]

Exogenous compounds. Various drugs and toxic substances can act as an analogue of NADPH oxidase and transfer an electron from NADPH to molecular oxygen. The best example of this is paraquat which can, in effect, insert itself into an electron transport chain, alternating between its singly and doubly ionized form. This process is accelerated at high levels of Po_2 and so there is a synergistic effect between paraquat and oxygen. Paraquat is concentrated in the alveolar epithelial type II cell where the Po_2 is as high as anywhere in the body. Because of the very short half-life of the oxygen-derived free radicals, damage is confined to the lung. Bleomycin and some antibiotics (e.g. nitrofurantoin) can act in a similar manner. Reactions usually occur at high dose levels, are again potentiated by increased oxygen levels or radiation and eventually lead to pulmonary fibrosis.

Biochemical targets of oxygen-derived free radicals

The three main targets are deoxyribonucleic acid (DNA), lipids and sulphydryl-containing proteins. All three are also sensitive to ionizing radiation. The mechanisms of both forms of damage have much in common and synergism occurs.

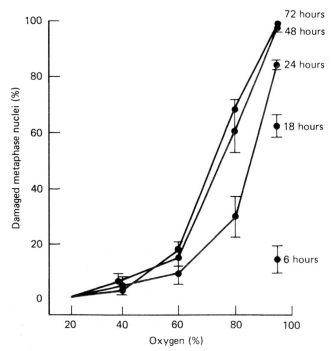

Figure 25.6 Breakage of chromosomes in a culture of Chinese hamster lung fibroblasts by oxygen at various concentrations and for varying durations of exposure. (Reproduced from reference 29 by courtesy of the Editors of *Mutation Research.*)

DNA. Breakage of chromosomes in cultures of animal lung fibroblasts by high concentrations of oxygen was demonstrated by Sturrock and Nunn in 1978[29] (Figure 25.6). The same authors showed that 48 hours' exposure to 95% oxygen increased the rate of mutations by a factor of 25. It is not yet clear to what extent damage to DNA is responsible for pulmonary oxygen toxicity.

Lipids. There is little doubt that lipid peroxidation is a major mechanism of tissue damage by oxygen-derived free radicals. The interaction of a free radical with an unsaturated fatty acid not only disrupts that particular lipid molecule but also generates another free radical so that a chain reaction ensues until stopped by an antioxidant.[18] Lipid peroxidation disrupts cell membranes and accounts for the loss of integrity of the alveolar/capillary barrier in pulmonary oxygen toxicity.

Proteins. Damage to sulphydryl-containing proteins results in the formation of disulphide bridges, which inactivate a range of enzymes including some that may be involved in oxygen convulsions (see below).

Interference with these fundamental cellular processes, particularly DNA, has widespread biological implications. Once damaged, lipids, DNA or proteins must either be replaced or repaired, and, though repair mechanisms are poorly understood, they are known to exist for DNA.[1] Inevitably, cell dysfunction will occur and may take the form of inflammation, malignancy or cell death. Oxygen-derived free radical damage is now closely linked with cardiovascular disease,[30] cancer[31] and the degenerative changes of ageing.[1]

Defences against oxygen-derived free radicals

Life in an oxidizing environment is possible only because of powerful antioxidant defences, which all aerobes have developed (see Chapter 1, page 8). The defensive systems are freely duplicated and operate in depth.

Antioxidant enzymes

These enzymes are widely distributed in different organs and different species but are deficient in most obligatory anaerobic bacteria. Young animals normally have increased levels of SOD and catalase, which confers greater resistance to oxygen toxicity. The reactions catalysed by antioxidant enzymes have been described above.

Superoxide dismutase activity has been described above. Three types of SOD exist, each derived from a separate gene:[17,32] extracellular SOD, cytoplasmic SOD containing manganese (MnSOD) and mitochondrial SOD containing both copper and zinc (CuZnSOD). Extra production of SOD may be induced by several mechanisms, of which hyperoxia is the most notable,[33] but inflammatory cytokines such as interferon,[34] TNF,[35] interleukin[35] and bacterial endotoxin[36] are almost certainly very important in the intact animal. A recent study of human bronchial epithelial cells exposed to 100% oxygen confirmed the induction of MnSOD by TNF but hyperoxia alone had no effect, indicating that changes in response to oxygen may be mediated by cytokines released from other cells. Production requires activation of the SOD gene and in animals takes 3 days or more to occur. Animal studies have also consistently shown that induction of SOD confers some protection against the toxic effects of oxygen.[17] In certain circumstances, induction may be feasible as a prophylactic measure and this must often have occurred during the early stages of treatment of severe acute lung injury (ALI), when the inspired oxygen concentration has been gradually increased to counter progressive failure of gas exchange. There are difficulties in the therapeutic use of SOD, because the most important forms are intracellular or mitochondrial enzymes which have very short half-lives in plasma. There is therefore little scope for their use by direct intravenous injection. It is possible for SOD to enter cells if it is administered in liposomes,[37] and extracellular SOD has been used by direct instillation into the lungs.[38]

Catalase has a cellular and extracellular distribution similar to that of SOD, with which it is closely linked in disposing of superoxide anion (Figure 25.2). Although studied less extensively, catalase production is believed to be induced by the same factors as SOD. Similarly, trials of exogenous antioxidant enzymes have usually given better results when both SOD and catalase are administered.

Glutathione peroxidase system scavenges not only the oxygen-derived free radicals themselves but also free radicals formed during lipid peroxidation. Two molecules of the tripeptide (glycine–cysteine–glutamic acid) glutathione (GSH) are oxidized to one molecule of reduced glutathione (GSSG) by the formation of a disulphide bridge linking the cysteine residues. GSH is re-formed from GSSG by the enzyme glutathione reductase, hydrogen being supplied by NADPH.

Endogenous antioxidants

Ascorbic acid is a small molecule with significant antioxidant properties, being particularly important for removal of the hydroxyl free radical. Humans, along with guinea-pigs and bats, lack the enzyme required for the production of ascorbate, and so must ingest sufficient vitamin C to compensate. In these mammals, SOD activity is markedly higher than in those able to produce endogenous ascorbate.[39]

Vitamin E (α-tocopherol) is a highly fat-soluble compound and is therefore found in high concentrations in cell membranes. Predictably, its main antioxidant role is in the prevention of lipid peroxidation chain reactions, described above.

Surfactant may act as an antioxidant in the lung. Animal studies have shown that administration of exogenous surfactant prolongs the duration of oxygen exposure required to cause lung damage.[40]

Over all, antioxidant activity from both enzymes and other endogenous antioxidants is very high in the fluid lining the pulmonary airways. Apart from the relatively high Po_2 in the inhaled gas, a whole range of other oxidizing substances may be inhaled, including common air pollutants and the constituents of cigarette smoke (Chapter 20).

Exogenous antioxidants

Allopurinol. Because xanthine oxidase plays a pivotal role in the reactions shown in Figures 25.4 and 25.5, it seemed logical to explore the use of allopurinol, which inhibits a range of enzymes, including xanthine oxidase. As may be expected, benefit is seen mainly after ischaemia–reperfusion injury.

Iron-chelating agents. Because ferrous iron is both a potent source of electrons for conversion of oxygen to the superoxide anion and a catalyst in the Fenton reaction, desferrioxamine has antioxidant properties *in vitro.*[41]

Steroids showed great promise as clinically useful antioxidants. Sturrock and Hulands in 1980[42] showed that maximal doses of methylprednisolone give considerable protection from the chromosome-breaking effect of oxygen described above. Similarly, dexamethasone in high dosage has been found to have therapeutic value in the late stage of pulmonary oxygen toxicity in rats but to decrease survival when used in the early stages of exposure.[43] It will be difficult if not impossible to confirm the value of steroids in the treatment of pulmonary oxygen toxicity in humans.

These compounds, along with other *in vitro* antioxidants such as *n*-acetyl cysteine, β-carotene and dimethylsulphoxide, have generally failed to live up to their expectations in human disease.[31] There are three possible explanations. First, studies of free radical production and antioxidants in human cells are relatively rare, and there is known to be considerable species variability.[17] Secondly, penetration of the exogenous antioxidant to the site of free radical generation (e.g. mitochondria) or damage (e.g. nuclear DNA) is likely to be poor. Finally, free radical production for bacterial killing is fundamental to mammalian defence systems, so any non-specific antioxidant activity may be detrimental. Their therapeutic role in oxygen toxicity or diseases known to involve excess production of oxygen-derived species is therefore far from fully clarified.

Clinical oxygen toxicity

The most important clinical conditions in which oxygen has been identified as the sole precipitating cause are oxygen convulsions, pulmonary oxygen toxicity and retrolental fibroplasia.

Oxygen convulsions (the Paul Bert effect)

It is well established that exposure to oxygen at a partial pressure in excess of 2 atmospheres absolute (2 ATA) may result in convulsions, which are usually lethal to divers. This limits the depth to which closed-circuit oxygen apparatus can be used. It is interesting that the threshold for oxygen convulsions is close to that at which brain tissue P_{O_2} is likely to be sharply increased (Table 25.1). The relationship to cerebral tissue P_{O_2} is supported by the observation that an elevation of P_{CO_2} lowers the threshold for convulsions. High P_{CO_2} increases cerebral blood flow and therefore raises the tissue P_{O_2} relative to the arterial P_{O_2}. Hyperventilation and anaesthesia each provide limited protection.

Convulsions result from poorly understood changes in cellular interactions between gamma-aminobutyric acid (GABA) and nitric oxide. GABA concentrations decrease in the brain prior to convulsion and the change correlates with the severity of the convulsion.[44] As GABA is an inhibitory neurotransmitter, it is not unreasonable to suggest that a reduced level might result in convulsions. Nitric oxide is known to sensitize neurones to the toxic effects of GABA in hypoxia (page 476), and is also involved in hyperoxic convulsions. Nitric oxide inhibitors delay the onset of convulsions in hyperoxia,[45,46] but paradoxically, the same effect is seen with some nitric oxide donors.[46] Whatever the role of nitric oxide, the final common pathway seems to be mediated by disturbed calcium fluxes and increased cyclic-GMP concentration.[45]

Incidence Hyperbaric oxygen used for the conditions described above – that is, intermittent exposure to less than 3 ATA – carries little risk of oxygen convulsions. At 2 ATA, a large series reported no convulsions in over 12 000 treatments.[47] Treatment for carbon monoxide poisoning is associated with a greater incidence of convulsions because of the higher pressures used (normally 2.8–3.0 ATA) and the toxic effects of carbon monoxide on the brain itself. In this case, 1–2 per cent of patients experience convulsions.[48]

Pulmonary oxygen toxicity

Pulmonary tissue P_{O_2} is the highest in the body and the lung is therefore the organ most vulnerable to oxygen toxicity. Pulmonary oxygen toxicity is unequivocal and lethal in laboratory animals such as the rat. Humans seem to be far less sensitive, but there are formidable obstacles to investigation of both human volunteers and patients. Study of oxygen toxicity in the clinical environment is complicated by the presence of the pulmonary pathology that necessitated the use of oxygen.

Symptoms.[49] High concentrations of oxygen cause irritation of the tracheobronchial tree, which gives rise initially to a sensation of retrosternal tightness. Continued exposure leads to chest pain, cough and an urge to take deep breaths. Reduced vital capacity is the first measurable change in lung function, occurring after about 24 hours of normobaric 100% oxygen. Oxygen exposure beyond this point leads to the widespread structural changes described below, which ultimately give rise to acute lung injury and possibly irreversible changes in lung function.

Cellular changes. Weibel reviewed the classic studies of his group in 1971.[50] Electron microscopy has revealed that, in rats exposed to 1 atmosphere of oxygen, the primary change is in the capillary endothelium, which becomes vacuolated and thin. Permeability is increased and fluid accumulates in the interstitial space. At a later stage, in monkeys, the epithelial lining is lost over large areas of the alveoli. This process affects the type I cell (page 29) and is accompanied by proliferation of the type II cell, which is relatively resistant to oxygen. The alveolar/capillary membrane is greatly thickened, partly because of the substitution of type II cells for type I and partly because of interstitial accumulation of fluid.

Limits of survival. Pulmonary effects of oxygen vary greatly between different species, probably because of different levels of provision of defences against free radicals. Most strains of rats will not survive for much more than 3 days in 1 atmosphere of oxygen. Monkeys generally survive oxygen breathing for about 2 weeks, and humans are probably even more resistant. Oxygen tolerance for normal humans has been investigated,[51,52] but these studies are based on reduction in vital capacity etc., which is a very early stage of oxygen toxicity. There is an approximately inverse relationship between P_{O_2} and duration of tolerable exposure. Thus 20 hours of 1 atmosphere had an effect similar to 10 hours of 2 atmospheres or 5 hours of 4 atmospheres.

Pulmonary oxygen toxicity seems to be related to P_{O_2} rather than inspired concentration. Early American astronauts breathed 100% oxygen at a pressure of about 0.3 atmosphere for many days (see Table 18.1) with no apparent ill effects. There is abundant evidence that prolonged exposure to this environment does not result in demonstrable pulmonary oxygen toxicity, thus establishing a P_{O_2} of 34 kPa (255 mmHg) as a safe level. It also confirms that the significant factor is partial pressure and not concentration. In contrast, the concentration of oxygen rather than its partial pressure is the important factor in absorption collapse of the lung (see below).

Clinical studies. Some limited information on human pulmonary oxygen toxicity has been obtained from patients in the course of therapeutic administration of oxygen. In 1967, a review of 70 patients who died after prolonged artificial ventilation reported a greater number of pulmonary abnormalities (fibrin membranes, oedema and fibrosis) in those who had received more than 90% oxygen.[53] However, the higher concentrations of oxygen would probably have been used in the patients with more severe defects in gas exchange, and it is therefore difficult to distinguish between the effects of oxygen itself and the conditions that required its use. A similar group of patients ventilated for long periods with high concentrations of oxygen were reviewed in 1980,[54] and these authors concluded that adverse effects of oxygen on the alveolar epithelium were rarely of practical importance in hypoxaemic patients. An elegant attempt to avoid the complicating factor of pre-existing pulmonary disease was made by Singer et al. in 1970,[55] who ventilated a group of patients with 100% oxygen for 24 hours after cardiac surgery. Two further patients received oxygen for 5 and 7 days respectively. Various indices of pulmonary function (V_D/V_T ratio, shunt and compliance) were not significantly different from a control group receiving less than 42% oxygen.

In contrast to these essentially negative findings, a study in 1987 obtained positive findings in a randomized trial involving patients ventilated after coronary artery bypass grafting.[56] Venous admixture was significantly greater and arterial P_{O_2} less in patients receiving 50% oxygen compared with the group receiving less than 30%. There are many possible causes for these changes but the authors concluded that unnecessary elevation of inspired oxygen concentration should be avoided, a view from which few would dissent in the present state of knowledge.

Pulmonary absorption collapse. Whatever the uncertainties about the susceptibility of humans to pulmonary oxygen toxicity, there is no doubt that high concentrations of oxygen in zones of the lung with low ventilation/perfusion ratios will result in collapse. This probably occurs routinely during anaesthesia (page 434), and may be demonstrated in the healthy but middle-aged awake volunteer. A few minutes of breathing oxygen at residual lung volume results in radiological evidence of collapse, a reduced arterial P_{O_2} and substernal pain on attempting a maximal inspiration.[57]

Balancing the risks. Prevention of dangerous hypoxia is always the first priority and must be treated in spite of the various hazards associated with the use of oxygen.[54] A reasonably safe arterial P_{O_2} is 10 kPa (75 mmHg), normally giving a saturation of 95% but, if this cannot be maintained without resorting to dangerous levels of inspired oxygen concentrations (in excess of 60%), it may be necessary to settle for a lower arterial P_{O_2}. The safe lower level of arterial P_{O_2} for an individual patient depends on many factors (page 477) and no general rule can be formulated.

The cornerstone of avoiding the potentially harmful effects of oxygen in the clinical environment is prevention. Although brief periods of exposure to 100% oxygen seem safe, inspired oxygen concentrations should be titrated against arterial P_{O_2}. This is particularly important in patients exposed to paraquat or bleomycin.

Retrolental fibroplasia (RLF)[58]

Shortly after RLF was first described in 1942, it became established that hyperoxia was the major aetiological factor and led to the use of oxygen being strictly curtailed in the management of neonates. This resulted in an increase in morbidity and mortality attributable to hypoxia, and thereafter oxygen was carefully monitored and titrated in the hope of steering the narrow course between the Scylla of hypoxia and the Charybdis of RLF. This policy has not eradicated the condition, and there is some evidence that RLF may occur in infants who have never received additional oxygen. Vitamin E has been used in the attempt to prevent RLF but it is currently believed that hyperoxia is but one of a variety of factors that may cause RLF by changes in the retinal oxygen supply. RLF is increasingly likely to occur with greater degrees of prematurity, and there is a well-established inverse relationship between birth weight and its incidence.

References

1. Beckman KB, Ames BN. The free radical theory of aging matures. *Physiol Rev* 1998; **78**: 547–81.
2. Down RHL, Castleden WM. Oxygen therapy for pneumatosis coli. *BMJ* 1975; **1**: 493–4.
3. Sharp GR, Ledingham IMcA, Norman JN. The application of oxygen at 2 atmospheres pressure in the treatment of acute anoxia. *Anaesthesia* 1962; **17**: 136–44.
4. Thom SR. Hyperbaric oxygen therapy. *Intensive Care Med* 1989; **4**: 58–63.
5. Marx RE, Ehler WJ, Tayapongsak P, Pierce LW. Relationship of oxygen dose to angiogenesis induction in irradiated tissue. *Am J Surg* 1990; **160**: 519–24.
6. Mandell G. Bactericidal activity of aerobic and anaerobic polymorphonuclear neutrophils. *Infect Immun* 1974; **9**: 337–41.
7. Tibbles PM, Edelsberg JS. Hyperbaric-oxygen therapy. *N Engl J Med* 1996; **334**: 1642–8.
8. Kindwall EP. Hyperbaric oxygen – more indications than many doctors realise. *BMJ* 1993; **307**: 515–6.
9. Seger D, Welch L. Carbon monoxide controversies: neuropsychologic testing, mechanism of toxicity, and hyperbaric oxygen. *Ann Emerg Med* 1994; **24**: 242–8.
10. Ernst A, Zibrak JD. Carbon monoxide poisoning. *N Engl J Med* 1998; **339**: 1603–7.
11. Brown SD, Piantadosi CA. *In vivo* binding of carbon monoxide to cytochrome *c* oxidase in rat brain. *J Appl Physiol* 1990; **68**: 604–10.
12. Thom SR. Dehydrogenase conversion to oxidase and lipid peroxidation in brain after carbon monoxide poisoning. *J Appl Physiol* 1992; **73**: 1584–9.
13. Staples J, Clement D. Hyperbaric oxygen chambers and the treatment of sports injuries. *Sports Med* 1996; **22**: 219–27.
14. Fischer BH, Marks M, Reich T. Hyperbaric-oxygen treatment of multiple sclerosis. A randomized, placebo controlled, double blind study. *N Engl J Med* 1983; **308**: 181–4.
15. Kleijnen J, Knipschild P. Hyperbaric oxygen for multiple sclerosis. Review of controlled trials. *Acta Neurol Scand* 1995; **91**: 330–4.
16. Royston D. Free radicals. Formation, function and potential relevance to anaesthesia. *Anaesthesia* 1988; **43**: 315–20.
17. Kinnula VL, Crapo JD, Raivio KO. Generation and disposal of reactive oxygen metabolites in the lung. *Lab Invest* 1995; **73**: 3–19.
18. Webster NR, Nunn JF. Molecular structure of free radicals and their importance in biological reactions. *Br J Anaesth* 1988; **60**: 98–108.
19. Nunn JF. Oxygen – friend or foe. *J Roy Soc Med* 1985; **78**: 618–22.
20. Fantone JC, Ward PA. Role of oxygen-derived free radicals and metabolites in leukocyte-dependent inflammatory reactions. *Am J Pathol* 1982; **107**: 397–418.
21. Gerschman R, Gilbert DL, Nye SW, Dwyer P, Fenn WO. Oxygen poisoning and X-irradiation: a mechanism in common. *Science* 1954; **119**: 623–6.
22. Capellier G, Maupoil V, Biollot A, Kantelip JP, Rochette L, Regnard J. L-NAME aggravates pulmonary oxygen toxicity in rats. *Eur Respir J* 1996; **9**: 2531–6.

23. McCord JM, Fridovich I. The reduction of cytochrome c by milk xanthine oxidase. *J Biol Chem* 1968; **243**: 5753–60.

24. Traystman RJ, Kirsch JR, Koehler RC. Oxygen radical mechanisms of brain injury following ischaemia and reperfusion. *J Appl Physiol* 1991; **71**: 1185–95.

25. Blake DR, Hall ND, Bacon PA, Dieppe PA, Halliwell B, Gutteridge JMC. The importance of iron in rheumatoid disease. *Lancet* 1981; **2**: 1142–4.

26. Larrick JW, Wright SC. Cytotoxic mechanism of tumor necrosis factor-α. *FASEB J* 1990; **4**: 3215–23.

27. Freeman BA, Topolsky MK, Crapo JD. Hyperoxia increases oxygen radical production in rat lung homogenates. *Arch Biochem Biophys* 1982; **216**: 477–84.

28. Kantner M. Free radicals, exercise and antioxidant supplementation. *Proc Nutrit Soc* 1998; **57**: 9–13.

29. Sturrock JE, Nunn JF. Chromosomal damage and mutations after exposure of Chinese hamster cells to high concentrations of oxygen. *Mutat Res* 1978; **57**: 27–31.

30. Rapola JM. Should we prescribe antioxidants to patients with coronary heart disease. *Eur Heart J* 1998; **19**: 530–2.

31. Hennekens CH, Buring JE, Manson JE, Stampfer M, Rosner B, Cook NR et al. Lack of effect of long-term supplementation with beta carotene on the incidence of malignant neoplasms and cardiovascular disease. *N Engl J Med* 1996; **334**: 1145–9.

32. Tsan MF. Superoxide dismutase and pulmonary oxygen toxicity. *Proc Soc Exp Biol Med* 1997; **214**: 107–13.

33. Crapo JD, Tierney DF. Superoxide dismutase and pulmonary oxygen toxicity. *Am J Physiol* 1974; **226**: 1401–7.

34. Harris CA, Derbin KS, Hunte-McDonough B, Krauss MR, Chen KT, Smith DM, Epstein LB. Manganese superoxide dismutase is induced by IFN-γ in multiple cell types. Synergistic induction by IFN-γ and tumor necrosis factor or IL-1. *J Immunol* 1991; **147**: 149–54.

35. Tsan MF, White JE, Del Vecchio PJ, Shaffer JB. IL-6 enhances TNF-alpha- and IL-1-induced increase of Mn superoxide dismutase mRNA and O_2 tolerance. *Am J Physiol* 1992; **263**: L22–6.

36. Frank L, Summerville J, Massaro D. Protection from oxygen toxicity with endotoxin: role of the endogenous antioxidant enzymes of the lung. *J Clin Invest* 1980; **65**: 1104–10.

37. Freeman BA, Turrens JF, Mirza Z, Crapo JD, Young SL. Modulation of oxidant lung injury by using liposome-entrapped superoxide dismutase and catalase. *Fed Proc* 1985; **44**: 2591–5.

38. Barnard ML, Baker RR, Matalon S. Mitigation of oxidant injury to lung microvasculature by intratracheal instillation of antioxidant enzymes. *Am J Physiol* 1995; **265**: L340–67.

39. Nandi A, Mukhopadhyay CK, Ghosh MK, Chattopadhyay DJ, Chatterjee IB. Evolutionary significance of vitamin C biosynthesis in terrestrial vertebrates. *Free Radic Biol Med* 1997; **22**: 1047–54.

40. Ghio AJ, Fracica PJ, Young SL, Piantadosi CA. Synthetic surfactant scavenges oxidants and protects against hyperoxic lung injury. *J Appl Physiol* 1994; **77**: 1217–23.

41. Gutteridge JMC, Rowley DA, Griffiths E, Halliwell B. Low-molecular-weight iron complexes and oxygen radical reactions in idiopathic haemochromatosis. *Clin Sci* 1985; **68**: 463–7.

42. Sturrock JE, Hulands GH. Protective effect of steroids on cultured cells damaged by high concentrations of oxygen. *Br J Anaesth* 1980; **52**: 567–72.

43. Koizumi M, Frank L, Massaro D. Oxygen toxicity in rats: varied effect of dexamethasone treatment depending on duration of hyperoxia. *Am Rev Respir Dis* 1985; **131**: 907–11.

44. Wood JD, Watson WJ. Gamma-aminobutyric acid levels in the brain of rats exposed to oxygen at high pressures. *Can J Biochem Physiol* 1963; **41**: 1907–13.

45. Wang WJ, Ho XP, Yan YL, Yan TH, Li CL. Intrasynaptosomal free calcium and nitric oxide metabolism in central nervous system toxicity. *Aviat Space Environ Med* 1998; **69**: 551–5.

46. Bitterman N, Bitterman H. L-Arginine–NO pathway and CNS oxygen toxicity. *J Appl Physiol* 1998; **84**: 1633–8.

47. Hill RK. Is more better? A comparison of different clinical hyperbaric treatment pressures – a preliminary report. *Undersea Hyperb Med* 1993; **20** (Supp): 12.

48. Hampson NB, Simonson SG, Kramer CC, Piantadosi CA. Central nervous system oxygen toxicity during hyperbaric treatment of patients with carbon monoxide poisoning. *Undersea Hyperb Med* 1996; **23**: 215–19.

49. Montgomery AB, Luce JM, Murray JF. Retrosternal pain is an early indicator of oxygen toxicity. *Am Rev Respir Dis* 1989; **139**: 1548–50.

50. Weibel ER. Oxygen effect on lung cells. *Arch Intern Med* 1971; **128**: 54–6.

51. Clark JM, Lambertsen CJ. Pulmonary toxicity – a review. *Pharmacol Rev* 1971; **23**: 37–133.

52. Clark JM, Lambertsen CJ, Gelfand R, Flores ND, Pisarello JB, Rossman MD, Elias JA. Effects of prolonged oxygen exposure at 1.5, 2.0, or 2.5 ATA on pulmonary function in men (Predictive studies V). *J Appl Physiol* 1999; **86**: 243–59.

53. Nash G, Blennerhassett JB, Pontoppidan H. Pulmonary lesions associated with oxygen therapy and artificial ventilation. *N Engl J Med* 1967; **276**: 368–74.

54. Gilbe CE, Salt JC, Branthwaite MA. Pulmonary function after prolonged mechanical ventilation with high concentrations of oxygen. *Thorax* 1980; **35**: 907–11.

55. Singer MM, Wright F, Stanley LK, Roe BB, Hamilton WK. Oxygen toxicity in man. A prospective study in patients after open-heart surgery. *N Engl J Med* 1970; **283**: 1473–8.

56. Register SD, Downs JB, Stock MC, Kirby RR. Is 50% oxygen harmful? *Crit Care Med* 1987; **15**: 598–601.

57. Nunn JF, Williams IP, Jones JG, Hewlett AM, Hulands GH, Minty BD. Detection and reversal of pulmonary absorption collapse. *Br J Anaesth* 1978; **50**: 91–100.

58. Lucey JF, Dangman B. A reexamination of the role of oxygen in retrolental fibroplasia. *Pediatrics* 1984; **73**: 82–96.

Part 3

Physiology of Pulmonary Disease

Chapter 26

Ventilatory failure

Definitions

Respiratory failure is defined as a failure of maintenance of normal arterial blood gas tensions. Hypoxia as a result of cardiac and other extrapulmonary forms of shunting are excluded from this definition. Respiratory failure may be subdivided according to whether the arterial Pco_2 is normal or low (type 1) or elevated (type 2). Mean of the normal arterial Pco_2 is 5.1 kPa (38.3 mmHg) with 95% limits (2 s.d.) of ±1 kPa (7.5 mmHg). The normal arterial Po_2 is more difficult to define because it decreases with age (page 276) and is strongly influenced by the concentration of oxygen in the inspired gas. Mechanisms that contribute to respiratory failure include ventilatory failure (reduced alveolar ventilation) and venous admixture as a result of either pure intrapulmonary shunt or ventilation/perfusion mismatch (Chapter 8).

Ventilatory failure is defined as a pathological reduction of the alveolar ventilation below the level required for the maintenance of normal alveolar gas tensions. Because arterial Po_2 (unlike arterial Pco_2) is so strongly influenced by shunting, the adequacy of ventilation is conveniently defined by the arterial Pco_2, although it is also reflected in end-expiratory Pco_2 and Po_2. This chapter is concerned mainly with pure ventilatory failure; other causes of respiratory failure are described in the next four chapters.

Pattern of changes in arterial blood gas tensions

Figure 26.1 shows, on a Po_2/Pco_2 diagram, the typical patterns of deterioration of arterial blood gas tensions in respiratory failure. The shaded area indicates the normal range of tensions with increasing age corresponding to a leftward shift. Pure ventilatory failure in a young person with otherwise normal lungs would result in changes along the broken line. Chronic obstructive airway disease, the commonest cause of predominantly ventilatory failure, occurs in older people, and the observed pattern of change is shown within the upper arrow in Figure 26.1. The limit of survival, while breathing air, is reached at a Po_2 of about 2.7 kPa (20 mmHg) and Pco_2 of 11 kPa (83 mmHg). The limiting factor is not Pco_2 but Po_2. This prevents the rise of Pco_2 to higher levels except when the patient's inspired oxygen concentration is increased. It may also be raised above 11 kPa by the inhalation of carbon dioxide. In either event, a Pco_2 in excess of 11 kPa may be

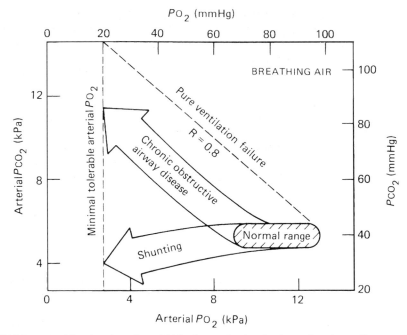

Figure 26.1 Pattern of deterioration of arterial blood gases in chronic obstructive airway disease and pulmonary shunting. The shaded area indicates the normal range of arterial blood gas tensions in which P_{O_2} decreases with age. The oblique broken line shows the theoretical changes in alveolar P_{O_2} and P_{CO_2} resulting from pure ventilatory failure. In chronic obstructive airway disease, the arterial P_{O_2} is always less than the value that would be expected in pure ventilatory failure at the same P_{CO_2} value. Discussion of shunting is to be found in Chapter 8 and further discussion of chronic obstructive airway disease in Chapter 27.

considered an iatrogenic disorder. Figure 26.1 also shows the pattern of blood gas changes caused by shunting or pulmonary venous admixture (Chapter 8).

In general, the arterial P_{O_2} indicates the severity of respiratory failure (assuming that the patient is breathing air), while the P_{CO_2} indicates the differential diagnosis between ventilatory failure and shunting as shown in Figure 26.1. In respiratory disease it is, of course, common for ventilatory failure and shunting to coexist in the same patient.

Time course of changes in blood gas tensions in acute ventilatory failure

Although the upper arrow in Figure 26.1 shows the effect of established ventilatory failure on arterial blood gas tensions, short-term deviations from this pattern occur in acute ventilatory failure. This is because the time courses of changes of P_{O_2} and P_{CO_2} in response to acute changes in ventilation are quite different.

Body stores of oxygen are small, amounting to about 1550 ml while breathing air. Therefore, following a step change in the level of alveolar ventilation, the alveolar and arterial P_{O_2} rapidly reach the new value (as shown in Figure 6.12) and the half-time for the change is only 30 seconds (see page 289 and Figure 11.20). In contrast, the body stores of carbon dioxide are very large – of the order of 120 litres. Therefore, following a step change in the level of alveolar ventilation, the alveolar and arterial $P\text{co}_2$ only slowly attain the value determined by the new alveolar ventilation as shown in Figure 6.12. Furthermore, the time course is slower following a reduction of ventilation than an increase (Figure 10.10) and the half-time of rise of $P\text{co}_2$ following a step reduction of ventilation is of the order of 16 minutes.

The practical point is that, during the transient phase of acute hypoventilation, there may be a low $P\text{o}_2$ while the $P\text{co}_2$ is increasing but is still within the normal range. Thus the pulse oximeter may, under certain circumstances such as when breathing air, give an earlier warning of hypoventilation than the capnograph. This breaks the rule that the $P\text{co}_2$ is the essential index of alveolar ventilation, and it may be erroneously believed that the diagnosis is shunting rather than hypoventilation.

Causes of ventilatory failure

The causes of ventilatory failure may be conveniently considered under the headings of the anatomical sites where they arise. These sites are indicated in Figure 26.2. Lesions or malfunctions at sites A to E result in a reduction of input to the respiratory muscles. Dyspnoea may not be apparent and the diagnosis of ventilatory failure may be overlooked on superficial inspection of the patient. Lesions or malfunctions at sites G to J result in evident dyspnoea and no one is likely to miss the diagnosis of hypoventilation. The various sites are now considered individually.

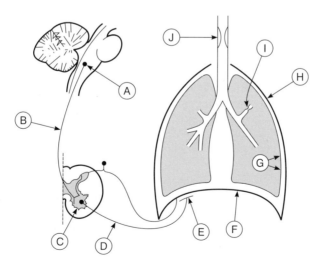

Figure 26.2 Summary of sites at which lesions, drug action or malfunction may result in ventilatory failure. (A) Respiratory centre. (B) Upper motor neurone. (C) Anterior horn cell. (D) Lower motor neurone. (E) Neuromuscular junction. (F) Respiratory muscles. (G) Altered elasticity of lungs or chest wall (H) Loss of structural integrity of chest wall and pleural cavity. (I) Increased resistance of small airways. (J) Upper airway obstruction.

A. The respiratory neurones of the medulla are depressed by hypoxia and also by very high levels of P_{CO_2}, probably of the order of 40 kPa (300 mmHg) in the healthy unanaesthetized subject, but at a lower P_{CO_2} in the presence of some drugs (see below). Reduction of P_{CO_2} below the apnoeic threshold results in apnoea in the unconscious subject but not usually in the conscious subject. Loss of respiratory sensitivity to carbon dioxide occurs in various types of long-term ventilatory failure, particularly chronic obstructive pulmonary disease; this is discussed further on page 533.

A wide variety of drugs may cause central apnoea or respiratory depression, and these include opioids, barbiturates and most anaesthetic agents, whether intravenous or inhalational. The respiratory neurones may also be affected by anything that reduces their blood supply, including pressure, trauma, neoplasm or vascular catastrophe. Localized lesions elsewhere in the brain may also cause ventilatory disturbances, which are presumed to result from interference with the many central nervous system connections with the central pattern generator of the respiratory centre (page 84).[1]

B. The upper motor neurones serving the respiratory muscles are most likely to be interrupted by trauma. Only lesions above third or fourth cervical vertebrae will affect the phrenic nerve and result in total apnoea. However, fracture dislocations of the lower cervical vertebrae are relatively common and result in loss of action of the intercostal and expiratory muscles while sparing the diaphragm. Upper motor neurones may be involved in various disease processes, including tumours, demyelination and, occasionally, in syringomyelia.

C. The anterior horn cell may be affected by various disease processes, of which the most important is poliomyelitis. Fortunately, this condition is now rare in the developed world but it can produce any degree of respiratory involvement up to total paralysis of all respiratory muscles.

D. Lower motor neurones supplying the respiratory muscles are prone to normal traumatic risks and, in former times, the phrenic nerves were surgically interrupted for the treatment of pulmonary tuberculosis. The later stages of motor neurone disease may cause ventilatory failure at this level. Idiopathic polyneuritis (Guillain–Barré syndrome) remains a relatively common neurological cause of ventilatory failure. The syndrome is characterized by a rapidly ascending motor nerve paralysis, which may progress to quadriplegia and total respiratory muscle paralysis, and is believed to result from an immune-mediated aetiology. With modern ventilatory support death is fortunately rare, and 85 per cent of sufferers make a complete neurological recovery.

E. The neuromuscular junction is affected by several causes including botulism, neuromuscular blocking agents used in anaesthesia, certain organophosphorus compounds and nerve gases. However, myasthenia gravis is by far the most common cause of ventilatory failure at this site, marked respiratory muscle weakness occurring in seemingly mild cases.[2] Myasthenia gravis is an autoimmune disease in which the acetylcholine receptors on the neuromuscular junction are destroyed, leading to progressive weakness. Administration of an anticholinesterase drug such as edrophonium increases acetylcholine levels at the neuromuscular junction and causes an immediate improvement in symptoms. Immunosuppression or thymectomy are very effective current therapies, but almost 90 per cent of patients with generalized myasthenia still require long-term treatment.[3]

F. The respiratory muscles themselves are unlikely to be involved in any disease process that results in ventilatory failure. However, the efficiency of contraction of the diaphragm may be severely affected by 'splinting' due to abdominal distension or by flattening of the domes due, for example, to tension pneumothorax. The respiratory muscles may also become fatigued as a result of working against excessive impedance (page 128), but this is not thought to occur until very late in the course of most acute respiratory problems.[4] However, there are some exceptions to this. After a long period of artificial ventilation, respiratory muscles develop 'disuse atrophy', which makes weaning from ventilation difficult (page 604). Cardiac failure may result in respiratory muscle weakness due to reduced blood supply,[5] often coupled with low compliance lungs due to pulmonary oedema (Chapter 28). In animal studies, it has been shown that the administration of *Escherichia coli* endotoxin causes ventilatory failure in the presence of increased electrical activity in the respiratory muscles and unaltered respiratory impedance,[6] though the implications of this in human sepsis remain unclear.

Assessment of respiratory muscle strength is described on page 134.

G. Loss of elasticity of the lungs or chest wall is a potent cause of ventilatory failure. It may arise in the lungs (e.g. pulmonary fibrosis, Hamman–Rich syndrome and acute lung injury), in the pleura (e.g. chronic empyema with fibrinous covering of the pleura), in the chest wall (e.g. kyphoscoliosis) or in the skin (e.g. contracted burn scars in children). It is frequently forgotten that seemingly mild pressures applied to the outside of the chest may seriously embarrass the breathing and even result in total apnoea. A sustained pressure of only 6 kPa (45 mmHg or a depth of 2 feet of water) is sufficient to prevent breathing. This is prone to occur when crowds get out of control and people fall on top of one another, or when either children or adults become accidentally buried under sand or other heavy materials.

H. Loss of structural integrity of the chest wall may result in ventilatory failure, for example from multiple fractured ribs. A condition known as flail chest arises when multiple ribs are broken in two places, allowing the middle, 'flail', rib section to move independently of the anterior and posterior 'fixed' sections. Movement of the flail segment is then determined by changes in intrathoracic pressure; with spontaneous breathing, a paradoxical respiratory movement of the flail segment develops, which if large enough will compromise tidal volume. This condition, resulting from blunt trauma such as impact on the steering wheel, has become less common in the UK since the use of car seat belts became compulsory. Flail chest may be successfully treated by artificial ventilation with intermittent positive pressure, although some centres prefer conservative treatment with good analgesia sometimes assisted by rib fixation.

Closed pneumothorax causes interference with ventilation in proportion to the quantity of air in the chest. With a tension pneumothorax, the pressure rises above atmospheric, collapsing the ipsilateral lung, displacing the mediastinum and partially collapsing the contralateral lung. Convexity of the diaphragm is lost and ventilation may be critically impaired. The diagnosis and correction of the condition is a matter of great urgency. In the case of open pneumothorax the reduction in overall minute volume is further complicated by pendulum breathing between the two lungs.

I. Small airway resistance remains the commonest and most important cause of ventilatory failure. The physiology of diseases affecting airway resistance are described in Chapter 27 and will not be further discussed here. However, the relationship between airway resistance and ventilatory failure is a complex subject, which is considered below. In the clinical field, airway resistance is seldom measured but is most often inferred from measurement of ventilatory capacity.

J. Upper airway obstruction occurs in a wide range of conditions such as airway and pharyngeal tumours, upper respiratory tract infections, inhaled foreign bodies and tumour or bleeding in the neck causing external compression of the airway. Stridor is common, and should quickly alert the clinician to the cause of respiratory distress. A smaller airway diameter in babies and children makes them more susceptible than adults to upper airway obstruction, as airway oedema from infections such as croup or epiglottitis quickly causes dramatic stridor. The excellent ability of the respiratory system to overcome increased airway resistance (page 73) is such that ventilatory failure is normally a late development.

Increased dead space

Very rarely, a large increase in the respiratory dead space may be the cause of ventilatory failure. Minute volume may be increased but the alveolar ventilation is reduced and the patient presents with a high P_{CO_2} accompanied by a high minute volume. This may be distinguished from a hypermetabolic state by measurement of either carbon dioxide output or dead space (page 194). The dead space/tidal volume ratio should be above 65 per cent in this condition. An increase in the arterial/end-expiratory P_{CO_2} gradient (more than 2 kPa or 15 mmHg) indicates an increase in the alveolar dead space. This condition may be caused by ventilation of large unperfused areas of the lungs (e.g. an air cyst communicating with the bronchus), pulmonary emboli or pulmonary hypotension. External or apparatus dead space also tends to reduce alveolar ventilation and may be added either intentionally or accidentally.

Relationship between ventilatory capacity and ventilatory failure

Tests for the measurement of ventilatory capacity are described on pages 133 *et seq.* However, a severe reduction in ventilatory capacity does not necessarily mean that a patient will be in ventilatory failure. Figure 26.3 shows the lack of correlation between FEV_1 and P_{CO_2} in the grossly abnormal range of FEV_1 0.3–1 litre from a series of patients with chronic obstructive pulmonary disease (COPD; Chapter 27).[7]

It should again be stressed that the usual tests of ventilatory capacity depend on the expiratory muscles while the work of breathing is normally achieved by the inspiratory muscles.

The relationship between metabolic demand and ventilatory failure

In renal failure, protein intake is a major factor in the onset of uraemia. Similarly, in ventilatory failure, the onset of hypoxia and hypercapnia is directly related to the metabolic demand. Just as a patient with renal failure may benefit from a low protein diet, so a patient with a severe reduction of ventilatory capacity protects himself by limiting the exercise which he takes.

As COPD progresses, the ventilatory capacity decreases and the minute volume of breathing required for a particular level of activity increases. The increased ventilatory requirement is because both the dead space and the oxygen cost of breathing increase. The patient is thus trapped in a pincer movement of decreasing ventilatory capacity and increasing ventilatory requirement. As the jaws of the pincer close, there is first a

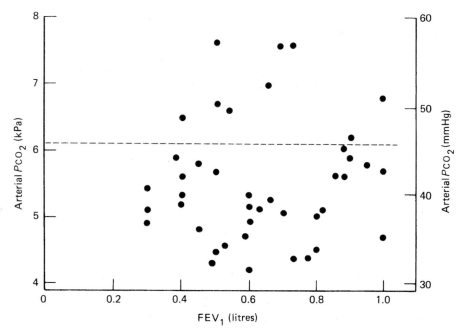

Figure 26.3 Lack of correlation between arterial P_{CO_2} and forced expiratory volume in one second (FEV$_1$) in 44 patients with chronic obstructive airway disease. The broken line indicates the upper limit of normal for P_{CO_2}. (Data from reference 7.)

limitation on heavy exercise, then on moderate exercise and so on until the patient is dyspnoeic at rest. At any time his work capacity is limited by the fraction of his ventilatory capacity that he is able to maintain for a given level of oxygen uptake.

The complex interaction between these factors is demonstrated in Figure 26.4, where the upper part shows the normal state. Assuming that an untrained subject can comfortably maintain a minute volume equal to about 30 per cent of his maximal breathing capacity (MBC) without dyspnoea, he has a reserve of ventilatory capacity that is adequate for rest and a power output of 100 watts. However, a power output of 200 watts requires a ventilation that exceeds a third of his MBC, and he becomes aware of his breathing at this level of exercise.

The middle section of Figure 26.4 shows moderately severe obstructive airway disease with the following changes:

1. MBC reduced from 150 to 60 l.min⁻¹.
2. Dead space/tidal volume ratio increased from 30 per cent to 40 per cent.
3. Oxygen cost of breathing increased by 10 per cent = for each level of activity.

Factors 2 and 3 together result in an increased minute volume for each level of activity.

Again, on the assumption that dyspnoea will not be apparent until the minute volume is 30 per cent of MBC, the reserve of ventilation is now sufficient for rest, but 100 watts of power output will result in dyspnoea.

Finally, in Figure 26.4c the changes have progressed to the point where resting minute volume exceeds 30 per cent of MBC and the patient is dyspnoeic at rest.

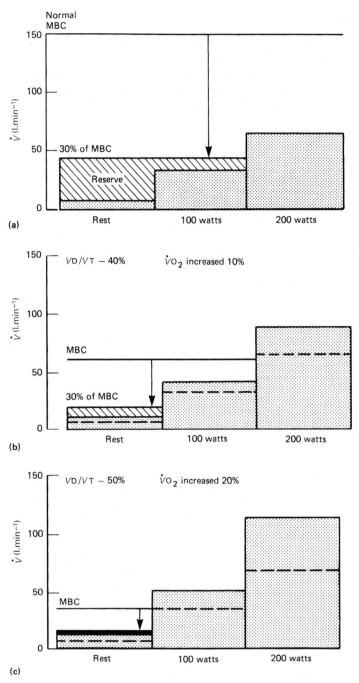

Figure 26.4 Relationship between maximal breathing capacity (MBC) and ventilatory requirements at rest and work at 100 and 200 watts. The tips of the arrows indicate 30 per cent of MBC which can usually be maintained without dyspnoea. Ventilatory reserve is between this level and the various ventilatory requirements. (a) Normal. (b) Moderate loss of ventilatory capacity with some increase in oxygen cost of breathing. (c) Severe loss of ventilatory capacity with considerable increase in the oxygen cost of breathing.

Breathlessness[8]

Breathlessness or dyspnoea has been defined as 'undue awareness of breathing or awareness of difficulty in breathing'.[9] This definition applies to both the awareness of breathing during severe exercise in the healthy subject and the dyspnoea of the patient with respiratory failure or heart failure. In the first case the sensation is normal and to be expected. However, in the latter, it is pathological and should be considered as a symptom.

The origin of the sensation

Hypoxia and hypercapnia may force the patient to breathe more deeply but they are not by themselves responsible for the sensation of dyspnoea, which arises from the ventilatory response rather than the stimulus itself. Patients with respiratory paralysis caused by poliomyelitis are not usually dyspnoeic in spite of abnormal blood gas tensions. Campbell and Guz[9] advanced their reasons for believing that dyspnoea is not akin to pain, though a sensation of 'air-hunger' can be induced with hypercapnia and there is some evidence of sensory activation of higher cerebral centres under these conditions.[10] Neither is dyspnoea strictly related to the work of breathing. Some patients have dyspnoea at relatively low levels of work of breathing, whereas others show no dyspnoea at high levels of work. Fatigue of the respiratory muscles (page 128) may be a factor in some cases but is clearly not the only cause of dyspnoea.

Campbell and Howell in 1963[11] suggested that a major factor in the origin of dyspnoea was an 'inappropriateness' between the tension generated in the respiratory muscles and the resultant shortening of the muscle fibres. This sensory input from muscle spindles would indicate to the brain that breathing was in some way hindered, but is again unlikely to be the full explanation of breathlessness.[12]

Breath holding (pages 105 et seq.) provides some insight into the origin of the sensation of breathlessness. Blood gas tensions are by no means the only factor limiting breath-holding time, though Po_2 is more important than Pco_2. The sensation that terminates breath holding can be relieved by ventilation without change of blood gas tensions, by bilateral vagal block and by curarization. Diaphragmatic afferents seem to be more important than those from the intercostals.

There is now little doubt that breathlessness involves a psychological component.[13] Dyspnoea arising from respiratory disease, particularly acutely, is often associated with anxiety and panic, which exacerbate the symptom. Conversely, many patients with primary psychological complaints such as panic disorder present with dyspnoea in the absence of any respiratory disease.

It cannot be said that the problem of breathlessness is completely understood at the present time.[14] It is, however, clear that there is no single and simple mechanism comparable to the sensations of touch, pain or temperature. The origin may well be multifactorial and the mechanisms of its generation are clearly complex.

Treatment of ventilatory failure

Many patients go about their business with arterial Pco_2 levels as high as 8 kPa (60 mmHg). Higher levels are associated with increasing disability, largely due to the accompanying hypoxaemia when the patient is breathing air (see Figure 26.1). Treatment may be divided into symptomatic relief of hypoxaemia and attempts to improve the alveolar ventilation.

Treatment of hypoxaemia due to hypoventilation by administration of oxygen

Hypoxia must be treated as the first priority, and administration of oxygen is the fastest and most effective method. However, it must be remembered that this will do nothing to improve the Pco_2 and may make it worse. It is therefore essential to ensure that palliative relief of hypoxia does not result in hypercapnia, and arterial Pco_2 should be checked if there is any doubt.

The relationship between alveolar Po_2, alveolar ventilation and inspired oxygen concentration is explained on pages 251 *et seq.* and illustrated in Figure 6.12. If other factors remain constant, an increase in inspired gas Po_2 will result in an equal increase in alveolar gas Po_2. Therefore, only small increases in inspired oxygen concentration are required for the relief of hypoxia *due to hypoventilation*. Figure 26.5 shows the rectangular hyperbola relating Pco_2 and alveolar ventilation (as in Figure 6.12), but superimposed are the concentrations of inspired oxygen required to restore a normal alveolar Po_2 for different degrees of alveolar hypoventilation. It will be seen that 30 per cent is sufficient for the degree of alveolar hypoventilation that will result in an alveolar Pco_2 of 13 kPa (almost 100 mmHg). Clearly this is an unacceptable Pco_2, and therefore 30 per cent can be regarded as the upper limit of inspired oxygen concentration to be used in the palliative relief of hypoxia due to ventilatory failure, without attempting to improve the alveolar ventilation.

The use of very high concentrations of inspired oxygen will prevent hypoxia even in gross alveolar hypoventilation which carries the risk of dangerous hypercapnia. Although this is itself a strong contraindication to the use of high concentrations of oxygen under these circumstances, an even graver risk exists in patients who have lost their ventilatory sensitivity to carbon dioxide and rely upon their hypoxic drive to maintain ventilation. High concentrations of oxygen will abolish the hypoxic drive and may precipitate acute-on-chronic ventilatory failure (see Figure 27.2). In 1949 Donald

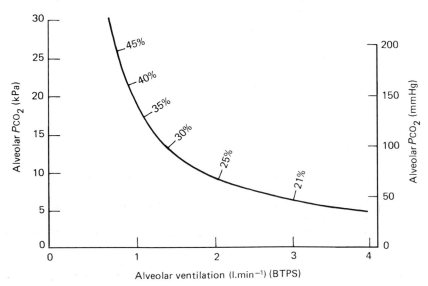

Figure 26.5 Alveolar Pco_2 as a function of alveolar ventilation at rest. The percentages indicate the inspired oxygen concentration that is then required to restore normal alveolar Po_2.

drew attention to the problem,[14] but this unfortunately resulted in a tendency to withhold oxygen for fear of causing hypercapnia. The rule is that hypoxia must be treated first, because hypoxia kills quickly whilst hypercapnia kills slowly. However, it must always be remembered that administration of oxygen to a patient with ventilatory failure will do nothing to improve the P_{CO_2} and may make it worse. The arterial P_{CO_2} must be checked if there is any doubt.

Symptomatic relief of hypoxaemia due to shunting, in patients who have probably retained their sensitivity to carbon dioxide, requires a completely different policy for estimating the optimal inspired oxygen concentration; this is discussed on page 260.

Improvement of alveolar ventilation

The only way to reduce the arterial P_{CO_2} is to improve the alveolar ventilation. The first line of therapy is to improve ventilatory capacity by treatment of the underlying cause while simultaneously providing carefully controlled oxygen therapy and avoiding the use of drugs that depress breathing.

The second line is chemical stimulation of breathing. Doxapram stimulates breathing via an action on the peripheral chemoreceptors (page 99) and is capable of prolonged stimulation of ventilation with little tachyphylaxis. It may be conveniently administered by a continuous intravenous infusion at a dose of 1.5–4 mg.min^{-1}.

The third line of treatment is by tracheal intubation or tracheostomy, which may improve alveolar ventilation by reducing dead space and facilitating the control of secretions.

The fourth line of therapy is the institution of artificial ventilation (considered in detail in Chapter 31). It is difficult to give firm guidelines for instituting artificial ventilation, and the arterial P_{CO_2} should not be considered in isolation. Nevertheless, a P_{CO_2} in excess of 10 kPa (75 mmHg) that cannot be reduced by other means in a patient who is deemed recoverable is generally considered as a firm indication. However, artificial ventilation may be required at much lower levels of P_{CO_2} if there is actual or impending respiratory fatigue as a result of increased work of breathing. This may be difficult to diagnose or predict. Although it is now well recognized that intense activity by the respiratory muscles results in fatigue, as in the case of other skeletal muscles under similar conditions, it is also thought that ventilatory failure from this cause occurs only very late in the course of most respiratory diseases. For example, it has been mentioned above that the P_{CO_2} rises only late in acute asthma, and artificial ventilation may be required before the arterial P_{CO_2} has risen much above the normal range.

A difficult decision may be required on whether to ventilate patients with untreatable progressive ventilatory failure. Great difficulties and much distress may arise from instituting artificial ventilation from which it proves impossible to wean the patient. However, it may be useful to ventilate a patient with chronic obstructive airway disease to tide him over a period of infection that has resulted in acute-on-chronic ventilatory failure. However, in the absence of a transient factor of this nature, it is unlikely that a period of artificial ventilation can influence the long-term progress of the disease.[15,16]

Artificial ventilation may be required for treatment of hypoxaemia that is not directly attributable to ventilatory failure. The benefit is often related to the increased tidal volume opening up closed airways and alveoli, and so reducing shunting. This effect can be augmented by the use of positive end-expiratory pressure (page 605).

References

1. Mier A. Respiratory muscle weakness. *Respir Med* 1991; **84**: 351–9.
2. Mier A, Brophy C, Green M. Respiratory muscle function in myasthenia gravis. *Am Rev Respir Dis* 1988; **138**: 867–74.
3. Grob D, Arsura EL, Brunner NG, Namba T. The course of myasthenia gravis and therapies affecting outcome. *Ann N Y Acad Sci* 1987; **505**: 472–99.
4. Roussos C, Zakynthinos S. Fatigue of the respiratory muscles. *Intensive Care Med* 1996; **22**: 134–55.
5. Hammond MD, Bauer KA, Sharp JT, Rocha RD. Respiratory muscle strength in congestive heart failure. *Chest* 1990; **98**: 1091–4.
6. Hussain SNA, Simkus G, Roussos C. Respiratory muscle fatigue: a cause of ventilatory failure in septic shock. *J Appl Physiol* 1985; **58**: 2033–40.
7. Nunn JF, Milledge JS, Chen D, Doré C. Respiratory criteria of fitness for surgery and anaesthesia. *Anaesthesia* 1988; **43**: 543–51.
8. Meek PM, Schwartzstein RM, Adams L, Altose MD, Breslin EH, Carrieri-Kohlman V et al. Dyspnea. Mechanisms, assessment, and management: a consensus statement. *Am J Respir Crit Care Med* 1999; **159**: 321–40.
9. Campbell EJM, Guz A. Breathlessness. In: Hornbein TF, ed. *Regulation of breathing,* Part II. New York: Marcel Dekker, 1981.
10. Guz A. Brain, breathing and breathlessness. *Respir Physiol* 1997; **109**: 197–204.
11. Campbell EJM, Howell JBL. The sensation of breathlessness. *Br Med Bull* 1963; **19**: 36–40.
12. Howell JBL. Breathlessness. In: Brewis RAL, Corrin B, Gedded DM, Gibson GJ, eds. *Respiratory medicine.* London: WB Saunders, 1995; 258–63.
13. Smoller JW, Pollack MH, Otto MW, Rosenbaum JF, Kradin RL. Panic anxiety, dyspnea, and respiratory disease – theoretical and clinical considerations. *Am J Respir Crit Care Med* 1996; **154**: 6–17.
14. Donald KW. Neurological effects of oxygen. *Lancet* 1949; **2**: 1056–7.
15. Nunn JF, Milledge JS, Sigaraya J. Survival of patients ventilated in an intensive care unit. *BMJ* 1979; **1**: 1525–7.
16. Petheram IS, Branthwaite MA. Mechanical ventilation for pulmonary disease. *Anaesthesia* 1980; **35**: 467–73.

Chapter 27

Airways disease

This chapter considers the physiological changes seen in the three most common diseases of the pulmonary airways: asthma, chronic obstructive pulmonary disease (COPD) and cystic fibrosis. The first two of these have many clinical and physiological features in common, and together constitute the vast majority of respiratory disease seen in clinical practice.

Asthma

Lung diseases resulting from air pollution and infection have decreased dramatically in recent decades, but have been almost entirely replaced by asthma. The prevalence of asthma has now reached dramatic proportions in many areas of the world, though the causes of this differ between the 'developed' and 'developing' world (see below).[1] In contrast to many respiratory diseases, the onset of asthma is usually in early childhood or young adulthood. The prevalence of asthma among children is now between 15 and 30 per cent in developed countries, and has approximately doubled in the last 20 years.[1,2,3] For many years, mortality from asthma increased in parallel with the prevalence of the disease. However, deaths from asthma seem to have peaked in many countries in the late 1980s (UK, Australia, Germany, New Zealand)[4] and are now decreasing, though this has not been observed in the USA where mortality rates are lower than other countries but continuing to rise.[5]

Clinical features

Asthma causes recurrent episodes of chest 'tightness', wheezing, breathlessness and coughing as a result of airway narrowing from both inflammation of the small airways and contraction of bronchial smooth muscle in the lower airway. The term 'asthma' includes a wide spectrum of illnesses, varying from a wheezy 6-month-old baby with a viral infection to a young adult with multiple allergies manifested as wheeze or an older patient with chronic lung disease. In the last case, clinical features of asthma merge with those of COPD, and differentiation between the two is difficult. Changing diagnostic criteria[3] have almost certainly contributed to the apparent increase in asthma prevalence, which is nevertheless still a real increase.[1] Whatever the clinical presentation, there are three closely related phases of an episode of asthma, as follows.

Bronchospasm occurs early in an asthma 'attack'. This is particularly prominent in atopic asthma when, within minutes of exposure to an allergen, wheezing develops. Narrowing of small airways occurs because of contraction of airway smooth muscle in response to the cellular mechanisms described below. Airway closure begins during expiration, gas trapping occurs and the lungs become hyperinflated.[6] Eventually, the patient is attempting to breath in when the lungs are almost at total lung capacity, and a sensation of inspiratory dyspnoea results, even though the defect is with expiration. Physiological effects of hyperinflation are discussed below.

The immediate response may quickly subside, either spontaneously or with treatment, but more commonly progresses to a late phase reaction.

Late-phase reactions are characterized by inflammation of the airway, and develop a few hours after the acute bronchospasm. Airway obstruction continues, and cough with sputum production develops. Asthma precipitated by respiratory tract infection may 'bypass' the acute bronchospasm phase and the onset of symptoms is then more gradual.

Airway hyperresponsiveness (AHR) describes the observation that asthmatic subjects become wheezy in response to a whole range of stimuli that have little effect on normal individuals. Stimuli include such things as cold air, exercise, pollution (page 416) or inhaled drugs, and occur via the neural pathways present in normal lungs (page 71). Methacholine or histamine can be used to measure AHR accurately by determining the inhaled concentration that gives rise to a 20 per cent reduction in forced expiratory volume in one second (FEV_1).[7] The degree of AHR seen in patients with asthma is highly variable. Severe asthma is associated with continuous AHR, whilst in mild asthma the patient's response will be normal between wheezy episodes.

Cellular mechanisms of asthma[1,2,8]

Many cell types are involved in the pathophysiology of asthma. A summary of the interactions between these cells is given in Figure 27.1, which also shows the principal cytokines that facilitate communication between the cells.

Mast cells are plentiful in the walls of airways and alveoli, and also lie free in the lumen of the airways where they may be recovered by bronchial lavage. Mast cell activation is the main cause of the immediate bronchospasm seen in allergen-provoked asthma. The surface of the mast cell contains a very large number of binding sites for the immunoglobulin IgE. Activation of the cell results from antigen bridging of only a small number of these receptors, and may also be initiated by a wide range of compounds, including the complement fractions C3a, C4a and C5a, substance P, physical stimulation and many drugs and other organic molecules.

The triggering mechanism of the mast cell is thus extremely sensitive, and is mediated by an increase in inositol triphosphate and intracellular calcium ions.[1,9] Within 30 seconds of activation, there is degranulation with discharge of a range of preformed mediators listed in Table 27.1. Histamine acts directly on H_1 receptors in the bronchial smooth muscle fibres to cause contraction, on other H_1 receptors to increase vascular permeability and on H_2 receptors to increase mucus secretion. The granules also contain proteases, mainly tryptase, which detach epithelial cells from the basement membrane, resulting in desquamation and possibly activating neuronal reflexes (page 71), causing further bronchospasm.

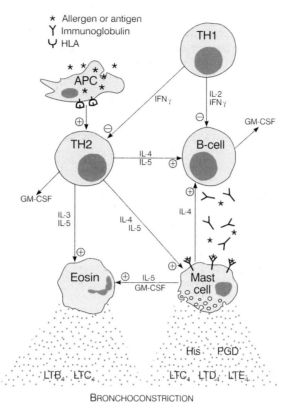

Figure 27.1 Inflammatory cells involved in the pathogenesis of asthma, and the cytokines by which they communicate with each other. For details see text. TH2 and TH1, subtypes of T-lymphocyte 'helper' cells; APC, antigen presenting cell; B-cell, B-lymphoctye; Eosin, eosinophil; GM-CSF, granulocyte/macrophage colony stimulating factor; His, histamine; HLA, human lymphocyte antigen; IFN, interferon; IL, interleukin; LT, leukotriene; PG, prostaglandin.

Table 27.1 Mediators released from mast cells when activated by IgE

Preformed mediators	Newly generated mediators	Cytokines
Histamine	Prostaglandin D_2	Interleukins 3,4,5,6 and 13
Heparin	Thromboxane A_2	Granulocyte/macrophage colony stimulating factor
Serotonin	Leukotrienes C_4, D_4 and E_4	Tumour necrosis factor
Lysosomal enzymes:		Platelet activating factor
Tryptase		
Chymase		
β-Galactosidase		
β-Glucuronidase		
Hexosaminidase		

The second major event after mast cell activation is the initiation of synthesis of arachidonic acid derivatives (see Figures 12.2 and 12.3). The most important derivative of the cyclo-oxygenase pathway is prostaglandin PGD_2, which is a bronchoconstrictor, although its clinical significance is still not clear. The lipoxygenase pathway results in the formation of LTC_4, from which two further peptide leukotrienes, LTD_4 and LTE_4, are formed. These three leukotrienes were known collectively as slow-reacting substance of anaphylaxis (SRS-A), until the constituents were identified.

Finally, mast cells also release a variety of cytokines, some of which are contained within the granules whilst others are generated *de novo* on activation of the cell. Interleukin-5 (IL-5) and granulocyte/macrophage colony stimulating factor (GM-CSF) are chemotactic for eosinophils whilst IL-4 stimulates IgE production by B-lymphocytes (Figure 27.1) and so amplifies the activation of mast cells.

Eosinophils are freely distributed alongside mast cells in the submucosa, and are now believed to be the principal cell involved in the late-phase reaction of asthma. In particular, they release leukotrienes B_4 and C_4, which are potent bronchoconstrictors with a prolonged action. They are attracted to the area by GM-CSF, which is released by many inflammatory cells, before being activated by IL-5 and IL-3 originating from mast cells and lymphocytes respectively (Figure 27.1).

Lymphocytes have an important role in the control of mast cell and eosinophil activation.[1] Activated B-lymphocytes are responsible for production of the antigen-specific IgE needed to cause mast cell degranulation. B-cells are in turn controlled by two subsets of T 'helper' lymphocytes, known as TH1 and TH2 cells. The latter releases many cytokines, which activate all the cells involved in promoting bronchoconstriction and inflammation (Figure 27.1). The TH2 cell is non-specific in its response, and relies on other 'antigen-presenting cells' (APCs) for its activation. It is unclear where APCs originate, but they are mostly located in lymphoid tissue near the site of inflammation. Antigens derived from almost any pathogen are ingested by the APCs and small peptide fragments of the antigen then expressed on the cell surface, in conjunction with human lymphocyte antigens, where they are potent activators of TH2 cells. TH1 cells are also activated in lymphoid tissue, but these cells produce interferon, which inhibits the activity of the TH2 and B-cells, and so represents a mechanism by which the inflammatory process is suppressed (Figure 27.1). Thus the relative activity of TH1 and TH2 lymphocytes seems to play an important role in the development and severity of asthma.

Nitric oxide (NO) is detectable in small concentrations in the expired air of normal subjects.[10] It is produced from the mucosa of the whole respiratory tract, including the nose and nasal sinuses, but its origin is unclear. Nitric oxide acts as the neurotransmitter for the non-adrenergic non-cholinergic (NANC) bronchodilator pathway in normal lungs (page 71), is involved in control of vascular tone in all tissues and is present in blood (page 274). In asthmatic patients with active disease, NO concentration in expired air is two to ten times greater than non-asthmatics.[11,12] In this situation, the extra NO is derived from inducible NO-synthase (iNOS, page 150) in the airway mucosa. Cytokines produced by the inflammatory cells already described are believed to result in increased production of iNOS[13] and, so, NO. This is likely to represent another means by which the inflammatory response is amplified, as NO may have an inhibitory effect on TH1 cells.[14] Although NO seems unlikely to have a major role in the development of asthma, its presence in expired air may in future provide a useful means of quantifying the inflammatory component of asthma.[11] In addition, the discovery of another mechanism involved in bronchospasm has opened further potential therapeutic avenues.[14]

Causes of airway obstruction in asthma[3]

Contraction of bronchial smooth muscle following stimulation by the substances shown in Figure 27.1 explains some of the airway narrowing seen in asthma, particularly during the acute and early stages. However, long-term airway obstruction seen in severe asthma or during the late phase response results from inflammation of the airway. Many cytokines released during asthma have effects on blood vessel permeability and therefore cause oedema of the epithelium and basement membrane.[3,15] Protease enzymes (Table 27.1) break down normal epithelial architecture and cause defects in the epithelial barrier, leading to further inflammation and eventually detachment of the epithelium from the basement membrane. Finally, hypersecretion of mucus and impaired mucociliary clearance are both recognized features of asthma,[16] and this correlates with the flow limitation seen in individual patients. These changes all contribute to a significant reduction in airway cross-sectional area, and thus a large increase in resistance (page 60). Mucus, inflammatory cells and epithelial debris cause obstruction of small airways, compounded by flow limitation preventing an effective cough. In severe asthma, obstruction of small airways gives rise to ventilation/perfusion mismatch, shunt and hypoxaemia, and has long been recognized as a significant pathological finding in fatal asthma.[17]

Recent studies using mathematical modelling and animal bronchi have reported interesting observations of the folding pattern of bronchial mucosa.[18,19] The external pressure that can be applied on a bronchus before collapse occurs ('buckling pressure') depends to some extent on the folding pattern of the mucosa in the bronchus. The more folds that develop in the mucosa, the greater the buckling pressure required. Chronically thickened mucosa is stiffer than normal and so helps to resist airway collapse when bronchospasm occurs, offering some degree of protection from airway obstruction. However, the authors also predict that airway oedema will change the folding properties of the mucosa, making it more likely to collapse with acute bronchospasm.[19]

Aetiology of asthma

Genetics. Asthma, along with other allergic diseases, has a substantial genetic component. Environmental factors invariably contribute to the development of clinical disease, but genetic susceptibility to asthma is strong. Two reasons explain this observation. First, the genes for most of the cytokines involved in asthma are found close together on chromosome 5, and asthmatic patients may have increased expression of these, so encouraging formation of TH2 cells and an allergic phenotype.[1,8] Secondly, human lymphocyte antigens (HLA) involved in sensitization of lymphocytes to specific antigens (Figure 27.1) are part of the major histocompatibility complex allowing immunological 'self-recognition', and so are inherited. It is possible that some HLA types are particularly active in the processing of common allergens and thus the stimulation of TH2 cells and allergy.[1]

Maternal allergic disease is more likely than paternal disease to be passed to offspring, though this may relate to modification of the fetal immune system *in utero* rather than a true genetic influence. During pregnancy, lymphocyte subsets TH1 and TH2 are closely involved in the prevention of maternal rejection, and abnormalities at this stage may influence the ratio of TH1 to TH2 cells in the offspring's immune system, leading to allergic diseases, including asthma, in later life.[20]

Allergy.[1] Changes in living conditions have undoubtedly contributed to the increase in asthma prevalence. In the developing world, population shifts from rural to urban environments have reduced exposure to parasitic infections and increased exposure to other allergens, and it seems likely that the extensive IgE and mast cell systems that formerly inactivated parasites now respond to urban allergens. In the developed world, changes in living conditions have resulted in a dramatic increase in allergen exposure, in particular house dust mite (HDM, *Dermatophagoides pteronyssinus*), domestic animals and fungi. Asthma is more common in affluent families, and correlates with exposure to HDM which thrives in warm, humid houses with extensive carpeting and bedding. These conditions are ideal for the HDM and its food supply of shed skin flakes. In some circumstances, up to 15 per cent of the contents of the vacuum cleaner bag are thought to be made up of HDM or their excretory products. Simply inhaling allergens is only part of the explanation of how allergen exposure causes asthma, and once again pregnancy plays a role. Allergen taken in by the mother is believed to cross the placenta and influence TH1 cells before birth. Neonatal T-lymphocytes taken from children who subsequently develop asthma already show a reduced production of interferon-γ in response to allergen, indicating an existing immunological susceptibility to asthma.[21]

Infection.[22] Viral respiratory tract infections cause wheezing in many asthmatics, and account for over half of acute exacerbations of asthma. In infants, respiratory syncytial or parainfluenza viruses are common, whilst in adults a 'common cold' rhinovirus is the most usual pathogen. Viral infection gives rise to an immune response involving many cells and cytokines, but T-lymphocytes are particularly important and undergo both virus-specific and generalized activation. Inevitably, TH2 activity is increased, giving rise to wheeze and airway inflammation by the mechanisms described above. In addition, stimulation of allergic mechanisms in susceptible individuals continues for some time after the viral symptoms have subsided. Thus, for example, after a simple rhinovirus infection, allergen-induced histamine production and eosinophil-induced late-phase reactions remain increased for 4–6 weeks.[23]

In contrast, viral and other infections may have a protective role in preventing the initiation of asthma in early childhood.[1,22] Children who are exposed to more infections in early life, such as those with older siblings, are less likely to develop allergic disease. This led to a suggestion that lower infection rates in the population at large and effective immunization programmes may have contributed to the rising incidence of asthma. Measles virus,[1] *Mycobacterium tuberculosis* and many other very common bacteria are all known to promote an increase in TH1 lymphocyte-type activity and secretion of IFN-γ.[24]

Pollution.[2] Trends in air pollution have not generally followed trends in asthma prevalence over recent decades, the levels of many pollutants declining while asthma becomes more common. Laboratory evidence described on page 417 describes how, in comparison with normal subjects, asthmatics develop wheeze when exposed to lower inhaled concentrations of nitrogen dioxide and sulphur dioxide. The levels required to cause wheezing are still higher than commonly encountered in the atmosphere, and though there is some evidence linking air pollution episodes to respiratory problems the effect is believed to be small.

A role for air pollution in the initiation of asthma has also remained elusive. Animal experiments indicate that common air pollutants can sensitize the airway to allergens, probably by disturbance of mucociliary clearance, leading to prolonged pulmonary retention of allergens in the airway[25] and allowing more time for sensitization of submucosal inflammatory cells.[2] There is no evidence that this contributes to asthma in humans.[2]

Gastric reflux.[26] Gastro-oesophageal reflux symptoms are common in asthmatics, and are involved in the production of cough or wheeze in up to a third of patients. Acid in the distal oesophagus can, via a vagally mediated reflex, provoke either bronchoconstriction itself or airway hypersensitivity to allergen. In more severe cases, oesophageal reflux leading to aspiration of small amounts of acid into the airway can provoke severe bronchospasm. In patients with asthma who are resistant to treatment or have mainly nocturnal symptoms, reflux should be considered as a cause. In the absence of symptoms of reflux, continuous monitoring of lower oesophageal pH is required to establish the diagnosis. Treatment of reflux leads to considerable improvement in asthma symptoms.

Principles of treatment

Detailed guidelines on the treatment of asthma are published for both the UK[27] and the USA,[28] and are beyond the scope of this book. Except in the most mild forms of asthma, treatment has moved away from the traditional bronchodilator inhaler 'when needed' approach of the past. The emphasis is now on continuous treatment with drugs and other strategies aimed at preventing exacerbations and suppressing airway inflammation.[29] Therapeutic approaches include the following.

Bronchodilators remain a common treatment for relief of acute bronchospasm. The β_2-adrenoceptor agonists are widely used, and recent developments include the introduction of longer acting drugs such as salmeterol.[30] A new group of drugs, including montelukast and zafirlukast, is now emerging; they act by inhibition of leukotriene receptors on bronchial smooth muscle,[31] blocking the effects of LTC_4, LTD_4 and LTE_4. They are effective in treating asthma, including the bronchospasm seen in the late-phase reaction, but their place in the overall management of asthma is currently unclear.

Corticosteroids,[32,33] either inhaled or oral, are an invaluable method of prophylaxis and treatment in asthma. Their mechanism of action remains incompletely understood, but suppression of cytokine gene expression seems likely.[8] With steroid treatment there are reductions in many indicators of airway inflammation, including eosinophil survival.

Allergen avoidance is an attractive strategy for the prevention of asthma in patients with known allergies. Low humidity is very effective in reducing HDM, and therefore at high altitude (above 1500 m or 5000 ft) HDM allergen is non-existent. Several studies have used this to compare asthma severity in normal and HDM-free high altitude environments, and have found improvements in both clinical and cellular measures of asthma severity.[34] However, the rather drastic intervention of moving to high altitude is clearly not practical, and reduction of allergen load in the home is considerably more difficult. Measures include removing carpets, reducing temperature and humidity, applying acaricides to kill HDM and encasing mattresses in allergen-impermeable membranes. Some studies have reported clinical benefits,[35] but a recent meta-analysis did not support this approach.[36]

Chronic obstructive pulmonary disease

Unlike asthma, where airways obstruction is usually intermittent, COPD is characterized by progressive chronic air-flow limitation along with intermittent (usually infective) exacerbations. Clinical features are similar to those of asthma, with wheeze, cough and dyspnoea but, though some degree of reversible airway obstruction is often present, bronchodilators rarely lead to complete resolution of symptoms. Patients affected by COPD are generally much older than those with asthma, and the progressive nature of the process leads to more serious interruption of normal activities and eventually respiratory failure (page 514). In the USA, COPD is now the fourth most common cause of death.[37]

Aetiology[38]

Smoking is the major aetiological factor in COPD. The accelerated decline in FEV_1 seen with smoking is shown in Figure 20.1, and the 15–20 per cent of smokers who develop COPD probably represent an extreme response to this effect of tobacco smoke.

Three pathophysiological changes give rise to COPD: emphysema, mucous hyper-secretion of larger airways and small airway obstruction. The last two of these are often collectively referred to as chronic bronchitis.

Emphysema may be defined as permanent enlargement of airspaces distal to the terminal bronchiole, accompanied by destruction of alveolar walls.[39] The process begins by enlargement of normal interalveolar holes, followed by destruction of the entire alveolar septum. Both ventilation and perfusion of the emphysematous area are therefore reduced, and, though some mismatch of ventilation and perfusion may occur in widespread emphysema, localized areas, as usually seen in COPD, have little effect. The loss of elastic tissue contained in the alveolar septa is, however, important, and reduces the elastic recoil of the pulmonary tissue, so contributing to closure of small airways, particularly during expiration.

Current views on the cellular defect responsible for emphysema involve the relationship between proteinase and antiproteinase activity in the lung. These enzymes are normally released following activation of neutrophils or macrophages in response to tobacco smoke or infection. A deficiency of the most well-known antiproteinase, α_1-antitrypsin, is a significant risk factor for early development of emphysema (page 308). Disturbances of less well understood proteinase–antiproteinase systems, particularly those with activity against elastin, are now believed to be involved in the generation of emphysema.[38] Elastin deposition in the lung occurs early in life, and is minimal beyond late adolescence. Later, any pulmonary elastin lost through disease is likely to be replaced with collagen, so reducing lung elasticity and probably explaining the general decline in lung recoil throughout life.[40]

Small airway obstruction plays a major role in COPD, but its aetiology is controversial.[38,41,42] Part of the expiratory airway obstruction results from emphysema as described above. It is also likely that changes in the airway wall itself contribute. Inflammatory changes in small airways are common in COPD,[42] and may lead to hypertrophy of bronchial smooth muscle and other tissues.

Large airway disease consists of goblet cell hyperplasia, mucosal oedema and production of excessive amounts of mucus. Recurrent respiratory tract infections and smoking (page 410) undoubtedly contribute, and a chronic productive cough is the result. This feature of COPD is not always present, and its contribution to overall airway obstruction is variable. In some patients, extensive and long-standing inflammation of the large airways gives rise to permanent thickening of the airway wall in the cartilaginous airways, and so causes clinically important degrees of obstruction.[42]

Hyperinflation.[43] Airway obstruction leads to prolonged expiratory time constants in affected lung units, and incomplete expiration (gas trapping). Acute bronchospasm is also associated with prolonged activity of inspiratory muscles that persists into expiration,[6] and so contributes to gas trapping. Hyperinflation of the lung will, in theory, tend to oppose airway closure (see Figure 4.5), but it also causes a significant reduction in the efficiency of the respiratory muscles. In particular, the diaphragm becomes displaced caudally and flattened, reducing the zone of apposition (see Figure 6.1) and causing much of the muscle activity to either oppose the opposite side of the diaphragm or pull the lower ribcage inwards rather than outwards (Figure 6.2). In time, lung hyperinflation becomes permanent, with expansion of the chest wall (barrel chest) and irreversible flattening of the diaphragm.

Oxygen therapy in COPD

Patients with advanced COPD may be broadly classified into 'pink puffers' and 'blue bloaters', which correspond to type 1 and type 2 respiratory failure respectively (page 513). 'Pink puffers', with predominantly emphysematous changes, maintain a considerable degree of respiratory sensitivity to carbon dioxide and struggle to keep a normal arterial Pco_2 for as long as possible, although with evident dyspnoea. On the other hand 'blue bloaters', mostly with airway disease (chronic bronchitis), have lost their sensitivity to carbon dioxide and allow their Pco_2 to increase above the normal reference range, usually without dyspnoea. Determinants of which pattern patients develop are uncertain. The underlying disease process (emphysema versus bronchitis) may determine the pattern, as may the patient's respiratory sensitivity to carbon dioxide before developing COPD.

Administration of oxygen to COPD patients may lead to hypercapnia. Two main mechanisms are believed to be responsible.

Ventilatory depression by oxygen. 'Blue bloaters' may be relying on their hypoxic drive to maintain ventilation. If this is abolished, as, for example, by the administration of 100% oxygen, hypoventilation or even apnoea may result. An extreme example of this is shown in Figure 27.2. However, studies investigating oxygen-induced hypercapnia in COPD have failed to find consistent changes in minute ventilation during either periods of stable respiratory symptoms[44] or acute exacerbations.[45] Reduction in minute volume in response to oxygen was either too small to explain adequately the changes in Pco_2 or only transient, returning towards baseline ventilation after a few minutes. Nevertheless, in one of these reports,[45] of 22 subjects studied, 2 developed severe respiratory depression leading to dangerous hypercapnia after just 15 minutes of breathing 100% oxygen. Some patients with COPD are therefore clearly susceptible to oxygen-induced respiratory depression, as illustrated in Figure 27.2.

Altered ventilation/perfusion relationships with oxygen have been proposed to explain hypercapnia seen in COPD patients in whom minute volume remains essentially unchanged.[44,45,46] Alveolar Po_2 is known to contribute to hypoxic pulmonary vasoconstriction (page 151) and so help to minimize $\dot{V}/\dot{Q}$ mismatch. Administration of oxygen may therefore abolish hypoxic pulmonary vasoconstriction in poorly ventilated areas and so increase alveolar dead space. If minute volume of ventilation remains constant, hypercapnia will ensue.

Which of these mechanisms predominates in an individual patient is currently difficult to predict. Administration of oxygen to patients with COPD must therefore be undertaken with great care, and accompanied by suitable monitoring of both oxygenation and arterial Pco_2.

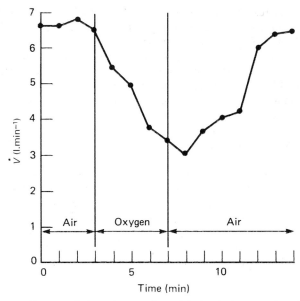

Figure 27.2 Rapid onset of hypoventilation when a patient with chronic hypercapnia and loss of chemoreceptor sensitivity to carbon dioxide breathed 100% oxygen. This patient had respiratory failure secondary to poliomyelitis, but a similar pattern may be seen with chronic obstructive pulmonary disease. (Nunn, unpublished data.)

Principles of treatment of COPD

As for asthma, detailed guidelines for the treatment of COPD have been published in several countries.[47]

Smoking cessation is central to all forms of treatment for COPD.[47,48] The progressive decline in lung function is halted (see Figure 20.1) and symptoms improve. Patients with COPD have often been heavy smokers for a considerable number of years, and they may therefore need great determination to stop smoking. On average, it will take patients more than three attempts before they become permanent non-smokers.[48]

Medical treatment. Inhaled bronchodilators may be used. Their efficacy depends on the reversibility of the airways disease in each patient, though recent advice indicates that symptoms may be relieved even if FEV_1 remains unchanged following inhaled β_2-agonists.[47] Corticosteroids are particularly effective in COPD. Medical treatment also involves active management of infective exacerbations of the underlying disease with antibiotics, oxygen and artificial ventilation if required.

Supplemental oxygen at low inspired concentrations for several hours a day is beneficial in the treatment of COPD. Indications for its use are a Pa_{O_2} of less than 7.3 kPa (55 mmHg) with evidence of long-term hypoxia such as cor pulmonale or poly-cythaemia.[48] Oxygen flow is titrated to achieve a Pa_{O_2} of 9–12 kPa (65–90 mmHg),[48] and under these conditions the long-term mortality from COPD is reduced.[38]

Surgical treatment is reserved for severe COPD as a result of extensive emphysema.[41] When the airspaces created in emphysema become larger than 1 cm in diameter, they are referred to as a 'bulla'. Nearby bullae can merge and result in extremely large airspaces, occupying up to one-third of the lung volume. Like emphysema, bullae have little effect on gas exchange, as both tidal ventilation and blood flow to the bulla are negligible. However, with giant bullae, the airspace acts in a similar fashion to a pneumothorax, and compresses surrounding normal lung tissue, causing further worsening of airways collapse and subsequently disturbing gas exchange. Early surgical treatment therefore focused on 'bullectomy', but complications relating to air leaks from the lung always limited success and caused considerable mortality (18 per cent in some series).[41] Advances in surgical techniques have led to a resurgence of interest in surgery for COPD. Rather than removing a single giant bulla, the current approach involves removing 20–30 per cent of lung volume, to include the most emphysematous areas. Early results are impressive, with bilateral lung volume reduction leading to substantial symptomatic relief[49] and an 82 per cent increase in mean FEV_1.[50] The physiological mechanisms of the improvement following surgery are poorly understood,[41] but probably include reducing pulmonary collapse adjacent to emphysema and greatly improved respiratory muscle function secondary to reduced hyperinflation.

Cystic fibrosis

Cystic fibrosis (CF) is an autosomal recessive genetic disorder affecting Caucasian individuals, of whom 1 in 25 carry the gene. The disease affects about 1 in 2500 births[51] and the gene can be identified prenatally, but there is a wide spectrum of clinical disease such that prediction of phenotype from genetic screening is complex.[52] Cystic fibrosis affects epithelial cell function in many body systems, but gastrointestinal and respiratory function are the most important; this chapter discusses only the latter.

Abnormalities of pulmonary airway defence mechanisms lead to lifelong colonization of the cystic fibrosis lung with bacteria. Recurrent airway infection produces hyper-secretion of mucus, cough and, over many years, destruction of normal lung architecture, including bronchiectasis. Initial infection normally occurs early in life, and progressive lung disease is the usual cause of death. Mortality from CF remains high, with a current median life expectancy of only 29 years.[53] This has improved considerably in recent years (Figure 27.3), though there continues to be a significant number of deaths in early infancy.[51] Thus, although the number of CF births is constant, improved survival means that the prevalence of CF is increasing steadily.

Aetiology

Biochemical abnormality. The molecular mechanisms of CF have been the focus of extensive research in recent years, which has led to CF being one of the most completely understood of inherited diseases. As long ago as 1989 the gene responsible for CF was identified.[54] It is located on chromosome 7, and codes for a protein named cystic fibrosis transmembrane conductance regulator (CFTR) found in epithelial cells. The CFTR proteins function as a membrane-bound active chloride channel, and play a major role in controlling salt concentration in epithelial secretions. Sweat production is influenced by CFTR function, allowing measurement of the sodium concentration in sweat to remain a relatively simple investigation for diagnosis, being over twice normal in CF patients.[55]

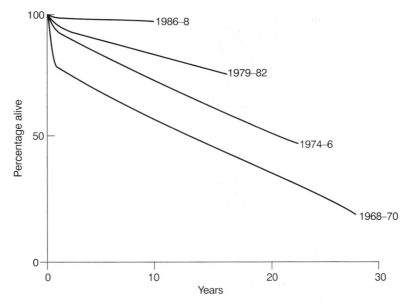

Figure 27.3 Mortality from cystic fibrosis in the UK over recent years. Each line shows the survival for successive cohorts of patients born in the three-year periods indicated. Improved survival has occurred at all ages, though there continues to be a slight excess of deaths in early infancy. (Redrawn from data in reference 51.)

The CFTR comprises three types of protein subunit.[56,57] A ring of membrane spanning domains form a channel through the lipid bilayer of the cell wall (Figure 27.4). Attached to the intracellular aspect of these are two nucleotide-binding domains (NBDs) that use ATP when the channel is activated. Finally, a single regulatory domain (R) protein is loosely attached to the nucleotide-binding domains and can move away from the membrane to 'open' the channel and allow chloride to pass into or out of the cell (Figure 27.4). Intracellular protein kinase A activates the channel by binding to the regulatory domain of CFTR, whilst ATP provides the energy and is dephosphorylated by nucleotide-binding domains. Several hundred different mutations of the CF gene have been identified, and can result in no CFTR being formed, failure of the different protein domains to align correctly or failure of the CFTR to become incorporated into the cell membrane.[53,56] Almost three-quarters of clinical CF cases result from a deletion of just three base pairs from the gene, which result in the loss of a single phenylalanine from one nucleotide-binding domain protein and failure to locate the CFTR in its transmembrane position.[52]

Causes of lung disease. Early opinions on this matter concentrated on the consistency of airway mucus, which was believed to be too viscous, leading to mucus retention and bacterial colonization, particularly with *Pseudomonas aeruginosa*. However, recent work has identified an endogenous antibiotic in the human lung, named human β-defensin (HBD), which is believed to play an important role in preventing pulmonary infection. Consisting of a 64 amino acid peptide, human β-defensin is inactivated by increased sodium chloride concentrations, so allowing proliferation of bacteria in CF lungs.[53,58] This has given rise to suggestions that bacterial colonization is the primary event, and hypersecretion of mucus occurs as a consequence of this rather than *vice versa*. Either

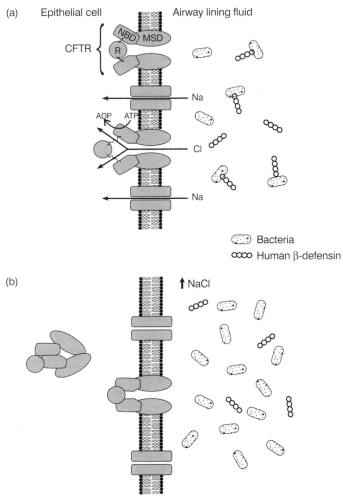

Figure 27.4 Sodium and chloride transport across the pulmonary epithelial cell wall in cystic fibrosis. (a) Normal lung. Cystic fibrosis transmembrane regulator (CFTR) chloride channel in the closed (upper) and open (lower) positions showing movement of the regulator domain (R). Sodium transport follows chloride via passive Na channels due to altered transmembrane potentials. Bacteria in the airway lining fluid are inactivated by human β-defensin. (b) Cystic fibrosis. The CFTR proteins are defective so do not locate in the membrane, or are non-functional when they do. Sodium and chloride concentration is therefore abnormally high in the airway, which inactivates human β-defensin and so allows bacterial proliferation. MSD, membrane spanning domain; NBD, nucleotide binding domain.

way, there is no doubt that a vicious cycle becomes established in which bacterial infection leads to airway inflammation, mucus production and more infection, associated with progressive lung tissue damage.[59]

Principles of treatment

Conventional treatment[59,60] involves assisting the clearance of airway secretions by physiotherapy and postural drainage. Thick secretions result in part from degradation of the numerous inflammatory cells found in infected airways, and it is DNA from these cells that tends to aggregate and increase viscosity. Treatment with inhaled recombinant human DNAase reduces the viscosity of sputum, and is a useful adjunct to physical methods of mucus clearance. Antibiotics, for both infective exacerbations and maintenance therapy, are used much more commonly nowadays than previously. Antibiotics undoubtedly improve CF in the short term, but emergence of bacterial resistance and patient hypersensitivity reactions may have serious long-term effects, and their contribution to the improved prognosis in CF is controversial.[60]

Lung transplantation is now a recognized treatment for CF; it is described in Chapter 33.

Gene therapy has held great potential for therapy ever since the CF gene was identified, but unfortunately this potential has not been realized.[61] A normal CFTR gene can be easily produced, but the problem arises in incorporating the gene into the airway cells and stimulating its expression into functioning CFTR *in vivo*.[62] Gene delivery, either in liposomes or genetically modified adenovirus vectors has been attempted, but the functional effect is poor, with only transient or small changes in CFTR expression. Viral vectors, which are the most effective technique for incorporating the new gene into the epithelial cell, are associated with significant, and possibly harmful, inflammatory reactions.[63] A more promising approach is to incorporate the normal gene into the fetus, which bypasses immunological reactions and should provide a permanent correction of the defective gene. This has been achieved in mice,[64] but studies of this type in humans are currently prohibited by international ethical convention.[61]

References

1. Holgate ST. Asthma and allergy – disorders of civilisation? *QJM* 1998; **91**: 171–84.
2. Committee on the Medical Effects of Air Pollutants. *Asthma and outdoor air pollution.* London: HMSO, 1995.
3. Nadel JA, Busse WW. Asthma. *Am J Respir Crit Care Med* 1998; **157**: S130–8.
4. Woolcock AJ. Learning from asthma deaths. *BMJ* 1997; **314**: 1427–8.
5. Sears MR. Changing patterns in asthma morbidity and mortality. *J Investig Allergol Clin Immunol* 1995; **5**: 66–72.
6. Cormier Y, Lecours R, Legris C. Mechanisms of hyperinflation in asthma. *Eur Respir J* 1990; **3**: 619–24.
7. Lötvall J, Inman M, O'Byrne P. Measurement of airway hyperresponsiveness: new considerations. *Thorax* 1998; **53**: 419–24.
8. Lee TH. Cytokine networks in the pathogenesis of bronchial asthma: implications for therapy. *J R Coll Physicians Lond* 1998; **32**: 56–64.
9. Robinson C, Holgate ST. Mast cell-dependent inflammatory mediators and their putative role in bronchial asthma. *Clin Sci* 1985; **68**: 103–12.
10. DuBois AB, Kelley PM, Douglas JS, Mohsenin V. Nitric oxide production and absorption in trachea, bronchi, bronchioles, and respiratory bronchioles of humans. *J Appl Physiol* 1999; **86**: 159–67.
11. Lundberg JON, Lundberg JM, Alving K, Weitzberg E. Nitric oxide and inflammation: the answer is blowing in the wind. *Nat Med* 1997; **3**: 30–1.
12. Frank TL, Adisesh A, Pickering AC, Morrison JFJ, Wright T, Francis H et al. Relationship between exhaled nitric oxide and childhood asthma. *Am J Respir Crit Care Med* 1998; **158**: 1032–6.
13. Hamid Q, Springall DR, Riveros-Moreno V, Chanez P, Howarth P, Redington A et al. Induction of nitric oxide synthase in asthma. *Lancet* 1993; **342**: 1510–13.
14. Barnes PJ. NO or no NO in asthma. *Thorax* 1996; **51**: 218–20.

15. Jeffery PK, Godfrey RW, Ädelroth E, Nelson F, Rogers A, Johansson S-A. Effects of treatment on airway inflammation and thickening of basement membrane reticular collagen in asthma. *Am Rev Respir Dis* 1992; **145**: 890–9.

16. O'Riordan TG, Zwang J, Smaldone GC. Mucociliary clearance in adult asthma. *Am Rev Respir Dis* 1992; **146**: 598–603.

17. Dunnill MS. The pathology of asthma, with special reference to changes in the bronchial mucosa. *J Clin Pathol* 1960; **13**: 27–33.

18. Lambert RK. Role of bronchial basement membrane in airway collapse. *J Appl Physiol* 1991; **71**: 666–73.

19. Lambert RK, Codd SL, Alley MR, Pack RJ. Physical determinants of bronchial mucosal folding. *J Appl Physiol* 1994; **77**: 1206–16.

20. Warner JA, Jones AC, Miles EA, Colwell BM, Warner JO. Maternofetal interaction and allergy. *Allergy* 1996; **51**: 447–51.

21. Tang MLK, Kemp AS, Thorburn J, Hill DJ. Reduced interferon-γ secretion in neonates and subsequent atopy. *Lancet* 1994; **344**: 983–5.

22. Folkerts G, Busse WW, Nijkamp FP, Sorkness R, Gern JE. Virus-induced airway hyperresponsiveness and asthma. *Am J Respir Crit Care Med* 1998; **157**: 1708–20.

23. Calhoun WJ, Dick EC, Schwartz LB, Busse WW. A common cold virus, rhinovirus 16, potentiates airway inflammation after segmental antigen bronchoprovocation in allergic subjects. *J Clin Invest* 1994; **94**: 2200–8.

24. Scott P. IL-12: initiation cytokine for cell-mediated immunity. *Science* 1993; **260**: 496–7.

25. Matsumura Y. The effects of ozone, nitrogen dioxide, and sulfur dioxide on the experimentally induced allergic respiratory disorder in guinea pigs. II. The effects of ozone on the absorption and the retention of antigen in the lung. *Am Rev Respir Dis* 1970; **102**: 438–43.

26. Harding SM, Richter JE. The role of gastroesophageal reflux in chronic cough and asthma. *Chest* 1997; **111**: 1389–402.

27. British Asthma Guidelines Coordinating Committee. British guidelines on asthma management: 1995 review and position statement. *Thorax* 1997; **52**: S1–S24.

28. National Heart, Lung and Blood Institute. *Expert Panel Report 2: Guidelines for the diagnosis and management of asthma*, Publication No 97–4051. Bethesda MD: National Institutes of Health, 1997.

29. Lipworth BJ. Modern drug treatment of chronic asthma. *BMJ* 1999; **318**: 380–4.

30. Moore RH, Khan A, Dickey BF. Long-acting inhaled beta$_2$-agonists in asthma therapy. *Chest* 1998; **113**: 1095–108.

31. Horwitz RJ, McGill KA, Busse WW. The role of leukotriene modifiers in the treatment of asthma. *Am J Respir Crit Care Med* 1998; **157**: 1363–71.

32. Barnes PJ. Inhaled glucocorticoids for asthma. *N Engl J Med* 1995; **332**: 868–75.

33. McFadden ER. Inhaled glucocorticoids and acute asthma. Therapeutic breakthrough or nonspecific effect. *Am J Respir Crit Care Med* 1998; **157**: 677–8.

34. Custovic A, Simpson A, Chapman MD, Woodcock A. Allergen avoidance in the treatment of asthma and atopic disorders. *Thorax* 1998; **53**: 63–72.

35. van der Heide S, Kauffman HF, Dubois AEJ, de Monchy JGR. Allergen-avoidance measures in homes of house-dust-mite-allergic asthmatic patients: effects of acaricides and mattress encasings. *Allergy* 1997; **52**: 921–7.

36. Gotzsche PC, Hammarquist C, Burr M. House dust mite control measures in the management of asthma: meta-analysis. *BMJ* 1998; **317**: 1105–10.

37. Madison JM, Irwin RS. Chronic obstructive pulmonary disease. *Lancet* 1998; **352**: 467–73.

38. Senior RM, Anthonisen NR. Chronic obstructive pulmonary disease (COPD). *Am J Respir Crit Care Med* 1998; **157**: S139–47.

39. Snider GL, Kleinerman J, Thurlbeck WM, Bengali ZH. The definition of emphysema: report of a National Heart, Lung, and Blood Institute, Division of Lung Diseases Workshop. *Am Rev Respir Dis* 1985; **132**: 182–5.

40. Pierce RA, Mariani TJ, Senior RM. Elastin in lung development and disease. *Ciba Found Symp* 1995; **192**: 199–214.

41. Davies L, Calverley PMA. Lung volume reduction surgery in chronic obstructive pulmonary disease. *Thorax* 1996; **51** (Supp 2); S29–34.

42. Tiddens HAWM, Paré PD, Hogg JC, Hop WCJ, Lambert R, De Jongste JC. Cartilaginous airway dimensions and airflow obstruction in human lungs. *Am J Respir Crit Care Med* 1995; **152**: 260–6.
43. Demedts M. Mechanisms and consequences of hyperinflation. *Eur Respir J* 1990; **3**: 617–18.
44. Sassoon CSH, Hassell KT, Mahutte CK. Hyperoxic-induced hypercapnia in stable chronic obstructive pulmonary disease. *Am Rev Respir Dis* 1987; **135**: 907–11.
45. Aubier M, Murciano D, Milic-Emili J, Touaty E, Daghfous J, Pariente R, Derenne JP. Effects of the administration of O_2 on ventilation and blood gases in patients with chronic obstructive pulmonary disease during acute respiratory failure. *Am Rev Respir Dis* 1980; **122**: 747–54.
46. Crossley DJ, McGuire GP, Barrow PM, Houston PL. Influence of inspired oxygen concentration on deadspace, respiratory drive, and $PaCO_2$ in intubated patients with chronic obstructive pulmonary disease. *Crit Care Med* 1997; **25**: 1522–6.
47. Taylor DR. Chronic obstructive pulmonary disease. *BMJ* 1998; **316**: 1475.
48. Chapman KR. Therapeutic approaches to chronic obstructive pulmonary disease: an emerging consensus. *Am J Med* 1996; **100** (1A): 5S–10S.
49. Wagner PD. Functional consequences of lung volume reduction surgery for COPD. *Am J Respir Crit Care Med* 1998; **158**: 1017–19.
50. Cooper JD, Trulock EP, Triantafillou AN, Patterson GA, Pohl MS, Deloney PA et al. Bilateral pneumectomy (volume reduction) for chronic obstructive pulmonary disease. *J Thorac Cardiovasc Surg* 1995; **109**: 106–19.
51. Dodge JA, Morison S, Lewis PA, Coles EC, Geddes D, Russell G et al. Incidence, population, and survival of cystic fibrosis in the UK, 1968–95. *Arch Dis Child* 1997; **77**: 493–6.
52. Davidson DJ, Porteus DJ. The genetics of cystic fibrosis lung disease. *Thorax* 1998; **53**: 389–97.
53. Rosenstein BJ, Zeitlin PL. Cystic fibrosis. *Lancet* 1998; **351**: 277–82.
54. Kerem B, Rommens JM, Buchanan JA, Markiewitz D, Cox TK, Chakravarti A et al. Identification of the cystic fibrosis gene: genetic analysis. *Science* 1989; **245**: 1073–80.
55. Wallis C. Diagnosing cystic fibrosis: blood, sweat, and tears. *Arch Dis Child* 1997; **76**: 85–91.
56. Welsh MJ, Ramsey BW. Research on cystic fibrosis. *Am J Respir Crit Care Med* 1998; **157**: S148–54.
57. Stern M, Geddes D. Cystic fibrosis: basic chemical and cellular mechanisms. *Br J Hosp Med* 1996; **55**: 237–40.
58. Goldman MJ, Anderson GM, Stolzenberg ED, Kari UP, Zasloff M, Wilson J. Human β-defensin-1 is a salt-sensitive antibiotic in lung that is inactivated in cystic fibrosis. *Cell* 1997; **88**: 553–60.
59. Bilton D, Mahadeva R. New treatments in adult cystic fibrosis. *J R Soc Med* 1997; **90** (Supp 31): 2–5.
60. Ramsey BW. Management of pulmonary disease in patients with cystic fibrosis. *N Engl J Med* 1996; **335**: 179–88.
61. Dodge JA. Gene therapy for cystic fibrosis. *Nat Med* 1995; **1**: 182.
62. Middleton PG, Alton EWFW. Gene therapy for cystic fibrosis: which postman, which box. *Thorax* 1998; **53**: 197–9.
63. McElvaney NG, Crystal RG. IL-6 release and airway administration of human CFTR cDNA adenovirus vector. *Nat Med* 1995; **1**: 182–4.
64. Larson JE, Morrow SL, Happel L, Sharp JF, Cohen JC. Reversal of cystic fibrosis phenotype in mice by gene therapy in utero. *Lancet* 1997; **349**: 619–20.

Chapter 28

Pulmonary vascular disease

Pulmonary oedema

Pulmonary oedema is defined as an increase in pulmonary extravascular water, which occurs when transudation or exudation exceeds the capacity of the lymphatic drainage. In its more severe forms there is free fluid in the alveoli.

Anatomical factors

The pulmonary capillary endothelial cells abut against one another at fairly loose junctions that are of the order of 5 nm (50 Å) wide.[1] These junctions permit the passage of quite large molecules and the pulmonary lymph contains albumin at about half the concentration in plasma. Epithelial cells meet at tight junctions with a gap of only about 1 nm.[1] The tightness of these junctions is crucial for preventing the escape of large molecules, such as albumin, from the interstitial fluid into the alveoli.

The lung has a well-developed lymphatic system draining the interstitial tissue through a network of channels around the bronchi and pulmonary vessels towards the hilum. Lymphatic vessels are seen in the juxtaseptal alveolar region (see below) and are commonly found in association with bronchioles. Down to airway generation 11 (see Table 2.1), the lymphatics lie in a potential space around the air passages and vessels, separating them from the lung parenchyma.

In the hilum of the lung, the lymphatic drainage passes through several groups of tracheobronchial lymph glands, where they receive tributaries from the superficial subpleural plexus. Most of the lymph from the left lung usually enters the thoracic duct, where it can be conveniently sampled in animals. The right side drains into the right lymphatic duct. However, the pulmonary lymphatics often cross the midline and pass independently into the junction of internal jugular and subclavian veins on the corresponding sides of the body.

The normal lymphatic drainage from human lungs is astonishingly small – only about 10 ml.h^{-1}. However, lymphatic flow can increase greatly when transudation into the interstitial spaces is increased. This presumably occurs when pulmonary oedema is threatened but it cannot be conveniently measured in humans.

Stages of pulmonary oedema

There is presumably a prodromal stage in which pulmonary lymphatic drainage is increased, but there is no increase in extravascular water. This may progress to the following stages.

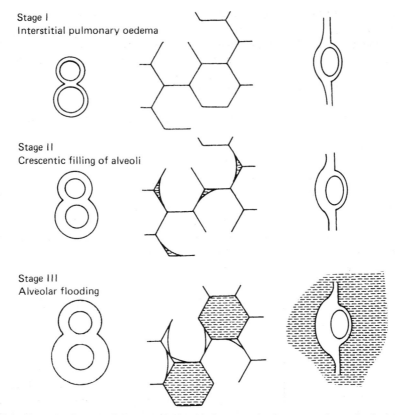

Figure 28.1 Schematic diagram of the stages in the development of pulmonary oedema. On the left is shown the development of the cuff of distended lymphatics around the branches of the bronchi and pulmonary arteries. In the middle is the appearance of the alveoli by light microscopy (fixed in inflation). On the right is the appearance of the pulmonary capillaries by electron microscopy. The active side of the capillary is to the right. See text for details.

Stage I. Interstitial pulmonary oedema. In its mildest form, there is an increase in interstitial fluid but without passage of oedema fluid into the alveoli. With the light microscope this is first detected as cuffs of distended lymphatics, typically '8'-shaped around the adjacent branches of the bronchi and pulmonary artery (Figure 28.1). Electron microscopy reveals fluid accumulation in the alveolar septa but this is characteristically confined to the 'service' side of the pulmonary capillary, which contains the stroma, leaving the geometry of the 'active' side unchanged (see page 27 and Figure 2.8). Thus, gas exchange is better preserved than might be expected from the overall increase in lung water.

Physical signs are generally minimal in stage I, except perhaps for mild dyspnoea, particularly with exercise. The alveolar/arterial Po_2 gradient is normal or only slightly increased. Diagnosis relies on the chest radiograph, in which Kerley B lines may be visible, and on the demonstration of causative factors such as an increased pulmonary capillary wedge pressure.

Stage II. Crescentic filling of the alveoli. With further increase in extravascular lung water, interstitial oedema of the alveolar septa is increased and fluid begins to pass into some alveolar lumina. It first appears as crescents in the angles between adjacent septa, at least in lungs that have been fixed in inflation (Figure 28.1). The centre of the alveoli and most of the alveolar walls remain clear, and gas exchange is not grossly abnormal, but dyspnoea at rest is likely and the characteristic butterfly shadow may be visible on the chest radiograph.

Stage III. Alveolar flooding. In the third stage, there is quantal alveolar flooding. Some alveoli are totally flooded while others, frequently adjacent, have only the crescentic filling or else no fluid at all in their lumina. It seems that fluid accumulates up to a point at which a critical radius of curvature results in surface tension sharply increasing the transudation pressure gradient. This produces flooding on an all-or-none basis for each individual alveolus. Owing to the effect of gravity on pulmonary vascular pressures (page 142), alveolar flooding tends to occur in the dependent parts of the lungs.

Clearly there can be no effective gas exchange in the capillaries of an alveolar septum that is flooded on both sides, and the overall defect of gas exchange may be considered as venous admixture or shunt. Râles can be heard during inspiration and the lung fields show an overall opacity superimposed on the butterfly shadow.

Stage IV. Froth in the air passages. When alveolar flooding is extreme, the air passages become blocked with froth, which moves to and fro with breathing. This effectively stops all gas exchange and is rapidly fatal unless treated.

The mechanism of pulmonary oedema[2]

Transudation of intravascular fluid into the alveoli must be considered in three stages. First, from the microcirculation into interstitial space (across the endothelium), secondly fluid dynamics within the interstitium and finally movement of fluid from the interstitial space into the alveoli (across the epithelium) (Figure 28.2).

Passage of fluid across the endothelium is promoted by the hydrostatic pressure differential between capillary and interstitium but counteracted by the osmotic pressure of the plasma proteins. The balance of pressures is normally sufficient to prevent any appreciable transudation but it may be upset in a wide variety of pathological circumstances.

It is customary to display the relationship between fluid flow and the balance of pressures in the form of the Starling equation. For the endothelial barrier this is as follows:

$$\dot{Q} = K[(Pmv - Ppmv) - \Sigma\,(\Pi mv - \Pi pmv)]$$

$\dot{Q}$ is the flow rate of transuded fluid which, in equilibrium, will be equal to the lymphatic drainage.

K is the hydraulic conductance (i.e. flow rate of fluid per unit pressure gradient across the endothelium.

Pmv is the hydrostatic pressure in the microvasculature.

$Ppmv$ is the hydrostatic pressure in the perimicrovascular tissue (i.e. the interstitium).

Σ is the reflection coefficient, in this case applying to albumin. It is an expression of the permeability of the endothelium to the solute (albumin). A value of unity indicates total reflection corresponding to zero concentration of the solute in the interstitial fluid. A value of zero indicates free passage of the solute across the

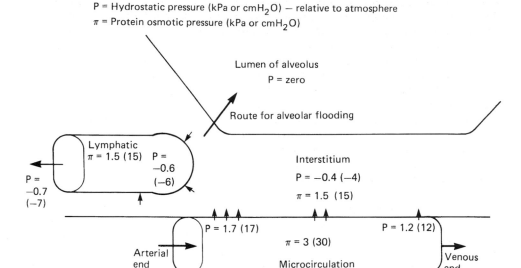

P = Hydrostatic pressure (kPa or cmH$_2$O) — relative to atmosphere

π = Protein osmotic pressure (kPa or cmH$_2$O)

Lumen of alveolus

P = zero

Route for alveolar flooding

Lymphatic

π = 1.5 (15)   P = −0.6 (−6)

P = −0.7 (−7)

Interstitium

P = −0.4 (−4)

π = 1.5 (15)

P = 1.7 (17)

π = 3 (30)

P = 1.2 (12)

Arterial end

Microcirculation

Venous end

Figure 28.2 Normal values for hydrostatic and plasma protein osmotic pressures in the pulmonary microcirculation and interstitium. (Values taken from reference 3.)

membrane and, with equal concentrations on both sides of the membrane, the solute could exert no osmotic pressure across the membrane. This normally applies to the crystalloids in plasma.

Πmv   is the osmotic pressure the solute exerts within the microvasculature.

Πpmv is the osmotic pressure the solute exerts in the perimicrovascular tissue.

Under normal circumstances in humans, the pulmonary lymph flow ($\dot{Q}$) is about $10\,ml.h^{-1}$ with a protein content about half that of plasma. The pulmonary microvascular pressure (*Pmv*) is in the range 0–2 kPa (0–15 mmHg), relative to atmosphere, depending on the vertical height in the lung field. Furthermore, there is a progressive decrease in capillary pressure from its arterial to its venous end, because about one-half the pulmonary vascular resistance is across the capillary bed (see Figures 7.2 and 28.2). In this context, it is meaningless to think of a single value for the mean pulmonary capillary pressure.

The hydrostatic pressure in the perimicrovascular tissue (*Ppmv*) is not easy to measure. An early study in 1968 using implanted pressure-measuring capsules in an isolated lung preparation found an average pressure of 1.3 kPa (10 mmHg or 13 cmH$_2$O) below atmospheric.[4] Later animal studies using micropuncture techniques confirmed the subatmospheric pressure of −0.40 to −1.25 kPa (−4 to −12.5 cmH$_2$O).[5,6] In the excised lung there was no vertical gradient in interstitial pressures such as might have been expected from the effect of gravity,[4] but this was observed when measurements were made with the chest and pleura intact.[6]

The reflection coefficient for albumin (Σ) in the healthy lung is about 0.5. The overall osmotic pressure gradient between blood and interstitial fluid is about 1.5 kPa (11.5 mmHg). Thus there is a fine balance between forces favouring and opposing transudation. There is a considerable safety margin in the upper part of the lung where the microvascular hydrostatic pressure is lowest. However, in the dependent part of the lung, where the hydrostatic pressure is highest, the safety margin is slender.

Fluid dynamics within the interstitium. Recent studies have challenged the long-held view that the interstitium simply acts as a passive conduit for fluid transfer to the lymphatics.[2,7] Proteoglycan and hyaluron molecules are present in the pulmonary interstitium of animals, and function like a gel to absorb water to minimize increase in interstitial pressure and prevent hydration of other extracellular structures such as collagen.[8] Regional differences in the properties of these molecules are believed to be responsible for the establishment of a pressure gradient between the septal interstitium and the juxtaseptal region where lymphatic channels originate. This gradient may promote, and allow some control of, fluid flow from the endothelium to the lymphatics in the normal lung.[7]

With increased fluid transfer across the endothelium, the interstitial space can accommodate large volumes of water with only small increases in pressure, the interstitial compliance being high. Some 500 ml can be accommodated in the interstitium and lymphatics of the human lungs with a rise of pressure of only about 0.2 kPa (2 cmH$_2$O).[3] Interstitial swelling is, however, not without risks, and swelling on the service side will eventually cause narrowing of the capillary lumen, though this does not occur until pulmonary oedema is very advanced. Eventually, the capacity of the molecules to absorb water is exceeded, and the proteoglycan structure breaks down, possibly leading to disturbances of nearby collagen molecules and therefore basement membrane function, producing alveolar oedema.[7] Alterations of interstitial proteoglycan structure during lung injury and repair may contribute to the greater likelihood of pulmonary oedema under these circumstances (Chapter 30).

Fluid exchange across the alveolar epithelium. The permeability of this membrane is considered in Chapter 9 (page 204). It is freely permeable to gases, water and hydrophobic substances but virtually impermeable to albumin.

It is possible to construct a Starling equation for the epithelium[9] but there are considerable uncertainties about the osmotic pressure of the alveolar lining fluid. It has even been suggested that the alveolar lining is largely dry,[10] which would make the concept meaningless, though evidence does exist for the presence of water at the epithelial surface.[11] Nevertheless, it does seem that transudation across the alveolar epithelium is virtually zero unless the integrity of the barrier is compromised or the interstitial pressure increases above a critical level.

Aetiology

On the basis of the Starling equations, it is possible to make a rational approach to the aetiology of pulmonary oedema. There are three groups of aetiological factors, classified according to their effect on factors in the Starling equation.

Increased capillary pressure (haemodynamic pulmonary oedema). This group comprises the commonest causes of pulmonary oedema. Basically the mechanism is an elevation of the hydrostatic pressure gradient across the pulmonary capillary wall, until it exceeds the osmotic pressure of the plasma proteins. Interstitial fluid accumulates until it overwhelms the ability of the interstitium to absorb fluid and transport it to the lymphatics. The oedema fluid has a protein content that is less than that of normal pulmonary lymph or plasma.[3] Apart from transudation in accord with the Starling equation, severe pulmonary capillary hypertension may result in loss of structural integrity (see below).

Causes of an increase in pulmonary capillary pressure are numerous:

Absolute hypervolaemia may result from overtransfusion, from excessive and rapid administration of other blood volume expanders or from accidental access of irrigation fluids through open venous channels in hollow organs, as for example during prostatectomy.

Relative pulmonary hypervolaemia may result from redistribution of the circulating blood volume into the lungs. This may be due to use of the Trendelenburg position or vasopressor drugs that act on the systemic circulation to a greater extent than on the pulmonary circulation and so redirect blood into the pulmonary circulation.

Raised pulmonary venous pressure will inevitably result in an increase in pulmonary capillary pressure. This may occur from any form of left heart failure, most commonly left ventricular failure or mitral valve lesions.

Increased pulmonary blood flow may raise the pulmonary capillary pressure sufficiently to precipitate pulmonary oedema. This may result from a left-to-right cardiac shunt, anaemia or, rarely, as a result of exercise.

Increased permeability of the alveolar/capillary membrane (permeability oedema). This group comprises the next commonest causes of pulmonary oedema. The mechanism is the loss of integrity of the alveolar/capillary membrane, allowing albumin and other macromolecules to enter the alveoli. The osmotic pressure gradient which opposes transudation is then lost. The oedema fluid has a protein content that approaches that of plasma.

The alveolar/capillary membrane can be damaged either directly or indirectly by many agents, which are reviewed in Chapter 30. Apart from the possibility of the condition progressing to the adult respiratory distress syndrome, permeability pulmonary oedema is always potentially very dangerous. The presence of protein in the alveoli tends to make the oedema refractory and the protein may become organized into a so-called hyaline membrane.

'Stress failure' of the pulmonary capillaries occurs when the pulmonary capillary pressure is increased in the range 3–5 kPa (30–50 cmH$_2$O). Discontinuities appear in the capillary endothelium and alveolar epithelium (type I cells), while the basement membrane often remains intact.[12,13] This would seem to result in increased permeability and leakage of protein into the alveoli. The gaps tend to occur in the cell body, rather than at the junctions between the cells.

Decreased osmotic pressure of the plasma proteins. The Starling equation indicates that the osmotic pressure of the plasma proteins is a crucial factor opposing transudation. Although seldom the primary cause of pulmonary oedema, a reduced plasma albumin concentration is very common in the seriously ill patient and it must inevitably decrease the microvascular pressure threshold at which transudation commences.

Miscellaneous causes of pulmonary oedema

Lymphatic obstruction. As in other tissues, obstruction of the pulmonary lymphatic drainage is a potential cause of pulmonary oedema. Because the pulmonary lymphatics drain into the great veins, raised systemic venous pressure has an adverse effect on pulmonary lymph flow and therefore the accumulation of lung water.[14] In the first few weeks after lung transplantation, lymph drains from the cut ends of the pulmonary lymphatics into the pleural cavity. Eventually the lymphatics re-form and normal drainage is resumed.

Neurogenic pulmonary oedema may follow head injuries or other cerebral lesions. Evidence for the existence of pulmonary venous sphincters has provided a possible mechanism for neurogenic pulmonary oedema.[15] Constriction of these sphincters, either due to circulating adrenaline or a neural response, could cause an abrupt increase in pulmonary capillary pressure. A study of neurogenic pulmonary oedema in humans supported this hypothesis by demonstrating that the oedema fluid often has a low protein content, suggesting a haemodynamic mechanism (see above).[15]

Re-expansion oedema. Sudden expansion of a collapsed lung may result in pulmonary oedema confined to the one side and probably caused by increased permeability.[16] The problem may arise after aspiration of a pneumothorax or a pleural effusion. Lungs that have been collapsed for some time should be re-expanded slowly and by not more than 1 litre at one time.

Pulmonary oedema occurring at high altitude is well documented, although the mechanism is still open to speculation. It is considered in Chapter 16.

Pathophysiology

The most important physiological abnormality caused by pulmonary oedema is venous admixture or shunt due to blood draining fluid-filled alveoli.[17] This results in an increased alveolar/arterial Po_2 gradient and hypoxaemia, which may be life threatening. Blood flow to the oedematous lung regions is slightly reduced by hypoxic pulmonary vasoconstriction (page 151), possibly in conjunction with interstitial swelling causing capillary obstruction (see above), but the shunt commonly remains substantial.

Hypercapnia is not generally a problem. In less severe pulmonary oedema, there is usually an increased respiratory drive, due partly to hypoxaemia and partly to stimulation of J-receptors (page 90). As a result the Pco_2 is usually normal or somewhat decreased.

Physiological principles of treatment

Immediate treatment aims to restore the arterial Po_2 to normal values. The inspired oxygen concentration should be increased, up to 100% if necessary. Sitting the patient up is a simple way to reduce the central blood volume. Treatment of the underlying cause of pulmonary oedema follows directly from the Starling equation and an understanding of the aetiology.

Haemodynamic pulmonary oedema. The essential feature of treatment is reduction of the left atrial pressure. Depending on the precise aetiology, treatment is directed towards improvement of left ventricular function and/or reduction of blood volume. The latter may be quickly and easily achieved by peripheral vasodilatation. Drugs that predominantly dilate the capacitance (venous) system, such as nitrates or angiotensin-converting enzyme inhibitors, will be most effective. This mechanism is probably also responsible for the beneficial effects of frusemide and diamorphine in the acute situation. Diuretics act more slowly but are useful for long-term treatment. Essentially the patient is titrated to the left along his Frank–Starling curve (Figure 28.3). In addition the curve is moved upwards and to the left, if this is possible, using positive inotropes as an adjunct to correction of left ventricular malfunction, for example from ischaemia. The further the curve can be moved, the greater will be that part of it lying in the safe quadrant between low cardiac output on one hand and pulmonary oedema on the other.

Permeability pulmonary oedema. Treatment should be directed towards restoration of the integrity of the alveolar/capillary membrane. Unfortunately, no particularly successful

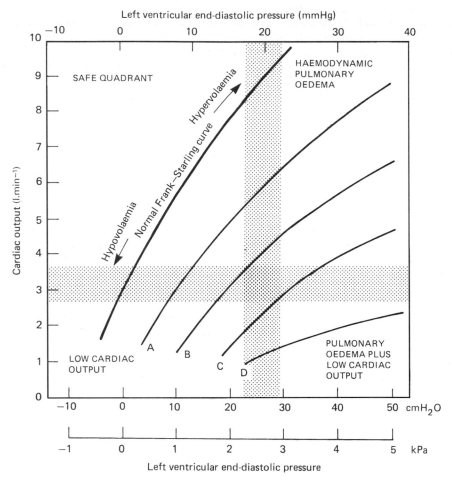

Figure 28.3 Quadrant diagram relating cardiac output to left ventricular end-diastolic pressure. The thick curve is a typical normal Frank–Starling curve. To the right are curves representing progressive left ventricular failure. *Top left* is the safe quadrant, which contains a substantial part of the normal curve but much less of the curves representing ventricular failure. *Top right* is the quadrant representing normal cardiac output but raised left atrial pressure, attained at the upper end of relatively normal Frank–Starling curves (e.g. hypervolaemia). There is a danger of haemodynamic pulmonary oedema. *Bottom left* is the quadrant representing normal or low left atrial pressure but low cardiac output, attained at the lower end of all curves (e.g. hypovolaemia). The patient is in shock. *Bottom right* is the quadrant representing both low cardiac output and raised left atrial pressure. There is simultaneous danger of pulmonary oedema and shock, and the worst Frank–Starling curves hardly leave this quadrant.

measures are available towards this end (see Chapter 30). It is, however, important to minimize left atrial pressure even though this is not the primary cause of the oedema. Attempts may be made to increase the plasma albumin concentration if it is reduced.

Artificial ventilation and positive end-expiratory pressure (PEEP). Severe pulmonary oedema causes degrees of hypoxia that may quickly be lethal. Tracheal intubation and positive pressure ventilation is therefore commonly required, and the results are often spectacular. Froth in the airways may be easily aspirated, and any areas of atelectasis occurring along with the oedema improved. Artificial ventilation is often combined with PEEP, resulting in further improvements in arterial P_{O_2}. It was originally thought that the positive pressures drove the fluid back into the circulation, but evidence that extravascular lung water is reduced by PEEP is contradictory, with few human studies. Animal models of pulmonary oedema indicate that, by increasing the lung volume, the capacity of the interstitium to hold liquid is increased.[18] Similarly, with haemodynamic pulmonary oedema in dogs, PEEP does not alter the total amount of lung water but a greater proportion is in the extra-alveolar interstitial space,[19] and lymphatic drainage is increased.[20] In addition to these theoretical benefits, the success of PEEP in patients probably depends on forcing airway liquid down the tracheobronchial tree and opening up alveoli that were previously not ventilated.

Clinical measurement

Pulmonary vascular pressures. As an indication of impending or actual haemodynamic pulmonary oedema, the most useful clinical measurement is the pulmonary artery occlusion (wedge) pressure, which equates to pulmonary venous pressure. Estimates of pulmonary capillary pressure itself may also be obtained with a Swan–Ganz catheter.[21,22,23,24] The decay curve seen on occluding a pulmonary artery branch is biphasic (Figure 28.4). The first, rapid, phase reflects the fall in pressure as the arterial compartment distal to the balloon empties across the precapillary resistance. The second, slower, phase represents the fall in pressure as the capillary compartment empties into the pulmonary veins across the postcapillary resistance. Thus, the inflection point of the curve should equate to mean capillary pressure.[22]

The Swan–Ganz catheter, though controversial,[25] continues to be widely used in managing patients with actual or potential pulmonary oedema.[21]

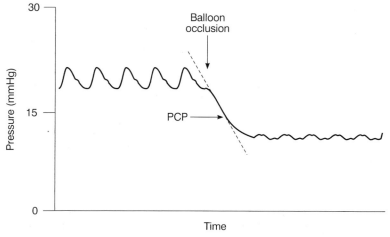

Figure 28.4 Estimation of pulmonary capillary pressure using the Swan–Ganz catheter. The pulmonary arterial trace has been slightly damped with air, and the occlusion balloon is inflated during a prolonged expiration to prevent pressure swings with respiration. The occlusion pressure decay curve is biphasic. Pulmonary capillary pressure (PCP) is estimated as the point at which the slow component causes the decay curve to depart from its initial steep decline, and may be measured manually as shown.

Permeability of the alveolar/capillary membrane. Laboratory methods are available for animals but the only practical approach for clinical use is measurement of the rate of loss of a gamma-emitting tracer molecule from the lung into the circulation. The most sensitive tracer is ^{99m}Tc-DTPA (metastable technetium-99-labelled diethylene triamine penta-acetate, molecular weight 492 daltons).[26] The half-time of clearance from the lung fields is usually in the range 40–100 minutes in the healthy non-smoker. The half-time is reduced below 40 minutes following a variety of lung insults. However, it is within the range 10–40 minutes in apparently healthy smokers and this limits its scope for the early detection of a damaged alveolar/capillary membrane.

Lung water. This would be an extremely valuable diagnostic and prognostic aid to the management of pulmonary oedema. It is easy enough to measure lung water gravimetrically at post-mortem in terms of the wet/dry difference or ratio, and there is usually sufficient protein in alveolar fluid for it to stain and be clearly visible by light microscopy.

   Measurement of lung water during life has proved elusive. A great deal of effort has been devoted to the double indicator method. This uses the techniques for the measurement of pulmonary or central blood volume by dye dilution but with two indicators. One indicator is chosen to remain within the circulation while the other (usually 'coolth' or tritiated water) diffuses into the interstitial fluid. Extravascular lung water is then derived as the difference between the volumes as measured with the two indicators. These methods are limited because a high level of accuracy is required to demonstrate small changes in lung water, though clinically acceptable results may now be obtained reasonably conveniently.[27]

Pulmonary embolism

The pulmonary circulation may be occluded by embolism, which may be gas, thrombus, fat, tumour or foreign body. The architecture of the microvasculature is well adapted to minimize the effects of embolism. Large numbers of pulmonary capillaries tend to arise from metarterioles at right angles and there are abundant anastomoses throughout the microcirculation. This tends to preserve circulation distal to the impaction of a small embolus. Nevertheless, a large pulmonary embolus is a serious and potentially lethal complication, causing some 50 000 deaths a year in the USA.[28]

Thromboembolism[29]

The commonest pulmonary embolus consists of detached venous thromboses, particularly from veins in the thigh and the pelvic venous plexuses. Smaller thrombi are filtered in the lungs without causing symptoms but larger emboli may impact in major vessels, typically at a bifurcation forming a saddle embolus. There may be a catastrophic increase in pulmonary vascular resistance, with acute right heart failure or cardiac arrest.

Diagnosis of pulmonary thromboembolus.[29,30] Massive pulmonary thromboembolus causes rapid cardiac arrest and death, and over half the cases are undiagnosed except at autopsy.[31] Similarly, small pulmonary emboli may be completely asymptomatic, but often precede more significant, or lethal, embolism later. For patients with intermediate-sized emboli, a combination of pleuritic chest pain, dyspnoea and tachypnoea is a highly sensitive indicator of pulmonary embolus.[32] Changes in the electrocardiogram following pulmonary embolus reflect disturbed cardiac function secondary to elevated pulmonary arterial pressure and are generally non-specific. Ischaemic changes, particularly T-wave inversion in the anterior leads, do correlate with the severity of the embolism.[33] The gold standard of diagnosis is pulmonary angiography, though this is not feasible in many hospitals. More use is made of pulmonary radioisotope perfusion or ventilation/perfusion scans,[33,34] but several investigations have demonstrated the relatively low sensitivity of the technique,[35] particularly ventilation scans. Data acquisition for computed tomography (CT) is now fast enough to enable imaging of thoracic structures,[36] including pulmonary emboli (Figure 28.5), and magnetic resonance imaging (MRI) can generate detailed images of the pulmonary vasculature.[37] Ultrasound investigations to detect clot in lower limb veins may aid diagnosis, and echocardiography of the heart is useful in patients with cardiac complications following pulmonary embolus.

Pathophysiology.[29,38,39] Three mechanisms give rise to the physiological changes seen in pulmonary embolism. First is physical occlusion of the pulmonary vascular system. Secondly, platelet activation in the thrombus leads to release of 5-hydroxytryptamine (5-HT, serotonin) and thromboxane A_2, causing a further increase in pulmonary vascular resistance.[38] Finally, the right ventricle commonly is unable to overcome the raised pulmonary vascular resistance and cardiac output falls, eventually culminating in heart failure.[40]

The primary respiratory lesion is an increase in alveolar dead space with an increased arterial/end-tidal P_{CO_2} gradient. Carbon dioxide elimination is therefore reduced and if ventilation remains unchanged arterial P_{CO_2} slowly climbs, until elimination is restored in spite of the large dead space.[41] However, in awake patients hypercapnia is unusual because hyperventilation is almost always present and arterial P_{CO_2} is usually below the normal range.[39] The cause of respiratory stimulation is unclear, but may involve stimulation of J-receptors as in air embolism (see below), or hypoxia if present.

Arterial P_{O_2} is also decreased. This results from derangement of normal ventilation/perfusion relationships, coupled with low mixed venous oxygen content because of poor cardiac output (page 185).[39]

Bronchospasm is a well-recognized complication[42] and has been attributed to the 5-HT released from platelets[38] and also to local hypocapnia in the part of the lung without effective pulmonary circulation. Pulmonary compliance may be reduced with large pulmonary emboli, but the mechanism of this change is unknown. Pulmonary infarction, which might be expected to occur, is rarely a problem. The lung can obtain oxygen direct from air in the airways and alveoli, from backflow along pulmonary veins and from the bronchial circulation. Only when these sources are also impaired does infarction occur, for example when localized pulmonary oedema or pulmonary haemorrhage into the airways occurs in conjunction with embolism.

Principles of treatment.[29,30] Anticoagulation with intravenous heparin is the mainstay of treatment and prevents further clot from forming, either in lung or elsewhere, and allows endogenous fibrinolysis to proceed. In more severe cases such as patients with cardiovascular compromise, thrombolysis via a pulmonary artery catheter may be required. In the past, thrombolytic regimens were associated with very high complication rates, such that thrombolysis developed a reputation as a heroic measure reserved for almost fatal cases. Contemporary treatment is however much improved, and believed to be underused in many hospitals.[43] Surgical embolectomy is now reserved for patients with significant pulmonary embolism who are unable to receive, or are unresponsive to, other forms of treatment.

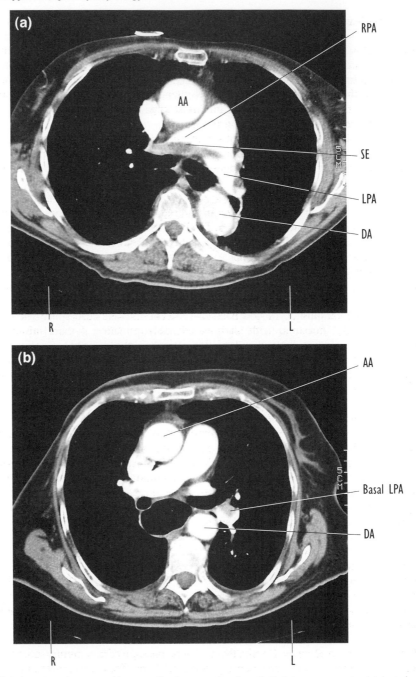

Figure 28.5 Spiral computed tomographic scan of pulmonary thomboemboli. Intravenous contrast injected immediately before scanning makes the blood vessels appear white. Emboli then appear as darker areas within the blood vessel lumen. (a) Saddle embolus (SE) situated mainly in the right pulmonary artery (RPA). (b) Pulmonary embolus in the basal branch of the left pulmonary artery (LPA). AA, ascending aorta; DA, descending aorta. (I am indebted to Celia Craven, Superintendent Radiographer, St James's Hospital, Leeds, for supplying the scans.)

Air embolism

An embolus may arise from pneumothorax and pulmonary barotrauma but is most commonly iatrogenic. In neurosurgery, the usual cause of air embolism is the use of the sitting position for posterior fossa surgery. This results in a subatmospheric venous pressure at the operative site and air may enter dural veins, which are held open by their structure. In open cardiac surgery, it is almost impossible to remove all traces of air from the cardiac chambers before closing the heart.

Some small degree of air embolism is almost inevitable in all types of intravenous therapy, but catastrophic air embolism can occur when compression bags are used to accelerate the flow rate of intravenous fluids or blood bags that already contain air.

Detection of air embolism. Early diagnosis of air embolism is essential in neurosurgery, and there are three principal methods in routine use. Bubbles in circulating blood give a very characteristic sound with a precordial Doppler probe. The method is, if anything, too sensitive, because a shower of very small bubbles produces a particularly large signal. The second method is based on the appearance of nitrogen in the expired air. There should be no significant exhaled nitrogen after the first 15 minutes of an anaesthetic in which the patient breathes a mixture of oxygen and nitrous oxide. The appearance of nitrogen is easily detected with a mass spectrometer and is diagnostic of air entering the circulation. The third and simplest method is based on the end-expired carbon dioxide concentration which is easily measured with an infrared analyser. Many factors influence the end-expiratory concentration but a sudden decrease is likely to be either cardiac arrest or air embolism. Transoesophageal echocardiography is an efficient method of detecting air embolism[44] and, furthermore, is the only practicable method of detecting paradoxical air embolism (see below).

Pathophysiology of air embolus. Provided there is no major intracardiac right-to-left shunt, small quantities of air are filtered out by the lungs where they are gradually excreted and no harm results. Alveolar dead space is increased according to the proportion of the pulmonary circulation that is occluded.[45] The resultant increase in arterial/end-tidal P_{CO_2} gradient is the basis of detection of air embolism by infrared carbon dioxide, as described above. Pulmonary arterial pressure is increased by a large embolus due to the right ventricle working against an increased pulmonary vascular resistance. Finally, in animal studies, airway resistance is increased following air embolism, an effect mediated by arachidonate metabolites, possibly in conjunction with platelet activation and stimulation of pulmonary irritant receptors.[46]

Massive air embolism (probably in excess of 100 ml) may cause cardiac arrest by accumulation in the right ventricle, where compression of the air bubble prevents ventricular ejection of blood. Treatment then requires aspiration of air through a cardiac catheter, which is difficult. In lesser degrees of embolization during surgery, reduced cardiac output probably also contributes to the sudden reduction in end-tidal P_{CO_2}.

Paradoxical air embolism. Rarely, there may be passage of air emboli from the right to left heart without there being an overt right-to-left shunt. This is important because air then enters the systemic arterial circulation where there may be embolism and infarction, particularly of the brain. It is possible to pass a probe through such a foramen ovale in 20–35 per cent of the adult population[47] but paradoxical embolism does not usually occur because pressure is slightly higher in the left atrium than the right. However, under many circumstances, such as following pulmonary embolism, right atrial pressure may be elevated to the point that a transient right-to-left shunt occurs. Performing a Valsalva manoeuvre, for example, causes echocardiographic evidence of right-to-left shunting in 18 per cent of normal individuals.[48] Anaesthesia in the sitting position is associated with elevated right atrial pressure, which exceeds the pulmonary capillary wedge pressure in about half of patients.[49]

The role of paradoxical embolism in neurological damage in divers is described on page 384.

Fat embolism

Fracture of long bones or major orthopaedic surgery may be associated with fat embolism.[50] This term is not strictly correct, as the features of 'fat embolism syndrome' result from embolization of fragments of bone marrow, which are found embedded in the lung at post-mortem. Fat embolism occurs in almost all patients having hip and knee replacement surgery, but clinical sequelae occur in only a small percentage of these.

Microscopic intravascular bone marrow fragments promote intravascular coagulation and platelet adherence, particularly under the conditions of venous stasis present during surgery, and so develop into larger 'mixed' emboli. There is initially an increase in physiological dead space[51] but this is soon accompanied by an increase in shunt,[52] which is probably caused by the release of substances in the lung which cause spasm of the airways and open up anastomotic channels between pulmonary artery and vein.

Lipid seems to pass through the pulmonary circulation to invade the systemic circulation. Surface forces between blood and lipid are much less than between blood and air, and so would not offer the same hindrance to passage through the lungs. In the systemic circulation, fat emboli cause characteristic petechiae in the anterior axillary folds. In addition, fat may be found in the urine and there is often evidence of cerebral involvement.

Amniotic fluid embolism[53]

Amniotic fluid embolism occurs rarely during delivery, but is fatal in half of cases. Death normally results from cardiovascular disturbances and haemorrhage secondary to coagulopathy. Pulmonary vascular resistance is increased, but the reasons for this are very unclear. Amniotic fluid and fetal cells in the circulation may cause no cardiovascular changes, and either an immune-mediated response or intravascular meconium have been suggested as mechanisms causing the clinical syndrome.

Pulmonary hypertension

There are many causes of pulmonary hypertension, which are classified as either primary or secondary (Table 28.1). The latter is much more common, and is therefore considered first.

Secondary pulmonary hypertension

Pulmonary vascular resistance is increased by almost any pulmonary disease that results in chronic hypoxia (Table 28.1). Similar changes occur with intermittent hypoxia caused, for example, by sleep apnoea (Chapter 15). The change is initially temporary and reversible but progresses to become permanent.

Table 28.1 Causes of pulmonary hypertension

Primary	*Secondary*		
	Respiratory	*Cardiac*	*Other*
Primary pulmonary hypertension	COPD	Left heart failure	Sleep apnoea
Hepatopulmonary syndrome	Emphysema	Valvular disease	Lupus
	Pulmonary fibrosis	Congenital disease	Scleroderma
	Cystic fibrosis		Rheumatoid arthritis
	Chronic embolism		HIV infection
			Vasculitis

Valvular disease of the left heart leads to an elevation of pressure in the left atrium. The maintenance of the pulmonary driving pressure requires a corresponding increase of the pulmonary arterial pressure. This may progress to a secondary increase in pulmonary vascular resistance, resulting in further elevation of the pulmonary arterial pressure. A low cardiac output results in reduction of mixed venous Po_2, which also causes increased pulmonary vascular resistance.

Whatever the cause, pulmonary hypertension will ultimately lead to dyspnoea and right ventricular hypertrophy, which may progress to right heart failure (cor pulmonale) and an increase in systemic venous pressure.

Mechanism of hypoxia-induced pulmonary hypertension.[54] Nitric oxide production by pulmonary endothelium contributes to the normal low resistance of the pulmonary vasculature (page 150). Hypoxia has been shown to reduce this basal nitric oxide secretion,[55] and further work has identified reduced production of constitutive nitric oxide synthase as the mechanism.[56]

Treatment should first be directed towards relief of chronic or intermittent hypoxia by improving the underlying condition. The long-term administration of oxygen to such patients, during the day and during sleep, retards the development of pulmonary hypertension, partially reverses established hypertension and improves survival (page 534).[57,58] Vasodilator therapy is complicated by the lack of drugs with specific action on the pulmonary circulation, and is discussed below.

Primary pulmonary hypertension[59,60]

Pulmonary hypertension occurring in the absence of hypoxia is termed primary pulmonary hypertension (PPH), and has a prevalence of approximately 1300 per million. It is a progressive disease, which normally presents in early adulthood with worsening shortness of breath and eventually right heart failure. There is a familial contribution to PPH, and it may rarely be associated with advanced liver disease or the use of some older appetite-suppressant drugs. Prognosis is poor, most patients dying within a few years of diagnosis.

Pathophysiology. The disease is characterized by proliferation of endothelial cells, hypertrophy of pulmonary arterial smooth muscle, and by thrombosis in pulmonary vessels.[61] Abnormal endothelial function is believed to be where the primary defect occurs, and nitric-oxide-related functions are abnormal. The defect seems to arise in communication between endothelial and smooth muscle cells, though this has yet to be fully characterized.

Treatment. The only truly specific pulmonary vasodilator drugs are acetylcholine (infused into the pulmonary artery) and nitric oxide (by inhalation), but both require continuous administration. Calcium channel blockers such as nifedipine and diltiazem are potent pulmonary vasodilators, and though they also have effects on the systemic circulation these are minimal. Prostacyclin is a pulmonary vasodilator in normal subjects (page 148), and recent trials of low dose intravenous prostacyclin in PPH have been promising.

PPH remains a common indication for lung transplantation (Chapter 33).

References

1. DeFouw DO. Ultrastructural features of alveolar epithelial transport. *Am Rev Respir Dis* 1983; **127** (Supp 5): S9–13.
2. Lai-Fook SJ. Mechanical factors in lung liquid distribution. *Annu Rev Physiol* 1993; **55**: 155–79.
3. Staub NA. Pathophysiology of pulmonary oedema. In: Staub NA, Taylor AE, eds. *Edema.* New York: Raven Press, 1984.
4. Meyer BJ, Meyer A, Guyton AC. Interstitial fluid pressure. V. Negative pressure in the lungs. *Circ Res* 1968; **22**: 263–71.
5. Bhattacharya J, Gropper MA, Staub NA. Interstitial fluid pressure gradient measured by micropuncture in excised dog lung. *J Appl Physiol* 1984; **56**: 271–7.
6. Miserocchi G, Negrini D, Gonano C. Direct measurement of interstitial pulmonary pressure in in situ lung with intact pleural space. *J Appl Physiol* 1990; **69**: 2168–74.
7. Bhattacharya J. The microphysiology of lung liquid clearance. *Adv Exp Med Biol* 1995; **381**: 95–108.
8. Negrini D, Passi A, De Luca G, Miserocchi G. Pulmonary interstitial pressure and proteoglycans during development of pulmonary oedema. *Am J Physiol* 1996; **270**: H2000–7.
9. Staub NA. Alveolar flooding and clearance. *Am Rev Respir Dis* 1983; **127** (Supp 5): S44–51.
10. Colacicco G. Arguments against and alternatives for an extracellular surfactant layer in the alveoli of mammalian lung. *J Theor Biol* 1985; **114**: 641–6.
11. Hills BA. The role of lung surfactant. *Br J Anaesth* 1990; **65**: 13–29.
12. West JB, Tsukimoto K, Mathieu-Costello O, Prediletto R. Stress failure in pulmonary capillaries. *J Appl Physiol* 1991; **70**: 1731–42.
13. Tsukimoto K, Mathieu-Costello O, Prediletto R, Elliott AR, West JB. Ultrastructural appearances of pulmonary capillaries at high transmural pressures. *J Appl Physiol* 1991; **71**: 573–82.
14. Laine GA, Allen SJ, Katz J, Gabel JC, Drake RE. Effect of systemic venous pressure elevation on lymph flow and lung edema formation. *J Appl Physiol* 1986; **61**: 1634–8.
15. Smith WS, Matthay MA. Evidence for a hydrostatic mechanism in human neurogenic pulmonary edema. *Chest* 1997; **111**: 1326–33.
16. Pavlin DJ, Nessly ML, Cheney FW. Increased pulmonary vascular permeability as a cause of re-expansion edema in rabbits. *Am Rev Respir Dis* 1981; **124**: 422–7.
17. Schumacker PT. Pulmonary edema, shunt and blood flow distribution. *Intensive Care Med* 1993; **19**: 183–4.
18. Gee MH, Williams DO. Effect of lung inflation on perivascular cuff fluid volume in isolated dog lung lobes. *Microvasc Res* 1979; **17**: 192–6.
19. Paré PD, Warriner B, Baile EM, Hogg JC. Redistribution of pulmonary extravascular water with positive end-expiratory pressure in canine pulmonary edema. *Am Rev Respir Dis* 1983; **127**: 590–3.
20. Mondéjar EF, Mata GV, Càrdenas A, Mansilla A, Cantalejo F, Rivera R. Ventilation with positive end-expiratory pressure reduces extravascular lung water and increases lymphatic flow in hydrostatic pulmonary oedema. *Crit Care Med* 1996; **24**: 1562–7.
21. Gómez CMH, Palazzo MGA. Pulmonary artery catheterization in anaesthesia and intensive care. *Br J*

Anaesth 1998; **81**: 945–56.

22. Cope DK, Grimbert F, Downey JM, Taylor AE. Pulmonary capillary pressure: a review. *Crit Care Med* 1992; **20**: 1043–56.
23. Baconnier PF, Eberhard A, Grimbert FA. Theoretical analysis of occlusion techniques for measuring pulmonary capillary pressure. *J Appl Physiol* 1992; **73**: 1351–9.
24. Cope DK, Allison RC, Parmentier JL, Miller JN, Taylor AE. Measurement of effective pulmonary capillary pressure using the pressure profile after pulmonary artery occlusion. *Crit Care Med* 1986; **14**: 16–22.
25. Soni N. Swan song for the Swan–Ganz catheter. *BMJ* 1996; **313**: 763–4.
26. Jones JG, Royston D, Minty BD. Changes in alveolar–capillary barrier function in animals and humans. *Am Rev Respir Dis* 1983; **127** (Supp 5): S51–9.
27. Godje O, Peyerl M, Seebauer T, Dewald O, Reichart B. Reproducibility of double indicator dilution measurements of intrathoracic blood volume compartments, extravascular lung water, and liver function. *Chest* 1998; **113**: 1070–7.
28. Moser KM. Venous thromboembolism. *Am Rev Respir Dis* 1990; **141**: 235–49.
29. Goldhaber SZ. Pulmonary embolism. *N Engl J Med* 1998; **339**: 93–104.
30. British Thoracic Society. Suspected pulmonary embolism: a practical approach. *Thorax* 1997; **52** (Supp 4): S1–24.
31. Ryu JH, Olson EJ, Pellikka PA. Clinical recognition of pulmonary embolism: problem of unrecognized and asymptomatic cases. *Mayo Clin Proc* 1998; **73**: 873–9.
32. Stein PD, Terrin ML, Hales CA, Palevsky HI, Saltzman HA, Thompson BT, Weg JG. Clinical, laboratory, roentgenographic, and electrocardiographic findings in patients with acute pulmonary embolism and no pre-existing cardiac or pulmonary disease. *Chest* 1991; **100**: 598–603.
33. Bone RC. Ventilation/perfusion scan in pulmonary embolism. *JAMA* 1990; **263**: 2794–5.
34. Morrell NW, Seed WA. Diagnosing pulmonary embolism. *BMJ* 1992; **304**: 1126–7.
35. PIOPED investigators. Value of the ventilation/perfusion scan in acute pulmonary embolism: results of the Prospective Investigation of Pulmonary Embolism Diagnosis (PIOPED). *JAMA* 1990; **263**: 2753–9.
36. Hansell DM, Flower CDR. Imaging pulmonary embolism. *BMJ* 1998; **316**: 490–1.
37. Meaney JFM, Weg JG, Chenevert TL, Stafford-Johnson D, Hamilton BH, Prince MR. Diagnosis of pulmonary embolism with magnetic resonance imaging. *N Engl J Med* 1997; **336**: 1422–7.
38. Elliott CG. Pulmonary physiology during pulmonary embolism. *Chest* 1992; **101**: 163S–71S.
39. Santolicandro A, Prediletto R, Fornai E, Formichi B, Begliomini E, Giannella-Neto A, Giuntini C. Mechanisms of hypoxemia and hypocapnia in pulmonary embolism. *Am J Respir Crit Care Med* 1995; **152**: 336–47.
40. Lualdi JC, Goldhaber SZ. Right ventricular dysfunction after acute pulmonary embolism: pathophysiologic factors, detection, and therapeutic implications. *Am Heart J* 1995; **130**: 1276–82.
41. Breen PH, Mazumdar B, Skinner SC. How does experimental pulmonary embolism decrease CO_2 elimination? *Respir Physiol* 1996; **105**: 217–24.
42. Windebank WJ, Boyd G, Moran F. Pulmonary thromboembolism presenting as asthma. *BMJ* 1973; **1**: 90–4.
43. Goldhaber SZ. Contemporary pulmonary embolism thrombolysis. *Chest* 1995; **107**: 45S–51S.
44. Furuya H, Okumura F. Detection of paradoxical air embolism by transesophageal echocardiography. *Anesthesiology* 1984; **60**: 374–7.
45. Severinghaus JW, Stupfel M. Alveolar dead space as an index of distribution of blood flow in pulmonary capillaries. *J Appl Physiol* 1957; **10**: 335–48.
46. Chen HF, Lee BP, Kou YR. Mechanisms underlying stimulation of rapidly adapting receptors during pulmonary air embolism in dogs. *Respir Physiol* 1997; **109**: 1–13.
47. Hagen PT, Scholz DG, Edwards WD. Incidence and size of patent foramen ovale during the first 10 decades of life: an autopsy study of 965 normal hearts. *Mayo Clin Proc* 1984; **59**: 17–20.
48. Lynch JJ, Schuchard GH, Gross CM, Wann LS. Prevalence of right-to-left shunting in the healthy population: detection by Valsalva maneuver contrast echocardiography. *Am J Cardiol* 1984; **53**: 1478–80.
49. Perkins-Pearson NAK, Marshall WK, Bedford RF. Atrial pressures in the seated position. *Anesthesiology* 1982; **57**: 493–7.
50. Hofmann S, Huemer G, Salzer M. Pathophysiology and management of the fat embolism syndrome. *Anaesthesia* 1998; **53** (Supp 2): 35–7.
51. Greenbaum R, Nunn JF, Prys-Roberts C, Kelman GR, Silk FF. Cardiopulmonary function after fat

embolism. *Br J Anaesth* 1965; **37**: 554–5.

52. Prys-Roberts C, Greenbaum R, Nunn JF, Kelman GR. Disturbances of pulmonary function in patients with fat embolism. *J Clin Pathol* 1970; **23** (Supp 4): 143–9.

53. McDougall RJ, Duke GJ. Amniotic fluid embolism syndrome: case report and review. *Anaesth Intensive Care* 1995; **23**: 735–40.

54. Higenbottam T, Cremona G. Acute and chronic hypoxic pulmonary hypertension. *Eur Respir J* 1993; **6**: 1207–12.

55. Adnot S, Raffestin B. Pulmonary hypertension: NO therapy? *Thorax* 1996; **51**: 762–4.

56. McQuillan L, Leung G, Marsden P, Kostyk S, Kourembanas S. Hypoxia inhibits expression of NOS via transcriptional and posttranscriptional mechanisms. *Am J Physiol* 1994; **36**: H1921–7.

57. Timms RM, Khaja FU, Williams GW. Hemodynamic response to oxygen therapy in chronic obstructive pulmonary disease. *Ann Intern Med* 1985; **102**: 29–34.

58. Flenley DC. Long-term home oxygen therapy. *Chest* 1985; **87**: 99–102.

59. Rubin LJ. Primary pulmonary hypertension. *N Engl J Med* 1997; **336**: 111–17.

60. Gaine SP, Rubin LJ. Primary pulmonary hypertension. *Lancet* 1998; **352**: 719–25.

61. Rich S. Clinical insights into the pathogenesis of primary pulmonary hypertension. *Chest* 1998; **114**: 237S–41S.

Chapter 29

Parenchymal lung disease

Pulmonary collapse

Pulmonary collapse may be defined as an acquired state in which the lungs or part of the lungs become airless. Atelectasis is strictly defined as a state in which the lungs of a newborn have never been expanded, but the term is often used loosely as a synonym for collapse.

Pulmonary collapse during anaesthesia is described in Chapter 21.

Collapse may be caused by two different mechanisms. The first of these is loss of the forces opposing the elastic recoil of the lung, which then decreases in volume to the point at which airways are closed and gas is trapped behind the closed airways. The second is obstruction of airways at normal lung volume, which may be due to many different causes. This also results in trapping of gas behind the obstructed airway. Whatever the cause of the airway closure, there is rapid absorption of the trapped gas because the total partial pressure of gases in mixed venous blood is always less than atmospheric (page 493). This generates a subatmospheric pressure more than sufficient to overcome any force tending to hold the lung expanded.

Loss of forces opposing retraction of the lung

The lungs are normally prevented from collapse by the outward elastic recoil of the ribcage and any resting tone of the diaphragm. The pleural cavity normally contains no gas but, if a small bubble of gas is introduced, its pressure is subatmospheric (see Figure 3.4). Pulmonary collapse due to loss of forces opposing lung retraction may be considered under five headings as follows.

Voluntary reduction of lung volume. It seems unlikely that voluntary reduction of lung volume below closing capacity will cause overt collapse of lung in a subject breathing air. However, in older subjects, there is an increase in the alveolar/arterial P_{O_2} gradient, suggesting trapping of alveolar gas (see Figure 21.11). If the subject has been breathing 100% oxygen, absorption collapse may follow reduction of lung volume (see below).

Excessive external pressure. Ventilatory failure is the more prominent aspect of an external environmental pressure in excess of about 6 kPa (60 cmH$_2$O), which is not communicated to the airways (page 517). However, some degree of pulmonary collapse could also occur and this is a normal consequence of the great depths attained by diving mammals while breath holding. An approximately normal lung volume is maintained during conventional diving operations when respired gas is kept at the surrounding water pressure, though this does not occur with surface diving or snorkelling (page 378).

Loss of integrity of the ribcage. Multiple rib fractures or the old operation of thoracoplasty may impair the elastic recoil of the ribcage to the point at which partial lung collapse results. This depends entirely on the extent of the injury to the ribcage, but six or more ribs fractured in two places will usually result in collapse. However, extensive trauma to the ribcage also causes interference with the mechanics of breathing that is generally more serious than collapse (page 517).

Intrusion of abdominal contents into the chest. Extensive atelectasis results from a congenital defect of the diaphragm. Abdominal contents may completely fill one-half of the chest with total atelectasis of that lung. In adults, similar changes may occur with a large hiatus hernia. Paralysis of one side of the diaphragm causes the diaphragm to lie higher in the chest, with a tendency to basal collapse on that side. An extensive abdominal mass (e.g. tumour or ascites) may force the diaphragm into the chest.

Space occupation of the pleural cavity. Air introduced into the pleural cavity reduces the forces opposing retraction of the lung and this is a potent cause of collapse. A *closed pneumothorax* is a fixed volume of air in the pleural cavity causing collapse in relation to the volume of air introduced. The intrapleural pressure rises in proportion to the volume of air in the cavity and is above atmospheric in a *tension pneumothorax*. The affected lung is then totally collapsed and the mediastinum is displaced towards the opposite side. This is a life-threatening condition requiring immediate relief of the pressure. An *open pneumothorax* communicates with the atmosphere and results in pendulum breathing in addition to collapse. The pleural cavity may also be occupied by an effusion, empyema or a haemothorax. All of these may result in collapse.

Absorption of trapped gas

Absorption of alveolar gas trapped beyond obstructed airways may be the consequence of reduction in lung volume by the mechanisms described above. However, it is the primary cause of collapse when there is total or partial airway obstruction at normal lung volume. Obstruction is commonly due to secretions, pus, blood or tumour but may be due to intense local bronchospasm or mucosal oedema.

Gas trapped beyond the point of airway closure is absorbed by the pulmonary blood flow. The total of the partial pressures of the gases in mixed venous blood is always less than atmospheric (see Table 25.2), although pressure gradients for the individual component gases between alveolar gas and mixed venous blood may be quite different.

The effect of respired gases. If the patient has been breathing 100% oxygen prior to obstruction, the alveoli will contain only oxygen, carbon dioxide and water vapour. Because the last two together normally amount to less than 13.3 kPa (100 mmHg), the alveolar Po_2 will usually be in excess of 88 kPa (660 mmHg). However, the Po_2 of the mixed venous blood is unlikely to exceed about 6.7 kPa (50 mmHg), so the alveolar/mixed venous Po_2 gradient will be of the order of 80 per cent of an atmosphere. Absorption collapse will thus be rapid and there will be no nitrogen in the alveolar gas to maintain

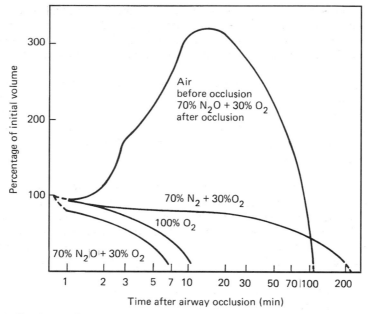

Figure 29.1 Predicted rates of absorption from alveoli of differing gas mixtures. The lower curves show the rate of absorption of the contents of sections of the lung whose air passages are obstructed, resulting in sequestration of the contents. The upper curve shows the expansion of the sequestered gas when nitrous oxide is breathed by a patient who has recently developed regional airway obstruction while breathing air. In all other cases, it is assumed that the inspired gas is not changed after obstruction has occurred. Similar considerations apply to closed gas cavities elsewhere in the body. (Reproduced from reference 2 by permission of the authors and the Editor of *Anaesthesia*.)

inflation. This has important implications during anaesthesia, when 100% oxygen is commonly administered (page 434).

The situation is much more favourable in a patient who has been breathing air, as most of the alveolar gas is then nitrogen which is at a tension only about 0.5 kPa (4 mmHg) below that of mixed venous blood.[1] Alveolar nitrogen tension rises above that of mixed venous blood as oxygen is absorbed and eventually the nitrogen will be fully absorbed. Collapse must eventually occur but the process is much slower than in the patient who has been breathing oxygen. Figure 29.1 shows a computer simulation of the time required for collapse with various gas mixtures.[2] Nitrous oxide/oxygen mixtures may be expected to be absorbed almost as rapidly as 100% oxygen. This is partly because nitrous oxide is much more soluble in blood than nitrogen, and partly because the mixed venous tension of nitrous oxide is usually much less than the alveolar tension, except after a long period of inhalation.

When the inspired gas composition is changed *after* obstruction and trapping occur, complex patterns of absorption may ensue. The inhalation of nitrous oxide, after airway occlusion has occurred while breathing air, results in temporary expansion of the trapped volume (Figure 29.1). This is caused by large volumes of the more soluble nitrous oxide passing from blood to alveolus in exchange for smaller volumes of the less soluble nitrogen passing in the reverse direction. This phenomenon also applies to any closed air space in the body, such as closed pneumothorax, gas emboli, bowel, and the middle ear with a blocked pharyngotympanic (eustachian) tube. It is potentially dangerous and may contraindicate the use of nitrous oxide as an anaesthetic.

Magnitude of the pressure gradients. It must be stressed that the forces generated by the absorption of trapped gases are very large. The total partial pressure of gases in mixed venous blood is normally 87.4 kPa (656 mmHg). The corresponding pressure of the alveolar gases is 95.1 kPa (713 mmHg), allowing for water vapour pressure at 37°C. The difference, 7.7 kPa (57 mmHg or 77 cmH$_2$O), is sufficient to overcome any forces opposing recoil of the lung. Absorption collapse after breathing air may therefore result in drawing the diaphragm up into the chest, reducing ribcage volume or displacing the mediastinum. If the patient has been breathing oxygen, the total partial pressure of gases in the mixed venous blood is barely a tenth of an atmosphere (see Table 25.2) and absorption of trapped alveolar gas generates enormous forces.

Effect of reduced ventilation/perfusion ratio. Absorption collapse may still occur in the absence of total airway obstruction provided that the ventilation/perfusion ($\dot{V}/\dot{Q}$) ratio is sufficiently reduced. It is now well established that older subjects as well as those with a pathological increase in scatter of $\dot{V}/\dot{Q}$ ratios may have substantial perfusion of areas of lung with $\dot{V}/\dot{Q}$ ratios in the range 0.01–0.10. This shows as a characteristic 'shelf' in the plot of perfusion against $\dot{V}/\dot{Q}$ (Figure 29.2). These grossly hypoventilated areas are liable to collapse if the patient breathes oxygen (Figure 29.2b). If the $\dot{V}/\dot{Q}$ ratio is less than 0.05, ventilation even with 100% oxygen cannot replace the oxygen that is removed (assuming the normal arterial/mixed venous oxygen content difference of 0.05 ml.ml^{-1}). As the $\dot{V}/\dot{Q}$ ratio decreases below 0.05, so the critical inspired oxygen concentration necessary for collapse also decreases (Figure 29.2c). The flat part of the curve between $\dot{V}/\dot{Q}$ ratios of 0.001 and 0.004 means that small differences in inspired oxygen concentration in the range 20–30% may be very important in determining whether collapse occurs. There is no difficulty in demonstrating that pulmonary collapse may be induced in healthy middle-aged subjects breathing oxygen close to residual volume.[3,4]

Perfusion through the collapsed lung[7]

Perfusion through collapsed lung tissue is one of the most important causes of intrapulmonary shunting. At least in the short term, some perfusion continues through the collapsed area and this is regulated mainly by hypoxic pulmonary vasoconstriction. In the absence of alveolar gas, the P_{O_2} that governs pulmonary vascular resistance is the mixed venous P_{O_2} (page 151). It has been observed that, in the presence of collapse, the shunt fraction of the pulmonary blood flow is directly proportional to the cardiac output (page 185), and this has been attributed to the effect of cardiac output on the mixed venous P_{O_2}. Thus, with a reduced cardiac output, the mixed venous P_{O_2} will be reduced and hypoxic pulmonary vasoconstriction in the area of the collapse will be increased. Therefore the shunt fraction will be decreased. However, the blood flowing through the shunt is more desaturated and these two effects counteract each other, so the arterial P_{O_2} is little changed (page 185).

Diagnosis of pulmonary collapse

The diagnosis may be made on physical signs of decreased air entry and chest dullness but reliance is usually placed on chest radiography. Pulmonary opacification is seen, along with indirect signs of thoracic volume loss such as displacement of interlobular fissures,

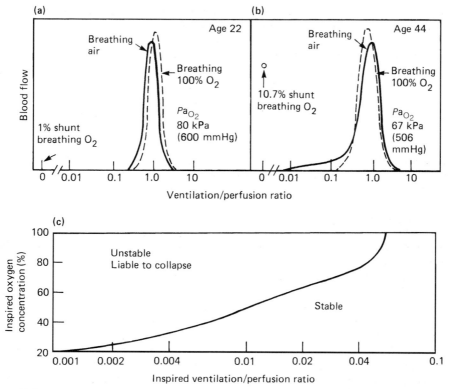

Figure 29.2 Inspiration of 100% oxygen causes collapse of alveoli with very low $\dot{V}/\dot{Q}$ ratios. (a) The minor change in the distribution of blood flow (in relation to $\dot{V}/\dot{Q}$ ratio) when a young subject breathes oxygen. Collapse is minimal and a shunt of 1% develops. (b) The changes in an older subject with a 'shelf' of blood flow distributed to alveoli with very low $\dot{V}/\dot{Q}$ ratios. Breathing oxygen causes collapse of these alveoli and this is manifested by disappearance of the shelf and development of an intrapulmonary shunt of 10.7%. (c) The inspired oxygen concentration relative to the inspired $\dot{V}/\dot{Q}$ ratio that is critical for absorption collapse. (Redrawn from reference 5 by permission of the authors and the Editor of the *Journal of Clinical Investigation*, and from reference 6 by permission of the authors and the Editor of *Journal of Applied Physiology*.)

raised diaphragms and displaced hilar or mediastinal structures.[8] In the upright position, collapse is commonest in the basal segments, often concealed behind the cardiac shadow unless the exposure is appropriate. Collapse in the supine position may well occur in the dorsal parts of the lung, which are then dependent. This is not easy to detect radiologically, because the collapsed areas may form a thin sheet parallel to the X-ray plate in an anteroposterior exposure. Areas of atelectasis are clearly seen with computed tomography (see Figure 21.10).

Collapse results in a reduction in pulmonary compliance, but its value in diagnosis is limited by the wide scatter in normal values. A sudden reduction may give an indication of collapse, provided, of course, that control measurements were available before collapse.

Collapse also reduces the functional residual capacity and arterial Po_2. However, in a study of absorption collapse, there was little to choose between these measurements and changes in the chest radiograph for the detection of minimal collapse.[4] When present, it was detected by all three methods. In patients undergoing intensive care, a reduction in arterial P_{O_2} cannot distinguish between the three very common conditions of pulmonary collapse, consolidation and oedema.

Treatment

This should be directed at the cause. Factors opposing the elastic recoil of the lung should be removed wherever possible. For example, pneumothorax, pleural effusion and ascites may be corrected. In other cases, particularly impaired integrity of the chest wall, it may be preferable to treat the patient with intermittent positive pressure ventilation. Re-expansion of collapsed lung often requires high pressures to be applied (page 434), but it is usually possible to restore normal lung volume.

When collapse is caused by regional airway obstruction, the most useful methods in both treatment and prevention are by chest physiotherapy, combined when necessary with tracheobronchial toilet through either a tracheal tube or a bronchoscope. Fibreoptic bronchoscopy alone will often clear an obstructed airway and permit re-expansion.

A logical approach is hyperinflation of the chest or an artificial 'sigh'. Some ventilators were designed to provide an intermittent 'sigh' but evidence of its efficacy is elusive. However, voluntary maximal inspirations have been effective in clearing areas of absorption collapse in subjects who had been breathing oxygen near residual volume.[4] The process imparted a distinctive tearing sensation in the chest, but rapidly restored to normal both chest radiograph and arterial P_{O_2}. This process is the basis of the 'incentive spirometer' as a means of preventing postoperative lung collapse.

Pulmonary consolidation (pneumonia)

Inflammation of areas of lung parenchyma, usually due to infection, can lead to the accumulation of exudate in the alveoli and small airways, causing consolidation. Areas of consolidation may be patchy, and referred to as bronchopneumonia, or confined to discrete areas of the lung, forming lobar pneumonia. Pulmonary collapse frequently occurs in conjunction with pneumonia as a result of airway narrowing in surrounding lung areas. Clinical features of pyrexia, cough, sputum production and dyspnoea occur with signs of consolidation such as bronchial breathing, chest dullness and inspiratory crackles, though physical signs may be absent in bronchopneumonia. Diagnosis again relies on chest radiography, where consolidation appears as pulmonary shadowing, sometimes accompanied by an 'air bronchogram'. Presence or absence of radiographic signs of reduced chest volume (see above) helps to differentiate between collapse and consolidation. With resolution of the infection, cough becomes more productive, and the lung returns to normal within a few weeks.

Effects on gas exchange.[9] Patients with pneumonia are commonly hypoxic. Consolidated areas of lung behave in a fashion similar to collapse, forming an intrapulmonary shunt through which mixed venous blood flows. In addition, there is an increase in areas with low $\dot{V}/\dot{Q}$ ratio (<0.1), but the contribution of these areas to impaired oxygenation is believed to be small because of hypoxic pulmonary vasoconstriction. Administration of oxygen to patients with pneumonia causes a further widening of the scatter of $\dot{V}/\dot{Q}$ ratios (page 173), implying a reduction in hypoxic pulmonary vasoconstriction,[9] but nevertheless results in a considerable improvement in arterial P_{O_2}. In comparison with collapsed lung, consolidation is commonly associated with a worse pulmonary shunt and therefore more severe hypoxia. Many of the inflammatory mediators released as part of the response to infection act as local pulmonary vasodilators, in effect overriding hypoxic pulmonary vasoconstriction.[7]

Pathophysiology of pneumonia

Airway inflammation was described in detail in Chapter 27. Invasion of the lower respiratory tract with viruses and bacteria leads to further inflammatory changes characterized by migration of neutrophils from the circulation into the lung tissue. These cells, along with alveolar macrophages, provoke the production of an inflammatory exudate that leads to consolidation of the lung tissue. The exudate is a complex mixture of invading organisms, inflammatory cells (dead and alive), immunoglobulins and other immune mediators, fluid transudate from increased capillary permeability, and products resulting from destruction of lung tissue as a result of proteolytic enzyme release.

Margination of neutrophils. Before a neutrophil can contribute to the inflammatory response it must stick to the blood vessel wall (margination), migrate across the endothelium, interstitium and epithelium, and become activated ready to contribute to pathogen removal (see Figure 30.3). These activities are controlled by an extensive, and incompletely understood, series of cytokines in a fashion very similar to airway inflammation (see Figure 27.1). Lymphocytes again play an important role, but in parenchymal inflammation macrophages have an important control function instead of eosinophils and mast cells as in the airway.

High blood flow through the pulmonary circulation provides a plentiful supply of neutrophils for margination. Adhesion molecules on the endothelial cell (e.g. intercellular adhesion molecule-1, ICAM-1) bind to specific receptors on the neutrophil surface (e.g. β_2-integrins CD11/CD18).[10] Once 'caught' by the endothelial cell, cytokines are released and neutrophil activation begins. The way in which neutrophils are marginated in the lung differs from elsewhere in the body.[11] Adhesion to endothelial cells occurs in the pulmonary capillary, rather than in venules as in the systemic circulation. Adhesion is facilitated by a slow transit time for neutrophils across pulmonary capillaries. Human neutrophils are of similar size to red blood cells, but are much less deformable such that the neutrophils takes up to 120 seconds to traverse a capillary compared with less than 1 second for an erythrocyte.[11]

Interstitial lung disease and pulmonary fibrosis

Diffuse pulmonary inflammation occurs in a wide variety of conditions, which are summarized in Table 29.1. Pneumonitis may simply resolve, as in pneumonia, leaving no permanent damage, but with long-term inflammation pulmonary fibrosis develops.

Clinical features vary according to the aetiology. Pneumonitis alone (i.e. without fibrosis) may be asymptomatic at first, progressing to a cough and dyspnoea, and in severe cases gives rise to systemic symptoms such as fever. When accompanied by fibrosis, dyspnoea becomes worse, and basal inspiratory crackles are present on examination. Lung function tests show a typical 'restrictive' pattern with similar reductions in both forced vital capacity and forced expiratory volume in 1 second (page 134). Diffuse reticular shadows develop on chest radiography, and CT scanning of the lungs shows either 'ground glass'

Table 29.1 Causes of interstitial pneumonitis and pulmonary fibrosis[12,13]

Causes	Subgroups	Examples
Drug induced	Anti-cancer	Bleomycin, busulphan, cyclophosphamide, methotrexate
	Antibiotics	Isoniazid, nitrofurantoin, sulphonamides
	Others	Amiodarone
Dust	Inorganic	Silicosis Asbestosis
	Organic	Farmer's lung
Infections	Viral	Viral pneumonia HIV
	Other	*Mycoplasma* Opportunistic infections
Systemic disease	Connective tissue disease	Rheumatoid arthritis, scleroderma, systemic lupus erythematosus, ankylosing spondylitis
	Others	Sarcoidosis, histiocytosis, uraemia
Miscellaneous	Acute inflammation	Acute lung injury, adult respiratory distress syndrome
	Inhalation injury	Smoke, cadmium, sulphur dioxide
	Radiation lung damage	
	Cryptogenic fibrosing alveolitis	

appearances, which correlate with pneumonitis, or 'honeycombing', which represents more advanced fibrosis.[10]

Pathophysiology of pulmonary fibrosis

Lung inflammation has been described earlier in this chapter as well as in Chapters 27 and 30. Progression to pulmonary fibrosis is not inevitable, but predicting which patients, and which underlying diseases, do so is important clinically. Being male and smoking both indicate a worse prognosis from pulmonary fibrosis, as does increased numbers of inflammatory cells in bronchoalveolar lavage fluid.[10] These observations contributed to extensive research into the mechanisms of fibrosis, though, so far, a useful prognostic test remains a distant prospect.

Inflammation anywhere in the body is naturally succeeded by a cellular healing process that involves the laying down of new collagen. The lung is no exception, and pulmonary fibrosis is a result of excessive deposition of collagen in the lung extracellular matrix. In a similar fashion to emphysema (page 532), repeated repair of lung tissue leads to a reduction in the amount of elastin present. Synthesis of elastin in normal lung is minimal in adults, and, though there is some evidence of increased production in pulmonary fibrosis, the elastic fibres formed are abnormal and probably non-functional.[14] Loss of elasticity by this mechanism causes collapse of both alveolar and small airway walls, leading to a reduction in compliance and the area available for gas exchange.

In pulmonary fibrosis the initial disease process is diverse (Table 29.1), and may cause changes in type II pneumocytes (page 30), pulmonary macrophages, neutrophils or T-lymphocytes.[15,16] Interactions between these cells produce numerous cytokines, of which transforming growth factor β (TGF-β) is believed to be the most important. This cytokine probably acts as the final common pathway for most mechanisms leading to fibrosis.[15] Unknown chemoattractant substances recruit fibroblasts into the lung interstitium, following which tumour necrosis factor α (TNF-α) and TGF-β cause *in situ* fibroblast proliferation. Collagen synthesis is then stimulated by TGF-β, which also inhibits the activity of collagenase.

Smoking will stimulate fibrosis by continuous activation of inflammatory cells (page 412). Other individual variations in fibrotic potential presumably relate to both genetic and disease-specific differences in patterns of cytokine production and cellular activity.

Causes of pulmonary fibrosis

These have been summarized in Table 29.1.

Drug-induced fibrosis may follow lung injury induced by oxygen toxicity (page 502) precipitated by, for example, bleomycin, but for many drugs the mechanism is unknown.

Inorganic dusts.[17] Occupational exposure to asbestos fibres (asbestosis) or silica (silicosis) for many years leads to pulmonary fibrosis. Inhaled dust particles between 1 and 3 μm in diameter reach the alveoli and are ingested by macrophages.[18] Different dust types have variable persistence in the lung, some being rapidly cleared and others persisting in the pulmonary macrophage for many years. In addition, the total (lifetime) fibre burden probably correlates with the degree of resulting fibrosis. Macrophages containing silica dust particles mediate the stimulation of fibroblasts by production of interleukin-1 and TGF-β,[19] though other cells and cytokines are also involved.[17]

Organic dusts may cause lung inflammation by an immune mechanism, a condition referred to as extrinsic allergic alveolitis. The allergen is normally derived from a fungus to which the patient has occupational exposure, giving rise to a host of disease names such as farmer's lung, malt worker's lung, etc. Bird fancier's lung differs in that it is precipitated by exposure to IgA derived from domestic birds. In extrinsic allergic alveolitis, pneumonitis results from activation of T-lymphocytes and IgG-mediated inflammation. If caught early enough, and avoidance measures are taken, allergic alveolitis resolves completely, but fibrosis develops with continued exposure.

Systemic diseases that lead to fibrosis are numerous and the mechanisms obscure. Many of the diseases associated with lung fibrosis have an immunological basis. For example, sarcoidosis results from T-lymphocyte activation in response to an unknown stimulus, whilst many connective tissue diseases are well known to have an autoimmune aetiology. These immune changes are therefore likely to cause activation of the pulmonary inflammatory cells already described.[18] Recurrent lung infections and some drugs used for treating systemic diseases may also contribute to the pulmonary complications seen.

Radiation lung damage[20] is seen after radiotherapy for tumours in or near the chest. Radiation pneumonitis develops over several weeks following radiotherapy, whilst fibrosis may take up to two years to develop. Cellular radiation damage occurs when cell division occurs, so susceptible cells in the lung are those with the greatest rate of turnover. Thus radiation injury begins with damage to type II pneumocytes and capillary endothelial cells, which results in altered surfactant and interstitial pulmonary oedema (page 542) respectively. A cascade of inflammatory cell activation will again follow, including increased macrophage production of TGF-β, and may persist for several months after a relatively short period of irradiation.[21]

Cryptogenic fibrosing alveolitis (CFA),[12,13,22] synonymous with idiopathic pulmonary fibrosis, includes all cases of pulmonary fibrosis in which no cause can be found. It is the most common type of pulmonary fibrosis and occurs almost exclusively in males.[12] The aetiology is uncertain, but with a genetic susceptibility, viral infection and environmental influences all being involved.[13] Patients with CFA have extensive activation of pulmonary inflammatory cells and cytokines described above, as well as a reduced production of interferon-γ which normally suppresses T-lymphocyte activity.[23] There is also accumulation of neutrophils, and this indicates a role for pulmonary oxidant injury (page 500) in CFA. Whatever the cause, CFA is rapidly progressive, with a median survival from diagnosis of just a few years.

Treatment of pulmonary fibrosis[12,13]

Where feasible, removal of the stimulant for lung inflammation or fibrosis is vital. Although this may not halt the development of fibrosis, for example following irradiation, it may limit the degree of pulmonary damage that occurs. Less than a fifth of patients with CFA gain any benefit from treatment with steroids, and predicting who will respond is difficult. More specific immunosuppression of T-lymphocytes with cyclosporin provides some benefit.

Recent elucidation of the cytokines involved in pulmonary fibrosis, particularly TGF-β, has led to optimism about future therapeutic approaches.[24,25] Antibodies to TGF-β do attenuate fibrosis in experimental models, but there are considerable potential risks involved in non-specific removal of a fundamental inflammatory cytokine.[26]

References

1. Klocke FJ, Rahn H. The arterial–alveolar inert gas ('N$_2$') difference in normal and emphysematous subjects, as indicated by the analysis of urine. *J Clin Invest* 1961; **40**: 286–94.
2. Webb SJS, Nunn JF. A comparison between the effect of nitrous oxide and nitrogen on arterial Po$_2$. *Anaesthesia* 1967; **22**: 69–81.
3. Nunn JF, Coleman AJ, Sachithanandan T, Bergman NA, Laws JW. Hypoxaemia and atelectasis produced by forced expiration. *Br J Anaesth* 1965; **37**: 3–12.
4. Nunn JF, Williams IP, Jones JG, Hewlett AM, Hulands GH, Minty BD. Detection and reversal of pulmonary absorption collapse. *Br J Anaesth* 1978; **50**: 91–100.
5. Wagner PD, Laravuso RB, Uhl RR, West JB. Continuous distributions of ventilation–perfusion ratios in normal subjects breathing air and 100% O$_2$. *J Clin Invest* 1974; **54**: 54–68.
6. Dantzker DR, Wagner PD, West JB. Instability of lung units with low V$_A$/Q ratios during O$_2$ breathing. *J Appl Physiol* 1975; **38**: 886–95.
7. Marshall BE, Hanson CW, Frasch F, Marshall C. Role of hypoxic pulmonary vasoconstriction in pulmonary gas exchange and blood flow distribution. 2. Pathophysiology. *Intensive Care Med* 1994; **20**: 379–89.
8. Woodring JH, Reed JC. Types and mechanisms of pulmonary atelectasis. *J Thorac Imaging* 1996; **11**: 92–108.

9. Gea J, Roca J, Torres A, Agusti AGN, Wagner PD, Rodriguez-Roisin R. Mechanisms of abnormal gas exchange in patients with pneumonia. *Anesthesiology* 1991; **75**: 782–9.

10. Ward PA, Hunninghake GW. Lung inflammation and fibrosis. *Am J Respir Crit Care Med* 1998; **157**: S123–9.

11. Hogg JC, Walker BA. Polymorphonuclear leucocyte traffic in lung inflammation. *Thorax* 1995; **50**: 819–20.

12. Egan JJ, Hasleton PS. Cryptogenic fibrosing alveolitis: diagnosis and treatment. *Hosp Med* 1998; **59**: 364–8.

13. Chan-Yeung M, Müller NL. Cryptogenic fibrosing alveolitis. *Lancet* 1997; **350**: 651–6.

14. Pierce RA, Mariani TJ, Senior RM. Elastin in lung development and disease. *Ciba Found Symp* 1995; **192**: 199–214.

15. Bienkowski RS, Gotkin MG. Control of collagen deposition in mammalian lung. *Proc Soc Exp Biol Med* 1995; **209**: 118–40.

16. Kumar RK, Lykke AWJ. Messages and handshakes: cellular interactions in pulmonary fibrosis. *Pathology* 1995; **27**: 18–26.

17. Mossman BT, Churg A. Mechanisms in the pathogenesis of asbestosis and silicosis. *Am J Respir Crit Care Med* 1998; **157**: 1666–80.

18. Greenberger PA. Immunological aspects of lung diseases and cystic fibrosis. *JAMA* 1997; **278**: 1924–30.

19. Jagirdar J, Begin R, Dufresne A, Goswami S, Lee TC, Rom WN. Transforming growth factor-β (TGF-β) in silicosis. *Am J Respir Crit Care Med* 1996; **154**: 1076–81.

20. Movsas B, Raffin TA, Epstein AH, Link CJ. Pulmonary radiation injury. *Chest* 1997; **111**: 1061–76.

21. Rubin P, Johnston CJ, Williams JP, McDonald S, Finkelstein JN. A perpetual cascade of cytokines postirradiation leads to pulmonary fibrosis. *Int J Radiat Oncol Biol Phys* 1995; **33**: 99–109.

22. Katzenstein AA, Myers JL. Idiopathic pulmonary fibrosis: clinical relevance of pathologic classification. *Am J Respir Crit Care Med* 1998; **157**: 1301–15.

23. Prior C, Haslam PL. *In vivo* levels and *in vitro* production of interferon-gamma in fibrosing interstitial lung diseases. *Clin Exp Immunol* 1992; **88**: 280–7.

24. Goldstein RH, Fine A. Potential therapeutic initiatives for fibrogenic lung diseases. *Chest* 1995; **108**: 848–55.

25. Phan SH. New strategies for treatment of pulmonary fibrosis. *Thorax* 1995; **50**: 415–21.

26. Shull MM, Ormsby I, Kier AB, Pawlowski S, Diebold RJ, Yin M et al. Targeted disruption of the mouse transforming growth factor-β1 gene results in multifocal inflammatory disease. *Nature* 1992; **359**: 693–9.

Chapter 30

Acute lung injury

Acute lung injury has features in common with several of the pulmonary diseases described in the preceding four chapters, but is considered separately here. The topic has been reviewed often in recent years.[1,2,3,4,5]

Terminology. Acute lung injury (ALI) describes a characteristic form of parenchymal lung disease, and represents a wide range of severity from short-lived dyspnoea to a rapidly terminal failure of the respiratory system, when the term acute respiratory distress (ARDS) is normally used. This was first described in 1967 when Ashbaugh et al.[6] reported a condition in adults that seemed similar to the respiratory distress syndrome in infants. Later the same group introduced the term 'adult respiratory distress syndrome'.[7] One of the subjects reported in 1967 was aged only 11 years, and, in recognition of the fact that respiratory distress syndrome is known to occur in children, the current recommended term is *acute* respiratory distress syndrome.[8] There are a great many other synonyms for ARDS, including acute respiratory failure, shock lung, respirator lung, pump lung and Da Nang lung.

Definition

There is no single diagnostic test, and much confusion has arisen in the past from differing diagnostic criteria. This has greatly complicated comparisons of incidence, mortality, aetiology and efficacy of therapy in different centres. To address this problem, recent European–American consensus conferences have now produced widely accepted definitions.[8]

Acute lung injury diagnosis requires the presence of four criteria:

1. Acute onset of impaired oxygenation.
2. Severe hypoxaemia defined as a ratio of Pa_{O_2} to $F_{I_{O_2}}$ of ≤ 40 kPa (300 mmHg).
3. Bilateral diffuse infiltration on the chest radiograph.
4. Pulmonary artery wedge pressure of ≤ 18 mmHg to exclude cardiogenic causes of pulmonary oedema.

Acute respiratory distress syndrome is defined in almost identical terms except that the impairment of gas exchange is worse with a Pa_{O_2} to $F_{I_{O_2}}$ ratio of ≤ 26.7 kPa (200 mmHg).

These definitions have clarified many previous discrepancies, and will be extremely helpful in future research of ALI, particularly epidemiological studies. However, there are several provisos to their use in the clinical situation. For example, it is possible for patients with diseases that elevate left atrial pressure to have ALI, but they would fall outside the strict definition. Also, many earlier definitions suggest that one or more of the known predisposing conditions should have been present and that the clinical course has followed the recognized pattern (see below). Finally, it is noted that the histology is usually diagnostic but it is seldom indicated or advisable to take a lung biopsy. There is no reliable laboratory test to confirm the diagnosis (see below).

In part, the diagnosis of ALI depends on the exclusion of other conditions. Sometimes it is not easy to separate it from other diseases such as pulmonary embolus, pulmonary oedema, fibrosing alveolitis, or diffuse pneumonia, which may present many similar features.

Scoring systems

Various attempts have been made to derive a single numerical value to assess the severity of the condition. This greatly facilitates comparison of incidence and therapeutic trials, as well as helping in the prognosis and assessment of progress in an individual patient.

Table 30.1 Lung injury score[10]

Chest radiograph appearance	No alveolar consolidation		0
	Alveolar consolidation confined to 1 quadrant		1
	Alveolar consolidation confined to 2 quadrants		2
	Alveolar consolidation confined to 3 quadrants		3
	Alveolar consolidation in all 4 quadrants		4
Hypoxaemia score $Pa_{O_2}:F_{I_{O_2}}$	$\geq$40 kPa	$\geq$300 mmHg	0
	30–39.9 kPa	225–299 mmHg	1
	23.3–29.9 kPa	175–224 mmHg	2
	13.3–23.2 kPa	100–174 mmHg	3
	<13.3 kPa	<100 mmHg	4
Positive end-expiratory pressure (when ventilated)	$\leq$0.5 kPa	$\leq$5 cmH$_2$O	0
	0.6–0.8 kPa	6–8 cmH$_2$O	1
	0.9–1.1 kPa	9–11 cmH$_2$O	2
	1.2–1.4 kPa	12–14 cmH$_2$O	3
	$\geq$1.5 kPa	$\geq$15 cmH$_2$O	4
Respiratory system compliance (when available)	$\geq$0.8 l.kPa^{-1}	$\geq$80 ml.cmH$_2$O^{-1}	0
	0.6–0.79 l.kPa^{-1}	60–79 ml.cmH$_2$O^{-1}	1
	0.4–0.59 l.kPa^{-1}	40–59 ml.cmH$_2$O^{-1}	2
	0.2–0.39 l.kPa^{-1}	20–39 ml.cmH$_2$O^{-1}	3
	$\leq$0.19 l.kPa^{-1}	$\leq$19 ml.cmH$_2$O^{-1}	4

$Pa_{O_2}:F_{I_{O_2}}$ is the arterial Po_2 divided by the fractional concentration of oxygen in the inspired gas. The final lung injury score is the mean of the individual scores for each of the components which are included in the assessment.

Score	
0	No lung injury
0.1–2.5	Mild to moderate ALI
>2.5	Severe ALI (ARDS)

APACHE III (acute physiology and chronic health evaluation) is widely used.[9] Murray et al.[10] have proposed an expanded three-part definition comprising distinction between acute and chronic phases, identification of aetiological and associated conditions, and a numerical lung injury score. The lung injury score is based on all or some of the following (Table 30.1):

1. The extent of alveolar consolidation seen on the chest radiograph.
2. The Pa_{O_2} to FI_{O_2} ratio.
3. The level of positive end-expiratory pressure (PEEP) in use.
4. Compliance of the respiratory system.

Predisposing conditions and risk factors for ALI

Although the clinical and histopathological picture of ALI are remarkably consistent, they have been described as the sequel to a very large range of predisposing conditions (Table 30.2). There are, however, very important differences in the progression of ALI and its response to treatment, depending on the underlying cause and associated pathology.[10] Nevertheless, recognition of the predisposing conditions is crucially important for predicting which patients are at risk and the establishment of early diagnosis.

By no means are all the conditions in Table 30.2 equally likely to proceed to ALI. Analysis of some of the more important risk factors has been undertaken by several groups. Two consecutive studies from the same institution involved 315 patients in total.[11,12] Sepsis syndrome (see below) was clearly identified as the condition most likely to result in development of ARDS, with 38–43 per cent of patients being affected.[12,13] The incidence was 30 per cent in patients who aspirated gastric contents, 24 per cent in patients with multiple emergency transfusions (more than 22 units in 12 hours) and 17 per cent in patients with pulmonary contusions. Over all, 25 per cent of patients with a single risk factor developed ARDS but this rose to 42 per cent with two factors and 85 per cent with three. Other studies have also found that multiple risk factors give rise to a greater occurrence of ARDS. A study of 116 patients with septicaemia found an 18 per cent incidence of ARDS but this was greatly increased if the patient also had thrombocytopenia (46 per cent incidence) or severe hypotension (64 per cent incidence). Age and gender did not affect the likelihood of development of ARDS. A further large study followed 993 patients considered to be at risk of ARDS as a result of cardiopulmonary bypass surgery,

Table 30.2 Some predisposing conditions for ALI

Direct lung injury	Indirect lung injury
Aspiration of gastric contents	Sepsis
Diffuse pulmonary infection	Shock or prolonged hypotension
Lung contusion	Severe non-thoracic trauma
Near-drowning	Pancreatitis
Inhalation of toxic gases or vapours	Diabetic ketoacidosis
Fat or amniotic fluid embolus	Massive blood transfusion
	Excessive fluid replacement
	Cardiopulmonary bypass
	Severe burns
	Disseminated intravascular coagulation

burns, bacteraemia, transfusions of 10 or more units of blood, major fractures, disseminated intravascular coagulation (DIC), aspiration of gastric contents or pneumonia.[14] As a single factor, aspiration had the highest incidence of ARDS (36 per cent) followed by DIC (22 per cent) and pneumonia (12 per cent). Other factors, including isolated bacteraemia, all showed an incidence of less than 6 per cent. Patients with multiple risk factors had an incidence of 25 per cent compared with 6 per cent for a single risk factor.

The sepsis syndrome

The sepsis syndrome is defined as a systemic response to proven or presumed infection, with hyper- (or hypo-) thermia, tachycardia, tachypnoea, and one or more organs exhibiting signs of hypoperfusion or dysfunction.[15] There is usually altered cerebral function, arterial hypoxaemia, lactacidosis and oliguria. Many cases of ARDS represent the pulmonary manifestation of the multi-organ dysfunction syndrome (MODS) that is a feature of this condition, and ARDS is frequently associated with circulatory failure (septic shock). Bacteraemia may or may not be present, and has little effect on outcome. In a study of 191 patients with the sepsis syndrome, 25 per cent developed ARDS and 36 per cent septic shock.[15]

Clinical aspects of ALI and ARDS

Incidence and mortality

The much-quoted American Lung Program study of 1972 estimated the incidence in the USA to be 150 000 cases per year, which equates to 71 cases per year per 100 000 population.[16] Several studies subsequently found much lower incidences. In 1984 the incidence in the Canary Islands was calculated to be around 2.5 cases per 100 000,[17] whilst in a region of the UK in 1985 the corresponding figure was 4.5.[18] More recently, in 1989 in Utah the incidence was found to be between 5 and 8 per 100 000 population.[19] The reasons for this discrepancy relate mainly to diagnostic criteria, and the first study probably represented the incidence of ALI generally rather than ARDS specifically.[2] Furthermore, the studies were separated by at least 12 years, during which there was increasing awareness of how to prevent the predisposing conditions.

There is, however, considerable agreement that the overall mortality of ARDS is of the order of 50 per cent whatever the criteria of diagnosis,[1,2] and often higher in cases that follow septicaemia.[14] Some more recent studies have indicated improvements in survival.[2] A comprehensive survey of mortality in one area of the USA has recently reported a substantial improvement in survival, from a mortality rate of 53–68 per cent for the period 1983–1987 to only 36 per cent in 1993.[3] The improvement occurred in all groups of patients regardless of risk factors, and the reason for this apparently sudden decline is difficult to explain.

Clinical course

Four phases may be recognized in the development of ALI. In the first the patient is dyspnoeic and tachypnoeic but there are no other abnormalities. The chest radiograph is normal at this stage, which lasts for about 24 hours. In the next phase there is hypoxaemia but the arterial P_{CO_2} remains normal or subnormal. There are minor abnormalities of the chest radiograph. This phase may last for 24–48 hours. Diagnosis is easily missed in these prodromal stages and is very dependent on the history of one or more predisposing conditions.

It is only in phase three that the diagnostic criteria of true ALI become established. There is severe arterial hypoxaemia due to an increased alveolar/arterial P_{O_2} gradient, and the P_{CO_2} may be slightly elevated. The lungs become stiff and the chest radiograph shows the characteristic bilateral diffuse infiltrates. Artificial ventilation is usually instituted at this stage.

The fourth phase is often terminal and comprises massive bilateral consolidation with unremitting hypoxaemia, the arterial P_{O_2} characteristically being less than 7 kPa (52.5 mmHg) when the inspired oxygen concentration is 100%. Dead space is substantially increased and the arterial P_{CO_2} is only with difficulty kept in the normal range by the use of a large minute volume.

Not every patient progresses through all these phases and the condition may resolve at any stage. It is difficult to predict whether the condition will progress and there is currently no useful laboratory test, though measurement of cytokine levels has some potential in this area.[20] Serial observations of the chest radiograph, the alveolar/arterial P_{O_2} gradient and function of other compromised organs are the best guides to progress. The more systems in failure, the worse is the outlook.

Pathophysiology

Oxygen consumption by the lung. Measurement of pulmonary oxygen consumption (as the difference between spirometry and the reversed Fick method – see page 300) has repeatedly shown very high values for lungs with ARDS.[21,22] It is quite possible that some of this represents free radical formation (see Chapter 25), but the increase in pulmonary oxygen consumption does not seem to correlate with various markers of pulmonary inflammation at the time the measurement is made.[22]

Maldistribution of ventilation and perfusion.[23] Computed tomography (CT) of patients with ARDS shows that opacities representing collapsed areas are distributed throughout the lungs in a heterogeneous manner but predominantly in the dependent parts.[24] After a change in posture, the opacities move to the newly dependent zones within a few minutes.[25,26] The most conspicuous functional disability is the shunt[23] (Figure 30.1), which is usually so large (often more than 40%) that increasing the inspired oxygen concentration cannot produce a normal arterial P_{O_2} (see the isoshunt chart, Figure 8.12). CT scans of patients with ALI also demonstrate substantial areas of lung overdistension.[27] These areas contribute to the increased dead space, which may exceed 70 per cent of tidal volume and requires a large increase in minute volume to attempt to preserve a normal arterial P_{CO_2}. Both shunt and dead space correlate strongly with the non-inflated lung tissue seen with CT (Figure 30.1).

Lung mechanics. In established ARDS, lung compliance is greatly reduced and the static compliance of the respiratory system (lungs + chest wall) is of the order of 300 ml.kPa^{-1} (30 ml.cmH$_2$O^{-1}).[28,29] A recent study has found differences in respiratory mechanics between severe ALI resulting from intrapulmonary and extrapulmonary disease (Table 30.2).[30] Respiratory system compliance was reduced to a similar extent in both groups, but the abnormality was mostly with lung compliance, when lung disease was the cause, and chest wall compliance with extrapulmonary causation.

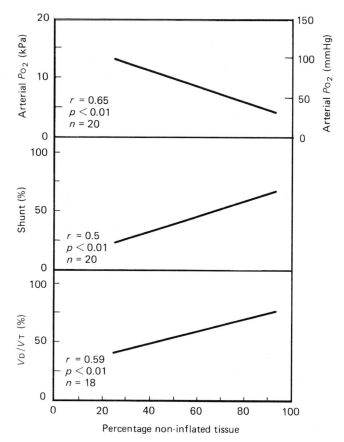

Figure 30.1 Relationship of arterial P_{O_2}, shunt and physiological dead space (V_D/V_T) to the percentage of non-inflated lung tissue seen by computed tomography in patients with adult respiratory distress syndrome, artificially ventilated with positive end-expiratory pressure of 0.5 kPa (5 cmH$_2$O). (Redrawn from data of reference 24.)

Functional residual capacity is reduced by collapse, tissue proliferation and increased elastic recoil.

Mean total resistance to air flow was found to be 1.5–2 kPa.l^{-1}.s (15–20 cmH$_2$O.l^{-1}.s),[28,29] or about three times those of anaesthetized patients with normal lungs, measured by the same techniques. Using the model shown in Figure 4.4c, some two-thirds of the total resistance in patients with ARDS could be assigned to viscoelastic resistance of tissue, although the airway resistance was still about twice normal.

Alveolar/capillary permeability is increased substantially throughout the course of ALI.[31] This may be demonstrated by the enhanced transit of various tracer molecules across the alveolar/capillary membrane (page 218),[32] which is becoming a feasible bedside investigation.

Mechanisms of ALI

Histopathology

Although of diverse aetiology, the histological appearances of ARDS are remarkably consistent and this lends support for ARDS being considered a discrete clinical entity. Histological changes at autopsy may be divided into two stages: acute and subacute or chronic.[33]

The acute stage. The acute stage is characterized by damaged integrity of the blood/gas barrier. The changes are primarily in the interalveolar septa and cannot be seen satisfactorily with light microscopy. Electron microscopy reveals extensive damage to the type I alveolar epithelial cells (page 29), which may be totally destroyed (Figure 30.2). Meanwhile the basement membrane is usually preserved and the endothelial cells still tend to form a continuous layer with apparently intact cell junctions. Endothelial permeability is nevertheless increased and interstitial oedema is found, predominantly on the 'service' side of the capillary (page 27). Fortunately, the oedema tends to spare the 'active' side of the capillary where endothelium and epithelium are in close apposition. This differentiation between the two sides of the pulmonary capillary is also seen in cardiogenic oedema.

Protein-containing fluid leaks into the alveoli, which also contain erythrocytes and leucocytes in addition to amorphous material comprising strands of fibrin (Figure 30.2). The exudate may form into sheets that line the alveoli as the so-called hyaline membrane. Intravascular coagulation is common at this stage and, in patients with septicaemia, capillaries may be completely plugged with leucocytes, and the underlying endothelium may then be damaged.

The subacute or chronic stage. Attempted repair and proliferation predominate in the chronic stage of ARDS. Within a few days of the onset of the condition, there is a thickening of endothelium, epithelium and the interstitial space. The type I epithelial cells are destroyed and replaced by type II cells, which proliferate but do not differentiate into type I cells as usual. They remain cuboidal and about ten times the thickness of the type I cells they have replaced. This seems to be a non-specific response to damaged type I cells, and is similar to that which results from exposure to high concentrations of oxygen (page 506).

The interstitial space is greatly expanded by oedema fluid, fibres and a variety of proliferating cells. Fibrosis commences after the first week and ultimately fibrocytes predominate: extensive fibrosis is seen in resolving cases.

Cellular mechanisms[1,2,34]

The diversity of predisposing conditions suggests that there may be several possible mechanisms, at least in the early stages of development of ALI, but the end-result is remarkably similar. In all cases, lung injury seems to begin with damage to the alveolar/capillary membrane. This is followed by progressive inflammation, leading to alveolar transudation, pulmonary vasoconstriction and capillary obstruction.

Cells that seem capable of damaging the alveolar/capillary membrane include neutrophils, basophils, macrophages and platelets. Damage may be inflicted by a large number of substances, including bacterial endotoxin, oxygen-derived free radicals, tumour necrosis factor (TNF), proteases, thrombin, fibrin, fibrin degradation products, histamine, bradykinin, 5-hydroxytryptamine (serotonin), platelet-activating factor (PAF) and some

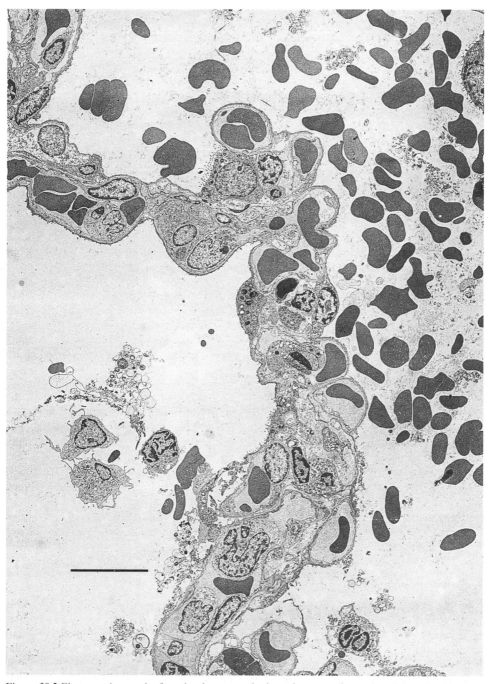

Figure 30.2 Electron micrograph of an alveolar septum in the early stages of acute lung injury. On the right-hand side of the septum there are many examples of damage to alveolar epithelium but the endothelium tends to remain intact. The alveolar gas spaces to the left and right contain many erythrocytes, leucocytes, cell debris and fibrin strands. The scale bar (bottom left) is 10 μm. (Reproduced from reference 33 by permission of the authors and the Editors of *Chest Medicine*.)

arachidonic acid metabolites. It seems improbable that any one mechanism is responsible for all cases of ALI. It is more likely that different mechanisms operate in different predisposing conditions and in different animal models of ALI.

Neutrophils are now accepted as having a key role in human ALI.[35] Although ALI can still be induced in neutrophil-depleted animals, patients with ARDS have large numbers of neutrophils and associated cytokines in samples of bronchoalveolar lavage (BAL) fluid.[2] Neutrophil activation may occur in response to a large number of substances, some of which are illustrated in Figure 30.3. Which of these are important in ALI is unknown, but likely to depend on the predisposing condition; for example, complement component C5a is known to be involved in sepsis-related ALI. Margination of neutrophils from the pulmonary capillary into the lung parenchyma is the first stage of neutrophil activation, and has been described on page 565. Many molecules are involved in this process, as shown in Figure 30.3, and bacterial wall fragments are also potent activators of

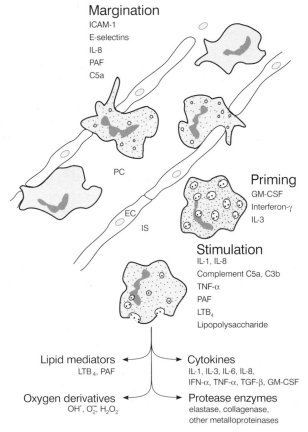

Figure 30.3 Neutrophil activation in acute lung injury and the main cytokines and mediators involved. This takes place in three stages: *margination*, when neutrophils adhere to the pulmonary capillary (PC) wall and migrate between endothelial cells (EC) into the interstitial space (IS); *priming*, when the cells generate preformed mediators and lysosomal contents; and *stimulation*, when neutrophils release the various mediators shown. Note that several of the mediators released also promote margination, priming and stimulation of other neutrophils to amplify the response. For explanation of abbreviations, see text.

margination.[35,36] Very large numbers of neutrophils may accumulate in the pulmonary circulation without any resultant pulmonary damage.[37] This occurs, for example, during the early stages of an anaphylactoid reaction and also during haemodialysis with a cellophane membrane. However, under other circumstances such as ALI, neutrophils marginated in the pulmonary circulation continue to become activated. During margination and once in the interstitium, the neutrophil is 'primed' – that is, stimulated to produce preformed mediators ready for release and to establish the bactericidal contents of their lysosomes. Finally, stimulation results from a whole host of cytokines, some derived from other inflammatory cells (macrophages, lymphocytes or endothelial cells) and some from other neutrophils, so amplifying the process. Stimulation causes release of a whole host of inflammatory mediators (Figure 30.3), and is also associated with inappropriate release of lysosomal contents. Instead of being released into phagocytic vesicles containing bacteria, they come into direct contact with the endothelium, which is thereby damaged.

Four groups of substances released from neutrophils (Figure 30.3) have been considered as contributing to lung damage, as follows.

1. Cytokines.[35,38] Neutrophils are capable of producing numerous cytokines,[35] most of which are pro-inflammatory. Tumour necrosis factor-α (TNF-α) and interleukin-1 (IL-1) activate endothelial cells to up-regulate the adhesion molecules ICAM-1 (intercellular adhesion molecule) and E-selectin which initiate margination, whilst C5a, platelet-activating factor (PAF) and IL-8 accelerate the process. Granulocyte macrophage colony stimulating factor (GM-CSF) and IL-3 contribute to priming of further neutrophils along with interferon-γ released from other inflammatory cells. Finally, IL-1, IL-8 and TNF-α all exert positive feedback on neutrophils, causing further stimulation. Transforming growth factor-β (TGF-β) is the principal anti-inflammatory cytokine produced by neutrophils, and is responsible for fibroblast stimulation and the development of pulmonary fibrosis (page 567). IL-8 is involved in most stages of neutrophil activation (Figure 30.3), and the serum concentration of IL-8 in ALI may help predict those patients with a poor prognosis.[20]
2. Protease enzymes lead to extensive tissue damage in the lung. The most damaging is elastase which, unlike what its name suggests, is very non-specific, with proteolytic activity against collagen, fibrinogen and many other proteins as well as elastin. A group of enzymes referred to as metalloproteinases are more specific for individual substrates such as collagen. In addition to directly damaging the endothelium, proteases also produce elastin fragments that are chemotactic for inflammatory cells.[39]
3. Oxygen-derived free radicals and related compounds (see Chapter 25). These are powerful and important bactericidal agents, which also have the capacity to damage the endothelium by lipid peroxidation and other means. In addition, they inactivate α_1-antitrypsin, an important antiprotease enzyme (page 308).
4. Lipid-derived mediators include prostaglandins, thromboxanes and leukotrienes (LT), but LTB_4 and PAF are the most important in ALI. These two act in the same way as other cytokines to amplify neutrophil activation, and, in addition, PAF damages endothelial cells directly and promotes intravascular coagulation.

Macrophages and basophils. Macrophages are already present in the normal alveolus (page 31) but their numbers increase greatly in ARDS. They produce a wide range of bactericidal agents and cytokines similar to those of the neutrophil. Lung macrophages produce IL-10, which suppresses gene expression of many cytokines, and so acts as one of the very few anti-inflammatory cytokines so far identified in lung inflammation.[38]

Platelets are present in the pulmonary capillaries in large number in ARDS. Aggregation in that site is associated with increased capillary hydrostatic pressure, possibly due to release of arachidonic acid metabolites. Platelet function may well be implicated in the formation of the 'hyaline' membrane that lines the alveoli in ARDS.[34]

Besides giving rise to pulmonary oedema, many of the mediators released by these inflammatory cells have other effects that contribute to the pulmonary changes seen in ALI. For example, arachidonic acid metabolites cause pulmonary venoconstriction, which will raise pulmonary capillary pressure and compound the effect of increased permeability. Accumulation of platelets and neutrophils along with intravascular coagulation will occlude pulmonary vessels, producing pulmonary hypertension and unperfused lung units. It has also been noted that many proteins, including albumin but particularly fibrin monomer, can antagonize the action of surfactant, thus fundamentally altering lung mechanics.[40]

The potential contribution to ALI of lung damage secondary to artificial ventilation is described on page 615.

Principles of management[1,3,4,5,41,42]

Treatment of the underlying cause in conjunction with supportive therapy remains the mainstay of current management. Optimal management of the cardiovascular and renal systems is a vital component in ALI treatment, because any increase in pulmonary capillary pressure (e.g. from fluid overload) may lead to catastrophic pulmonary oedema. Respiratory support requires artificial ventilation in all but the most minor degrees of ALI.

Artificial ventilation in ARDS

General principles of artificial ventilation and the resulting physiological effects are described in detail in the next chapter. In this section, only the problems associated with ventilation of patients with ALI are described.

The lungs of patients with severe ALI may be conveniently divided into three hypothetical sections.[43] First, there will be some 'normal' areas, usually in the non-dependent region. Second, there will be areas of lung, usually in dependent regions, with such severe collapse and alveolar flooding that ventilation of these areas will be impossible. Finally, there will be an intermediate area with poorly ventilated or collapsed alveoli that are capable of being 'recruited' by appropriate artificial ventilation, with a resultant improvement in gas exchange. Although the relative amounts of each section will vary greatly according to the severity of the ALI, there will always be *some* lung in the final area, and so capable of recruitment.

Tidal volume. The recognition that positive pressure ventilation can lead to lung damage (page 615) has led to a change in ventilatory technique used in patients with ALI. Overdistension of alveoli by application of large tidal volumes is now believed to be a significant factor in lung damage. In particular, a typical patient with ARDS may have only about one-third of the lung being ventilated. Thus use of a normal tidal volume $(10–12\,ml.kg^{-1})$ will, for the few alveoli being ventilated in the patient, equate to a tidal volume of three times usual in normal healthy lungs, which is over 2 litres in a 70 kg subject. Initial tidal volumes used for ventilation should therefore be between 6 and $10\,ml.kg^{-1}$.[3] If airway pressure exceeds values of $30–35\,cmH_2O$, tidal volume should be reduced or an alternative ventilatory strategy used.

Pressure-controlled ventilation (page 590) is now the preferred technique in many centres to prevent the problems outlined in the previous paragraph. However, with pressure-controlled ventilation in lungs with low compliance, such as ALI, the delivery of an adequate minute volume may be difficult. Two techniques are advocated to deal with this problem. First, inverse *I/E* ratios may be used, in which expiratory time is shorter than inspiratory time, allowing the delivery of a larger tidal volume. Secondly, the hypercapnia that results from the inadequate minute volume may be partially ignored. Known as 'permissive hypercapnia',[44,45] arterial P_{CO_2} is allowed to increase until such time as the

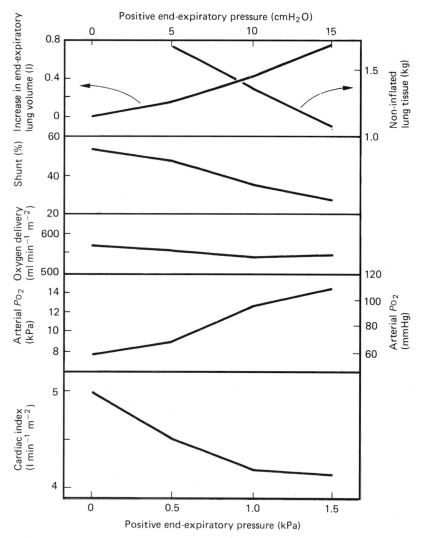

Figure 30.4 Effect of positive end-expiratory pressure on various factors influencing oxygen delivery in patients with severe acute lung injury (ALI). Although arterial P_{O_2} is increased, cardiac output is decreased and there is no significant change in oxygen transport. (Data on non-inflated lung tissue are from reference 24; remaining data from reference 48.)

respiratory acidosis is deemed detrimental, which will usually depend on the patient's cardiovascular function.

Positive end-expiratory pressure (PEEP). At one time it seemed that the early use of PEEP might prevent the development of ARDS,[46] but it now seems unlikely that there is any such effect. PEEP does, however, reduce the amount of non-inflated lung tissue seen at CT scan,[24] particularly in dependent lung regions.[47] Shunt fraction and therefore the arterial P_{O_2} (Figure 30.4) also improve. Reduced pulmonary compliance means that cardiac output is better maintained than might be expected (page 613), with a reduction of the order of 20 per cent with PEEP of 1.5 kPa (15 cmH_2O) (Figure 30.4). The resultant reduction in oxygen delivery is insignificant.[48] Inspiratory resistance is unaffected but, surprisingly, expiratory resistance of the respiratory system is increased, particularly by high levels of PEEP.

The ideal PEEP value to use has been controversial for decades.[4] Differing end-points (in parentheses) have given rise to numerous terms such as 'optimal' PEEP (lowest physiological shunt fraction), 'best' PEEP (optimal static lung compliance), 'preferred' PEEP (best oxygen delivery), and 'least' PEEP ('acceptable' values for Pa_{O_2}, inspired oxygen and cardiac output).[4,49] High levels of PEEP will probably result in increased alveolar recruitment and improved oxygenation, but normal alveoli can only enlarge in response to PEEP to a certain extent, above which dramatic increases in alveolar pressure, and possible damage, occur (page 615 *et seq.*). Identifying this point has vexed intensivists

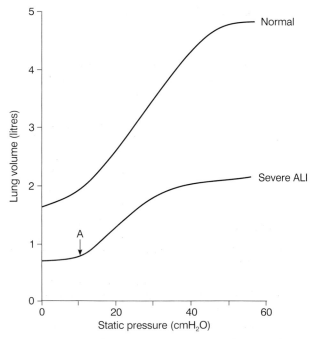

Figure 30.5 Static pressure versus lung volume curves for patients receiving positive pressure ventilation. Note the severely reduced lung volume and compliance in acute lung injury. Point A indicates the lower inflection of the curve, above which compliance is considerably improved. Application of positive end-expiratory pressure of approximately 12 cmH_2O in this patient will therefore improve tidal volume relative to the ventilatory pressure required.

for some time. It is now recommended that PEEP be increased until the lower inflection of the patient's respiratory system static compliance curve is reached (A in Figure 30.5), which is normally between 10 and 15 cmH$_2$O.[5,50] The pressure seen at the lower point of inflection is also believed to represent the pressure at which most recruitable alveoli have been opened.[4]

Other ventilatory strategies. Satisfactory gaseous exchange may be impossible by conventional means, and both high frequency ventilation and extracorporeal techniques have been used (see Chapters 31 and 32).

Inspired oxygen concentration should be carefully controlled to prevent dangerous hypoxia, on the one hand, and the possibility of pulmonary oxygen toxicity on the other. Most clinicians regard an inspired concentration of less than 65% as acceptable.[41]

Other therapeutic options

Specific therapy is the goal of much research, which is directed particularly towards the control of infection and the development of antagonists to the various mediators considered above.[41] In most cases it has proved difficult to demonstrate their efficacy, and the financial implications of their widespread use have caused grave concern in some cases, such as the monoclonal antibody to endotoxin. These, and several other pharmacological approaches to the treatment of ALI, are summarized in Table 30.3. Detailed description of all these therapeutic options is beyond the scope of this book, but two techniques are of particular physiological interest.

Table 30.3 Summary of pharmacological interventions suggested for the treatment of ALI or ARDS

Therapy	Examples	Proposed mechanism
Pulmonary vasodilators	Prostacyclin	Non-specific pulmonary vasodilator
	Nitric oxide	Regional pulmonary vasodilator (see text)
Surfactant	Artificial surfactants	Replaces depleted alveolar surfactant, may also have anti-inflammatory properties
Anti-inflammatory	Steroids	General anti-inflammatory
	Ketoconazole	Inhibits thromboxane synthesis
	Ibuprofen/indomethacin	Inhibits prostaglandin production
	Prostaglandin E$_1$	Inhibits platelet aggregation, vasodilator
	Pentoxifylline	Reduces neutrophil chemotaxis and activation
	Endotoxin/TNF/IL-1 antagonists	Inhibition of specific aspects of inflammatory response
Antioxidants	N-Acetylcysteine	Increased glutathione activity (page 504)
	Recombinant human manganese SOD	Replaces epithelial extracellular SOD (page 503)
Antibiotics	Numerous	Reduces inflammation from bacterial infections

NB. All the therapies listed have been shown to have beneficial effects in *in vitro* or *in vivo* animal studies of ALI. There is insufficient evidence of improved outcome for any of the therapies listed to be recommended for routine use in human ALI. For further details see the recent reviews on therapy of ALI.[1,3]

IL-1, interleukin 1; SOD, superoxide dismutase (page 503); TNF, tumour necrosis factor.

Patient position. Pulmonary collapse in dependent lung areas raised the possibility of alveolar recruitment by changing the patient's position. The prone position is the most widely studied,[51,52] though the lateral decubitus position is also recommended,[3] and much less complicated to use in patients receiving intensive care. There is little doubt that oxygenation improves on turning the patient from supine to prone,[53] and the improvement may be sustained for many hours in some patients.[52] When prone, areas of pulmonary collapse quickly redistribute,[25,26] and ventilation and perfusion become more homogenous throughout the lung and gas exchange improves.[23]

Inhaled nitric oxide. Pulmonary hypertension is a frequent observation in ALI; the pathophysiology has been described above. Inhalation of nitric oxide (5–80 ppm) reduces pulmonary artery pressure, and causes selective vasodilatation in the *ventilated* alveoli and so reduces intrapulmonary shunt.[54] Once in the blood, nitric oxide is rapidly bound by haemoglobin (page 273), which prevents it exerting an effect on the systemic vasculature. Some of its beneficial effects may be only transient, and there are concerns that prolonged inhalation of nitric oxide may contribute to pulmonary toxicity from oxygen-derived species (page 499).[1] Nevertheless, inhalation of nitric oxide remains a useful addition to therapy when more conventional techniques are failing.

References

1. Fulkerson WJ, MacIntyre N, Crapo JD. Pathogenesis and treatment of the adult respiratory distress syndrome. *Arch Intern Med* 1996; **156**: 29–38.
2. Luce JM. Acute lung injury and the acute respiratory distress syndrome. *Crit Care Med* 1998; **26**: 369–76.
3. Kolleff MH, Schuster DP. The acute respiratory distress syndrome. *N Engl J Med* 1995; **332**: 27–37.
4. Peruzzi WT, Franklin ML, Shapiro BA. New concepts and therapies of adult respiratory distress syndrome. *J Cardiothorac Vasc Anesth* 1997; **11**: 771–86.
5. Bigatello LM, Zapol WM. New approaches to acute lung injury. *Br J Anaesth* 1996; **77**: 99–109.
6. Ashbaugh DG, Bigelow DB, Petty TL, Levine BE. Acute respiratory distress in adults. *Lancet* 1967; **2**: 319–23.
7. Petty TL, Ashbaugh DG. The adult respiratory distress syndrome. *Chest* 1971; **60**: 233–8.
8. Bernard GR, Artigas A, Brigham KL, Carlet J, Falke K, Hudson L et al. The American–European consensus conference on ARDS: definitions, mechanisms, relevant outcomes, and clinical trial coordination. *Am J Respir Crit Care Med* 1994; **149**: 818–24.
9. Knaus WA, Wagner DP, Draper EA, Zimmerman JE, Bergner M, Bastos PG et al. The APACHE III prognostic system. Risk prediction of hospital mortality for critically ill hospitalized adults. *Chest* 1991; **100**: 1619–36.
10. Murray JF, Matthay MA, Luce JM, Flick MR. An expanded definition of the adult respiratory distress syndrome. *Am Rev Respir Dis* 1988; **138**: 720–3.
11. Pepe PE, Potkin RT, Reus DH, Hudson LD, Carrico CJ. Clinical predictors of the adult respiratory distress syndrome. *Am J Surg* 1982; **144**: 124–30.
12. Hudson LD, Millberg JA, Anardi D, Maunder RJ. Clinical risks for development of the acute respiratory distress syndrome. *Am J Respir Crit Care Med* 1995; **151**: 293–301.
13. Milberg JA, Davis DR, Steinberg KP, Hudson LD. Improved survival of patients with acute respiratory distress syndrome (ARDS): 1983–1993. *JAMA* 1995; **273**: 306–9.
14. Fowler AA, Hamman RF, Good JT, Benson KN, Baird M, Eberle DJ et al. Adult respiratory distress syndrome: risk with common predispositions. *Ann Intern Med* 1983; **98**: 593–7.
15. Bone RC, Fisher CJ, Clemmer TP, Slotman GJ, Metz CA, Balk RA. Sepsis syndrome: a valid clinical entity. *Crit Care Med* 1989; **17**: 389–93.

16. National Heart and Lung Institute. *Respiratory distress syndromes: task force on problems, research approaches, needs*, DHEW Publication No. (NIH) 73–432. Washington DC: US Government Printing Office, 1973.

17. Villar J, Slutsky AS. The incidence of the adult respiratory distress syndrome. *Am Rev Respir Dis* 1989; **140**: 814–16.

18. Webster NR, Cohen AT, Nunn JF. Adult respiratory distress syndrome – how many cases in the UK? *Anaesthesia* 1988; **43**: 923–6.

19. Thomsen GE, Morris AH. Incidence of the adult respiratory distress syndrome in the state of Utah. *Am J Respir Crit Care Med* 1995; **152**: 965–71.

20. Pittet JF, Mackersie RC, Martin TR, Matthay MA. Biological markers of acute lung injury: prognostic and pathogenic significance. *Am J Respir Crit Care Med* 1997; **155**: 1187–205.

21. Smithies MN, Royston B, Makita K, Konieczko K, Nunn JF. Comparison of oxygen consumption measurements: indirect calorimetry versus the reversed Fick method. *Crit Care Med* 1991; **19**: 1401–6.

22. Jolliet P, Thorens JB, Nicod L, Pichard C, Kyle U, Chevrolet JC. Relationship between pulmonary oxygen consumption, lung inflammation, and calculated venous admixture in patients with acute lung injury. *Intensive Care Med* 1996; **22**: 277–85.

23. Sinclair SE, Albert RK. Altering ventilation–perfusion relationships in ventilated patients with acute lung injury. *Intensive Care Med* 1997; **23**: 942–50.

24. Gattinoni L, Pesenti A, Bombino M, Baglioni S, Rivolta M, Rossi F et al. Relationships between lung computed tomographic density, gas exchange, and PEEP in acute respiratory failure. *Anesthesiology* 1988; **69**: 824–32.

25. Gattinoni L, Pelosi P, Vitale G, Pesenti A, D'Andrea L, Mascheroni D. Body position changes redistribute lung computed-tomographic density in patients with acute respiratory failure. *Anesthesiology* 1991; **74**: 15–23.

26. Gattinoni L, Pelosi P, Pesenti A, Brazzi L, Vitale G, Moretto A et al. CT scan in ARDS: clinical and physiopathological insights. *Acta Anaesthesiol Scand* 1991; **35** (Supp 95): 87–96.

27. Vieira SRR, Puybasset L, Richecoeur J, Lu Q, Cluzel P, Gusman PB et al. A lung computed tomographic assessment of positive end-expiratory pressure-induced lung overdistension. *Am J Respir Crit Care Med* 1998; **158**: 1571–7.

28. Tantucci C, Corbeil C, Chassé M, Robatto FM, Nava S, Braidy J et al. Flow and volume dependence of respiratory system flow resistance in patients with adult respiratory distress syndrome. *Am Rev Respir Dis* 1992; **145**: 355–60.

29. Eissa NT, Ranieri VM, Corbeil C, Chassé M, Robatto FM, Braidy J, Milic-Emili J. Analysis of behavior of the respiratory system in ARDS patients: effects of flow, volume, and time. *J Appl Physiol* 1991; **70**: 2719–29.

30. Gattinoni L, Pelosi P, Suter PM, Pedoto A, Vercesi P, Lissoni A. Acute respiratory distress syndrome caused by pulmonary and extrapulmonary disease. Different syndromes? *Am J Respir Crit Care Med* 1998; **158**: 3–11.

31. Sinclair DG, Braude S, Haslam PL, Evans TW. Pulmonary endothelial permeability in patients with severe lung injury: clinical correlates and natural history. *Chest* 1994; **106**: 535–9.

32. Rocker GM. Bedside measurement of pulmonary capillary permeability in patients with acute lung injury. What have we learned? *Intensive Care Med* 1996; **22**: 619–21.

33. Bachofen M, Weibel ER. Structural alterations and lung parenchyma in the adult respiratory distress syndrome. *Clin Chest Med* 1982; **3**: 35–43.

34. Wiener-Kronish JP, Gropper MA, Matthay MA. The adult respiratory distress syndrome: definition and prognosis, pathogenesis and treatment. *Br J Anaesth* 1990; **65**: 107–29.

35. Fujishima S, Aikawa N. Neutrophil-mediated tissue injury and its modulation. *Intensive Care Med* 1995; **21**: 277–85.

36. Albert RK. Mechanisms of the adult respiratory distress syndrome: selectins. *Thorax* 1995; **50** (Supp 1): S49–52.

37. Glauser FL, Fairman RP. The uncertain role of the neutrophil in increased permeability pulmonary edema. *Chest* 1985; **88**: 601–7.

38. Ward PA. Role of complement, chemokines, and regulatory cytokines in acute lung injury. *Ann N Y Acad Sci* 1996; **796**: 104–12.

39. Senior RM, Griffin GL, Mecham RP. Chemotactic activity of elastin-derived peptides. *J Clin Invest* 1980; **66**: 859–62.

40. Seeger W, Stöhr G, Wolf HRD, Neuhof H. Alteration of surfactant function due to protein leakage. *J Appl Physiol* 1985; **58**: 326–38.

41. Artigas A, Bernard GR, Carlet J, Dreyfus D, Gattinoni L, Hudson L et al. The American–European consensus conference on ARDS, Part 2: Ventilatory, pharmacologic, supportive therapy, study design strategies and issues related to recovery and remodelling. *Intensive Care Med* 1998; **24**: 378–98.

42. Lessard MR. New concepts in mechanical ventilation for ARDS. *Can J Anaesth* 1996; **43**: R50–4.

43. Gattinoni L, Pesenti A. ARDS: the non-homogenous lung: facts and hypotheses. *Intensive Crit Care Digest* 1987; **6**: 1–4.

44. Hickling KG, Joyce C. Permissive hypercapnia in ARDS and its effect on tissue oxygenation. *Acta Anaesthesiol Scand* 1995; **39** (Supp 107): 201–8.

45. Lewandowski K. Permissive hypercapnia in ARDS: just do it? *Intensive Care Med* 1996; **22**: 179–81.

46. Schmidt GB, O'Neill WW, Koth K, Hwang KK, Bennett EJ, Bombeck CT. Continuous positive airway pressure in the prophylaxis of the adult respiratory distress syndrome. *Surg Gynecol Obstet* 1976; **143**: 613–20.

47. Gattinoni L, D'Andrea L, Pelosi P, Vitale G, Pesenti A, Fumagalli R. Regional effects and mechanism of positive end-expiratory pressure in early adult respiratory distress syndrome. *JAMA* 1993; **269**: 2122–7.

48. Ranieri VM, Eissa NT, Corbeil C, Chassé M, Braidy J, Matar N, Milic-Emili J. Effects of positive end-expiratory pressure on alveolar recruitment and gas exchange in patients with the adult respiratory distress syndrome. *Am Rev Respir Dis* 1991; **144**: 544–51.

49. Carroll GC, Tuman KJ, Braverman B, Logas WG, Wool N, Ivankovich AD. Minimal positive end-expiratory pressure (PEEP) may be 'best PEEP'. *Chest* 1988; **93**: 1020–5.

50. Rupie E, Dambrosio M, Servillo G, Mentec H, El Atrous S, Beydon L et al. Titration of tidal volume and induced hypercapnia in acute respiratory distress syndrome. *Am J Respir Crit Care Med* 1995; **152**: 121–8.

51. Albert RK. The prone position in acute respiratory distress syndrome: where we are, and where do we go from here. *Crit Care Med* 1997; **25**: 1453–4.

52. Mure M, Martling C-R, Lindahl SGE. Dramatic effect on oxygenation in patients with severe acute lung insufficiency treated in the prone position. *Crit Care Med* 1997; **25**: 1539–44.

53. Pelosi P, Tubiolo D, Mascheroni D, Vicardi P, Crotti S, Valenza F, Gattinoni L. Effects of the prone position on respiratory mechanics and gas exchange during acute lung injury. *Am J Respir Crit Care Med* 1998; **157**: 387–93.

54. Rossaint R, Falke KJ, López F, Slama K, Pison U, Zapol WM. Inhaled nitric oxide for the adult respiratory distress syndrome. *N Engl J Med* 1993; **328**: 399–405.

Artificial ventilation

Artificial ventilation is defined as the provision of the minute volume of respiration by external forces. This is usually required when there is impaired action of the patient's respiratory muscles or a severe dysfunction of the mechanics of breathing. It may also be used to improve oxygenation of arterial blood even when Pco_2 is within normal limits. It is used in four main situations:

1. *Resuscitation following acute apnoea.* It is agreed that in the absence of equipment the best method of artificial ventilation during resuscitation is inflation of the lungs with the expired air of the rescuer; the physiology of this technique is considered below.
2. *Anaesthesia with paralysis.* Much the commonest application of artificial ventilation is during anaesthesia with paralysis. It would normally be applied to some 2–5 per cent of the population of a developed country each year. Almost without exception it is achieved by the application of intermittent positive pressure ventilation (IPPV) to the airway of the patient.
3. *Intensive care.* Artificial ventilation during intensive care is also undertaken almost exclusively by IPPV. However, in this environment, a proportion of patients present problems in ventilation, and there is a requirement for more sophisticated ventilators with increased control of the manner and pattern of ventilation.
4. *Treatment of chronic ventilatory failure.* Once again, the commonest method is by the intermittent development of a positive pressure gradient between airways and the air surrounding the trunk. Until quite recently, this required tracheostomy or prolonged periods of tracheal intubation to ensure the necessary airtight fit to the airways. However, the development of clinically acceptable tight-fitting facemasks has facilitated the prolonged use of non-invasive ventilation in chronic respiratory failure. Alternatively, ventilation may be achieved by generating the intermittent pressure differential by phasic reduction of pressure in the air around the trunk by means of a tank or cuirass ventilator.

For most of these applications, clinical practice has moved more towards respiratory 'support' or 'assist' in which the patient's breathing is assisted, but not replaced, by a variety of techniques described throughout this chapter.[1] Provision of the whole minute ventilation by artificial means, or 'controlled' ventilation, is now seen only during anaesthesia with paralysis and in the most critically ill of intensive care patients.

Extracorporeal gas exchange is considered separately in Chapter 32.

Methods used for resuscitation

Until about 1960, artificial ventilation was usually attempted by application of mechanical forces directly to the trunk. Methods were based on the rescuer manipulating the trunk and arms of the victim to achieve changes in lung volume which, when performed in sequence, could produce some degree of pulmonary ventilation. These methods, which undoubtedly saved many lives in the past, are now largely obsolete; they were described in earlier editions of this book.

Expired air resuscitation

Recognition of the inadequacy of the manual methods of artificial ventilation led directly to a radical new approach to artificial ventilation in an emergency. Around 1960 there was vigorous re-examination of the concept of the rescuer's expired air being used for inflation of the victim's lungs. Elisha has been credited with use of this technique on the son of the Shunammite woman (2 Kings 4:32) but the first clear and unequivocal account of the method was by Herholdt and Rafn in 1796.[2]

At first sight, it might appear that expired air would not be a suitable inspired air for the victim. However, if the rescuer doubles his ventilation he is able to breathe for two. If neither party had any respiratory dead space, the simple relationship shown in Table 31.1 would apply. In fact, the rescuer's dead space improves the situation. At the start of inflation, the rescuer's dead space is filled with fresh air and this is the first gas to enter the victim's lungs. If the rescuer's dead space is artificially increased by apparatus dead space, this will improve the freshness of the air that the victim receives and will also prevent hypocapnia in the rescuer.

Expired air resuscitation has now displaced the manual methods in all except the most unusual circumstances. Its success depends on the following factors:

1. It is normally possible to achieve adequate ventilation for long periods of time without fatigue.[3]
2. The hands of the rescuer are free to control the patency of the victim's airway.
3. The rescuer can monitor the victim's chest expansion visually and can also hear any airway obstruction and sense the tidal exchange from the proprioceptive receptors in his own chest wall.

Table 31.1 Alveolar gas concentrations during expired air resuscitation

	Normal spontaneous respiration	Expired air resuscitation with doubled ventilation	
		Donor	Recipient
Alveolar CO_2	6%	3%	6%
Alveolar O_2	15%	18%	15%

Doubling the donor's ventilation increases his alveolar O_2 concentration to a value midway between the normal alveolar oxygen concentration and that of room air.

4. The method is extremely adaptable and has been used, for example, before drowning victims have been removed from the water, and on linesmen electrocuted while working on pylons. No manual method would have any hope of success in such situations.
5. The method seems to come naturally, and many rescuers have achieved success with the minimum of instruction.

There have been few new developments in recent years, although there is now increased fear of infection from the victim, which has led to renewed interest in mechanical methods of ventilation as an alternative to techniques requiring more intimate contact.[4]

Intermittent positive pressure ventilation

Phases of the respiratory cycle

Inspiration. During IPPV, the mouth (or airway) pressure is intermittently raised above ambient pressure. The inspired gas then flows into the respiratory system in accord with the resistance and compliance of the respiratory system. If inspiration is slow, the distribution is governed mainly by regional compliance. If inspiration is fast, there is preferential ventilation of parts of the lungs with short time constants (see Figure 3.6). Different temporal patterns of pressure may be applied, as discussed below.

Expiration. During IPPV, expiration results from allowing mouth pressure to fall to ambient. Expiration is then passive, and differs from expiration during spontaneous breathing in which diaphragmatic tone is gradually reduced (page 85). Expiration may be impeded by the application of positive end-expiratory pressure (PEEP). In the past, expiration was sometimes accelerated by the application of a subatmospheric pressure, termed negative end-expiratory pressure (NEEP), though this technique is no longer used. Expiration to ambient pressure is termed zero end-expiratory pressure (ZEEP).

If the inflating pressure is maintained for several seconds, the resulting tidal volume will be indicated by the following relationship:

$$\text{tidal volume} = \text{sustained inflation pressure} \times \text{total static compliance.}$$

Thus, for example, a sustained inflation pressure of $10\,\text{cmH}_2\text{O}$ with a static compliance of $0.5\,\text{l.kPa}^{-1}$ $(0.05\,\text{l.cmH}_2\text{O}^{-1})$ would result in a lung volume $500\,\text{ml}$ above functional residual capacity (FRC).

Time course of inflation and deflation

Equilibration according to the above equation usually takes several seconds. When the airway pressure is raised during inspiration, it is opposed by the two forms of impedance – the elastic resistance of lungs and chest wall (Chapter 3) and resistance to air flow (Chapter 4). At any instant, the inflation pressure equals the sum of the pressures required to overcome these two forms of impedance. The pressure required to overcome elastic resistance equals the lung volume above FRC divided by the total (dynamic) compliance, while the pressure required to overcome air flow resistance equals the air flow resistance multiplied by the instantaneous flow rate.

The effect of applying a constant pressure (or square wave inflation) is shown in Figure 31.1. The two components of the inflation pressure vary during the course of inspiration while their sum remains constant. The component overcoming air flow resistance is

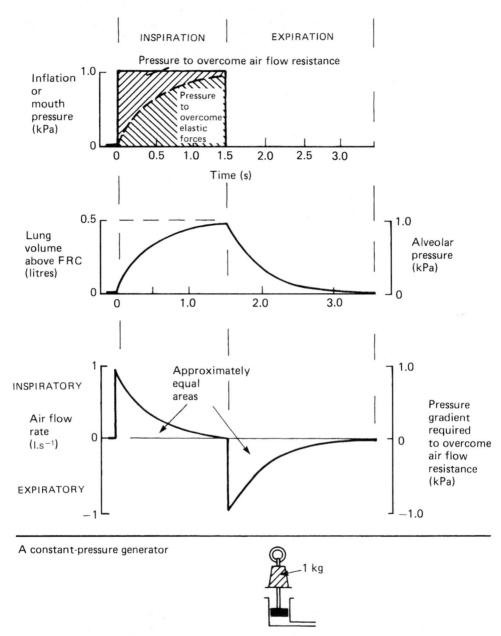

Figure 31.1 Artificial ventilation by intermittent application of a constant pressure (square wave) followed by passive expiration. Inspiratory and expiratory flow rates are both exponential. Assuming that air flow resistance is constant, it follows that flow rate and pressure gradient required to overcome resistance may be shown on the same graph. Lung volume and alveolar pressure may be shown on the same graph if compliance is constant. Values are typical for an anaesthetized supine paralysed patient: total dynamic compliance, $0.5\,l.kPa^{-1}$ ($50\,ml.cmH_2O^{-1}$); pulmonary resistance $0.3\,kPa.l^{-1}.s$ ($3\,cmH_2O.l^{-1}.s$); apparatus resistance $0.7\,kPa.l^{-1}.s$ ($7\,cmH_2O.l^{-1}.s$); total resistance, $1\,kPa.l^{-1}.s$ ($10\,cmH_2O.l^{-1}.s$); time constant, $0.5\,s$.

maximal at first and declines exponentially with air flow as inflation proceeds. The component overcoming elastic resistance increases with the lung volume. With normal respiratory mechanics in the unconscious patient, the change in lung volume should be 95 per cent complete in about 1.5 seconds, as in Figure 31.1.

The approach of the lung volume to its equilibrium value is according to an exponential function of the wash-in type (see Appendix F). The time constant, which is the time required for inflation to 63 per cent of the equilibrium value, equals the product of resistance and compliance. Normal values for an unconscious patient are:

$$\text{time constant} = \text{resistance} \times \text{compliance}$$

$$0.5 \text{ second} = 1 \text{ kPa.l}^{-1}.\text{s} \times 0.5 \text{ l.kPa}^{-1}$$

(or, in non-SI units, $10 \text{ cmH}_2\text{O.l}^{-1}.\text{s} \times 0.05 \text{ l.cmH}_2\text{O}^{-1}$, which also equals 0.5 second).

The time constant is the time that would be required to reach equilibrium if the initial inspiratory flow rate were maintained. It is sometimes more convenient to use the half-time, which is 0.69 times the time constant. The inflation curve is shown in full with further mathematical detail in Appendix F.

It is normal practice for the inspiratory phase to be terminated after 1 or 2 seconds, at which time the lung volume will still be increasing. Inflation pressure is not then the sole arbiter of tidal volume but must be considered in relation to the duration of the inspiratory phase.

If expiration is passive and mouth pressure remains at ambient, the driving force is the elevation of alveolar pressure above ambient, caused by elastic recoil of lungs and chest wall. This pressure is dissipated in overcoming air flow resistance during expiration. In Figure 31.1, during expiration the alveolar pressure (proportional to the lung volume above FRC) is directly proportional to expiratory flow rate, and all three quantities decline according to a wash-out exponential function with a time constant, which is again equal to the product of compliance and resistance.

The effect of changes in inflation pressure, resistance and compliance

The heavy line in Figure 31.2 shows the inflation curve for the normal parameters of an unconscious paralysed patient as listed in Table 31.2. These are the same values that were considered above. The basic curve is a single exponential approaching a lung volume 0.5 litre above FRC with a time constant of 0.5 second.

Changes in inflation pressure do not alter the time constant of inflation, but directly influence the amount of air introduced into the lungs in a given number of time constants. In Figure 31.2, each point on the curve labelled 'inflation pressure doubled' is twice the height of the corresponding point on the basic curve for the same time.

Effect of changes in compliance and resistance. If the compliance is doubled, the equilibrium tidal volume is also doubled. However, the time constant (product of compliance and resistance) is also doubled and therefore the equilibrium volume is approached more slowly (Figure 31.2). Conversely, if the compliance is halved, the equilibrium tidal volume is also halved and so is the time constant.

Changes in resistance have a direct effect on the time constant of inflation but do not affect the equilibrium tidal volume. Thus the effect of an increased resistance on tidal volume is through the reduction in inspiratory flow rate. Within limits, this can be counteracted by prolonging inspiration or by increasing the inflation pressure and the degree of overpressure (explained below). The effects, shown in Figure 31.2, apply not

Table 31.2 Parameters for inflation curves shown in Figure 31.2

	Basic curve	Pulmonary resistance doubled	Inflation pressure doubled	Compliance doubled	Compliance halved
Inflation pressure					
(kPa)	1	1	2	1	1
(cmH$_2$O)	10	10	20	10	10
Compliance					
(l.kPa^{-1})	0.5	0.5	0.5	1	0.25
(ml.cmH$_2$O^{-1})	50	50	50	100	25
Final tidal volume (l)	0.5	0.5	1	1	0.25
Pulmonary resistance					
(kPa.l^{-1}.s)	1	2	1	1	1
(cmH$_2$O.l^{-1}.s)	10	20	10	10	10
Time constant					
(s)	0.5	1	0.5	1	0.25

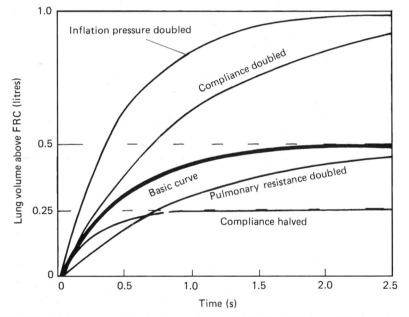

Figure 31.2 Effect of changes in various factors on the rate of inflation of the lungs. Fixed relationships: final tidal volume achieved = inflation pressure × compliance; time constant = compliance × resistance. (See also Table 31.2.)

only to the whole lung but also to regions that may have different compliances, resistances and time constants (page 167).

Overpressure. Increasing the inflation pressure has a major effect on the time required to achieve a particular lung volume above FRC. In Figure 31.3, the lung characteristics are the same as for the basic curve in Figure 31.2. If the required tidal volume is 475 ml, this is achieved in 1.5 seconds with an inflation pressure of 10 cmH$_2$O. However, the same lung volume is achieved in only 0.3 second by doubling the inflation pressure. The application of a pressure that, if sustained, would give a tidal volume higher than that which is intended, is known as overpressure; it is used extensively to increase the inspiratory flow rate and so to shorten the inspiratory phase. The use of a subatmospheric pressure to increase the rate of passive expiration is similar in principle but is complicated by airway trapping (Figure 31.3b).

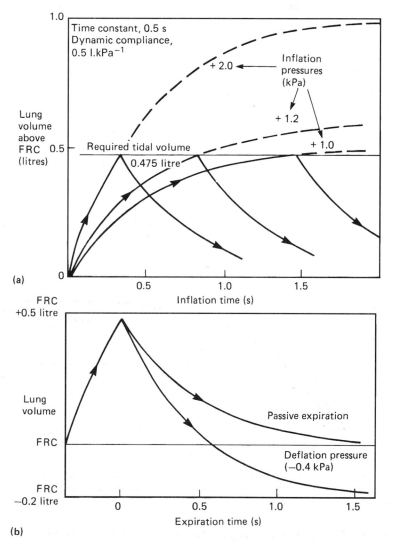

Figure 31.3 (a) How the duration of inflation may be shortened by the use of overpressure. Inflation curves are shown for +2 kPa (+20 cmH$_2$O) (equilibrium 1 litre), +1.2 kPa (+12 cmH$_2$O) (equilibrium 0.6 litre) and +1 kPa (+10 cmH$_2$O) (equilibrium 0.5 litre). With a required tidal volume of 0.475 litre note the big reduction in duration of inflation needed when the inflation pressure is increased from 1 to 2 kPa (10 to 20 cmH$_2$O). (b) How expiration is influenced by the use of a subatmospheric pressure or 'negative phase'. Expiration may be terminated at the FRC after 0.6 s, or may be prolonged, in which case the lung volume will fall to 0.2 litre below FRC.

Deviations from true exponential character of expiration. It is helpful to assume that the patterns of air flow described above are exponential in character, as this greatly assists our understanding of the situation. However, there are many reasons why air flow should not be strictly exponential in character. Air flow is normally partly turbulent (see Chapter 4) and therefore resistance cannot be considered as a constant. Furthermore, as expiration proceeds, the calibre of the air passages decreases and there is also a transition to more laminar flow as the instantaneous flow rate decreases. Approximation to a single exponential function is nevertheless good enough for many practical purposes.

Alternative patterns of application of inflation pressure

Constant pressure or square wave inflation has been considered above because it is the easiest for mathematical analysis. There are, however, an almost infinite number of pressure profiles that may be applied for IPPV. There is no very convincing evidence of the superiority of one over the other, except that distribution of inspired gas is improved if there is a prolongation of the period during which the applied pressure is maximal. This permits better ventilation of the 'slow' alveoli and is not very important in patients with relatively healthy lungs.

Constant flow rate ventilators are used extensively, and Figure 31.4 shows pressure, volume and flow changes in a manner analogous to Figure 31.1. This pattern of air flow is conveniently achieved with electronically controlled ventilators.[5]

Sine wave generators were popular in the days of mechanical ventilators. The pattern of inspiratory flow rate was a direct consequence of the mechanical linkage used in these ventilators, which are now employed only rarely. Figure 31.5 shows the pattern of pressure, volume and flow rate changes with a sine wave generator.

Control of duration of inspiration

Three methods are in general use.

Time cycling terminates inspiration after a preset time. With mechanical ventilators delivering a sine pressure wave, the inspiratory time usually derives directly from the system itself. However, with constant pressure generators and constant flow generators, a separate and variable timing device is incorporated. With constant flow generators, inspiratory time has a direct effect on the tidal volume. With constant pressure generators the relationship is more complex, as described above (see Figure 31.3).

Volume cycling terminates inspiration when a preset volume has been delivered. In the absence of a leak, this should guarantee the tidal volume even if the compliance or resistance of the patient changes within limits. Formerly, volume-cycled ventilators were usually based on a reciprocating pump of preset tidal volume. Nowadays they are more likely to be flow generators with an inspiratory flow sensor that terminates inspiration when the required volume (integral of flow rate) has entered the lungs.

Pressure cycling terminates inspiration when a particular mouth pressure is achieved. This in no way guarantees the tidal volume. Increased airway resistance, for example, would

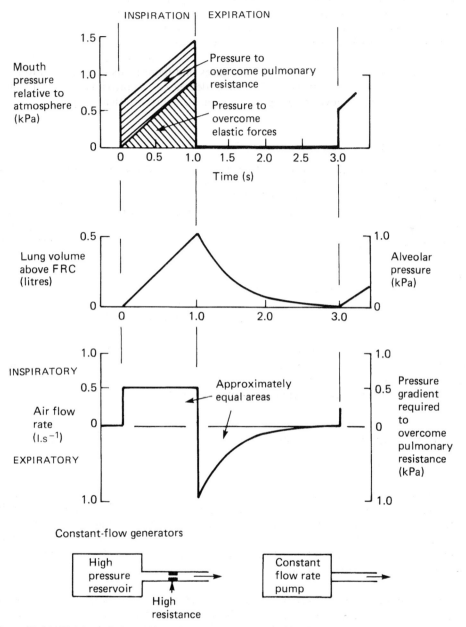

Figure 31.4 Artificial ventilation by intermittent application of a constant-flow generator, with passive expiration. Note that inspiratory flow rate is constant. Assuming that pulmonary resistance is constant, it follows that a constant amount of the inflation pressure is required to overcome flow resistance. Lung volume and alveolar pressure may be shown on the same graph if compliance is constant. Values are typical for an anaesthetized supine paralysed patient: total dynamic compliance, $0.5\,\mathrm{l.kPa^{-1}}$ ($50\,\mathrm{ml.cmH_2O^{-1}}$); pulmonary resistance $0.3\,\mathrm{kPa.l^{-1}.s}$ ($3\,\mathrm{cmH_2O.l^{-1}.s}$); apparatus resistance $0.7\,\mathrm{kPa.l^{-1}.s}$ ($7\,\mathrm{cmH_2O.l^{-1}.s}$); total resistance, $1\,\mathrm{kPa.l^{-1}.s}$ ($10\,\mathrm{cmH_2O.l^{-1}.s}$); time constant, $0.5\,\mathrm{s}$.

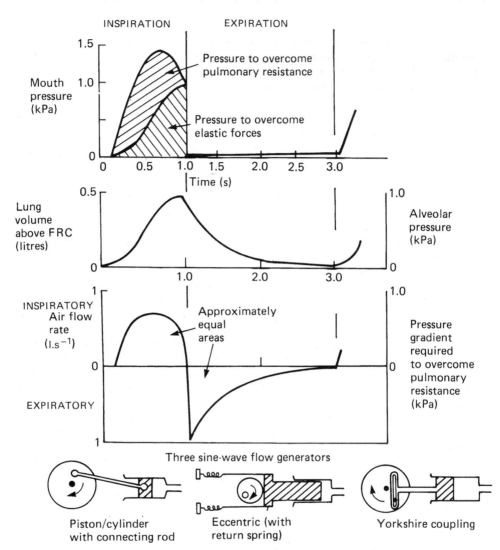

Figure 31.5 Artificial ventilation with inspiratory gas flow conforming to a sine wave, with passive expiration. Note that inspiratory gas flow rate is out of phase with the change in lung volume. (The latter conforms to a sine wave and the former to the differential of the sine which is the cosine.) Assuming that air flow resistance is constant, it follows that flow rate and pressure gradient required to overcome resistance may be shown on the same graph. Lung volume and alveolar pressure may be shown on the same graph if compliance is constant. Peak inspiratory flow rate = $\pi \times$ minute volume $\times 1.5$. (The factor 1.5 is used because in this example inspiration does not last half the respiratory cycle.) Values are typical for an anaesthetized supine paralysed patient: total dynamic compliance, $0.5 \, \text{l.kPa}^{-1}$ ($50 \, \text{ml.cmH}_2\text{O}^{-1}$); pulmonary resistance $0.3 \, \text{kPa.l}^{-1}.\text{s}$ ($3 \, \text{cmH}_2\text{O.l}^{-1}.\text{s}$); apparatus resistance $0.7 \, \text{kPa.l}^{-1}.\text{s}$ ($7 \, \text{cmH}_2\text{O.l}^{-1}.\text{s}$); total resistance, $1 \, \text{kPa.l}^{-1}.\text{s}$ ($10 \, \text{cmH}_2\text{O.l}^{-1}.\text{s}$); time constant, $0.5 \, \text{s}$.

limit inspiratory flow rate and cause a more rapid increase in mouth pressure, thus terminating the inspiratory phase. Pressure-cycled ventilators are almost invariably flow generators.

Limitations on inspiratory duration. Whatever the means of cycling, it is possible to add a limitation on inspiratory duration, usually as a safety precaution. For example, a pressure limitation can be added to a time-cycled or a volume-cycled ventilator. This can either function as a pressure relief valve or it can terminate the inspiratory phase.

The inspiratory/expiratory (*I/E*) ratio

For a given minute volume of ventilation, it is possible to vary within wide limits the duration of inspiration and expiration and the ratio between the two. A common pattern is about 1 second for inspiration, followed by 2–4 seconds for expiration (*I/E* ratio 1:2–1:4), giving respiratory frequencies in the range 12–20 breaths per minute. The problem is whether changes from this pattern confer any appreciable benefit in terms of gas exchange. There is no guarantee that studies in animals or healthy anaesthetized patients are relevant to patients with pulmonary dysfunction in whom some benefit might be expected to accrue. Several studies in the 1960s[6,7,8,9] demonstrated an increase in dead space when the duration of inspiration was reduced below 1 second. There seems to be no convincing evidence in any of these studies that the duration of inspiration (in the range 0.5–3 seconds) has any appreciable effect on the alveolar/arterial Po_2 gradient. Thus the consensus view seems to be that 1 second is a reasonable minimal time for inspiration.

Inverse I/E ratio ventilation has the effect of increasing the mean lung volume and so may be expected to achieve some of the advantages of PEEP as considered below. It may be achieved either by slowing the inspiratory flow rate (shallow ramp) or by holding the lung volume at the end of inspiration (inspiratory pause), the latter seeming to be more logical. *I/E* ratios as high as 4:1 have been used but 2:1 is generally preferable. The degree of inverse *I/E* ratio used is limited by the cardiovascular disturbances seen with the technique (see below) and the time available for expiration. If the latter is unduly curtailed, FRC will be increased – so-called intrinsic-PEEP (see below).

Gas redistribution during an inspiratory hold reduces the dead space (page 179) and so results in a lower Pco_2 for the same minute volume.[10] This permits the use of a lower peak inflation pressure. Shunting is also reduced,[11] presumably because of the increased fraction of the respiratory cycle during which airways tend to be open.

Interaction of ventilator controls

The commonest controls that are provided on an artificial ventilator are drawn from the following list:

tidal volume
inspiratory flow rate
duration of inspiration
duration of expiration
I/E ratio
respiratory frequency
minute volume

It will be found that the maximum possible number of independent controls is three. A setting of any three on this list will determine the values for all the remaining variables. Opinion is divided on which of these controls the clinician likes to operate directly. However, an excellent compromise is to display computed values corresponding to the variables that are not available as controls.

Clinical use of IPPV[12,13]

The previous section classifies ventilators according to the method of gas flow generation – for example, constant flow, constant pressure or sine wave generators – based on the mechanism by which the ventilator worked. Most ventilators in clinical use in the developed world are now microprocessor controlled. These allow accurate control of gas pressure and flow throughout the ventilator circuit, and can usually perform as either flow or pressure generators, usually with a variety of inspiratory flow patterns. In addition, they have given rise to a whole host of previously impossible ventilatory techniques, most of which depend on the ventilator responding appropriately to the patient's own respiratory efforts.

Interactions between patient and ventilator

For many years there have been ventilators in which the inspiratory phase could be triggered with a spontaneous breath, and mechanical ventilators could be modified to facilitate a mandatory minute volume of ventilation, as described below. Electronic ventilators continuously monitor tidal volume, whether generated by the patient (spontaneous breath) or artificially (ventilator breath). With this information available it is a simple task to achieve, by electronic means, a predetermined minute volume, number of breaths, etc. by introducing extra ventilator breaths when necessary. The challenge for ventilator design in recent years has been the speed and sensitivity with which ventilators can sense, and respond to, the patient's own respiratory efforts in order to synchronize ventilator and spontaneous breaths. Without this synchronization, a patient with any reasonable spontaneous respiratory effort begins to 'fight' against the ventilator,[14] leading to discomfort, poor gas exchange and even cardiovascular disturbance.

There are two ways by which a ventilator may detect the onset of a spontaneous breath: pressure sensing and flow sensing.[15]

Pressure sensing. At the onset of a respiratory effort, the patient will generate a reduction in pressure within the circuit, which may be detected in the ventilator. This pressure wave travels through the circuit at approximately the speed of sound, and so reaches the ventilator within 12 ms, following which the pressure sensor must respond, and flow into the circuit be increased to facilitate inspiration. Over all, these events take approximately 100 ms to occur, which is undetectable by the patient. The pressure drop required to trigger inspiration is now always measured relative to circuit (not atmospheric) pressure, to allow the use of continuous positive airway pressure (CPAP) during ventilation. The time taken to trigger the ventilator increases with decreased sensitivity settings – that is, when a greater pressure drop is required for triggering. Pressure triggering is also affected by the circuit compliance, which is function of the circuit volume and the stiffness of the tubing.

Flow sensing. Detection of inspiratory flow may trigger a ventilator breath or some type of respiratory assist (see below). Many current intensive care ventilators provide a continuous base flow around the ventilator circuit of $2–20\,l.min^{-1}$. Any difference between ventilator inflow and outflow represents the patient's respiration. Flow triggering occurs in approximately 80 ms, irrespective of the sensitivity setting. A high base flow provides adequate inspiratory flow for the patient at the start of inspiration and the flow rate is increased when the ventilator is triggered. Flow sensing can also detect the end of inspiration, and is used in pressure support ventilation (see below).

Ventilatory modes in common use

In addition to control mode ventilation (CMV), there are now a bewildering range of ventilation patterns. Many of these are essentially the same but have different nomenclature owing to their development by rival ventilator manufacturers. Those in common use are described below and shown graphically in Figure 31.6.

Mandatory minute volume (MMV). Hewlett, Platt and Terry in 1977[16] described a simple technique for controlling the volume of artificial ventilation so that the total of spontaneous and artificial ventilation did not fall below a preset value. If the patient is able to achieve the preset level of MMV, ventilator breaths do not occur. Electronic ventilators allow MMV to be used, and can coordinate the mandatory breaths with patient respiration to a greater degree than the original mechanical technique, including provision for the spontaneous ventilation to exceed the MMV. Achievement of the preset MMV by a rapid, shallow respiratory pattern commonly seen in intensive care patients was a major disadvantage of MMV, which has now been almost entirely replaced by other techniques.

Assist-control ventilation or synchronized IPPV (Figure 31.6c). This was one of the earlier ventilatory modes, which depended on patient triggering of the ventilator breaths. It is essentially the same as volume preset IPPV except that breaths are triggered by the patient, normally as a result of reduced circuit pressure. A maximum time delay between breaths is incorporated, following which a breath will be generated by the ventilator if spontaneous 'triggering' has ceased. There is no provision for spontaneous breathing between ventilator breaths.

Airway pressure release ventilation (Figure 31.6d). This technique is essentially the reverse of intermittent positive pressure ventilation. It consists of CPAP that is released intermittently to cause the patient to *exhale* to FRC with a subsequent inspiration when CPAP is reapplied.[17] The patient is able to breathe as he wishes during the periods when CPAP is applied, but this is from the lung volume following an inspiration after reapplication of CPAP. Artificial breaths are thus within the conventional tidal range set by his FRC, whilst spontaneous inspirations are within his inspiratory reserve. The CPAP release valve is controlled to provide mandatory ventilation as necessary. The pattern of the imposed breaths is basically similar to that of reversed *I/E* ratio. Dead space was found to be significantly less, but intrapulmonary shunt more, than with assist-control ventilation.[18]

Synchronized intermittent mandatory ventilation (SIMV) (Figure 31.6e). Intermittent mandatory ventilation was introduced by Downs and his colleagues in 1974,[19] followed in the 1980s by the ability to synchronize ventilator breaths with the patient's own respiratory effort as described above. The essential feature of SIMV is to allow the patient to take a spontaneous breath between artificial breaths. This confers three major advantages. First, a spontaneous inspiration is not obstructed by a closed inspiratory valve

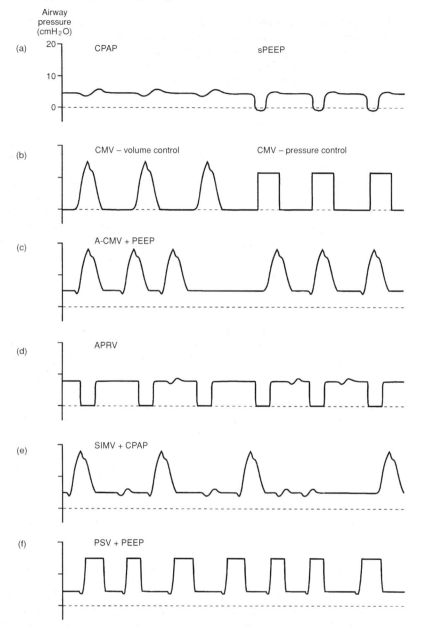

Figure 31.6 Airway pressure curves with a variety of commonly used modes of ventilation. (a) CPAP, continuous positive airway pressure, and sPEEP, true positive end-expiratory pressure applied during spontaneous breathing. (b) CMV, control mode ventilation showing volume and pressure-controlled breaths. (c) A-CMV, assist-control mode ventilation where breaths are triggered by a fall in circuit pressure. When apnoea occurs, ventilator breaths occur without triggering. (d) APRV, airway pressure release ventilation when a CPAP of 8 cmH₂O is intermittently removed to allow expiration, spontaneous breaths occurring between. (e) SIMV, synchronized intermittent mandatory ventilation, as for A-CMV except that spontaneous breathing can occur between ventilator breaths. (f) PSV, pressure support ventilation in which pressure-controlled breaths are triggered by the patient, who also controls the duration of the breath. In practice, many ventilators allow combinations of these modes, such as SIMV, PSV and PEEP together.

and this helps to prevent the patient fighting the ventilator. The second advantage is the facilitation of weaning, which is considered further below. Thirdly, the patient is able to breathe spontaneously at any time during prolonged ventilation; this may prevent respiratory muscle atrophy and helps to reduce the mean intrathoracic pressure. Most ventilators now provide SIMV as a normal feature, and it is used extensively in many parts of the world, often in conjunction with pressure support ventilation (see below).

Inspiratory pressure support ventilation (PSV) (Figure 31.6f).[20,21] In this system a spontaneous inspiration triggers a rapid flow of gas that increases until airway pressure reaches a preselected level. Flow sensing by the ventilator is also then able to detect when the spontaneous inspiration ends, at which point the pressure support ceases and expiration occurs. The purpose is not to provide a prescribed tidal volume, but to assist the patient in making an inspiration of a pattern that lies largely in his own control; patients usually find this very acceptable.[22] The level of support may be increased until the pressure is sufficient to provide the full tidal volume (maximal pressure support), and may be gradually reduced as the patient's ventilatory capacity improves. The amount of pressure support provided does seem to be inversely related to the work of breathing.[21]

High frequency ventilation[12,23]

Öberg and Sjöstrand (1967, unpublished) made the surprising observation that effective respiration could be maintained in dogs during artificial ventilation at a respiratory frequency of 80 breaths per minute (breath.min^{-1}) with a tidal volume that did not seem to be sufficient to wash out the dead space.[24] It was soon found that similar techniques could be applied to patients.[25]

High frequency ventilation may be classified into the following categories: high frequency positive pressure ventilation (HFPPV), high frequency jet ventilation (HFJV) and high frequency oscillation (HFO).

High frequency positive pressure ventilation (HFPPV) is applied in the frequency range 1–2 Hz (60–120 breath.min^{-1}) and can be considered as an extension of conventional IPPV techniques. Although many conventional ventilators will operate within this frequency range, specially designed ventilators have been used. The method has enjoyed limited application for endoscopy and airway surgery but the advantages of HFPPV have not been proven.

High frequency jet ventilation (HFJV) covers the frequency range 1–5 Hz. Inspiration is driven by a high velocity stream of gas from a jet, which may or may not entrain gas from a secondary supply. Humidification with HFJV is technically difficult, and if done properly requires equipment as complex as the ventilator itself. The position of the jet may be proximal to the patient, in the hope of avoiding dead space, or more distal, which is safer in terms of mucosal trauma and thermal injury from cooling due to the Joule–Kelvin effect.[23] A unique advantage is the ability to ventilate through a narrow cannula, as for example through the cricothyroid membrane.

HFJV has been used extensively both in the operating theatre and during intensive therapy. Jet systems are extremely versatile. Jets may face towards or away from the patient and may thus power inspiration, retard expiration, assist expiration or provide PEEP. It has been proposed that purely passive expiration be designated by the suffix -P and actively assisted expiration by the suffix -A.[26]

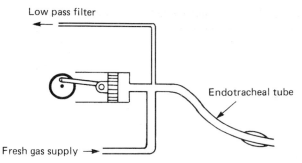

Figure 31.7 Circuit for provision of high frequency oscillation.

High frequency oscillation (HFO) covers the frequency range 3–50 Hz, and the flows are usually generated by an oscillating pump or diaphragm making a fourth connection to a T-piece with a low pass filter on the open limb (Figure 31.7). At these high frequencies, the respiratory waveform is usually sinusoidal, including active expiration. Tidal volumes are inevitably small and are difficult to measure.

Studies in dogs have shown that satisfactory gas exchange may be maintained by this technique, for periods up to at least 36 hours, with oscillator frequencies in the range 13–28 Hz. There were no important differences in respiratory or cardiovascular function when high frequency was compared with conventional artificial ventilation.[27] In another study by the same group it was shown that oxygenation and the uniformity of distribution of ventilation and perfusion were somewhat better at 5.8 Hz than at 15 or 29.8 Hz or with conventional artificial ventilation.[28] Similar results have been obtained in humans, with adequate gas exchange and little difference in cardiac output between IPPV and HFO.[29,30] In one of these studies, mean shunt was decreased with HFO in all 8 patients in whom the measurement was made, the benefit being greatest in the patients thought to have an extensive mismatch of ventilation and perfusion.[29]

The relationship between tidal volume and dead space during high frequency ventilation is crucial to an understanding of the technique. It is useless to infer values for tidal volume and dead space from measurements made under other circumstances, yet it is very difficult to make direct measurements of these variables under the actual conditions of high frequency ventilation, especially in humans. Chakrabarti and colleagues[31] studied anaesthetized humans during HFPPV up to frequencies of 2 Hz, holding arterial Pco_2 approximately constant at about 5 kPa (37.5 mmHg). As frequency increased from conventional ventilation at 15 breath.min^{-1} to HFPPV at 2 Hz it was necessary to double the minute volume (Table 31.3). The actual volume of the physiological dead space decreased with decreasing tidal volume, to reach a minimal value of about 90 ml at about 1 Hz. However, the normal proportionality between dead space and tidal volume (page 179) was not maintained. Dead space/tidal volume ratio increased from 37 per cent at 15 breath.min^{-1} to 75 per cent at 2 Hz, which explains the requirement for the increased minute volume. The situation is more complex at higher frequencies. Butler et al.[29] found that tidal volumes of at least 100 ml were still required at frequencies of 15 Hz, corresponding to an *applied* minute volume of 90 l.min^{-1}, which would indicate a dead space/tidal volume ratio of over 90 per cent. There are severe technical difficulties in the measurement of the actual delivered tidal volumes which, though undoubtedly less than the pump settings, are probably much larger than the external movements of the thorax would suggest.

Table 31.3 Gas exchange during high frequency ventilation

		Respiratory frequency		
		15 b.p.m. 0.25 Hz	60 b.p.m. 1 Hz	120 b.p.m. 2 Hz
Arterial P_{CO_2}	kPa	4.8	4.8	4.9
	mmHg	36	36	37
$\dot{V}$	l.min^{-1}	6.8	10.2	14
V_T	ml	454	170	117
V_D (physiol.)	ml	165	96	88
V_D/V_T ratio	%	36	56	75

b.p.m, breaths per minute.
(Data from reference 31.)

End-expiratory pressure is inevitably raised at high frequencies because the duration of expiration will be inadequate for passive exhalation to FRC, the time constant of the normal respiratory system being about 0.5 second (see above). Therefore, the use of respiratory frequencies above about 2 Hz will usually result in 'intrinsic-PEEP',[32] and hence an increased end-expiratory lung volume, which is likely to be a major factor promoting favourable gas exchange.

Gas mixing and streaming is likely to be modified at high frequencies. The sudden reversals of flow direction are likely to set up eddies that blur the boundary between dead space and alveolar gas, thus improving the efficiency of ventilation. It has been suggested that such 'enhanced diffusion' or 'augmented dispersion' plays a major role in gas exchange during HFO.[29] Air passages dilated by intrinsic-PEEP may contribute to this effect. Furthermore, cardiac mixing of gases becomes relatively more important at small tidal volumes.[33] It has also been suggested that high frequency ventilation causes 'accelerated diffusion', but this is difficult to demonstrate.

The clinical indications for high frequency ventilation are still not clear. The techniques have been used mainly for weaning from artificial ventilation in adults and for respiratory support in babies. HFJV seems to have a wider acceptance than HFPPV or HFO, but randomized trials have generally failed to demonstrate any clear clinical advantage over conventional methods of ventilation.[34,35] There is no doubt that effective gas exchange is usually possible with high frequency ventilation but the advantages over conventional artificial ventilation are less clear. Although there are enthusiasts, others believe that it is merely a technique in search of an application. There is agreement on its special role for patients with bronchopleural fistula, and the technique is particularly convenient when there is no airtight junction between ventilator and the tracheobronchial tree, at laryngoscopy, for example. Another attractive feature is the avoidance of high *peak* inspiratory pressures. However, *mean* airway pressure may still be high if exhalation is impeded, as it must be at very high frequencies. Whether high frequency ventilation is less likely to produce pulmonary barotrauma than conventional techniques of ventilation will be difficult to determine in humans but animal experiments suggest this may be so. It may prove valuable to combine high frequency ventilation with conventional artificial ventilation. A recently developed non-invasive form of high frequency ventilation is described below.

Weaning[36,37]

'Weaning' describes the process by which artificial ventilation is gradually withdrawn and the patient returned to normal respiration. In practice it is useful to think of two stages – the withdrawal of ventilatory support and the removal of any artificial airway, usually a tracheal tube or tracheostomy. Only the first of these stages is considered here.

Predicting successful weaning. Before weaning can be attempted, the balance between ventilatory load and capacity must be favourable. Extra demands on the respiratory system may originate from increased oxygen consumption, commonly as a result of sepsis, but also occasionally from thyrotoxicosis, convulsions or shivering. Reduced respiratory system compliance or increased airway resistance also impose additional loads on the respiratory system. The capacity of the respiratory system to wean depends on having, first, adequate ventilation perfusion matching and, secondly, low intrapulmonary shunt and respiratory dead space. Finally, good respiratory muscle function must be achieved, including correction of any metabolic disturbance and provision of adequate blood supply to the muscles; that is, the patient must have reasonable cardiovascular function. Some of the criteria that have been used to predict successful weaning are shown in Table 31.4.

Table 31.4 Criteria used to assess suitability for weaning from artificial ventilation

Criteria	Value for successful weaning
Tests of respiratory muscle function	
VC	$\geq 10-15$ ml.kg^{-1}
FEV$_{1.0}$	≥ 10 ml.kg^{-1}
Maximum inspiratory pressure	-20 to -30 cmH$_2$O
Airway occlusion pressure P$_{0.1}$	<6 cmH$_2$O
Resting minute volume	<10 l.min^{-1}
Maximum voluntary ventilation	$>2 \times$ resting $\dot{V}$
Tests of lung function	
(A/a) Po$_2$ difference	$<40-47$ kPa (300–350 mmHg)
Shunt	$<10-20\%$
V$_D$/V$_T$ ratio	$<50-60\%$

(After references 37 and 38.)

No single variable is a reliable indicator of success, most having very low predictive values.[37] This has led to the development of more complex scoring systems, which include:

Compliance, Rate, Oxygenation, Pressure (CROP) score, calculated as:

$$\text{CROP} = \text{dynamic } Crs \times Pi_{max}, \times (Pa_{O_2}/PA_{O_2})/\text{respiratory rate}$$

(Crs, respiratory system compliance; Pi_{max} maximum inspiratory pressure).

Rate:volume ratio (RVR) score is respiratory rate (breath.min^{-1}) divided by tidal volume (litres) measured over 1 minute without artificial ventilation.

A CROP score of ≥ 13 ml.breath^{-1}.min or a RVR score ≤ 105 breath.min^{-1}.l^{-1} are both reasonable predictors of successful weaning,[39] but are by no means infallible.[40]

Techniques for weaning. The commonest technique for weaning is the abrupt cessation of artificial ventilation for periods of 2–3 minutes, with gradual prolongation of these periods depending on the performance of the patient during the last period. Whereas this approach is satisfactory for an uncomplicated case and for healthy patients recovering from neuromuscular block, it may well be unsatisfactory for patients in whom ventilatory capacity and gas exchange function are marginal.

Ventilation strategies now all focus on gradual withdrawal of respiratory support using the techniques described above. Control mode ventilation is usually replaced by either SIMV or A-CMV until the patient has established adequate respiratory effort, following which the number of ventilator breaths can be gradually reduced. While breathing via an artificial airway, some respiratory support is normally required, and this is most commonly provided with PSV, the level of which can again be reduced gradually.

Excessive reliance on modern ventilator systems for weaning has recently been challenged.[36] In a group of 40 patients who had proved difficult to wean by conventional methods, a multidisciplinary approach to weaning was highly successful.[41] The programme included close attention to nutrition, psychological care such as establishment of normal night:day sleep patterns, and the use of non-invasive ventilation (see below) following early extubation.

Positive end-expiratory pressure

A great variety of pathological conditions, as well as general anaesthesia, result in a decrease in FRC. The deleterious effect of this on gas exchange has been considered elsewhere in Chapter 21, and it is reasonable to consider increasing the FRC by the application of PEEP, first described by Hill et al. in 1965.[42]

Expiratory pressure can be raised during both artificial ventilation and spontaneous breathing, and these forms are best considered together. The terminology is confusing and this chapter adheres to the definitions illustrated in Figure 31.6. Note in particular sPEEP in which a patient inhales spontaneously from ambient pressure but exhales against PEEP. This involves him in a considerable amount of additional work of breathing because he must raise his entire minute volume to the level of PEEP that is applied. This is undesirable and CPAP is much to be preferred to sPEEP.

True CPAP is more difficult to achieve than sPEEP. Biased demand valves may be used but usually result in a pronounced dip in inspiratory pressure, increasing the total work of breathing. Loaded bellows are better but less convenient to manufacture. A high degree of constancy of airway pressure may be achieved with a weighted inspiratory bellows and balanced PEEP valve, with which the inspiratory/expiratory pressure difference was only about 0.1 kPa (1 cmH$_2$O) during spontaneous breathing.[16] The simplest approach is a T-piece with a high fresh gas flow venting through a PEEP valve at the expiratory limb throughout the respiratory phase.[43] Electronic ventilators produce CPAP in a similar fashion by circulating high flows of gas around the ventilator circuit at the required positive pressure.

PEEP may be achieved by many techniques. The simplest is to exhale through a preset depth of water but more convenient methods are spring-loaded valves or diaphragms pressed down by gas, a column of water or a spring. It is also possible to use venturis and fans opposing the direction of expiratory gas flow.

Intrinsic-PEEP[13,14]

If a passive expiration is terminated before the lung volume has returned to FRC, there will be residual end-expiratory raised alveolar pressure, known variously as dynamic hyperinflation, auto-PEEP or intrinsic PEEP (PEEPi).[44] The elevated alveolar pressure will not be transmitted back to the ventilator pressure sensors, so PEEPi may go undetected,[45] but simple methods to measure it have been described.[44] Artificial ventilation with inverse *I/E* ratio may result in PEEPi, but it is more commonly a result of increased expiratory flow resistance due to airway disease or retention of mucus, or from the tracheal tube (Figure 31.8). Eventually, alveolar pressure and lung volume increase sufficiently to cause reduction in both lung compliance and airway resistance (pages 42 and 67); expiratory flow rate then increases and so the degree of PEEPi stabilizes.

At first sight PEEPi may be perceived as beneficial – for example, leading to increased FRC and alveolar recruitment – and it is likely that improved gas exchange seen with inverse *I/E* ratio results, at least in part, from this mechanism. However, the first hazard of PEEPi is its variability. Small changes in airway resistance (e.g. with mucus retention) can lead to rapid increases in the level of PEEPi. The cardiovascular consequences of PEEPi are significant (see below), and have been described as 'applying a tourniquet to the right heart'.[45] Finally, the presence of PEEPi will impede the ability of the patient to trigger ventilators, by necessitating a greater fall in alveolar pressure to initiate respiratory support.[14]

Application of external PEEP will, to some extent, attenuate the generation of PEEPi by maintaining airway patency in late expiration and so improving expiratory flow.

Physiological effects of artificial ventilation

A positive pressure in the chest cavity is a significant physiological insult that normally occurs only transiently with coughing, straining, etc., although the pressure achieved in these situations may be very high. Most physiological effects of IPPV are related to the mean pressure throughout the whole respiratory cycle, which is in turn influenced by a large number of ventilatory settings such as mode of ventilation, tidal volume, respiratory rate and *I/E* ratio. PEEP results in large increases in mean intrathoracic pressure. For example, IPPV in a patient with normal lungs using 10 breaths of 10 ml.kg^{-1} and an *I/E* ratio of 1:2 will generate mean airway pressures of approximately 5 cmH$_2$O. Addition of a modest 5 cmH$_2$O of PEEP will therefore double the mean airway pressure, and thus the physiological insult associated with IPPV. For this reason, much research into the physiological effects of artificial ventilation has focused on PEEP.

Respiratory effects

Distribution of ventilation. Intermittent positive pressure ventilation results in a spatial pattern of distribution that is determined by inflation pressure, regional compliance and time constants. Based on external measurements the anatomical pattern of distribution of inspired gas is different from that of spontaneous breathing, there being a relatively greater expansion of the ribcage.[46] However, with spontaneous breathing regional differences in ventilation are small in the supine position (page 165) and, in spite of the altered ribcage motion, changes in regional ventilation with IPPV are minimal.[47] It thus seems that, although the spatial distribution of gas seems to be altered by IPPV, the functional effect

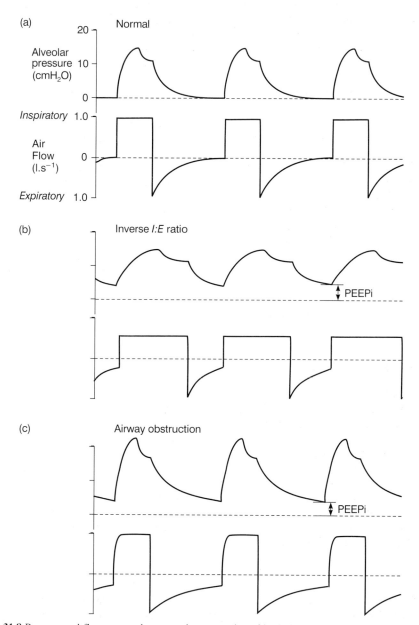

Figure 31.8 Pressure and flow curves demonstrating generation of intrinsic positive end-expiratory pressure (PEEPi). (a) Normal ventilation with both alveolar pressure and airway flow returning to zero before the next breath. (b) Inverse I/E ratio ventilation. Although the decline in pressure and flow is normal, there is insufficient time for complete expiration to occur. (c) Airway obstruction. Expiratory time is normal, but the decline in pressure and flow is retarded to such an extent that expiration is again incomplete.

is minimal. Application of PEEP increases lung volume and re-expands collapsed alveoli, which changes the compliance of dependent lung regions and so improves ventilation of these areas.

Apparatus dead space. Positive pressure ventilation, whether invasive or non-invasive, requires the provision of an airtight connection to the patient's airway. This inevitably involves the addition of some apparatus dead space. With orotracheal and tracheostomy tubes much of the normal anatomical dead space (page 179) is bypassed, such that overall anatomical dead space may be unchanged or reduced. With non-invasive ventilation using facemasks, apparatus dead space may be substantial. Ventilator tubing used to deliver IPPV is normally corrugated, and expands longitudinally with each inspiration. For an average ventilator circuit, this expansion may amount to $2-3\,ml.cmH_2O^{-1}$ of positive pressure,[1] and this volume will constitute dead space ventilation.

Physiological dead space. In normal lungs, IPPV alone seems to have little effect on the V_D/V_T ratio compared with the value obtained during anaesthesia with spontaneous breathing.[48] There is a slight widening of the distribution of $\dot{V}/\dot{Q}$ ratios (page 173), mostly as a result of a reduction in pulmonary blood flow from depression of cardiac output (see below). These changes are normally not sufficient to alter gas exchange. The acute application of moderate amounts of PEEP causes only a slight increase in dead space/tidal volume ratio.[48]

The alveolar component of physiological dead space may be increased by ventilation of patients with widespread lung injury, or when mean intrathoracic pressure is high such as with significant amounts of PEEP. Under the latter conditions, lung volume is increased to such an extent that not only does cardiac output fall but pulmonary vascular resistance rises as well (see Figure 7.4).[49] Perfusion to overexpanded alveoli is reduced and areas of lung with high $\dot{V}/\dot{Q}$ ratios develop, which constitute alveolar dead space. In healthy lungs, this effect is not seen until PEEP levels exceed $10-15\,cmH_2O$.[48] However, with IPPV in lung injury there is now good evidence that overdistension occurs in the relatively small number of functional alveoli (page 580), and local perfusion to these lung units is likely to be impeded.

There is indirect evidence that long-term application of PEEP may cause a very large increase in the dead space, probably because of bronchiolar dilatation (see below).

Lung volume. IPPV and ZEEP will have no effect on FRC. However, with PEEP, end-expiratory alveolar pressure will equal the level of applied PEEP and this will reset the FRC in accord with the pressure/volume curve of the respiratory system (see Figure 3.8). For example, PEEP of $10\,cmH_2O$ will increase FRC by 500 ml in a patient with a compliance of $0.5\,l.kPa^{-1}$ ($50\,ml.cmH_2O^{-1}$). In many patients this may be expected to raise the tidal range above the closing capacity (page 53) and so reduce pulmonary collapse. Opening of previously closed alveoli is probably the greatest single advantage of PEEP. It will also reduce airway resistance according to the inverse relationship between lung volume and airway resistance (see Figure 4.5). It may also change the relative compliance of the upper and lower parts of the lung (Figure 31.9), thereby improving the ventilation of the dependent overperfused parts of the lung.

Permeability. It has been found that PEEP increases the permeability of the lung to DTPA, a tracer molecule that does not readily cross the alveolar/capillary membrane.[50] However, it seems that this effect may be related to lung volume rather than to any damage to the

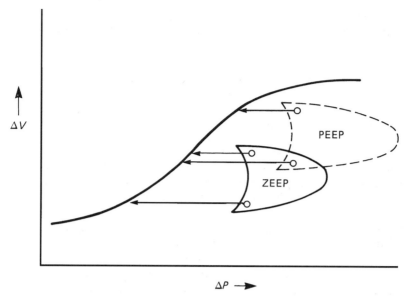

Figure 31.9 Effect of positive end-expiratory pressure (PEEP) on the relationship between regional pressure and volume in the lung (supine position). Note that compliance is greater in the upper part of the lung with zero end-expiratory pressure (ZEEP) and in the lower part of the lung with PEEP, which thus improves ventilation in the dependent zone of the lung. (Diagram kindly supplied by Professor J Gareth Jones.)

membrane. The effect of PEEP on extravascular lung water distribution is discussed on page 549.

Arterial Po_2. Neither IPPV nor PEEP will improve arterial oxygenation appreciably in patients with healthy lungs. It has been repeatedly observed that PEEP during anaesthesia does little to improve arterial oxygenation in the patient with sound lungs. Pulmonary shunting is decreased, but the accompanying decrease in cardiac output reduces the mixed venous oxygen saturation, which counteracts the effect of a reduction in the shunt, resulting in minimal increase in arterial Po_2.[48] There is, however, no doubt that positive pressure ventilation improves arterial Po_2 in a wide range of pathological situations. In most cases, the improvement in Po_2 relates to the mean airway pressure achieved,[13] and, as described above, PEEP provides an easy way of elevating airway pressures. Re-expansion of collapsed lung units, improved ventilation of alveoli with low $\dot{V}/\dot{Q}$ ratios, and redistribution of extravascular lung water will all contribute to the observed improvement in oxygenation. The use of PEEP for preventing atelectasis in anaesthesia is described on page 434, whilst its contribution to the treatment of pulmonary oedema and acute lung injury are described on pages 548 and 582 respectively.

The Valsalva effect

It has long been known that an increase in intrathoracic pressure has complex circulatory effects, characterized as the Valsalva effect, which is the circulatory response to a subject increasing his airway pressure to about 5 kPa (50 cmH$_2$O) against a closed glottis for about 30 seconds. The normal response is in four parts (Figure 31.10a). Initially the raised intrathoracic pressure alters the base line for circulatory pressures, and the arterial

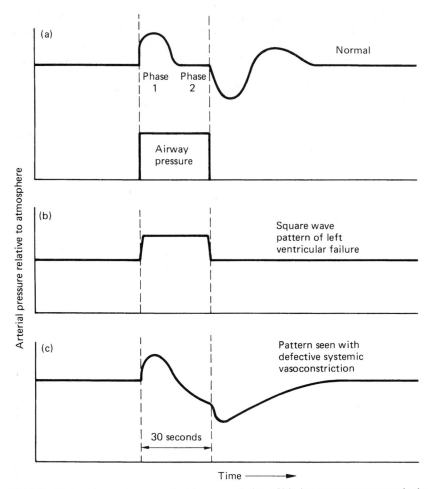

Figure 31.10 Qualitative changes in mean arterial pressure during a Valsalva manoeuvre as seen in the normal subject and for two abnormal responses. See text for explanation of the changes.

pressure (measured relative to atmosphere) is consequently increased (phase 1). At the same time, ventricular filling is decreased by the adverse pressure gradient from peripheral veins to the ventricle in diastole, and cardiac output therefore decreases. The consequent decline in arterial pressure in phase 2 is normally mitigated by three factors – tachycardia, increased systemic vascular resistance (afterload) and an increase in peripheral venous pressure, which tends to restore the venous return. As a result of these compensations, the arterial pressure normally settles to a value fairly close to the level before starting the Valsalva manoeuvre. When the intrathoracic pressure is restored to normal, there is an immediate decrease in arterial pressure due to the altered base line. Simultaneously the venous return improves and therefore the cardiac output increases within a few seconds. However, the arteriolar bed remains constricted temporarily, and there is therefore a transient overshoot of arterial pressure.

Figure 31.10b shows the abnormal 'square wave' pattern that occurs with raised end-diastolic pressure or left ventricular failure or both. The initial increase in arterial pressure (phase 1) occurs normally, but the decline in pressure in phase 2 is missing because the output of the congested heart is not usually limited by end-diastolic pressure. Because the cardiac output is unchanged, there is no increase in pulse rate or systemic vascular resistance. Therefore, there is no overshoot of pressure when the intrathoracic pressure is restored to normal.

Figure 31.10c shows a different abnormal pattern, which may be seen with defective systemic vasoconstriction (e.g. autonomic neuropathy or a spinal anaesthetic). Phase 1 is normal, but in phase 2 the decreased cardiac output is not accompanied by an increase in systemic vascular resistance and the arterial pressure therefore continues to decline. The normal overshoot is replaced by a slow recovery of arterial pressure as the cardiac output returns to control values.

Cardiovascular effects of positive pressure ventilation[51,52]

Initially there was great reluctance to use PEEP, partly because of the well-known Valsalva effect and partly because of the circulatory hazard that had been described in the classic paper of Cournand et al. in 1948.[53] Not many papers in this field have two Nobel prize winners among their authors. The cardiovascular effects of IPPV and PEEP continue to

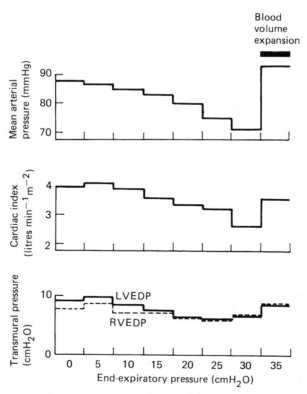

Figure 31.11 Cardiovascular responses as a function of positive end-expiratory pressure (PEEP) in patients with acute lung injury. Left and right ventricular end-diastolic pressure (LVEDP and RVEDP) were measured relative to intrapleural pressure. (Drawn from data of reference 54 and reproduced from reference 55 by permission of the Editors of *International Anesthesiology Clinics*.)

cause problems in clinical practice and, after another half century of investigation, the effects remain incompletely elucidated.[52]

Cardiac output.[52] Bindslev et al.[48] reported a progressive decrease in cardiac output with IPPV and PEEP in anaesthetized patients without pulmonary pathology. Compared with when anaesthetized and breathing spontaneously, cardiac output was reduced by 10 per cent with IPPV and ZEEP, 18 per cent with 9 cmH$_2$O of PEEP, and 36 per cent with 16 cmH$_2$O of PEEP. Another study, this time in patients with severe acute lung injury, also demonstrated a progressive reduction in cardiac output for PEEP in the range 5–30 cmH$_2$O, but the effect was partially reversed by blood volume expansion (Figure 31.11).

There is general agreement that the main cause of the reduction in cardiac output is obstruction to filling of the right atrium, caused by the elevated intrathoracic pressure. With spontaneous respiration, the negative intrathoracic pressure during inspiration draws blood into the chest from the major veins, known as the 'thoracic pump'. Positive intrathoracic pressure abolishes this effect and also imposes a further reduction in driving pressure for flow between extra- and intrathoracic vessels. Reduced right ventricle filling pressures quickly lead to reduced left ventricle filling, and cardiac output falls.[56] These changes will clearly be more pronounced with hypovolaemia. A second cause for reduced cardiac output may come into play with high airway pressures, moderate PEEP, or lung hyperinflation such as occurs with PEEPi. As described above, increasing lung volume leads to elevated pulmonary vascular resistance, which will cause an increase in right ventricle volume[49] and further reduce left ventricle filling. There is now good evidence that dilation of the right ventricle has profound effects on left ventricular function, preventing adequate filling of the left ventricle and reducing left ventricle compliance, both of which lead to a fall in cardiac output.[52] Contractility of the left ventricle is not thought to change with positive intrathoracic pressure, though plasma from animals subjected to PEEP will depress contractility of isolated heart muscle preparations, suggesting the release of a negative inotrope.[57] Interactions of some of the factors by which PEEP may influence cardiac output and systemic arterial pressure are shown in Figure 31.12.

Oxygen flux. In many patients with pulmonary disease, PEEP tends to improve the arterial Po_2 while decreasing the cardiac output. As PEEP is increased the oxygen delivery (the product of cardiac output and arterial oxygen content; page 283) tends to rise to a maximum and then falls.[58] Assuming that a normal or high oxygen flux is desirable, use of IPPV or PEEP therefore requires optimization of cardiac output with fluid replacement (see Figure 31.11) or with positive inotropes, and this is now standard practice in intensive care.

Arterial blood pressure. Figure 31.11 shows the decline in arterial pressure closely following the change in cardiac output with increasing PEEP. Although there was some increase in systemic vascular resistance, this was only about half that required for maintenance of the arterial pressure in the face of the declining cardiac output. It has been suggested that this is due to PEEP causing inhibition of the cardiovascular regulatory centres.[59]

Interpretation of vascular pressures. Atrial pressures are normally measured relative to atmospheric pressure. With positive pressure ventilation, atrial pressures tend to be increased relative to atmospheric. However, relative to intrathoracic pressure, they are

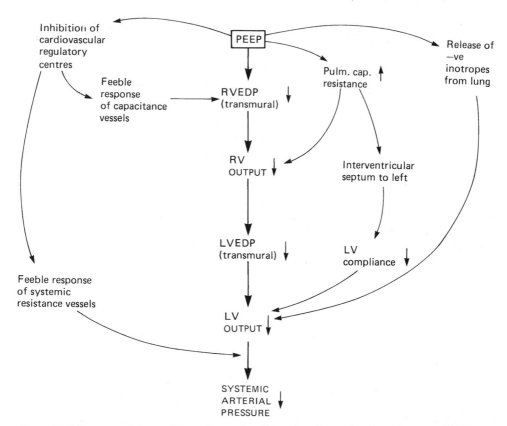

Figure 31.12 Summary of the possible cardiovascular effects of positive end-expiratory pressure (PEEP). See text for full explanation. RVEDP and LVEDP, right and left ventricular end-diastolic pressure; RV and LV, right and left ventricle.

reduced at higher levels of PEEP (Figure 31.11). It is the transmural pressure gradient and not the level relative to atmosphere that is relevant to atrial filling.

An additional problem arises if the tip of a Swan–Ganz catheter lies in zone 1 of the lung where there is no pulmonary blood flow (page 147). It is possible that the application of PEEP increases the extent of zone 1, and an artefact may thus be introduced into the measurement of pulmonary capillary wedge pressure.[51,60]

Transmission of airway pressure to other intrathoracic structures. The intrapleural pressure is protected from the level of PEEP by the transmural pressure gradient of the lungs. Animal studies have shown that reduced pulmonary compliance is the main factor governing the transmission of airway pressure to other thoracic structures. With reduced compliance the effect of mean intrathoracic pressure on cardiac output is greatly reduced.[61] Patients with diseased lungs tend to have reduced pulmonary compliance, which limits the rise in intrapleural pressure (Figure 31.13). Therefore, their cardiovascular systems are better protected against the adverse effects of IPPV and PEEP.

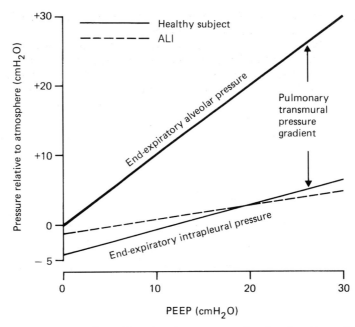

Figure 31.13 End-expiratory alveolar and intrapleural pressures as a function of positive end-expiratory pressure (PEEP). The lower unbroken line shows intrapleural pressure in the relaxed healthy subject. The broken line shows values of intrapleural pressure in patients with severe acute lung injury (ALI) taken from reference 54. Absolute values of pressure probably reflect experimental technique and cannot be compared between studies. (Reproduced from reference 55 by permission of the Editor of *International Anesthesiology Clinics.*)

Haemodynamic response in heart failure. The cardiovascular responses described thus far apply only to patients with normal cardiac function, and, like the Valsalva response, are very different in patients with raised ventricular end-diastolic pressure with or without ventricular failure. Cardiac performance is then on the flat part of the cardiac output/filling pressure curve, and a reduction in end-diastolic volume may not be deleterious and may even be favourable. This corresponds to the square wave pattern of Valsalva response (Figure 31.10b) and is probably a factor in the success of continuous positive airway pressure in the treatment of cardiogenic pulmonary oedema.[62,63]

Other physiological effects

Renal effects. Patients undergoing IPPV tend to become oedematous. Protein depletion and inappropriate fluid loading may be factors but there is also evidence that PEEP itself reduces glomerular filtration.[64] Arterial pressure tends to be reduced as described above, while central venous pressure is raised. Therefore, the pressure gradient between renal artery and vein is reduced, and this has a direct effect on renal blood flow. In addition, PEEP causes elevated levels of antidiuretic hormone, possibly due to activation of left atrial receptors, although this is insufficient to fully explain the changes in urinary flow rate.

Pulmonary neutrophil retention. Neutrophils have a diameter close to that of a pulmonary capillary, and this is important in slowing their transit time through the lung to facilitate margination for pulmonary defence mechanisms (page 565). Any reduction in pulmonary capillary diameter may therefore be expected to increase pulmonary neutrophil retention, which has indeed been demonstrated in humans following a Valsalva manoeuvre[65] or with the application of PEEP.[66] In animals, the pattern of artificial ventilation used can also influence pulmonary neutrophil influx, with high frequency ventilation causing less activation than conventional IPPV.[67] If the neutrophils trapped in this way have already been activated – for example, following cardiopulmonary bypass – lung injury could result (page 578).

Ventilator-induced lung injury (VILI)[68]

Artificial ventilation may damage *normal* lungs only after prolonged ventilation with high airway pressures or large tidal volumes, and is very rarely a problem in clinical practice. However, in abnormal lungs such as acute lung injury (Chapter 30), VILI may contribute not only to further lung damage but also to multisystem organ failure affecting other body systems.[69]

Barotrauma

A sustained increase in the transmural pressure gradient can damage the lung.[70] The commonest forms of barotrauma attributable to artificial ventilation with or without PEEP are subcutaneous emphysema, pneumomediastinum and pneumothorax. Tension lung cysts and hyperinflation of a lung or lobe have also been reported but the incidence of these complications is variable. Pulmonary barotrauma probably starts as disruption of the alveolar membrane, with air entering the interstitial space and tracking back to the mediastinum along the bronchovascular bundles into the mediastinum from which it can reach the peritoneum, the pleural cavity or the subcutaneous tissues. Radiological demonstration of pulmonary interstitial gas may provide an early warning of barotrauma.

In patients who died following a prolonged period of exposure to PEEP, Slavin and his colleagues[71] in 1982 demonstrated at autopsy a gross dilatation of terminal and respiratory bronchioles, which they termed bronchiolectasis (Figure 31.14). Another more recent study described similar changes in 26 of 30 patients who died following artificial ventilation.[72] These studies found development of the condition to be increased by high PEEP levels, high peak airway pressures, large tidal volumes and the duration of artificial ventilation. Indirect evidence suggested barotrauma that resulted in a large increase in dead space. Follow-up of a group of patients who had survived the use of PEEP indicated a return to normal pulmonary function with normal values for dead space.[73] The condition of bronchiolectasis seems to be analogous to bronchopulmonary dysplasia described in infants ventilated for respiratory distress syndrome.[74]

Volutrauma[75]

Many animal studies have demonstrated pulmonary oedema following artificial ventilation with high inflation pressures. In one of these studies, lung damage with high inflation pressures was attenuated by restricting chest movement to prevent overdistension of the lungs, indicating that alveolar size rather than pressure was responsible for lung

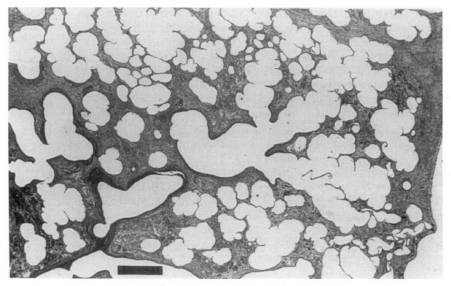

Figure 31.14 Histological appearance of bronchiolectasis in a patient who died after 16 days of artificial ventilation with positive end-expiratory pressure of 5 cmH$_2$O. Terminal and respiratory bronchioles are grossly dilated, and surrounding alveoli are collapsed. Diameter of normal terminal bronchiole is 0.5 mm. Scale bar is 1 mm. (Reproduced from reference 55 by permission of the Editor of *International Anesthesiology Clinics.*)

injury.[70] Termed volutrauma, this is now believed to contribute significantly to lung damage in patients with acute lung injury, in whom only a small proportion of alveoli may receive the entire tidal volume (page 580).

This form of VILI most commonly manifests itself as interstitial or alveolar pulmonary oedema. There are several possible underlying mechanisms, all of which are closely interrelated.

Alveolar distension causes permeability pulmonary oedema (page 546).[68] With extreme lung distension in animal studies, this occurs quickly and probably results from direct trauma to alveolar structures. In larger animals and humans, the permeability changes occur more slowly (several hours) and are more likely to result from the alterations in surfactant and inflammatory mediators described below.

Airway trauma occurs with repeated closure and reopening of small airways with each breath. Eventually, mucosal oedema will develop and the airways become progressively more difficult to open until collapse occurs. Recruitment of lung units with positive pressure ventilation has beneficial effects on gas exchange, and so encourages the use of higher pressures and volumes to recruit more airways, leading to further VILI.

Surfactant function is affected by artificial ventilation. Animal studies have demonstrated that surfactant release is increased by artificial ventilation, but there is also ample evidence that surfactant function is reduced.[68] Cyclical closure of airways during expiration causes surfactant to be drawn from the alveoli into the airway,[76] whilst alveolar proteins seen with permeability oedema inactivate surfactant (page 580). The resultant increase in alveolar surface tension will not only affect lung compliance but may also increase local microvascular permeability and encourage alveolar collapse.

Lung inflammation occurs with VILI as a result of neutrophil activation; pulmonary retention of neutrophils has been described above. Once activated – for example, by exposure to the alveolar basement membrane – inflammatory mediators will contribute to permeability oedema and further loss of surfactant function.

Prevention of VILI

PEEP In spite of its contribution to mean airway pressure, animal studies show that modest amounts of PEEP are helpful in reducing VILI.[75] Reduction of interstitial oedema, prevention of cyclical airway closure and preservation of surfactant function are all possible mechanisms for this effect. Determination of an acceptable level of PEEP in injured lungs is discussed on page 582.

Tidal volume and airway pressure should be minimized as far as possible. Plateau pressure is the ventilator measurement that equates most closely to the degree of alveolar distension. It is currently recommended that in patients with normal chest wall compliance the plateau pressure should not be allowed to exceed 35 cmH$_2$O.[77] The use of smaller tidal volumes, possibly achieved by the use of pressure-controlled ventilation, with or without permissive hypercapnia, are suitable tactics for reducing airway pressure.

Non-invasive ventilation[78]

Non-invasive ventilation is defined as respiratory support without establishing a tracheal airway. It may be achieved either by negative pressure ventilation or by positive pressure ventilation via a mask or similar device.

Negative pressure ventilation[79]

This requires the application of subatmospheric pressure to the trunk. It was first reported in 1929[80] and widely used for the following 30 years during polio epidemics. Enthusiasm for the technique has varied since, but there continues to be interest in negative pressure ventilation for a small group of patients.[81]

Cabinet ventilators, often referred to as an 'iron lung', require the whole body except the head to be encased in a cabinet with an airtight seal around the neck. Negative pressure is then applied in the tank, causing inspiration, with passive expiration as normal. A superimposed continuous negative pressure may also be applied, which provides the negative pressure equivalent of PEEP. In terms of the airway-to-ambient pressure gradient, cabinet ventilators are identical in principle to positive pressure ventilation, with very similar effects on cardiovascular and respiratory physiology. Collapse of the extrathoracic upper airway during inspiration may occur, particularly during sleep. Vomiting or regurgitation of gastric contents exposes the patient to the danger of aspiration during the inspiratory phase, and fatalities have occurred under particularly distressing circumstances.

Cuirass and jacket ventilators are a simplified form of cabinet ventilators in which the application of subatmospheric pressure is confined to the trunk or anterior abdominal wall.

Function depends on a good airtight seal. They are less efficient than cabinet ventilators and suffer from the same disadvantages. However, they are much more convenient to use and may be useful to supplement inadequate spontaneous breathing.

Hayek oscillator is a form of cuirass that encircles the trunk and allows high frequency ventilation (0.25–5 Hz) with a continuous negative pressure.[82,83] It facilitates a wide range of tidal volumes, and some degree of control of the FRC. It may be used during surgery on the airway, so avoiding the need for any form of tracheal tube.[84]

Negative pressure ventilation continues to have a place in the management of respiratory failure due to neuromuscular disorders,[79] kyphoscoliosis[79] or central apnoeas,[78] or in paediatric intensive care.[81] In spite of the cumbersome and costly equipment required, long-term home ventilation may be highly successful. For other pulmonary diseases, in particular chronic obstructive pulmonary disease (COPD), early reports of benefit were not confirmed in a randomized controlled trial.[85]

Non-invasive positive pressure ventilation[78]

Positive pressure ventilation may be delivered using soft masks that fit over the mouth and nose or only the nose. With nasal ventilation, positive pressure in the nasopharynx normally displaces the soft palate anteriorly against the tongue, thus preventing escape of gas through the mouth. Many ventilator systems used are pressure generators and so are 'leak tolerant'; that is, flow automatically increases to compensate for a pressure drop due to gas leakage. Side effects of nasal ventilation include eye irritation, conjunctivitis and facial skin necrosis.

Techniques of ventilation are similar to invasive IPPV. Ventilator modes that use patient triggering are better tolerated than controlled ventilation, particularly in awake patients, but both techniques are used. Volume-controlled ventilation is poorly tolerated and does not compensate for leaks, so is rarely used. Pressure-controlled ventilation or PSV (see above) is commonly used, as is CPAP. In bilevel positive airway pressure (bilevel PAP) the ventilator pressure steps between two preset values for inspiration and expiration, and, except for the terminology used to describe the pressures, is similar to PSV.[78]

Ventilation may be provided continually during acute respiratory problems, or only at night for long-term respiratory disease.[86] The use of nasal CPAP for treating the sleep apnoea hypopnoea syndrome has been described on page 353. In this case, benefit occurs simply by displacing the soft palate away from the posterior pharyngeal wall. Benefit in other respiratory diseases is more difficult to explain. Resting the respiratory muscles, re-expansion of areas of atelectasis and reducing hypercapnia have all been suggested.

Clinical applications. Hypoventilation and hypercapnia associated with neuromuscular disorders or central hypoventilation syndromes may be readily treated with non-invasive ventilation, with good symptom relief. The case for long-term treatment of COPD is much less clear,[87] and benefit seems to be confined to patients with symptomatic hypercapnia. Similarly for congestive cardiac failure, improvement is seen only in patients with predominantly nocturnal symptoms. Acute pulmonary oedema may be treated success-fully with non-invasive positive pressure ventilation,[63] but in another reported study there were severe cardiovascular disturbances associated with the use of bilevel PAP in this group of patients.[88] At present, the most well-documented indication for non-invasive ventilation is for the treatment of acute exacerbations of COPD. Three randomized trials have all shown benefits, including reduced mortality and need for intubation.[89,90,91]

References

1. Shneerson JM. Techniques in mechanical ventilation: principles and practice. *Thorax* 1996; **51**: 756–61.
2. Herholdt JD, Rafn CG. Life-saving methods for drowning persons. Copenhagen: T Tikiob, 1796. Reprinted in 1960; Aarhuus, Denmark: Stiftsbogtrykkerie.
3. Cox J, Woolmer R, Thomas V. Expired air resuscitation. *Lancet* 1960; **1**: 727–9.
4. Idris AH. Reassessing the need for ventilation during CPR. *Ann Emerg Med* 1996; **27**: 569–75.
5. Nunn JF, Lyle DJR. Bench testing of the CPU-1 ventilator. *Br J Anaesth* 1986; **58**: 653–62.
6. Sykes MK, Lumley J. The effect of varying the inspiratory:expiratory ratios on gas exchange during anaesthesia for open-heart surgery. *Br J Anaesth* 1969; **41**: 374–80.
7. Watson WE. Observations on physiological dead space during intermittent positive pressure respiration. *Br J Anaesth* 1962; **34**: 502–8.
8. Fairley HB, Blenkarn GD. Effect on pulmonary gas exchange of variations in inspiratory flow rate during intermittent positive pressure ventilation. *Br J Anaesth* 1966; **38**: 320–8.
9. Bergman NA. Effects of varying respiratory waveforms on gas exchange. *Anesthesiology* 1967; **28**: 390–5.
10. Fuleihan S, Wilson RS, Pontoppidan H. Effect of mechanical ventilation with end-expiratory pause on blood-gas exchange. *Anesth Analg* 1976; **55**: 122–30.
11. Perez-Chada RD, Gardaz J-P, Madgwick RG, Sykes MK. Cardiorespiratory effects of an inspiratory hold and continuous positive pressure ventilation in goats. *Intensive Care Med* 1983; **9**: 263–9.
12. Slutsky AS. Nonconventional methods of ventilation. *Am Rev Respir Dis* 1988; **138**: 175–83.
13. Gammon RB, Strickland JH, Kennedy JI, Young KR. Mechanical ventilation: a review for the internist. *Am J Med* 1995; **99**: 553–62.
14. Rossi A, Appendini L. Wasted efforts and dyssynchrony: is the patient–ventilator battle back? *Intensive Care Med* 1995; **21**: 867–70.
15. Sassoon CSH, Gruer SE. Characteristics of the ventilator pressure- and flow-trigger variables. *Intensive Care Med* 1995; **21**: 159–68.
16. Hewlett AM, Platt AS, Terry VG. Mandatory minute volume. *Anaesthesia* 1977; **32**: 163–9.
17. Downs J, Stock MC. Airway pressure release ventilation: a new concept in ventilatory support. *Crit Care Med* 1987; **15**: 459–61.
18. Valentine DD, Hammond MD, Downs JB, Sears NJ, Sims WR. Distribution of ventilation and perfusion with different modes of mechanical ventilation. *Am Rev Respir Dis* 1991; **143**: 1262–6.
19. Downs JB, Perkins HM, Modell JH. Intermittent mandatory ventilation – an evaluation. *Arch Surg* 1973; **109**: 519–23.
20. Wahba RW. Pressure support ventilation. *J Cardiothorac Anesth* 1990; **4**: 624–30.
21. Dekel B, Segal E, Perel A. Pressure support ventilation. *Arch Intern Med* 1996; **156**: 369–73.
22. MacIntyre NR. Respiratory function during pressure support ventilation. *Chest* 1986; **89**: 677–83.
23. Smith BE. High frequency ventilation: past, present and future? *Br J Anaesth* 1990; **65**: 130–8.
24. Sjöstrand U. High-frequency positive-pressure ventilation (HFPPV): a review. *Crit Care Med* 1980; **8**: 345–64.
25. Heijman K, Heijman L, Jonzon A, Sedin G, Sjöstrand U, Widman B. High frequency positive pressure ventilation during anaesthesia and routine surgery in man. *Acta Anaesthesiol Scand* 1972; **16**: 176–87.
26. Froese AB, Bryan AC. High frequency ventilation. *Am Rev Respir Dis* 1987; **135**: 1363–74.
27. Rehder K, Schmid ER, Knopp TJ. Long-term high-frequency ventilation in dogs. *Am Rev Respir Dis* 1983; **128**: 476–80.
28. Brusasco V, Knopp TJ, Schmid ER, Rehder K. Ventilation–perfusion relationship during high-frequency ventilation. *J Appl Physiol* 1984; **56**: 454–8.
29. Butler WJ, Bohn DJ, Bryan AC, Froese AB. Ventilation by high-frequency oscillation in humans. *Anesth Analg* 1980; **59**: 577–84.
30. Crawford M, Rehder K. High-frequency small-volume ventilation in anesthetized humans. *Anesthesiology* 1985; **62**: 298–304.
31. Chakrabarti MK, Gordon G, Whitwam JG. Relationship between tidal volume and deadspace during high frequency ventilation. *Br J Anaesth* 1986; **58**: 11–17.
32. Beamer WC, Prough DS, Royster RL, Johnston WE, Johnson JC. High frequency jet ventilation produces auto-PEEP. *Crit Care Med* 1984; **12**: 734–7.

33. Nunn JF, Hill DW. Respiratory dead space and arterial to end-tidal CO_2 tension difference in anesthetized man. *J Appl Physiol* 1960; **15**: 383–9.
34. Carlon GC, Howland WS, Ray C, Miodownik S, Griffin JP, Groeger JJ. High frequency jet ventilation. A prospective randomized evaluation. *Chest* 1983; **84**: 551–9.
35. Hurst JM, Branson RD, Davis K, Barrette RR, Adams KS. Comparison of conventional mechanical ventilation and high-frequency ventilation. A prospective randomized trial in patients with respiratory failure. *Ann Surg* 1990; **211**: 486–91.
36. Shneerson JM. Are there new solutions to old problems with weaning? *Br J Anaesth* 1997; **78**: 238–40.
37. Manthous CA, Schmidt GA, Hall JB. Liberation from mechanical ventilation: a decade of progress. *Chest* 1998; **114**: 886–901.
38. Weisman IM, Rinaldo JE, Rogers RM, Sanders MH. Intermittent mandatory ventilation. *Am Rev Respir Dis* 1983; **127**: 641–7.
39. Yang KL, Tobin MJ. A prospective study of indexes predicting the outcome of trials of weaning from mechanical ventilation. *N Engl J Med* 1991; **324**: 1445–50.
40. Lee Kh, Hui KP, Chan TB, Tan WC, Lim TK. Rapid shallow breathing (frequency–tidal volume ratio) did not predict extubation outcome. *Chest* 1994; **105**: 540–3.
41. Smith IE, Shneerson JM. A progressive care programme for prolonged ventilatory failure: analysis of outcome. *Br J Anaesth* 1995; **75**: 399–404.
42. Hill JD, Main FB, Osborn JJ, Gerbode F. Correct use of respirator on cardiac patient after operation. *Arch Surg* 1965; **91**: 775–8.
43. Hillman DR, Finucane KE. A model of the respiratory pump. *J Appl Physiol* 1985; **63**: 951–61.
44. Gottfried SB, Reissman H, Ranieri M. A simple method for the measurement of intrinsic end-expiratory pressure during controlled and assisted modes of mechanical ventilation. *Crit Care Med* 1992; **20**: 621–9.
45. Conacher ID. Dynamic hyperinflation – the anaesthetist applying a tourniquet to the right heart. *Br J Anaesth* 1998; **81**: 116–17.
46. Vellody VPS, Nassery M, Balasaraswathi K, Goldberg NB, Sharp JT. Compliances of human rib cage and diaphragm–abdomen pathways in relaxed versus paralyzed states. *Am Rev Respir Dis* 1978; **118**: 479–91.
47. Hulands GH, Greene R, Iliff LD, Nunn JF. Influence of anaesthesia on the regional distribution of perfusion and ventilation in the lung. *Clin Sci* 1970; **38**: 451–60.
48. Bindslev LG, Hedenstierna G, Santesson J, Gottlieb I, Carvallhas A. Ventilation–perfusion distribution during inhalational anaesthesia. *Acta Anaesthesiol Scand* 1981; **25**: 360–71.
49. Biondi JW, Schulman DS, Soufer R, Matthay RA, Hines RL, Kay HR, Barash PG. The effect of incremental positive end-expiratory pressure on right ventricular hemodynamics and ejection fraction. *Anesth Analg* 1988; **67**: 144–51.
50. Rizk NW, Luce JM, Hoeffel JM, Price DC, Murray JF. Site of deposition and factors affecting clearance of aerosolized solute from canine lungs. *J Appl Physiol* 1984; **56**: 723–9.
51. Hurford WE. Effect of positive pressure ventilation on cardiovascular function. *Curr Opin Anaesthesiol* 1989; **2**: 789–95.
52. Pinsky MR. The hemodynamic consequences of mechanical ventilation: an evolving story. *Intensive Care Med* 1997; **23**: 493–503.
53. Cournand A, Motley HL, Werko L, Richards DW. Physiological studies of the effects of intermittent positive pressure breathing on cardiac output in man. *Am J Physiol* 1948; **152**: 162–74.
54. Jardin F, Farcot J-C, Boisante L, Curien N, Margairaz A, Bourdarias J-P. Influence of positive end-expiratory pressure on left ventricular performance. *N Engl J Med* 1981; **304**: 387–92.
55. Nunn JF. Positive end-expiratory pressure. *Int Anaesthesiol Clin* 1984; **22**: 149–64.
56. Mitaka C, Nagura T, Sakanishi N, Tsunoda Y, Amaha K. Two-dimensional echocardiographic evaluation of inferior vena cava, right ventricle, and left ventricle during positive-pressure ventilation with varying levels of positive end-expiratory pressure. *Crit Care Med* 1989; **17**: 205–10.
57. Grindlinger GA, Manny J, Justice R, Dunham B, Shepro D, Hechtman HB. Presence of negative inotropic agents in canine plasma during positive end-expiratory pressure. *Circ Res* 1979; **45**: 460–7.
58. Suter PM, Fairley HB, Isenberg MD. Optimum end-expiratory airway pressure in patients with acute pulmonary failure. *N Engl J Med* 1975; **292**: 284–9.
59. Cassidy SS, Gaffney FA, Johnson RL. A perspective on PEEP. *N Engl J Med* 1981; **304**: 421–2.

60. Roy R, Powers SR, Fuestel PJ, Dutton RE. Pulmonary wedge catheterization during positive end-expiratory pressure ventilation in the dog. *Anesthesiology* 1977; **46**: 385–90.

61. Traverse JH, Korvenranta H, Adams EM, Goldthwait DA, Carlo WA. Impairment of hemodynamics with increasing mean airway pressure during high-frequency oscillatory ventilation. *Ped Res* 1988; **23**: 628–31.

62. Räsänen J, Heikkilä J, Downs J, Nikki P, Väisänen I, Viitanen A. Continuous positive airway pressure by face mask in acute cardiogenic pulmonary edema. *Am J Cardiol* 1985; **55**: 296–301.

63. Bersten AD, Holt AW, Vedig AE, Skowronski GA, Baggoley CJ. Treatment of severe cardiogenic pulmonary edema with continuous positive airway pressure delivered by facemask. *N Engl J Med* 1991; **325**: 1825–30.

64. Marquez JM, Douglas ME, Downs JB, Wu W-H, Mantini EL, Kuck EJ, Calderwood HW. Renal function and cardiovascular responses during positive airway pressure. *Anesthesiology* 1979; **50**: 393–8.

65. Markos J, Hooper RO, Kavanagh-Gray D, Wiggs BR, Hogg JC. Effect of raised alveolar pressure on leukocyte retention in the human lung. *J Appl Physiol* 1990; **69**: 214–21.

66. Loick HM, Wendt M, Rötker J, Theissen JL. Ventilation with positive end-expiratory airway pressure causes leukocyte retention in human lung. *J Appl Physiol* 1993; **75**: 301–6.

67. Sugiura M, McCulloch PR, Wren S, Dawson RH, Froese AB. Ventilator pattern influences neutrophil influx and activation in atelectasis-prone rabbit lung. *J Appl Physiol* 1994; **77**: 1355–65.

68. Dreyfuss D, Saumon G. Ventilator-induced lung injury: lessons from experimental studies. *Am J Respir Crit Care Med* 1998; **157**: 294–323.

69. Slutsky AS, Tremblay LN. Multiple system organ failure – is mechanical ventilation a contributing factor. *Am J Respir Crit Care Med* 1998; **157**: 1721–5.

70. Dreyfuss D, Soler P, Basset G, Saumon G. High inflation pressure pulmonary edema. Respective effects of high airway pressure, high tidal volume and positive end-expiratory pressure. *Am Rev Respir Dis* 1988; **137**: 1159–64.

71. Slavin G, Nunn JF, Crow J, Doré CJ. Bronchiolectasis – a complication of artificial ventilation. *BMJ* 1982; **285**: 931–4.

72. Rouby JJ, Lherm T, de Lassale EM, Poète P, Bodin L, Finet JF et al. Histologic aspects of pulmonary barotrauma in critically ill patients with acute respiratory failure. *Intensive Care Med* 1993; **19**: 383–9.

73. Navaratnarajah M, Nunn JF, Lyons D, Milledge JS. Bronchiolectasis caused by positive end-expiratory pressure. *Crit Care Med* 1984; **12**: 1036–8.

74. Taghizadeh A, Reynolds EOR. Pathogenesis of bronchopulmonary dysplasia following hyaline membrane disease. *Am J Pathol* 1976; **82**: 241–64.

75. Hooper J. Advances in mechanical ventilation. *Can J Anaesth* 1998; **45**: R149–54.

76. Faridy EE. Effect of ventilation on movement of surfactant in airways. *Respir Physiol* 1976; **27**: 323–34.

77. Slutsky AS. Consensus conference on mechanical ventilation – January 28–30, 1993 at Northbrook, Illinois, USA. *Intensive Care Med* 1994; **20**: 64–79.

78. Hillberg RE, Johnson DC. Noninvasive ventilation. *N Engl J Med* 1997; **337**: 1746–52.

79. Hill NS. Clinical applications of body ventilators. *Chest* 1986; **90**: 897–905.

80. Drinker P, Shore LA. An apparatus for the prolonged administration of artificial respiration. *J Clin Invest* 1929; **7**: 229–47.

81. Thomson A. The role of negative pressure ventilation. *Arch Dis Child* 1997; **77**: 454–8.

82. Petros AJ, Fernando SSD, Shenoy VS, Al-Saady NM. The Hayek oscillator. Nomograms for tidal volume and minute ventilation using external high frequency oscillation. *Anaesthesia* 1995; **50**: 601–6.

83. Al-Saady NM, Fernando SSD, Petros AJ, Cummin ARC, Sidhu VS, Bennett ED. External high frequency oscillation in normal subjects and in patients with respiratory failure. *Anaesthesia* 1995; **50**: 1031–5.

84. Dilkes MG, McNeill JM, Hill AC, Monks PS, McKelvie P, Hollamby RG. The Hayek oscillator: a new method of ventilation in microlaryngeal surgery. *Ann Otol Rhinol Laryngol* 1993; **102**: 455–8.

85. Shapiro SH, Ernst P, Gray-Donald K, Martin JG, Wood-Dauphinee S, Beaupré A et al. Effect of negative pressure ventilation in severe chronic obstructive pulmonary disease. *Lancet* 1992; **340**: 1425–9.

86. Claman DM, Pipier A, Sanders MH, Stiller RA, Votteri BA. Nocturnal noninvasive positive pressure ventilatory assistance. *Chest* 1996; **110**: 1581–8.

87. Hill NS. Non-invasive ventilation – does it work, for whom, and how. *Am Rev Respir Dis* 1993; **147**: 1050–5.

88. Mehta S, Jay GD, Woolard RH, Hipona RA, Connolly EM, Cimini DM et al. Randomized, prospective trial of bilevel versus continuous positive airway pressure in acute pulmonary edema. *Crit Care Med* 1997; **25**: 620–8.
89. Bott J, Carroll MP, Conway JH, Keilty SEJ, Ward EM, Brown AM et al. Randomised controlled trial of nasal ventilation in acute ventilatory failure due to chronic obstructive airways disease. *Lancet* 1993; **341**: 1555–7.
90. Kramer N, Meyer TJ, Heharg J, Cece RD, Hill NS. Randomized, prospective trial of noninvasive positive pressure ventilation in acute respiratory failure. *Am J Respir Crit Care Med* 1995; **151**: 1799–806.
91. Brochard L, Mancebo J, Wysocki M, Lofaso F, Conti G, Rauss A et al. Noninvasive ventilation for acute exacerbations of chronic obstructive pulmonary disease. *N Engl J Med* 1995; **333**: 817–22.

Chapter 32

Extrapulmonary gas exchange

The development of an artificial lung remains only a distant possibility,[1] but techniques for short-term replacement of lung function or more prolonged partial respiratory support have existed for many years. Extracorporeal gas exchangers were first developed for cardiac surgery to facilitate cardiopulmonary bypass and so allow surgery on a motionless heart. Subsequently the use of extracorporeal, and more recently intracorporeal, gas exchange was extended into the treatment of respiratory failure.

Factors in design[2]

The lungs of an adult have an interface between blood and gas of the order of 126 m^2 (page 28). It is not possible to achieve this in an artificial substitute, and artificial lungs can be considered to have a very low 'diffusing capacity'. Nevertheless, they function satisfactorily within limits for many reasons.

Factors favouring performance

1. The real lung is adapted for maximal exercise, while patients requiring extrapulmonary gas exchange are usually close to basal metabolic rate or less if hypothermia is used, for example during cardiac surgery.
2. Under resting conditions at sea level, there is an enormous reserve in the capacity of the lung to achieve equilibrium between pulmonary capillary blood and alveolar gas (see Figure 9.2). Therefore, a subnormal diffusing capacity does not necessarily result in arterial hypoxaemia.
3. It is possible to operate an artificial lung with an 'alveolar' oxygen concentration in excess of 90%, compared with 14% for real alveolar gas under normal circumstances. This greatly increases the gas transfer for a given 'diffusing capacity' of the artificial lung.
4. There is no great difficulty in increasing the 'ventilation/perfusion ratio' of a membrane artificial lung above the value of about 0.8 in the normal lung at rest.
5. The 'capillary transit time' of an artificial lung can be increased beyond 0.75 second in the real lung. This facilitates the approach of blood Po_2 to 'alveolar' Po_2 (see Figure 9.2).
6. It is possible to use countercurrent flow between gas and blood. This does not occur in the lungs of mammals although it is used in the gills of fishes.

Carbon dioxide exchanges much more readily than oxygen because of its greater blood and lipid solubility. Therefore, in general, elimination of carbon dioxide does not present a major problem and the limiting factor of an artificial lung is oxygenation.

Unfavourable factors

Against these favourable design considerations, there are certain advantages of the real lung – apart from its very large surface area – that are difficult to emulate in an artificial lung.

1. The pulmonary capillaries have a diameter close to that of the erythrocyte. Therefore, each erythrocyte is brought into very close contact with the alveolar gas (see Figure 2.8). The diffusion distance for artificial lungs is considerably greater and this problem is considered further below.
2. The vascular endothelium is specially adapted to prevent undesirable changes in the formed elements of blood, particularly neutrophils and platelets. Most artificial surfaces cause clotting of blood, and artificial lungs therefore require the use of anticoagulants.
3. No artificial lung has the extensive non-respiratory functions of the real lung, which include uptake, synthesis and biotransformation of many constituents of the blood (see Chapter 12). This function is lost when the lungs are bypassed.
4. The lung is an extremely efficient filter with an effective pore size of about $10 \, \mu m$ for flow rates of blood up to about $25 \, l.min^{-1}$. This is difficult to achieve with any man-made filter.

Bubble oxygenators

The simplest design of extracorporeal oxygenator stems from the well-tried wash bottle of the chemist. By breaking up the gas stream into small bubbles, it is possible to achieve very large surface areas of interface. However, the smaller the bubbles, the greater the tendency for them to remain in suspension when the blood is returned to the patient. This is dangerous because of the direct access of the blood to the cerebral circulation. A compromise is to break the gas stream into bubbles ranging from 2 to 7 mm diameter, giving an effective area of interface of the order of $15 \, m^2$. With a mean red cell transit time of 1–2 seconds and a 'ventilation/perfusion ratio' of unity or slightly more and an oxygen concentration of more than 90%, this gives an acceptable outflow blood Po_2 with blood flow rates up to about $6 \, l.min^{-1}$. The Pco_2 of the outflowing blood must be controlled by admixture of carbon dioxide with the inflowing oxygen in the gas phase. Priming volumes range from 400 to 900 ml. Gas is passed through the blood in a reservoir of about 1 litre capacity in which foaming takes place. Blood is then passed to a second reservoir for 'debubbling' with the help of an antifoaming compound.

Cellular and protein damage (see below) at the blood/gas interface occurs in bubble oxygenators. This is not considered to have significant clinical effects during short-term use, as for example with cardiac surgery, but may become significant when used for prolonged periods in the treatment of respiratory failure.[2]

Membrane oxygenators

Diffusion properties. Unlike their predecessors, currently available membranes offer little resistance to the diffusion of oxygen and carbon dioxide. At 25–50 μm thick, artificial membranes are several times thicker than the active side of the alveolar/capillary membrane (see Figure 2.8), but they contain small (<1 μm) pores which increase gas transfer substantially. The hydrophobic nature of the membrane material prevents water entering the pores and in normal use membranes can withstand a hydrostatic pressure gradient of the order of normal arterial blood pressure. However, over time the pores tend to fill with protein, which slowly reduces the membrane efficiency.

Gas diffusion within the blood presents a considerable barrier to the efficiency of membrane oxygenators. Slow diffusion of gases through plasma is now thought to limit gas transfer in normal lung, in which the erythrocyte is almost in contact with the capillary wall (page 210). Streamline flow through much wider channels in a membrane oxygenator tends to result in a stream of erythrocytes remaining at a distance from the interface. It has been estimated that in membrane oxygenators the diffusion path for oxygen is about 25 times further than in lung. Much thought has been devoted to the creation of turbulent flow to counteract this effect by 'mixing' the blood. Unfortunately, this inevitably leads to a greater degree of cell damage (see below) and increased resistance to flow through the oxygenator.

Biocompatibility. Adsorption of proteins, particularly albumin, onto the membrane reduces platelet, neutrophil and complement activation (see below), and this technique may be used to 'prime' oxygenators before use. Attempts to mimic endothelial cell properties have led to the production of membranes with heparin bonded to the surface, which also reduces activation of most of the processes described below.

Damage to blood

Damage due to non-occlusive roller pumps and centrifugal pumps is almost negligible. Damage due to oxygenators is probably far less than that resulting from surgical suction in removing blood from the operative site; during cardiac surgery, this factor outweighs any differences attributable to the type of oxygenator. However, during prolonged extracorporeal oxygenation for respiratory failure, the influence of the type of oxygenator becomes important, and membrane oxygenators are then clearly superior to bubble oxygenators.

Protein denaturation. Contact between blood and either gas bubbles or plastic surfaces results in protein denaturation, and plastic surfaces become coated with a layer of protein. With membrane oxygenators this tends to be self-limiting, and the protein products remain bound to the membrane. Bubble oxygenators cause a continuous and progressive loss of protein, including the release of denatured proteins into the circulation where they may have biological effects.

Complement activation. Complement activation occurs when blood comes into contact with any artificial surface, and complement C5a is known to be formed after cardiopulmonary bypass surgery.[3] Heparin-bonded systems cause less complement activation.[4]

Erythrocytes. Shear forces, resulting from turbulence or foaming, may cause shortened survival or actual destruction of erythrocytes. However, surgical suction is generally more damaging than the oxygenator. Without suction, the damage to erythrocytes with membrane oxygenators remains within reasonable limits for many days. Released haemoglobin is initially bound to plasma proteins but eventually saturates the receptors and is excreted through the kidneys. Red cell ghosts are now believed to be more damaging than free haemoglobin, and they may need to be removed by filtration.

Leucocytes and platelets. Counts of these elements are usually reduced by an amount in excess of the changes attributable to haemodilution. Platelets are lost by adhesion and aggregation, and following cardiac surgery postoperative counts are commonly about half the preoperative value. Neutrophil activation may occur in the extracorporeal circuit, leading to pathological effects in distant organs.

Coagulation. No oxygenator can function without causing coagulation of the blood. Anticoagulation is therefore a *sine qua non* of the technique and heparin is usually employed for this purpose. This inevitably results in excess bleeding from any surgical incision. Heparin-bonded components have significantly reduced the systemic anticoagulant requirement and allowed more prolonged use of circuits, but coagulopathy remains the most common complication of extracorporeal circulation.[5]

Systems for extrapulmonary gas exchange

Cardiopulmonary bypass for cardiac surgery remains the most common situation in which patients are exposed to extrapulmonary gas exchange. The duration of such exposure is normally very short, and causes few physiological disturbances postoperatively. Providing longer term respiratory support is much less common, and also considerably more difficult, but three techniques exist.

Extracorporeal membrane oxygenation (ECMO)[6,7]

Provision of ECMO requires continuous blood flow from the patient to a reservoir system, from which a pump propels blood through an oxygenator and a heat exchanger back to the patient. Venovenous ECMO is acceptable for treatment of respiratory failure, and may be instituted via percutaneous venous catheters. If circulatory support is also required, venoarterial ECMO is used, which normally requires surgical access to the vessels. A typical adult ECMO circuit provides $7\,m^2$ of membrane for oxygenation using 100% oxygen,[6] with blood flows of approximately $2-4\,l.min^{-1}$. The technique is available only in specialized centres, so in recent years ECMO systems have been developed for use while transporting the patient to the ECMO facilities.[8]

Extracorporeal carbon dioxide removal (ECCO$_2$R)

A different approach to artificial gas exchange was developed by Gattinoni et al. in Milan.[9] In essence, they restricted an ECMO system to removal of carbon dioxide only, and maintained oxygenation by a modification of apnoeic mass-movement oxygenation (page 240). The lungs were either kept motionless or ventilated two to three times per minute (low-frequency positive-pressure ventilation with extracorporeal CO_2 removal – LFPPV-ECCO$_2$R).[10]

   The technique depends on two important differences between the exchange of carbon dioxide and oxygen. First, membrane oxygenators remove carbon dioxide 10–20 times more effectively than they take up oxygen. Secondly, the normal arterial oxygen content $(20\,ml.dl^{-1})$ is very close to the maximum oxygen capacity, even with 100% oxygen in the gas phase $(22\,ml.dl^{-1})$. Therefore, there is little scope for superoxygenation of a fraction

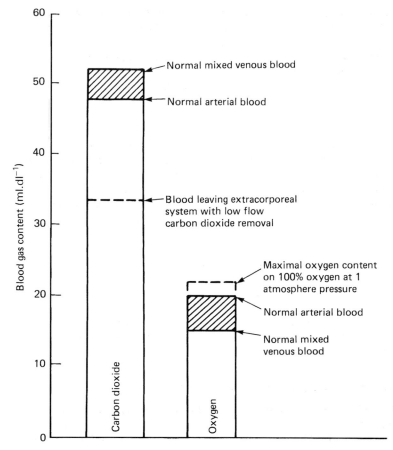

Figure 32.1 Comparison of absolute contents of carbon dioxide and oxygen in blood at 1 atmosphere pressure. Note that there is ample reserve potential for removing carbon dioxide below the level attained in normal arterial blood. In contrast, the maximal possible oxygen content of blood at 1 atmosphere is not greatly in excess of the level in normal arterial blood. This difference makes possible the extracorporeal removal of carbon dioxide (but not the supply of oxygen) by passing only a small fraction of the cardiac output through an extracorporeal gas exchanger.

of the pulmonary circulation to compensate for a larger fraction of the pulmonary circulation in which oxygenation does not take place. In contrast, the normal mixed venous carbon dioxide content is 52 ml.dl^{-1} compared with an arterial carbon dioxide content of 48 ml.dl^{-1}. There is therefore ample scope for removing a larger than normal fraction of carbon dioxide from part of the pulmonary circulation to compensate for the remaining fraction, which does not undergo any removal of carbon dioxide (Figure 32.1).

It is therefore possible to maintain carbon dioxide homoeostasis by diversion of only a small fraction of the cardiac output through an extracorporeal membrane oxygenator.[9] This is best illustrated by means of the Fick equation for carbon dioxide:

$$\frac{CO_2}{\text{removal}} = \frac{\text{pulmonary}}{\text{blood flow}} \left(\frac{\text{mixed venous}}{CO_2 \text{ content}} - \text{arterial } CO_2 \text{ content} \right)$$

Under normal circumstances, typical values might be:

$$240 = 6000 (52/100 - 48/100)$$

(values in ml and ml.min^{-1}).

With a flow through the membrane oxygenator of 1.3 l.min^{-1}, typical values might be:

$$240 = 1300 (52/100 - 33.5/100)$$

The outflow from the membrane oxygenator would thus be 1.3 l.min^{-1} with a carbon dioxide content of 33.5 ml.dl^{-1}, corresponding to a Pco_2 of about 2 kPa (15 mmHg). This would account for removal of the whole of the normal metabolic production of carbon dioxide. Furthermore, there is no necessity for the bypass to be venoarterial, and the far simpler venovenous bypass may be used. Therefore, there need be no reduction in pulmonary blood flow, and the non-respiratory functions of the lung are preserved.

With Pco_2 held constant by extracorporeal removal of carbon dioxide, there is no obstacle to the continued uptake of oxygen by mass-movement apnoeic oxygenation, a process that is otherwise terminated by progressive increase in Pco_2. All that is necessary is to replace the alveolar gas with oxygen and connect the trachea to a supply of oxygen, which is then drawn into the lungs at a rate equal to the metabolic consumption of oxygen, and this should continue indefinitely.

The technique would seem to expose the lungs to very high concentrations of oxygen and the possibility of oxygen toxicity (Chapter 25). In practice this does not appear to have been a problem, possibly due to induction of superoxide dismutase during an earlier stage of therapy (page 503). Furthermore, the air that flows through the membrane exchanger maintains the nitrogen tension of the body and this does not seem to interfere with the uptake of oxygen. Alternatively, the oxygen concentration of the gas passing through the membrane exchanger can be increased to make a contribution to oxygenation of the arterial blood.

Intravascular oxygenators (IVOX)[11]

Siting the gas exchange membrane in the patient's own circulation obviates the need for any extracorporeal circulation. In return, the size of the gas exchange surface is severely limited, and the blood flow around the membrane no longer controlled. However, the development of a heparin-bonded hollow fibre oxygenator suitable for use in humans has promoted great interest in the technique.[12] The device is inserted via surgical exposure of the femoral vein until it lies throughout the length of both inferior and superior venae cavae, through the right atrium. An IVOX device comes in different sizes, between 40 and 50 cm long with 600–1100 fibres through which oxygen flows, providing a surface area of 0.21–0.52 m^2 for gas exchange.[13] Blood flow in the venae cavae is thought to be mostly laminar, even with the IVOX in place, and gas exchange is again therefore limited by diffusion within the blood.[11] The available membrane surface area with IVOX is such that total extrapulmonary gas exchange is currently impossible, and the technique is suitable only for partial respiratory support. Even so, the modest improvement in blood gases seen with IVOX allows significant reductions in several ventilator settings such as inspiratory airway pressure and minute volume.[13,14]

Table 32.1 Aetiology of respiratory failure in infants treated with extracorporeal membrane oxygenation

Neonates (0–1 month old)	Other infants (over 1 month old)
Meconium aspiration syndrome	Viral pneumonia
Congenital diaphragmatic hernia	Bacterial pneumonia
Pneumonia/sepsis	Acute respiratory distress syndrome
Respiratory distress syndrome	Near-drowning
Persistent pulmonary hypertension	

(From references 6, 15, 16 and 17.)

Clinical applications

Neonates and infants[15]

It is estimated that, world-wide, 11 000 babies have received treatment involving ECMO.[16] The indication for treatment is acute respiratory failure of such severity that predicted survival is less than 20 per cent;[17] the causes are shown in Table 32.1. Though survival varies with the aetiology, there is general agreement that ECMO improves outcome substantially in infants, some centres achieving survival figures of almost 80 per cent.[6,18]

This benefit is not without costs. Vascular access in infants is difficult, and venoarterial ECMO using the carotid and jugular veins is often required, though venovenous ECMO with a double-lumen cannula is possible in some infants. In either case, there are believed to be significant disturbances to cerebral blood flow during ECMO, possibly exacerbated by altered cerebral autoregulation. As a result, up to one-quarter of ECMO treated infants develop clinical evidence of cerebral damage, which in some infants causes long-term disability.[17,18]

Adults

Extrapulmonary gas exchange is occasionally used as a therapeutic 'bridge' in patients waiting for lung transplantation, but its main indication is for management of severe acute lung injury (ALI, Chapter 30). Lung trauma as a result of artificial ventilation (page 615) contributes to respiratory failure in severe ALI, and the prospect of using extrapulmonary gas exchange to facilitate 'lung rest' is attractive. Unfortunately, the significant benefits of ECMO in infants have not been found in adults, and its place in treatment remains controversial. The invasive nature of extrapulmonary gas exchange and the serious potential complications mean that treatment is used only in the most severely ill patients. Even in specialist centres, recruitment of enough patients for randomized trials is difficult, and units have tended to simply publish results of uncontrolled case series.

IVOX as described above does allow some improvement in ventilator settings, which should alleviate the risk of lung trauma. Outcome studies have not yet been performed, but it is unlikely that the modest improvement in gas exchange seen with current systems will have significant effects.[19]

ECMO. A multicentre randomized prospective trial of ECMO for patients with severe ALI was published in 1979.[20] Entry criteria were based around arterial Po_2 values below 6.7 kPa (50 mmHg) on high inspired oxygen concentration and at least $5 \, cmH_2O$ PEEP. Patients were then randomly allocated to conventional artificial ventilation or ECMO. The study was terminated after treatment of the first 90 patients, when it was found that mortality was more than 90 per cent in both groups, with no statistically significant difference between the two forms of treatment. This trial effectively stopped ECMO use in adults for several years; in the meantime, significant advances were made in the causes and treatment of ALI by other means such as ventilator strategies to limit ventilator-induced lung injury (Chapter 31). In addition, since 1979 there have been major advances in the technology available for ECMO, in particular the advent of heparin-bonded and intravascular devices. Current ECMO techniques do seem to offer some patients substantial benefits,[21] particularly if instituted early in the course of severe ALI,[19] but comparative trials are still awaited.

ECCO₂R has been compared with currently accepted techniques of artificial ventilation and found to provide no improvement in mortality (67 per cent with $ECCO_2R$ versus 58 per cent for the control group).[22] This study has been criticized by the proponents of ECMO because of a high complication rate, mostly related to bleeding as a result of anticoagulation used for the non-heparin bonded circuit.[8]

References

1. Jack D. Artificial lungs on the way – but don't hold your breath. *Lancet* 1997; **349**: 260.
2. Wegner JA. Oxygenator anatomy and function. *J Cardiothorac Vasc Anaesth* 1997; **11**: 275–81.
3. Chenoweth DE, Cooper SW, Hugli TE, Stewart RW, Blackstone EH, Kirlin JW. Complement activation during cardiopulmonary bypass. Evidence for generation of C3a and C5a anaphylatoxins. *N Engl J Med* 1981; **304**: 497–503.
4. Videm V, Svennevig JL, Fosse E, Semb G, Osterud A, Mollnes TE. Reduced complement activation with heparin-coated oxygenator and tubings in coronary bypass operations. *J Thorac Cardiovasc Surg* 1992; **103**: 806–13.
5. Briegel J, Hummel T, Lenhart A, Heyduck M, Schelling G, Haller M. Complications during long-term extracorporeal lung assist (ECLA). *Acta Anaesthesiol Scand Supp* 1996; **109**: 121–2.
6. Peek GA, Killer MK, Sosnowski AW, Firmin RK. Extracorporeal membrane oxygenation: potential for adults and children? *Hosp Med* 1998; **59**: 304–8.
7. Zapol WM, Kolobow T. Extracorporeal membrane lung gas exchange. In: Crystal RG, West JB, eds. *The lung: scientific foundations.* New York: Raven Press, 1991; 2197.
8. Rossaint R, Pappert D, Gerlach H, Lewandowski K, Keh D, Falke K. Extracorporeal membrane oxygenation for transport of hypoxaemic patients with severe ARDS. *Br J Anaesth* 1997; **78**: 241–6.
9. Gattinoni L, Pesenti A, Rossi GP, Vesconi S, Fox U, Kolobow T et al. Treatment of acute respiratory failure with low-frequency positive-pressure ventilation and extracorporeal removal of CO_2. *Lancet* 1980; **2**: 292–4.
10. Gattinoni L, Pesenti A, Mascheroni D, Marcolin R, Funagalli R, Rossi F. Low-frequency positive-pressure ventilation with extracorporeal CO_2 removal in severe acute respiratory failure. *JAMA* 1986; **256**: 881–6.
11. Bidani A, Zwischenberger JB, Cardenas V. Intracorporeal gas exchange: current status and future development. *Intensive Care Med* 1996; **22**: 91–3.
12. Mortensen JD, Berry G. Conceptual and design features of a practical clinically effective intravenous mechanical blood oxygen/carbon dioxide exchange device (IVOX). *Int J Artif Organs* 1989; **12**: 384–9.
13. Conrad SA, Eggerstedt JM, Grier LR, Morris VF, Romero MD. Intravenacaval membrane oxygenation and carbon dioxide removal in severe acute respiratory failure. *Chest* 1995; **107**: 1689–97.
14. Mira JP, Brunet F, Belghith M, Soubrane O, Termignon JL, Renaud B et al. Reduction of ventilator settings allowed by intravenous oxygenator (IVOX) in ARDS patients. *Intensive Care Med* 1995; **21**: 11–17.

15. Soll RF. Neonatal extracorporeal membrane oxygenation – a bridging technique. *Lancet* 1996; **348**: 70–1.
16. Zobel G, Kuttnig-Hain M, Urlesberger B, Dacar D, Reiterer F, Riccabona M. Extracorporeal lung support in pediatric patients. *Acta Anaesthesiol Scand Supp* 1996; **109**: 122–5.
17. Mansfield RT, Parker MM. Cerebral autoregulation during venovenous extracorporeal membrane oxygenation. *Crit Care Med* 1996; **24**: 1945–6.
18. Field D, Davis C, Elbourne D, Grant A, Johnson A, Macrea D and UK Collaborative ECMO Trial Group. UK collaborative randomised trial of neonatal extracorporeal membrane oxygenation. *Lancet* 1996; **348**: 75–82.
19. Peek GJ, Firmin RK. Extracorporeal membrane oxygenation; a favourable outcome? *Br J Anaesth* 1997; **78**: 235–6.
20. Zapol WM, Snider MT, Hill JD, Fallat RJ, Bartlett RH, Edmunds LH et al. Extracorporeal membrane oxygenation in severe respiratory failure. *JAMA* 1979; **242**: 2193–6.
21. Lennartz H. Extracorporeal lung assist in ARDS: history and state of the art. *Acta Anaesthesiol Scand Supp* 1996; **109**: 114–16.
22. Morris AH, Wallace CJ, Menlove RL, Clemmer TP, Orme JF, Weaver LK et al. Randomized clinical trial of pressure-controlled inverse ratio ventilation and extracorporeal CO_2 removal for adult respiratory distress syndrome. *Am J Respir Crit Care Med* 1994; **149**: 295–305.

Chapter 33

Lung transplantation

Transplantation of a human lung was first performed in 1963,[1] but in the years following this few patients survived for longer than a month.[2] Improved immunosuppression led to a resurgence of interest in the early 1980s and the technique has now become an established form of treatment. Key developments included steps to ensure revascularization of the airway anastomosis and the use of cyclosporin A to prevent rejection. The function of a transplanted lung is important for the well-being of the recipient, but also furthers our understanding of certain fundamental issues of pulmonary physiology. The subject was reviewed recently.[3,4,5,6]

Clinical aspects

Indications

Patients who are considered for transplant have severe respiratory disease, and are receiving optimal therapy, but still have a life expectancy of less than two to three years. Uncontrolled respiratory infection, significant cardiac disease or continued smoking are normally contraindications. Precise selection criteria for recipients vary between transplant centres, but in general patients referred for transplant have a forced expiratory volume in one second (FEV_1) of less than 30 per cent predicted, resting hypoxia, hypercapnia and, commonly, pulmonary hypertension. The indications for lung transplant are given in Table 33.1, where it can be clearly seen that chronic obstructive pulmonary disease (COPD) is now by far the most common. Further discussion of the lung diseases shown in Table 33.1 may be found elsewhere (COPD, page 531; α_1-antitrypsin deficiency, page 307; idiopathic pulmonary fibrosis, page 568; cystic fibrosis (CF), page 535; and primary pulmonary hypertension, page 555).

In most countries with transplant programmes the number of patients awaiting transplant exceeds the number of donors,[8] and in the USA about 10–15 per cent of patients die while on the waiting list.

Types of transplant

Cadaveric donor lungs are taken from patients less than 65 years of age with limited smoking history and no evidence of lung disease, including asthma or lung infection. Only 20 per cent of organ donors are suitable for lung donation. Donor and recipient chest sizes

Table 33.1 Indications for lung transplantation and the type of operation performed

Indication	Total number	Operations performed for each indication		
		Heart–lung (%)	Bilateral (%)	Single (%)
COPD	2466	2.9	20.7	76.4
α_1-Antitrypsin deficiency	813	5.4	36.2	58.4
Idiopathic pulmonary fibrosis	1153	4.4	18.3	77.3
Cystic fibrosis	1321	22.3	71.2	6.5
Primary pulmonary hypertension	996	49.1	28.7	22.2
Congenital heart disease	522	100	–	–
Retransplantation	243	21.8	25.1	53.1

Bilateral lung transplant includes double lung and bilateral single lung procedures.
(Data are from the Registry of the International Society for Heart and Lung Transplantation,[7] and include lung transplants performed world-wide for the indications shown up to the end of 1997.)

are matched. With current organ preservation solutions, lung transplants must be performed within six to eight hours of organ removal.

Single-lung transplant (SLT) is the simplest procedure. The recipient's pneumonectomy is undertaken via a thoracotomy using one-lung ventilation (page 451), which presents a significant challenge in these patients.[9] The donor lung is implanted, with anastomoses of the main bronchus, the left or right pulmonary artery and a ring of left atrium containing both pulmonary veins of one side. Cardiopulmonary bypass is required in some cases: rarely in patients with COPD and in about one-third of patients with restrictive lung disease. The requirement for cardiopulmonary bypass usually results from right heart failure during clamping of the pulmonary artery and is related to preoperative pulmonary arterial pressure.

Bilateral lung transplant (BLT). Double lung transplant performed at a single operation is a more complex procedure, for which sternotomy and total cardiopulmonary bypass are required. The donor lungs are implanted with anastomoses of either the trachea or both bronchi, the main pulmonary artery and the posterior part of the left atrium containing all four pulmonary veins. Tracheal anastomoses have a high complication rate (see below), and the necessity for full anticoagulation causes problems with haemostasis. A simpler alternative is to transplant two lungs sequentially (termed a double single-lung transplant) through bilateral thoracotomies, and this has almost completely replaced double-lung transplant.

Heart–lung transplant (HLT) was originally used for patients with primary pulmonary hypertension and Eisenmenger's syndrome, and continues to be the operation of choice for the latter (Table 33.1). Total cardiopulmonary bypass is, of course, essential and the anastomoses involve the right atrium, the aorta and the trachea.

Choice of operation depends on the indication for the transplant, and types of surgery performed are shown in Table 33.1. Single-lung transplantation is favoured, partly because mortality seems to be lower after this operation but also because each suitable donor can be used to transplant two recipients. Congenital heart disease requires heart–lung transplant, whilst diseases associated with pulmonary hypertension normally need either heart–lung or bilateral lung transplant to normalize pulmonary arterial pressure. Lung disease alone is treated satisfactorily with single-lung transplant. Patients with cystic fibrosis have widespread pulmonary infection and so are rarely suitable for single-lung transplant if infection of the transplanted lung is to be avoided.

Living-related lung transplants are now being carried out at several centres in the world, but the majority have been performed at the University of Southern California.[10,11,12] Left or right lower lobes of the donor relative are transplanted into the whole hemithorax of the recipient, so the technique is suitable only for children or very small adults such as patients with cystic fibrosis. The same selection criteria apply as for cadaveric transplantation, so cystic fibrosis patients must have bilateral transplants and therefore two related donors. Early results show survival figures at least comparable with other forms of lung transplantation,[10] but the numbers involved are currently very small. The technique is in its infancy, and offers theoretical benefits in the availability of organs and attenuated organ rejection, but the ethical issues for donors are substantial.

Airway anastomosis. The tracheal or bronchial circulation of the donor lung is usually compromised, and the problem of stenosis, leakage or even occasional dehiscence of the airway anastomosis remains in up to 20 per cent of transplanted lungs. This is a particular problem for tracheal anastomoses, which seem to be in a watershed where both tracheal and bronchial blood supply is poor. The earliest approach was omentopexy, in which omentum was brought up through the diaphragm and wrapped round the anastomosis to provide collateral circulation. Later, 'telescoping' bronchial anastomoses or direct anastomosis of the internal mammary artery to the donor bronchial circulation were advocated. There is no agreement as to which, if any, of these techniques is the most useful.[13]

Outcome following transplant

Mortality. The actuarial survival of lung transplant recipients is shown in Figure 33.1. Given the nature of the surgery, it is not surprising that there is significant perioperative and early postoperative mortality. Thereafter, mortality rates are low when consideration is given to the two-year predicted survival of recipients prior to transplant. It can be seen from Figure 33.1 that the underlying disease has a large effect on survival rates, with COPD and cystic fibrosis having the best results and congenital heart disease the worst. Survival following single-lung transplant is generally better than with bilateral, which is in turn better than heart–lung transplant.

Ventilatory performance. After single-lung transplant, total lung capacity and vital capacity reach approximately 60 per cent of predicted value within two months.[15] FEV_1 is initially poor owing to the effects of the surgery, but then shows a gradual improvement from pretransplant values of 20–30 per cent of predicted normal to between 50 per cent and 80 per cent of predicted.[4] However, this measurement depends on many factors (page 134), and it would be difficult to define the precise reasons for the slow recovery. Following heart–lung or bilateral lung transplant, values close to normal are often attained[3] and this can be considered very satisfactory. These improvements in ventilatory performance contribute to the huge improvement in quality of life following lung transplant.

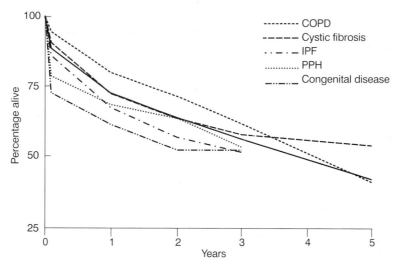

Figure 33.1 Actuarial survival following lung transplantation. The solid line shows results for all lung transplants, and the various broken lines show results for individual diseases as indicated. Data are from the US Scientific Registry[14] and include 2616 transplants carried out between 1987 and 1994. COPD, chronic obstructive pulmonary disease; IPF, idiopathic pulmonary fibrosis; PPH, primary pulmonary hypertension.

Exercise performance. The attainable level of exercise depends on many factors, which, in addition to pulmonary function, include circulation, condition of the voluntary muscles, motivation and freedom from pain on exertion. Improvement in performance does occur following lung transplantation, but exercise limitation remains common, with maximal oxygen uptake (page 335) of about half normal. There is no evidence that this limitation results from poor pulmonary function, and a muscular origin is more likely, possibly related to myopathy induced by immunosuppressant drugs.[3]

Rejection[3]

Acute rejection occurs following activation of cytotoxic T-lymphocytes by helper T-cells, which 'recognize' the foreign tissue. Acute lung inflammation ensues by mechanisms similar to those for other pulmonary diseases (page 576). Chronic rejection in the lung manifests itself as obliterative bronchiolitis syndrome, the origin of which is not clear but which occurs in up to half of patients, normally more than a year after transplantation.

Detection of rejection. There is a major difficulty in detecting the early stages of acute rejection, and it is difficult to distinguish rejection from infection on clinical evidence. Both conditions feature arterial hypoxaemia, pyrexia, leucocytosis, dyspnoea and a reduced capacity for exercise. These changes are followed by a decrease in diffusing capacity and FEV_1, and later by perihilar infiltration or graft opacification on the chest radiograph. Pulmonary blood flow through the threatened lung may then be reduced from the high levels noted above.

Chronic rejection can usually be detected from a deterioration in previously stable lung function. Bronchiolitis obliterans, as the name suggests, causes significant air-flow limitation; the FEV_1 is used as a screening test and also to stage the degree of rejection.

Nevertheless, none of the symptoms and signs described is truly diagnostic of either acute or chronic threatened rejection. The gold standard is the histopathology of an open-lung biopsy that shows perivascular lymphocytic infiltration or bronchiolitis obliterans. However, this procedure is unsuitable for routine screening. Transbronchial biopsy is less invasive, but unreliable in comparison with open-lung biopsy, and also not entirely free from hazard.

Immunosuppression. Except in the case of identical twins, survival of the transplanted lung depends on immunosuppression. Cyclosporin A made lung transplant possible and, in conjunction with azathioprine and corticosteroids, continues to be the mainstay of immunosuppressant therapy today, though new drugs such as tacrolimus are very promising.[3] The continued use of immunosuppression greatly reduces resistance to infection, and the transplanted lung is particularly vulnerable to *Cytomegalovirus, Herpes simplex* and *Pneumocystis carinii*. Cyclosporin A also has a wide variety of drug interactions and side effects, including nephrotoxicity and hepatotoxicity.[3,16]

Physiological effects of lung transplant

Transplantation inevitably disrupts innervation, lymphatics and the bronchial circulation. The condition of the recipient is further compromised by immunosuppressive therapy.

The denervated lung

The transplanted lung has no afferent or efferent innervation and there is, as yet, no evidence that reinnervation occurs in patients.[17] However, in dogs, vagal stimulation has been observed to cause bronchoconstriction three to six months after reimplantation,[18] and sympathetic reinnervation has been demonstrated after 45 months.[19]

Respiratory rhythm. In Chapter 5, attention was paid to the weakness of the Hering–Breuer reflex in humans. It was therefore to be expected that denervation of the lung, with block of pulmonary baroreceptor input to the medulla, would have minimal effect on the respiratory rhythm. This is in contrast to the dog and most other laboratory animals, in whom vagal block is well known to cause slow deep breathing. Bilateral vagal block in human volunteers was already known to leave the respiratory rhythm virtually unchanged,[20] and it was therefore no great surprise when it was shown that bilateral lung transplant had no significant effect on the respiratory rate and rhythm in patients, after the early postoperative period.[16] Breathing during sleep is also normal.[21] Chemical control of ventilation (Chapter 5) does not depend on either afferent or efferent innervation of the lung, and there is no evidence of any abnormality after lung transplant.

Bronchial hypersensitivity. Enhanced sensitivity to the bronchoconstrictor effects of inhaled methacholine and histamine can be demonstrated after heart–lung transplantation.[22] This is thought to be due to hypersensitivity of receptors in airway smooth muscle, following denervation of the predominantly constrictor autonomic supply, though not all studies have demonstrated this.[17] In spite of these findings, airway hyperresponsiveness (page 526) is rarely a problem in transplanted patients.[3]

The cough reflex, in response to afferents arising from below the level of the tracheal or bronchial anastomosis, is permanently lost after lung transplantation.[23] Following single-lung transplant, the remaining diseased lung will continue to stimulate coughing, which will facilitate clearance of secretions from the transplanted lung. Similarly, a double single-lung transplant (see above) may be preferable to a double-lung transplant, as the former will maintain intact the potent carinal cough reflex. The abnormality in cough reflex is a major contributor to lung infection following transplant, along with altered mucus clearance as described below.

Ventilation/perfusion ($\dot{V}/\dot{Q}$) relationships

Bilateral lung or heart–lung transplant usually result in normal $\dot{V}/\dot{Q}$ relationships, but following single-lung transplant the situation is more complex. For most indications, including COPD, the single transplanted lung receives the majority of pulmonary ventilation (60–80 per cent of the total) and a similar proportion of pulmonary blood flow, and so $\dot{V}/\dot{Q}$ relationships are acceptable, though not normal.[24,25] However, following single-lung transplant for primary pulmonary hypertension, ventilation to the two lungs remains approximately equal whilst the majority of blood flow (often >80 per cent) is to the transplanted lung. This $\dot{V}/\dot{Q}$ mismatch fortunately has little effect on arterial oxygenation at rest. During exercise in patients with a single-lung transplant, the already high blood flow to the transplanted lung seems not to increase further, and the normal recruitment of apical pulmonary capillaries (page 144) cannot be demonstrated.[24]

Hypoxic pulmonary vasoconstriction seems to be an entirely local mechanism and, as might be expected, has been shown to persist in the human transplanted lung,[26] though some studies have demonstrated abnormalities, particularly in patients with pulmonary hypertension.[24,25]

Pleural effusion[27]

The hilar lymphatics are severed at pneumonectomy and it is not feasible to anastomose with the lymphatics of the donor lung. In animals, restoration of pulmonary lymphatics occurs spontaneously within a few weeks, but this has not been demonstrated in humans. In the meantime, lymph drains from the severed ends of the donor lung into the recipient's pleural cavity and an effusion develops, which must be drained with a chest tube. Also, there is some degree of increased pulmonary capillary permeability in the first few days after transplantation, probably as a result of ischaemia–reperfusion injury (page 500) of the graft.[3] This will cause a substantial increase in lymph production, and further contribute to pleural fluid accumulation. Drainage of pleural fluid is minimal by nine days after the transplant.

Mucociliary clearance

Mucociliary clearance is defective after transplantation.[28] The cause seems to be defective production of mucus, rather than changes in the frequency of cilial beat. This, together with the absent cough reflex below the line of the airway anastomosis, means that the patient is at a disadvantage in clearing secretions. Side effects of immunosuppression compound these changes and lead to enhanced susceptibility to infection of the transplanted lung. Although these factors clearly do not preclude long-term survival of the graft, one-quarter of deaths following lung transplantation result from infection.[3]

References

1. Hardy JD, Webb WR, Dalton ML, Walker GR. Lung homotransplantation in man. *JAMA* 1963; **186**: 1065–74.
2. Blumenstock DA, Lewis C. The first transplantation of the lung in a human revisited. *Ann Thorac Surg* 1993; **56**: 1423–5.
3. Trulock EP. Lung transplantation. *Am J Respir Crit Care Med* 1997; **155**: 789–818.
4. Bracken CA, Gurkowski MA, Naples JJ. Lung transplantation: historical perspectives, current concepts, and anesthetic considerations. *J Cardiothorac Vasc Anesth* 1997; **11**: 220–41.
5. Grover FL, Fullerton DA, Zamora MR, Mills C, Ackerman B, Badesch D et al. The past, present, and future of lung transplantation. *Am J Surg* 1997; **173**: 523–33.
6. Yankaskas JR, Mallory GB. Lung transplantation in cystic fibrosis. Consensus conference statement. *Chest* 1998; **113**: 217–26.
7. International Society for Heart and Lung Transplantation. 15th Annual Data Report, April 1998. http://www.ishlt.org/registry.html
8. Keller CA. The donor lung: conservation of a precious resource. *Thorax* 1998; **53**: 506–13.
9. Singh H, Bossard RF. Perioperative anaesthetic considerations for patients undergoing lung transplantation. *Can J Anaesth* 1997; **44**: 284–99.
10. Starnes VA, Barr ML, Cohen RG, Hagen JA, Wells WJ, Horn MV, Schenkel FA. Living-donor lobar lung transplantation experience: intermediate results. *J Thorac Cardiovasc Surg* 1996; **112**: 1284–91.
11. Quinlan JJ, Gasior T, Firestone S, Firestone LL. Anesthesia for living-related (lobar) lung transplantation. *J Cardiothorac Vasc Anesth* 1996; **10**: 391–6.
12. Dark JH. Lung: living related transplantation. *Br Med Bull* 1997; **53**: 892–903.
13. Patterson GA. Airway revascularization: is it necessary. *Ann Thorac Surg* 1993; **56**: 807–8.
14. Trulock EP. Lung transplantation for COPD. *Chest* 1998; **113**: 269S–76S.
15. Egan TM, Kaiser LR, Cooper JD. Lung transplantation. *Curr Probl Surg* 1989; **26**: 673–751.
16. Shaw IH, Kirk AJB, Conacher ID. Anaesthesia for patients with transplanted hearts and lungs undergoing non-cardiac surgery. *Br J Anaesth* 1991; **67**: 772–81.
17. Stretton CD, Mak JCW, Belvisi MG, Yacoub MH, Barnes PJ. Cholinergic control of human airways *in vitro* following extrinsic denervation of the human respiratory tract by heart–lung transplantation. *Am Rev Respir Dis* 1990; **142**: 1030–3.
18. Edmunds LH, Graf PD, Nadel JA. Reinnervation of reimplanted canine lung. *J Appl Physiol* 1971; **31**: 722–7.
19. Lall A, Graf PD, Nadel JA, Edmunds LH. Adrenergic reinnervation of the reimplanted dog lung. *J Appl Physiol* 1973; **35**: 439–42.
20. Guz A, Noble MIM, Widdicombe JG, Trenchard D, Mushin WW, Makey AR. The role of the vagal and glossopharyngeal afferent nerves in respiratory sensation, control of breathing and arterial pressure regulation in conscious man. *Clin Sci* 1966; **30**: 161–70.
21. Sanders MH, Costantino JP, Owens GR, Sciurba FC, Rogers RM, Reynolds CF et al. Breathing during wakefulness and sleep after human heart–lung transplantation. *Am Rev Respir Dis* 1989; **140**: 45–51.
22. Glanville AR, Burke CM, Theodore J, Baldwin JC, Harvey J, Vankessel A, Robin ED. Bronchial hyper-responsiveness after human cardiopulmonary transplantation. *Clin Sci* 1987; **73**: 299–303.
23. Higenbottam T, Jackson M, Woolman P, Lowry R, Wallwork J. The cough response to ultrasonically nebulized distilled water in heart–lung transplantation patients. *Am Rev Respir Dis* 1989; **140**: 58–61.
24. Ross DJ, Waters PF, Waxman AD, Koerner SK, Mohsenifar Z. Regional distribution of lung perfusion and ventilation at rest and during steady-state exercise after unilateral lung transplantation. *Chest* 1993; **104**: 130–5.
25. Kuni CC, Ducret RP, Nakhleh RE, Boudreau RJ. Reverse mismatch between perfusion and aerosol ventilation in transplanted lungs. *Clin Nucl Med* 1993; **18**: 313–17.
26. Robin ED, Theodore J, Burke CM, Oesterle SN, Fowler MB, Jamieson SW et al. Hypoxic pulmonary vasoconstriction persists in the human transplanted lung. *Clin Sci* 1987; **72**: 283–7.
27. Judson MA, Handy JR, Sahn SA. Pleural effusions following lung transplantation: time course, characteristics, and clinical implications. *Chest* 1996; **109**: 1190–4.
28. Herve P, Silbert D, Cerrina J, Simonneau G, Dartevelle P, and the Paris–Sud Lung Transplant Group. Impairment of bronchial mucociliary clearance in long-term survivors of heart/lung and double-lung transplantation. *Chest* 1993; **103**: 59–63.

Appendix A

Physical quantities and units of measurement

SI units

A clean transition from the old to the new metric units has failed to occur. The old system was based on the centimetre–gram–second (CGS) and was supplemented with many non-coherent derived units such as the millimetre of mercury for pressure and the calorie for work, which could not be related to the basic units by factors which were powers of ten. The new system, the Système Internationale or SI, is based on the metre–kilogram–second (MKS) and comprises base and derived units that are obtained simply by multiplication or division without the introduction of numbers, not even powers of ten.[1]

Base units are metre (length), kilogram (mass), second (time), ampere (electric current), kelvin (thermodynamic temperature), mole (amount of substance) and candela (luminous intensity).

Derived units include newton (force: kilograms metre second^{-2}), pascal (pressure: newton metre^{-2}), joule (work: newton metre) and hertz (periodic frequency: second^{-1}).

Special non-SI units are recognized as having sufficient practical importance to warrant retention for general or specialized use. These include litre, day, hour, minute and the standard atmosphere.

Non-recommended units include the dyne, bar, calorie and gravity-dependent units such as the kilogram-force, centimetre of water and millimetre of mercury, the demise of which has been expected for many years.

The introduction of SI units into anaesthesia and respiratory physiology remains incomplete. The kilopascal is replacing the millimetre of mercury for blood gas tensions, the transition being almost complete in most European countries but barely started in the USA, where mmHg had been replaced by the almost identical torr. The introduction of the kilopascal for fluid pressures in the medical field is being delayed for what seems to be an entirely specious attachment to the mercury or water manometer. We appear to be condemned to a further period during which we record arterial pressure in mmHg, venous pressure in cmH$_2$O, cerebrospinal fluid pressure in mmH$_2$O and some suction pumps are

Table A.1 Conversion factors for units of measurement

Force
1 N (newton) $= 10^5$ dyn

Pressure
1 kPa (kilopascal) $= 7.50$ mmHg
                                                       $= 10.2$ cmH$_2$O
                                                       $= 0.009\,87$ standard atmosphere
                                                       $= 10\,000$ dyn.cm^{-2}

1 standard atmosphere $= 101.3$ kPa
                                                       $= 760$ mmHg
                                                       $= 1033$ cmH$_2$O
                                                       $= 10$ m of sea water (S.G. 1.033)

1 mmHg $= 1.36$ cmH$_2$O
                                                       $= 1$ torr (approx.)

Compliance
1 l.kPa^{-1} $= 0.098$ l.cmH$_2$O^{-1}

Flow resistance
1 kPa.l^{-1}.s $= 10.2$ cmH$_2$O.l^{-1}.s

Work
1 J (joule) $= 0.102$ kilopond metres
                                                       $= 0.239$ calories

Power
1 W (watt) $= 1$ J.s^{-1}
                                                       $= 6.12$ kp.m.min^{-1}

Surface tension
1 N.m^{-1} (newton/metre or pascal metre) $= 1000$ dyn.cm^{-1}
                                                       $= 1$ dyn.cm^{-1}

In the Figures, Tables and text of this book 1 kPa has been taken to equal
7.5 mmHg or 10 cmH$_2$O.

still calibrated in cmHg. This absurd situation would be less dangerous if all staff knew the relationship between a millimetre of mercury and a centimetre of water.

As in previous editions of this book, it has proved necessary to make text and figures bilingual, with both SI and CGS units for the benefit of readers who are unfamiliar with one or other of the systems. Some useful conversion factors are listed in Table A.l. There continue to be some areas of physiology and medicine where non-SI units continue to be extensively used, such as millimetres of mercury for most vascular pressures and centimetres of water for airway pressure, so these units are retained throughout this book to aid clarity.

Physical quantities relevant to respiratory physiology are defined below, together with their mass/length/time (MLT) units. These units provide a most useful check of the validity of equations and other expressions that are derived in the course of studies of respiratory function. Only quantities with identical MLT units can be added or subtracted, and the units must be the same on both sides of an equation.

Volume (dimensions: L^3)

In this book we are concerned with volumes of blood and gas. Strict SI units would be cubic metres and submultiples. However, the litre (l) and millilitre (ml) are recognized as special non-SI units and will remain in use. For practical purposes, we may ignore changes in the volume of liquids that are caused by changes of temperature. However, the changes in volume of gases caused by changes of temperature or pressure are by no means negligible and constitute an important source of error if they are ignored. These are discussed in detail in Appendix C.

Fluid flow rate (dimensions: L^3/T, or L^3T^{-1})

In the case of liquids, flow rate is the physical quantity of cardiac output, regional blood flow, etc. The strict SI units would be $metre^3.second^{-1}$, but litres per minute ($l.min^{-1}$) and millilitres per minute ($ml.min^{-1}$) are special non-SI units that may be retained. For gases, the dimension is applied to minute volume of respiration, alveolar ventilation, peak expiratory flow rate, oxygen consumption, etc. The units are the same as those for liquids except that litres per second are used for the high instantaneous flow rates that occur during the course of inspiration and expiration.

In the case of gas flow rates, just as much attention should be paid to the matter of temperature and pressure as when volumes are being measured (Appendix C).

Force (dimensions: MLT^{-2})

Force is defined as mass times acceleration. In respiratory physiology we are chiefly concerned with force in relation to pressure, which is force per unit area. An understanding of the units of force is essential to an understanding of the units of pressure. Force, when applied to a free body, causes it to change either the magnitude or the direction of its velocity.

The units of force are of two types. The first is the force resulting from the action of gravity on a mass and is synonymous with weight. It includes the kilogram-force and the pound-force (as in the pound per square inch). All such units are non-recommended under the SI and are expected to disappear. The second type of unit of force is absolute and does not depend on the magnitude of the gravitational field. In the CGS system, the absolute unit of force was the dyne and this has been replaced under the MKS system and the SI by the newton (N), which is defined as the force that will give a mass of 1 kilogram an acceleration 1 metre per second per second.

$$1 N = 1 kg.m.s^{-2}$$

Pressure (dimensions: MLT^{-2}/L^2, or $ML^{-1}T^{-2}$)

Pressure is defined as force per unit area. The SI unit is the pascal (Pa) which is 1 newton per square metre.

$$1 Pa = 1 N.m^{-2}$$

The pascal is inconveniently small (one hundred-thousandth of an atmosphere) and the kilopascal (kPa) has been adopted for general use in the medical field. Its introduction is simplified by the fact that the kPa is very close to 1% of an atmosphere. Thus a standard atmosphere is 101.3 kPa and the Po_2 of dry air is very close to 21 kPa: The kilopascal will eventually replace the millimetre of mercury and the centimetre of water, both of which are gravity based.

The standard atmosphere may continue to be used under SI. It is defined as $1.013\ 25 \times 10^5$ pascals.

The torr came into use only shortly before the move towards SI units. This is unfortunate for the memory of Torricelli, as the torr will disappear from use. The torr is defined as exactly equal to 1/760 of a standard atmosphere and it is therefore very close to the millimetre of mercury, the two units being considered identical for practical purposes. The only distinction is that the torr is absolute, while the millimetre of mercury is gravity based.

The bar is the absolute unit of pressure in the old CGS system and is defined as 10^6 dyn.cm^{-2}. The unit was convenient because the bar is close to 1 atmosphere (1.013 bars) and a millibar is close to 1 centimetre of water (0.9806 millibars).

Compliance (dimensions: $M^{-1}L^4T^2$)

The term 'compliance' is used in respiratory physiology to denote the volume change of the lungs in response to a change of pressure. The dimensions are therefore volume divided by pressure, and the commonest units have been litres (or millilitres) per centimetre of water. It is likely that this will change to litres per kilopascal (l.kPa^{-1}).

Resistance to fluid flow (dimensions: $ML^{-4}T^{-1}$)

Under conditions of laminar flow (see Figure 4.2) it is possible to express resistance to gas flow as the ratio of pressure difference to gas flow rate. This is analogous to electrical resistance, which is expressed as the ratio of potential difference to current flow. The dimensions of resistance to gas flow are pressure difference divided by gas flow rate, and typical units in the respiratory field have been cmH$_2$O/litre/second or dynes.sec.cm^{-5} in absolute units. Appropriate SI units will probably be kilopascals.litre^{-1}.second (kPa.l^{-1}.s).

Work (dimensions: ML^2T^{-2}, derived from $MLT^{-2} \times L$ or $ML^{-1}T^{-2} \times L^3$)

Work is done when a force moves its point of application or gas is moved in response to a pressure gradient. The dimensions are therefore either force times distance or pressure times volume, in each case simplifying to ML^2T^{-2}. The multiplicity of units of work has caused confusion in the past. Under SI, the erg, calorie and kilopond-metre will disappear in favour of the joule, which is defined as the work done when a force of 1 newton moves its point of application 1 metre. It is also the work done when 1 litre of gas moves in response to a pressure gradient of 1 kilopascal. This represents a welcome simplification.

$$1 \text{ joule} = 1 \text{ newton metre} = 1 \text{ litre kilopascal}$$
$$1 \text{ J} = 1 \text{ N m} = 1 \text{ l kPa}$$

The kilojoule replaces the kilocalorie in metabolism.

Power (dimensions: ML^2T^{-2}/T or ML^2T^{-3})

Power is the rate at which work is done and so has the dimensions of work divided by time. The SI unit is the watt, which equals 1 joule per second. Power is the correct dimension for the rate of continuous expenditure of biological energy, although one talks loosely about the 'work of breathing'. This is incorrect and 'power of breathing' is the correct term.

Surface tension (dimensions: MLT^{-2}/L or MT^{-2})

Surface tension has become important to the respiratory physiologist since the realization of the part it plays in the 'elastic' recoil of the lungs (Chapter 3). The CGS units of surface tension are dynes per centimetre (of interface). The appropriate SI unit would be the newton per metre. This has the following rather curious relationships:

$$1\,Nm^{-1} = 1\,Pa\,m = 1\,kg.s^{-2}$$

The unit for surface tension is likely to be called the pascal metre (Pa m), which is identical to the newton per metre. As an unexpected bonus, a millinewton per metre (or a millipascal metre) is identical in value to the old and familiar CGS unit, the dyn/cm.

Reference

1. Baron DN. *Units, symbols, and abbreviations. A guide for biological and medical editors*, 4th edn. London: Royal Society of Medicine Services, 1988.

Appendix B

The gas laws

A knowledge of physics is more important to the understanding of the respiratory system than of any other system of the body. Not only gas transfer but also ventilation and perfusion of the lungs occur largely in response to physical forces, with vital processes playing a less conspicuous role than is the case, for example, in brain, heart or kidney.

Certain physical attributes of gases are customarily presented under the general heading of the gas laws. These are of fundamental importance in respiratory physiology.

Boyle's law describes the inverse relationship between the volume and absolute pressure of a perfect gas at constant temperature:

$$PV = K \qquad \qquad \ldots(1)$$

where P represents pressure and V represents volume. At temperatures near their boiling point, gases deviate from Boyle's law. At room temperature, the deviation is negligible for oxygen and nitrogen, and of little practical importance for carbon dioxide or nitrous oxide.

Charles' law describes the direct relationship between the volume and absolute temperature of a perfect gas at constant pressure:

$$V = KT \qquad \qquad \ldots(2)$$

where T represents the absolute temperature. There are appreciable deviations at temperatures immediately above the boiling point of gases. Equations (1) and (2) may be combined as:

$$PV = RT \qquad \qquad \ldots(3)$$

where R is the universal gas constant, which is the same for all perfect gases and has the value of 8.1314 joules.degrees kelvin^{-1}.moles^{-1}. From this it may be derived that the mole volume of all perfect gases is 22.4 litres at standard temperature and pressure, dry (STPD). Carbon dioxide and nitrous oxide deviate from the behaviour of perfect gases to the extent of having mole volumes of about 22.2 litres at STPD.

Henry's law describes the solution of gases in liquids with which they do not react. The general principle of Henry's law is simple enough. The number of molecules of gas dissolving in the solvent is directly proportional to the partial pressure of the gas at the surface of the liquid, and the constant of proportionality is an expression of the solubility of the gas in the liquid. This is a constant for a particular gas and a particular liquid at a particular temperature but usually falls with rising temperature.

Unfortunately, confusion often arises from the multiplicity of units that are used. For example, when considering oxygen dissolved in blood, it has been customary to consider the amount of gas dissolved in units of vols% (ml of gas (STPD) per 100 ml blood) and the pressure in mmHg. Solubility is then expressed as vols% per mmHg, the value for oxygen in blood at 37°C being about 0.003. However, for carbon dioxide in blood, we tend to use units of mmol.l^{-1} of carbon dioxide per mmHg. The units are then mmol.l^{-1}.mmHg^{-1}, the value for carbon dioxide in blood at 37°C being 0.03. Both vols% and mmol.l^{-1} are valid measurements of the quantity (mass or number of molecules) of the gas in solution and are interchangeable with the appropriate conversion factor.

Physicists are more inclined to express solubility in terms of the *Bunsen coefficient*. For this, the amount of gas in solution is expressed in terms of volume of gas (STPD) per unit volume of solvent (i.e. one-hundredth of the amount expressed as vols%) and the pressure is expressed in atmospheres.

Biologists, on the other hand, prefer to use the *Ostwald coefficient*. This is the volume of gas dissolved, expressed as its volume under the conditions of temperature and pressure at which solution took place. It might be thought that this would vary with the pressure in the gas phase, but this is not so. If the pressure is doubled, according to Henry's law, twice as many molecules of gas dissolve. However, according to Boyle's law, they would occupy half the volume at double the pressure. Therefore, if Henry's and Boyle's laws are obeyed, the Ostwald coefficient will be independent of changes in pressure at which solution occurs. It will differ from the Bunsen coefficient only because the gas volume is expressed as the volume it would occupy at the temperature of the experiment rather than at 0°C. Conversion is thus in accord with Charles' law and the two coefficients will be identical at 0°C. This should not be confused with the fact that, like the Bunsen coefficient, the Ostwald coefficient falls with rising temperature.

The partition coefficient is the ratio of the number of molecules of gas in one phase to the number of molecules of gas in another phase when equilibrium between the two has been attained. If one phase is gas and the other liquid, the liquid/gas partition coefficient will be identical to the Ostwald coefficient. Partition coefficients are also used to describe partitioning between two media (e.g. oil/water, brain/blood, etc.).

Graham's law of diffusion governs the influence of molecular weight on the diffusion of a gas through a gas mixture. Diffusion rates through orifices or through porous plates are inversely proportional to the square root of the molecular weight. This factor is of importance only in the gaseous part of the pathway between ambient air and the tissues, and is, in general, of importance only when the molecular weight is greater than that of oxygen or carbon dioxide. Graham's law is not relevant to the process of 'diffusion' through the alveolar/capillary membrane (page 204).

Dalton's law of partial pressure states that, in a mixture of gases, each gas exerts the pressure that it would exert if it occupied the volume alone. This pressure is known as the partial pressure (or tension) and the sum of the partial pressures equals the total pressure of the mixture. Thus, in a mixture of 5% carbon dioxide in oxygen at a total pressure of

101 kPa (760 mmHg), the carbon dioxide exerts a partial pressure of $5/100 \times 101 = 5.05$ kPa (38 mmHg). In general terms:

$$P_{CO_2} = F_{CO_2} \times P_B$$

In the alveolar gas at sea level, there is about 6.2% water vapour, which exerts a partial pressure of 6.3 kPa (47 mmHg). The available pressure for other gases is therefore (P_B – 6.3) kPa or (P_B – 47) mmHg. Gas concentrations are usually measured in the dry gas phase, so it is necessary to apply this correction for water vapour in the lungs.

Tension is synonymous with partial pressure and is applied particularly to gases dissolved in a liquid such as blood. Molecules of gases dissolved in liquids have a tendency to escape, but net loss may be prevented by exposing the liquid to a gas mixture in which the partial pressure of the gas exactly balances the escape tendency. The two phases are then said to be in equilibrium, and *the tension of a gas in a liquid is defined as the tension of the gas in a gas mixture with which the liquid is in equilibrium*. Thus a blood P_{CO_2} of 5.3 kPa (40 mmHg) means that there would be no net exchange of carbon dioxide if the blood were exposed to a gas mixture that had a P_{CO_2} of 5.3 kPa (40 mmHg).

Appendix C

Conversion factors for gas volumes

Gas volumes are usually measured at ambient (or environmental) temperature and pressure, either dry (as from a cylinder passing through a rotameter) or saturated with water vapour at ambient temperature (e.g. an expired gas sample). Customary abbreviations are ATPD (ambient temperature and pressure, dry) and ATPS (ambient temperature and pressure, saturated).

Conversion factors for gas volume – ATPS to BTPS

Gas volumes measured by spirometry and other methods usually indicate the volume at ambient temperature and pressure, saturated (ATPS). Tidal volume, minute volume, dead space, lung volumes, ventilatory gas flow rates, etc. should be converted to the volumes they would occupy in the lungs of the patient at body temperature and pressure, saturated (BTPS).

Conversion from ATPS to BTPS is based on Charles' and Boyle's laws (Appendix B), and conversion factors are listed in Table C.1.

Derivation of conversion factors:

$$\text{volume}_{(BTPS)} = \text{volume}_{(ATPS)} \left(\frac{273 + 37}{273 + t} \right) \left(\frac{P_B - P_{H_2O}}{P_B - 6.3} \right)$$

P_B is barometric pressure (kPa) and the Table has been prepared for a barometric pressure of 100 kPa (750 mmHg): variations in the range 99–101 kPa (740–760 mmHg) have a negligible effect on the factors.

t is ambient temperature (°C). The Table has been prepared for a body temperature of 37°C: variations in the range 35–39°C are of little importance.

P_{H_2O} is the water vapour pressure of the sample (kPa) at ambient temperature (see Table C.1).

Conversion factors for gas volume – ATPS to STPD

In the measurement of absolute amounts of gases such as oxygen uptake, carbon dioxide output and the exchange of 'inert' gases, we need to know the actual quantity (i.e. number

647

Table C.1 Factors for conversion of gas volumes measured under conditions of ambient temperature and pressure, saturated (ATPS), to volumes which would be occupied under conditions of body temperature and pressure, saturated (BTPS)

Ambient temperature °C	Conversion factor	Saturated water vapour pressure	
		kPa	mmHg
15	1.129	1.71	12.8
16	1.124	1.81	13.6
17	1.119	1.93	14.5
18	1.113	2.07	15.5
19	1.108	2.20	16.5
20	1.103	2.33	17.5
21	1.097	2.48	18.6
22	1.092	2.64	19.8
23	1.086	2.80	21.0
24	1.081	2.99	22.4
25	1.075	3.16	23.7
26	1.069	3.66	25.2

Table C.2 Factors for conversion of gas volumes measured under conditions of ambient temperature and pressure, saturated (ATPS), to volumes which would be occupied under conditions of standard temperature and pressure, dry (STPD) – 0°C, 101.3 kPa (760 mmHg)

Ambient temperature °C	Barometric pressure, kPa (mmHg)			
	97.3 (730)	98.7 (740)	100 (750)	101.3 (760)
15	0.895	0.907	0.919	0.932
16	0.890	0.903	0.915	0.928
17	0.886	0.899	0.911	0.923
18	0.882	0.894	0.907	0.919
19	0.878	0.890	0.902	0.915
20	0.873	0.886	0.898	0.910
21	0.869	0.881	0.893	0.906
22	0.865	0.877	0.889	0.901
23	0.860	0.872	0.885	0.897
24	0.856	0.868	0.880	0.892
25	0.851	0.863	0.875	0.887
26	0.847	0.859	0.871	0.883

of molecules) of gas exchanged, and this is most conveniently expressed by stating the gas volume as it would be under standard conditions; i.e. 0°C, 101.3 kPa (760 mmHg) pressure and dry (STPD). Under these conditions, one mole of an ideal gas occupies 22.4 litres.

Conversion from ATPS to STPD is again by application of Charles' and Boyle's laws; it is described below, with conversion factors shown in Table C.2.

Derivation of conversion factors:

$$\text{volume}_{(STPD)} = \text{volume}_{(ATPS)} \left(\frac{273}{273 + t} \right) \left(\frac{P_B - P_{H_2O}}{101} \right)$$

P_B is barometric pressure (kPa).

t is ambient temperature (°C).

P_{H_2O} is the saturated water vapour pressure of the sample (kPa) at ambient temperature (see Table C.1).

Appendix D

Symbols, abbreviations and definitions

Symbols

Symbols used in this book are in accord with recommendations for editors of biological and medical publications in the UK.[1] There continues to be variation between journals, particularly between Europe and the USA. The use of these symbols is very helpful for an understanding of the quantitative relationships that are so important in respiratory physiology.

Primary symbols (large capitals) denoting physical quantities.

F fractional concentration of gas
P pressure, tension or partial pressure of a gas
V volume of a gas
Q volume of blood
C content of a gas in blood
S saturation of haemoglobin with oxygen
R respiratory exchange ratio (RQ)
D diffusing capacity

$\cdot$ denotes a time derivative; e.g. $\dot{V}$ ventilation
$\qquad\qquad\qquad\qquad\qquad\quad \dot{Q}$ blood flow

Secondary symbols denoting location of quantity.

in gas phase (small capitals)	*in blood* (lower case)
I inspired gas	a arterial blood
E expired gas	v venous blood
A alveolar gas	c capillary
D dead space	t total
T tidal	s shunt
B barometric (usually pressure)	

$^{-}$ denotes mixed or mean; e.g. $\bar{v}$ mixed venous blood
$\qquad\qquad\qquad\qquad\qquad\qquad \bar{E}$ mixed expired gas

$'$ denotes end; e.g. E$'$ end-expiratory gas
$\qquad\qquad\qquad\quad$ c$'$ end-capillary blood

Tertiary symbols indicating particular gases.

O_2 oxygen
CO_2 carbon dioxide
N_2O nitrous oxide
etc.

f denotes the respiratory frequency

BTPS, ATPS and STPD: see Appendix C.

Examples of respiratory symbols

$P_{A_{O_2}}$ alveolar oxygen tension
$C\bar{v}_{O_2}$ oxygen content of mixed venous blood
$\dot{V}_{O_2}$ oxygen consumption

Reference

1. Baron DN. *Units, symbols, and abbreviations. A guide for biological and medical editors*, 4th edn. London: Royal Society of Medicine Services, 1988.

Appendix E

Nomograms and correction charts

Blood gas correction nomograms for time

This nomogram (Figure E.1) is designed for the application of corrections for metabolism of blood occurring between sampling and analysis (page 243). The effect of temperature is based on the cooling curve when blood is drawn at 37°C into a 5 ml glass or 2 ml plastic syringe at room temperature, followed by storage at room temperature. Elapsed time between sampling and analysis is shown on the ordinate. Line charts indicate the change in P_{CO_2} (which rises), pH (which falls) and base excess (which falls). A graph is required for the change in P_{O_2} (which falls) because the rate of fall depends upon the P_{O_2}. For details, see reference 1.

Blood gas correction nomogram for temperature (Figure E.2)

Enter with the patient's temperature on the abscissa. *Multiply* the measured gas tension by the factor shown on the ordinate, using the appropriate curve for P_{O_2} based on the saturation of the sample. The broken line should be used for P_{O_2}, whatever the level of P_{CO_2}. The line chart at the top of the graph may be used for the pH correction which should be *added*. For details, see reference 1.

The Siggaard-Andersen curve nomogram

The *in vitro* relationship between pH and P_{CO_2} of oxygenated blood is indicated either by a line joining two points obtained after *in vitro* equilibration or by a line passing through the actual arterial values and with a slope dependent on the haemoglobin concentration. The slope is that of a line joining the normal arterial point (indicated by a small circle in the diagram) and the appropriate point on the haemoglobin scale (i.e. $14\,g.dl^{-1}$ in the example). Intersections of the buffer line indicate three indices of metabolic acid–base state: buffer base, standard bicarbonate and base excess which is the most commonly used. Interpolation of P_{CO_2} indicates corresponding (*in vitro*) pH values and *vice versa*.

The example in Figure E.3 is normal arterial blood (*in vitro* changes); other equilibration curves are shown in Figure 10.4.

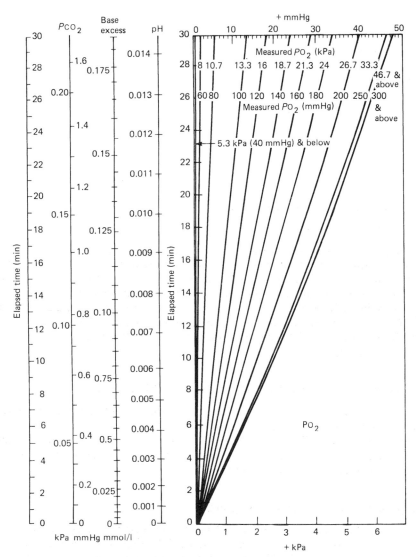

Figure E.1 Nomogram for correcting blood P_{CO_2}, P_{O_2}, pH and base excess for metabolic changes occurring between sampling and analysis. (Reproduced from reference 1 by permission of the Editors of the *Journal of Applied Physiology*.)

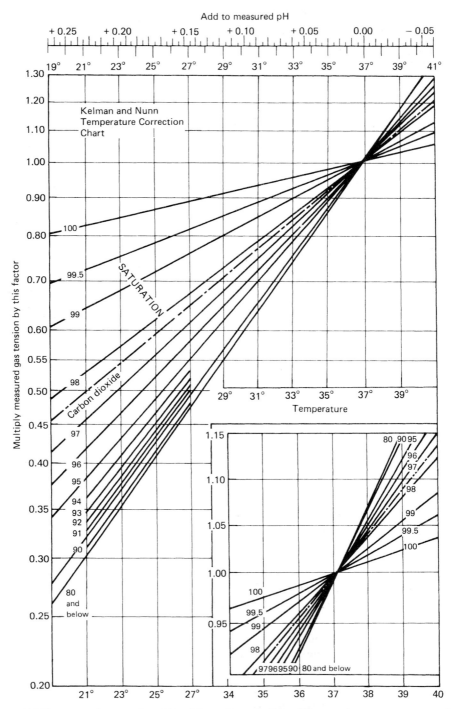

Figure E.2 Nomogram for correction of blood P_{CO_2}, P_{O_2} and pH for differences between temperature of patient and electrode system (assumed to be 37°C). (Reproduced from reference 1 by permission of the Editors of the *Journal of Applied Physiology*.)

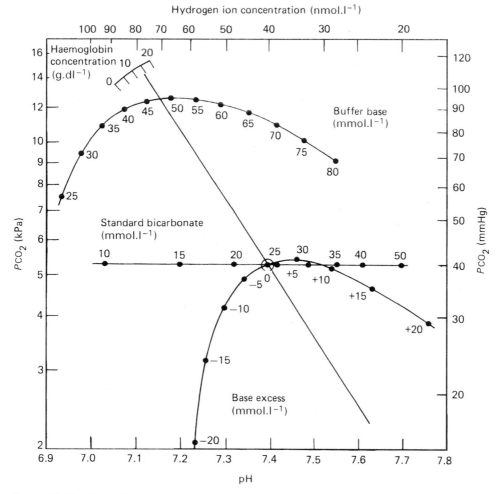

Figure E.3 The Siggaard-Andersen curve nomogram relating pH and P_{CO_2} for oxygenated blood *in vitro*. (Adapted from reference 2 by permission of the author and the Editors of the *Scandinavian Journal of Clinical and Laboratory Investigation*.)

The iso-shunt chart

Figure E.4 is a diagram of the theoretical relationship between arterial P_{O_2} and inspired oxygen concentration for different values of virtual shunt. It is based on assumed values as follows:

Arterial P_{CO_2} 5.3 kPa (40 mmHg)
Arterial/mixed venous oxygen content difference 5 ml.dl^{-1}
Haemoglobin concentration 14 g.dl^{-1}

Virtual shunt is defined as the shunt that gives the relationships depicted when the arterial/ mixed venous oxygen content difference is 5 ml.dl^{-1}. These curves include a small component for moderate non-uniformity of ventilation/perfusion ratios of the ventilated alveoli.[3,4] For further details, see page 185 *et seq*.

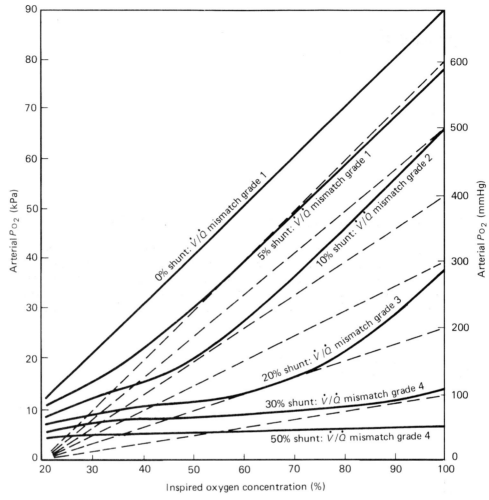

Figure E.4 Arterial P_{O_2} as a function of inspired oxygen concentration on a modified iso-shunt diagram (Figure 8.12), incorporating a factor for ventilation/perfusion mismatch (Table 8.3, Figure 8.15). Normal values are assumed for P_{CO_2}, haemoglobin concentration and arterial/mixed venous oxygen content difference. Note the reverse curves below an inspired oxygen concentration of 40% with mismatch grades of 2–4. The broken lines indicate arterial P_{O_2} expressed as a ratio of inspired oxygen concentration, as used for example in the calculations of lung injury score (Table 30.1).

References

1. Kelman GR, Nunn JF. Nomograms for correction of blood P_{O_2}, P_{CO_2}, pH and base excess for time and temperature. *J Appl Physiol* 1966; **21**: 1484–90.
2. Siggaard-Andersen O. The pH, log P_{CO_2} blood acid–base nomogram revisited. *Scand J Clin Lab Invest* 1962; **14**: 598–604.
3. Benator SR, Hewlett AM, Nunn JF. The use of iso-shunt lines for control of oxygen therapy. *Br J Anaesth* 1973; **45**: 711–18.
4. Petros AJ, Doré CJ, Nunn JF. Modification of the iso-shunt lines for low inspired oxygen concentrations. *Br J Anaesth* 1994; **72**: 515–22.

Appendix F

Mathematical functions relevant to respiratory physiology

This book contains many examples of mathematical statements, which relate respiratory variables under specified conditions. Appendix F is intended to refresh the memory of readers whose knowledge of mathematics has been attenuated under the relentless pressure of new information acquired in the course of study of the biological sciences.

The most basic study of respiratory physiology requires familiarity with at least four types of mathematical relationship:

1. The linear function.
2. The rectangular hyperbola or inverse function.
3. The parabola or squared function.
4. Exponential functions.

These four types of function will now be considered separately with reference to examples drawn from this book.

The linear function

Examples

1. Pressure gradient against flow rate with laminar flow (page 59). There is no constant factor and the pressure gradient is zero when flow rate is zero.
2. Respiratory minute volume against P_{CO_2} (page 95). In this case there is a constant factor corresponding to a 'negative' respiratory minute volume when P_{CO_2} is zero.
3. Over a limited range, lung volume is proportional to inflating pressure (page 42). The slope of the line is then the compliance.

Mathematical statement

A linear function describes a change in one variable (dependent or y variable) that is directly proportional to another variable (independent or x variable). There may or may not be a constant factor that is equal to y when x is zero. Thus:

$$y = ax + b$$

where a is the slope of the line and b is the constant factor. In any one particular relationship a and b are assumed to be constant but both may have different values in other circumstances. These are not therefore true constants (like π, for example) and are more precisely termed parameters, whilst y and x are variables.

Graphical representation

Figure F.1 shows a plot of a linear function, following the convention that the independent variable (x) is plotted on the abscissa and the dependent variable (y) on the ordinate. Note that the relationship is a straight line and simple regression analysis is based on the assumption that the relationship is of this type. If the slope (a) is positive, the line goes upwards and to the right. If the slope is negative, the line goes upwards and to the left.

The rectangular hyperbola or inverse function

Examples

1. The ventilatory response to hypoxia (expressed in terms of Po_2) approximates to a rectangular hyperbola, asymptotic on the horizontal axis to the respiratory minute volume at high Po_2 and, on the vertical axis, to the Po_2 at which it is assumed ventilation increases towards infinity.
2. The relationships of alveolar gas tensions to alveolar ventilation are conveniently described by rectangular hyperbolas (for carbon dioxide see page 236, and for oxygen see page 253). The curves are concave upwards for gases that are eliminated (e.g. carbon dioxide) and concave downwards for gases that are taken up from the lungs (e.g. oxygen). Curvature is governed by gas output (or uptake) and the asymptotes in each case are zero ventilation and partial pressure of the gas under consideration in the inspired gas. The relationship is extremely helpful for understanding the quantitative relationship between ventilation and alveolar gas tensions.
3. Airway resistance approximates to an inverse function of lung volume (page 67).

Mathematical statement

A rectangular hyperbola describes a relationship when the dependent variable y is inversely proportional to the independent variable x thus:

$$y = a/x + b$$

The asymptote of x is its value when y is infinity, and the asymptote of y is its value when x is infinity. If b is zero, the relationship may be simply represented as:

$$xy = a$$

Graphical representation

Figure F.2a shows rectangular hyperbolas with and without constant factors. Changes in the value of a alter the curvature but not the asymptotes. Figure F.2b shows the same relationships plotted on logarithmic coordinates. The relationship is now linear but with a negative slope of unity because, if:

$$xy = a$$

then:

$$\log y = -\log x + \log a$$

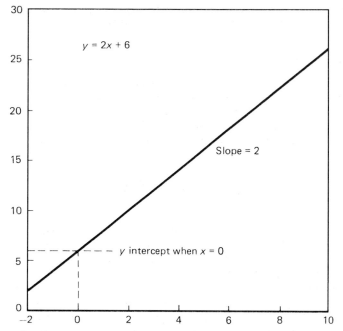

Figure F.1 A linear function plotted on linear coordinates. Examples include pressure/flow rate relationships with laminar flow (see Figure 4.2) and P_{CO_2}/ventilation response curves (see Figure 5.6).

The parabola or squared function

Example

With fully turbulent gas flow, pressure gradient changes according to the square of gas flow and the plot is a typical parabola (Chapter 4).

Mathematical statement

A parabola is described when the dependent variable (y) changes in proportion to the square of the independent variable (x), thus:

$$y = ax^2$$

Graphical representation

On linear coordinates, a parabola, with positive values of the abscissa, shows a steeply rising curve (Figure F.3a), which may be confused with an exponential function (see below) although it is fundamentally different. On logarithmic coordinates for both abscissa and ordinate, a parabola becomes a straight line with a slope of two (Figure F.3b) because $\log y = \log a + 2 \log x$ (a and $\log a$ are parameters).

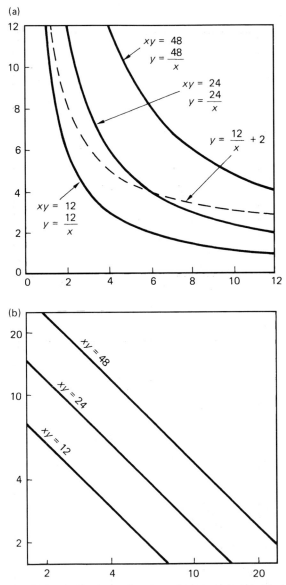

Figure F.2 Rectangular hyperbolas plotted on (a) linear coordinates and (b) logarithmic coordinates. Examples include the relationships between alveolar gas tensions and alveolar ventilation (see Figures 6.12, 10.8, 11.2), Po_2/ventilation response curves (see Figure 5.9) and the relationship between airway resistance and lung volume (see Figures 4.5 and 21.13).

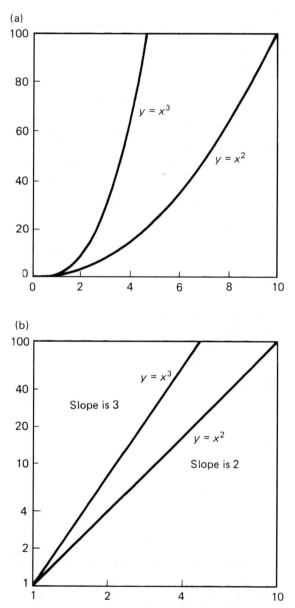

Figure F.3 Parabolas plotted on (a) linear coordinates and (b) logarithmic coordinates. An example is the pressure/volume relationship with turbulent flow (see Figure 4.3).

Exponential functions

General statement

An exponential function describes a change in which the rate of change of the dependent variable is proportional to the magnitude of the independent variable at that time. Thus, the rate of change of y with respect to x (i.e. dy/dx)* varies in proportion to the value of y at that instant. That is to say:

$$\frac{dy}{dx} = ky$$

where k is a constant or a parameter.

This general equation appears with minor modifications in three main forms. To the biological worker they may be conveniently described as the tear-away, the wash-out and the wash-in.

The tear-away exponential function

This must be described first, as it is the simplest form of the exponential function. It is, however, the least important of the three in relation to respiratory function.

Simple statement

In a tear-away exponential function, the quantity under consideration increases at a rate that is in direct proportion to its actual value – the richer one is, the faster one makes money.

Examples

Classic examples are compound interest, and the mythical water-lily that doubles its diameter every day (Figure F.4). A typical biological example is the free spread of a bacterial colony in which (for example) each bacterium divides every 20 minutes. The doubling time of this example would be 20 minutes.

Mathematical statement

In the case of exponential functions relevant to respiratory function, the independent variable x almost invariably represents time, and so we shall take the liberty of replacing x with t throughout. The tear-away function may thus be represented as:

$$\frac{dy}{dt} = ky$$

A little mathematical processing will convert this equation into a more useful form, which will indicate the instantaneous value of y at any time, t.

* dy/dx is the mathematical shorthand for the rate of change of y with respect to x. The 'd' means 'a very small bit of'. Therefore dy/dx means a very small bit of y divided by the corresponding very small bit of x. This is equal to the slope of the graph of y against x at that point. In the case of a curve, it is the slope of a tangent drawn to the curve at that point.

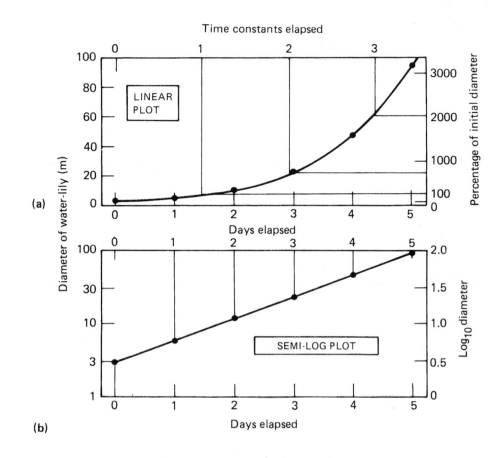

Elapsed time (days)	Diameter of water-lily	
	metres	percentage of initial diameter
0	3	100
1	6	200
1.44	8.2	272
2	12	400
2.88	22.2	739
3	24	800
4	48	1 600
4.32	60.3	2 009
5	96	3 200

Diameter of water-lily $= 3e^{t/1.44}$
(t is measured in days, diameter in metres)

Figure F.4 The growth of a water-lily that doubles its diameter every day – a typical tear-away exponential function. Initial diameter, 3 metres; size doubled every day (i.e. doubling time = 1 day). Compare the figures in the table with those in Table F.1.

First, multiply both sides by dt/y:

$$\frac{1}{y}\text{d}y = k\text{d}t$$

Next integrate both sides with respect to t:

$$\log_e y + C_1 = kt + C_2$$

(C_1 and C_2 are constants of integration and may be collected on the right-hand side.)

$$\log_e y = (C_2 - C_1) + kt$$

Finally, take antilogs of each side to the base e:

$$y = e^{(C_2 - C_1)} \times e^{kt}$$

At zero time, $t = 0$ and $e^{kt} = 1$. Therefore the constant $e^{(C_2 - C_1)}$ equals the initial value of y, which we may call y_0. Our final equation is thus:

$$y = y_0 e^{kt}$$

y_0 is the initial value of the variable y at zero time.

e is the base of natural or naperian logarithms (discovered in 1619 before the circulation of the blood was known). This constant (2.71828...) possesses many remarkable mathematical properties.

k is a constant that defines the speed of the particular function. For example, it will differ by a factor of two if our mythical water-lily doubles its size every 12 hours instead of every day. In the case of the wash-out and wash-in, we shall see that k is directly related to certain important physiological quantities, from which we may predict the speed of certain biological changes.

Instead of using e, it is possible to take logs to the more familiar base 10, thus:

$$y = y_0 \, 10^{k_1 t}$$

This is a perfectly valid way of expressing a tear-away exponential function, but you will notice that the constant k has changed to k_1. This new constant does not have the simple relationships of physiological variables mentioned above. It does, however, bear a constant relationship to k, as follows:

$$k_1 = 0.4343k \text{ (approx.)}$$

Graphical representation

On linear graph paper, a tear-away exponential functional rapidly disappears off the top of the paper (Figure F.4). If plotted on semi-logarithmic paper (time on a linear axis and y on a logarithmic axis), the plot becomes a straight line and this is a most convenient method of presenting such a function. The logarithmic plots in Figures F.4–F.6 are all plotted on semi-log paper.

The wash-out or die-away exponential function

The account of the tear-away exponential function has really been an essential introduction to the wash-out or die-away exponential function, which is of great importance to the biologist in general and to the respiratory physiologist in particular.

Simple statement

In a wash-out exponential function, the quantity under consideration falls at a rate that decreases progressively in proportion to the distance it still has to fall. It approaches but, in theory, never reaches zero.

Examples

Familiar examples are cooling curves, radioactive decay and water running out of the bath. In the last example, the rate of flow of bath water to waste is proportional to the pressure of water, which is proportional to the depth of water in the bath, which in turn is proportional to the quantity of water in the bath (assuming that the sides are vertical). Therefore, the flow rate of water to waste is proportional to the amount of water left in the bath, and decreases as the bath empties. The last molecule of bath water takes an infinitely long time to drain away. A similar example is the mountaineer who each day ate half of the food he carried. In this way he made his food last indefinitely.

In the field of respiratory physiology, examples include:

1. Passive expiration (Figure F.5).
2. The elimination of inhalational anaesthetics.
3. The fall of arterial P_{CO_2} to its new level after a step increase in ventilation.
4. The fall of arterial P_{O_2} to its new level after a step decrease in ventilation.
5. The fall of blood P_{CO_2} towards the alveolar level as it progresses along the pulmonary capillary.
6. The fall of blood P_{O_2} towards the tissue level as blood progresses through the tissue capillaries.

Mathematical statement

When a quantity *decreases* with time, the rate of change is *negative*. Therefore, the wash-out exponential function is written:

$$\frac{dy}{dt} = -ky$$

from which we may derive the following equations, which give the value of y at any time t:

$$y = y_0 e^{-kt}$$

which is simply another way of saying:

$$y = \frac{y_0}{e^{kt}}$$

y_0 is again the initial value of y at zero time. In Figure F.5, y_0 is the initial value of (lung volume – FRC) at the start of expiration; that is to say, the tidal volume inspired.

e is again the base of natural logarithms (2.71828. . .).

k is the constant that defines the rate of decay, and is the reciprocal of a most important quantity known as the *time constant*, represented by the Greek letter tau (τ). Three things should be known about the time constant:

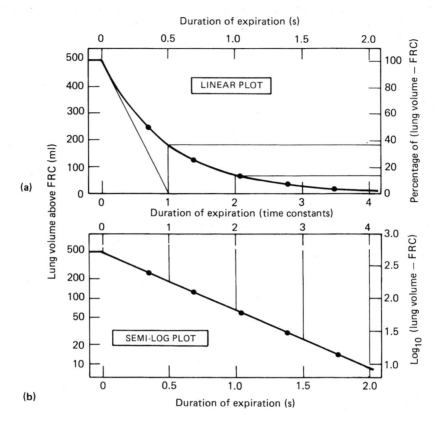

Figure F.5 Passive expiration – a typical wash-out exponential function. Tidal volume, 500 ml; compliance, 0.5 l.kPa^{-1} (50 ml.cmH$_2$O^{-1}); airway resistance, 1 kPa.l^{-1}.s (10 cmH$_2$O.l^{-1}.s); time constant, 0.5 s; half-life, 0.35 s. The points on the curve indicate the passage of successive half-lives.

	Elapsed time (constants)	Lung volume remaining above FRC	
		ml	percentage of tidal volume
Lung volume above FRC = $500e^{-(t/0.5)}$	0	500	100
	0.69	250	50
	1	184	36.8
	2	67.5	13.5
	3	25	5.0
	4	9	1.8

Note that the logarithmic coordinate has no zero. This accords with the lung volume approaching, but never actually equalling, the FRC.

1. Figure F.5 shows a tangent drawn to the first part of the curve. This shows the course events would take if the initial rate were maintained instead of slowing down in the manner characteristic of the wash-out curve. The time that would then be required for completion would be the time constant (τ) or $1/k$. The wash-out exponential function may thus be written:

$$y = y_0 e^{-t/\tau}$$

2. After 1 time constant, y will have fallen to $1/e$ of its initial value, or approximately 37 per cent of its initial value.
   After 2 time constants, y will have fallen to $1/e^2$ of its initial value, or approximately 13.5 per cent of its initial value.
   After 3 time constants, y will have fallen to $1/e^3$ of its initial value, or approximately 5 per cent of its initial value.
   After 5 time constants, y will have fallen to $1/e^5$ of its initial value, or approximately 1 per cent of its initial value.
   (More precise values are indicated in Table F.1).

3. The time constant is often determined by physiological factors. When air escapes passively from a distended lung, the time constant is governed by two variables: compliance and resistance (see Chapters 3, 4 and 31).

We may now consider the example of passive expiration. Let V represent the lung volume (above FRC), then $-dV/dt$ is the instantaneous expiratory gas flow rate. Assuming that Poiseuille's law is obeyed:

$$-\frac{dV}{dt} = \frac{P}{R}$$

when P is the instantaneous alveolar-to-mouth pressure gradient and R is the airway resistance. However, compliance $(C) = V/P$. Therefore:

$$-\frac{dV}{dt} = \frac{1}{CR} V$$

or:

$$\frac{dV}{dt} = -\frac{1}{CR} V$$

Then by integration and taking antilogs as described above:

$$V = V_0 e^{-(t/CR)}$$

By analogy with the general equation of the wash-out exponential function, it is clear that $CR = 1/k = \tau$ (the time constant). Thus the *time constant equals the product of compliance and resistance*.* This is analogous to the discharge of an electrical capacitor through a resistance, when the time constant of discharge equals the product of the capacitance and

---

* It is strange at first sight that two quantities as complex as compliance and resistance should have a product as simple as time. In fact, the MLT units (Appendix A) check perfectly well:

$$\text{compliance} \times \text{resistance} = \text{time}$$
$$M^{-1}L^4T^2 \times ML^{-4}T^{-1} = T$$

the resistance. Analysis of the passive expiration has been considered in greater detail on page 66.

Half-life. It is often convenient to use the half-life instead of the time constant. This is the time required for y to change to half its previous value. The special attraction of the half-life is its ease of measurement. The half-life of a radioactive element may be determined quite simply. First of all the degree of activity is measured and the time noted. Its activity is then followed and the time noted at which its activity is exactly half the initial value. The difference between the two times is the half-life and is constant at all levels of activity. Half-lives are shown in Figures F.4–F.6 as dots on the curves. For a particular exponential function there is a constant relationship between the time constant and the half-life.

$$Half\text{-}life = 0.69 \text{ times the } time\ constant$$

$$Time\ constant = 1.44 \text{ times the } half\text{-}life$$

Graphical representation

Plotting a wash-out exponential function is similar to the tear-away function (Figure F.5). A semi-log plot is particularly convenient, as the curve (being straight) may then be defined by far fewer observations. It is also easy to extrapolate backwards to zero time if the initial value is required but could not be measured directly for some reason. It is, for example, an essential step in the measurement of cardiac output with a dye that is rapidly lost from the circulation (page 158).

The wash-in exponential function

The wash-in function is also of special importance to the respiratory physiologist and is the mirror image of the wash-out function.

Simple statement

In a wash-in exponential function, the quantity under consideration rises towards a limiting value, at a rate that decreases progressively in proportion to the distance it still has to rise.

Examples

A typical example would be a mountaineer who each day manages to climb half the remaining distance between his overnight camp and the summit of the mountain. His rate of ascent declines exponentially and he will never reach the summit. A graph of his altitude plotted against time would resemble a 'wash-in' curve.
   Biological examples include the reverse of those listed for the wash-out function:

1. Inflation of the lungs of a paralysed patient by a sustained increase of mouth pressure (Figure F.6).
2. The uptake of inhalational anaesthetics.
3. The rise of arterial P_{CO_2} to its new level after a step decrease of ventilation.
4. The rise of arterial P_{O_2} to its new level after a step increase of ventilation.

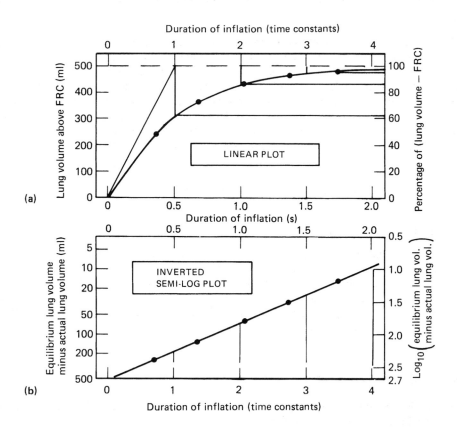

Figure F.6 Passive inflation of the lungs with a sustained mouth pressure – a typical wash-in exponential function. Final tidal volume, 500 ml; compliance, 0.5 l.kPa^{-1} (50 ml.cmH$_2$O^{-1}); airway resistance, 1 kPa.l^{-1}.s (10 cmH$_2$O.l^{-1}.s); time constant, 0.5 s; half-life, 0.35 s. The points on the curves indicate the passage of successive half-lives.

Lung volume above FRC $= 500\,(1 - e^{-(t/0.5)})$

Elapsed time (constants)	Lung volume attained above FRC	
	ml	percentage of tidal volume
0	0	0
0.69	250	50
1	316	63.2
2	433	86.5
3	475	95.0
4	491	98.2

Note that, for the semi-log plot, the log scale (ordinate) is from above downwards and indicates the difference between the equilibrium lung volume (inflation pressure maintained indefinitely) and the actual lung volume.

5. The rise of blood Po_2 to the alveolar level as it progresses along the pulmonary capillary.
6. The rise of blood Pco_2 to the venous level as blood progresses through the tissue capillaries.

Mathematical statement

With a wash-in exponential function, y increases with time and therefore the rate of change is positive. As time advances, the rate of change falls towards zero. The initial value of y is often zero and y approaches a final limiting value, which we may designate y_∞ – that is, the value of y when time is infinity (∞). A change of this type is indicated thus:

$$\frac{dy}{dt} = k(y_\infty - y)$$

As y approaches y_∞ so the quantity within the parentheses approaches zero, and the rate of change slows down. The corresponding equation that indicates the instantaneous value of y is:

$$y = y_\infty(1 - e^{-kt})$$

y_∞ is the limiting value of y (attained only at infinite time).

e is again the base of natural logarithms.

k is a constant defining the rate of build-up and, as is the case of the wash-out function, it is the reciprocal of the *time constant*, the significance of which is described above. It is the time that would be required to reach completion if the initial rate of change were maintained without slowing down.

After 1 time constant, y will have risen to approximately $100 - 37 = 63$ per cent of its final value.
After 2 time constants, y will have risen to approximately $100 - 13.5 = 86.5$ per cent of its final value.
After 3 time constants, y will have risen to approximately $100 - 5 = 95$ per cent of its final value.
After 5 time constants, y will have risen to approximately $100 - 1 = 99$ per cent of its final value.
(More precise values are indicated in Table F.1.)

As in the wash-out function representing passive exhalation, the time constant for the corresponding wash-in exponential function (passive inflation of the lungs) equals the product of compliance and resistance. For the wash-in of a substance into an organ, the time constant equals tissue volume divided by blood flow, or FRC divided by alveolar ventilation as the case may be. As above, the time constant is approximately 1.5 times the half-life.

    There are many situations in which the same parameters apply to both wash-in and wash-out functions of the same system. The time constant for each function will then be the same. A classic example is the charging of an electrical capacitor through a resistance and then allowing it to discharge to earth through the same resistor. The time constant is the same for each process and equals the product of capacitance and resistance. This is

Table F.1 Percentage change of y after lapse of different numbers of time constants

Time elapsed in time constants	Tear-away function $y = y_0 e^{kt}$ (expressed as percentage of y_0)	Wash-out function $y = y_0 e^{-kt}$ (expressed as percentage of y_0)	Wash-in function $y = y_\infty(1 - e^{-kt})$ (expressed as percentage of y_∞)
0	100	100	0
0.693*	200	50	50
1	272	36.8	63.2
2	739	13.5	86.5
3	2 009	4.98	95.02
4	5 460	1.83	98.17
5	14 841	0.67	99.33
10	2 202 650	0.004 5	99.9995 5
∞	∞	0	100

* Half-life or doubling time.
Note =   272 = $100 \times e$
             739 = $100 \times e^2$
            2009 = $100 \times e^3$

approximately true for passive deflation and inflation of the lungs (Figures F.5 and F.6), on the assumption that compliance and airway resistance remain the same.

Graphical representation

The wash-in function may be represented on linear paper as for the other types of exponential function. However, for the semi-log plot, the paper must be turned upside down and the plot made as indicated in Figure F.6. The curve will then be a straight line.

Index